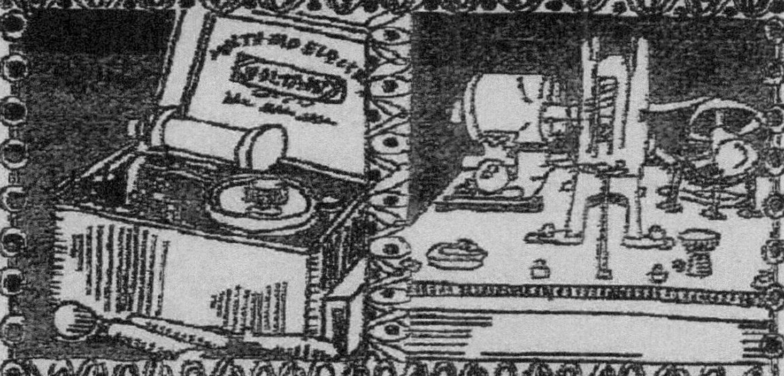

GUIDE TO ELECTROTHERAPY INSTRUMENTS AND HISTORY OF THEIR AMERICAN MAKERS

BY

DEAN P CURRIER

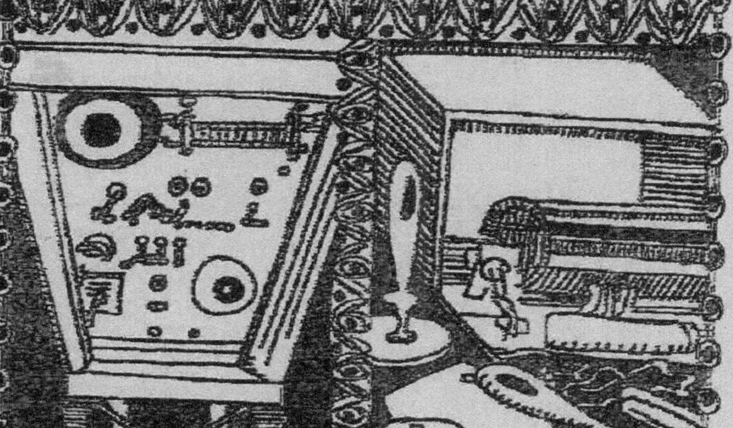

GUIDE TO ELECTROTHERAPY

INSTRUMENTS AND HISTORY OF

THEIR AMERICAN MAKERS

BY

DEAN P CURRIER

ISBN 978-0-7414-2232-3

Published by:

INFINITY
PUBLISHING.COM

1094 New Dehaven Street, Suite 100
West Conshohocken, PA 19428-2713
Info@buybooksontheweb.com
www.buybooksontheweb.com
Toll-free (877) BUY BOOK
Local Phone (610) 941-9999
Fax (610) 941-9959

Printed in the United States of America

Published June 2013

PREFACE

Collectors of medical electrical batteries often want information about the artifacts that they have gathered. Sellers of these artifacts most of the time know little about the artifacts that they sell unless they are collectors of that field of interest themselves. Turning to libraries and museums for help may be unrewarding except when these facilities are in possession of trade catalogs or the artifacts or both. Few museums exist that exhibit medical electrical batteries, but selective libraries hold scant editions of manufacturers' trade catalogs. Trade catalogs often contain vintage information about their companies, illustrations, and descriptions of products, and general information about electrotherapeutics. Trade catalogs have contributed much to the information gathered herein.

Many old books exist that provide illustrations, descriptions, and technology of medical electrical batteries. This resource of textbooks on medical electrotherapeutics has been used liberally to gather information.

Booklets and manuals that originally accompanied the purchase of medical electrical batteries have also provided valuable information. This resource was particularly helpful for information about the apparatuses aimed for home usage.

Bits and pieces of information were gathered through resources that were less concentrated than that of libraries and museums. The bits and pieces (eg, articles; correspondence, internet, newspapers) were also valuable contributions to the present information.

This book was written for educational purposes, and should assist collectors and those interested in the history of medical electrical batteries. This information provides a foundation for expansion and growth of what may be available about the American medical electrical battery industry and its product lines, and should be a reference for identifying and dating artifacts.

Despite the resources mentioned some histories of the apparatuses and their manufacturers are scant. Additional information is warranted if an inclusive resource is to be available for the serious collectors; therefore, the process of gathering information is ongoing. The medical electrical battery industry contained herein is limited to "La Americana" and mostly to the period of time from the 1870s to 1920s. Some content precedes 1870 and extends to 1932. Equal pagination of products for the home consumer with that used by the physician or professional is not possible. History and the market have dictated that physician use of medical electrical batteries occupy the most pages. The most favored period of use of the medical electrical battery in medicine was probably from 1871 to 1900, and then declined steadily to the mid 1930s when physical therapists became the dominant purveyors of the apparatus. The physical therapist became a legitimate practitioner of electrotherapeutics just before World War I so artifacts after that date until mid the 1930s were used by both the physician and physical therapist, while apparatuses for home consumers were prevalent during that period of time, also. The most favored period of use of the medical electrical battery for home use took place from the 1890s to the 1930s. Today, clinical (electrical stimulation) and home use (TENS for pain control) of electrical apparatus continues under regulations and scrutiny by professional medical caregivers.

The descriptions and illustrations included may not bear out the quality differences between medical electrical batteries used by the professional practitioner and that used by the home consumer. Cursory examination of the apparatuses easily reveals the quality differences to the serious collector. Whenever prices are listed the reader can detect the differences that reflect quality. Today, differences continue to exist in apparatuses used by professionals and that recommended and sold to public consumers. Today the apparatuses and quality are controlled by regulatory laws, but in yesteryear little or no control by regulatory law existed. Thus, the emphasis and purpose of the apparatuses are somewhat different today from that of yesteryear. Electrical stimulation is much better controlled as a treatment today than formerly.

Some manufacturers of physician apparatuses and of home apparatuses, and retailers of one or both apparatus are not included in this edition. There were many very small manufacturers during the late nineteenth and early twentieth centuries, and very little or nothing is known about them except a trade name assigned to an occasioned artifact. Retailers of medical electrical batteries were every where throughout the United States and are too numerous for detailed inclusion. Those firms included in this edition are the most numerously encountered in reviewed resources, and most often available for collecting their artifacts.

TABLE OF CONTENTS

ACKNOWLEDGEMENT

I would like to thank the kind people of these facilities that supplied valuable information for this book: Burton Historical Collection of Detroit Public Library, Detroit, MI; Eagle Herald of Marinette and Menominee, MI; Enock Pratt Free Library, Baltimore, MD; Free Library, Philadelphia, PA; Hagley Museum and Library, Wilmington, DE; Hammond Historical Society, Hammond, IN; Indiana Historical Society, Indianapolis, IN; JH Bunnell & Co, New York; Maryland Historical Society, Baltimore, MD; Menominee (MI) County Historical Society, Inc; New York Academy of Medicine, NY; Radiology Centennial, Inc; Spies Public Library, Menominee, MI; The Armed Forces Pathology Museum and Library, Washington, DC; The Bakken Museum and Library, Minneapolis, MN; The Medical Library of the University of Kentucky, Lexington, KY; The Public Library of Cincinnati, OH; The Public Library of Hammond, IN; The Public Library of Portland, ME; The Public Library of Providence, RI, and The Smithsonian Institute, Washington, DC.

I greatly appreciate the materials supplied by individuals that contributed much to the book, and wish to thank: Bob Alexander, Clarkston, MI; Jeff Behary, W Palm Beach, FL; Dr David Cofeen, Hastings-On-Hudson, NY; Dr Richard Elgin, Rolla, MO; Frank of Spirit Lake, Idaho; Dr Tom Greenslade, Kenyon College, Gambier, OH; Dr Joe Jacobs, Newport, NY; James Kreuzer of New Wireless Pioneers, Elma, NY; Alex Peck, Charleston, IL; David Rickert, Arlington, VA, and Pamela Warren, Westerville, OH.

The book is enhanced by its attractive cover that was illustrated by Wendy Currier Zumwalt, Georgetown, KY. Thanks especially to Brad Currier who freed the computer of its many bugs, to Joan who got me hooked on collecting, and to Tracey who provides fervor for my projects.

PART 1. COLLECTING MEDICAL ELECTRICAL BATTERIES

In Part 1 the reader is introduced to the general aspects of the medical electrical battery; that is, its manufactory and its early evolvement in the United States. Then a brief history of the medical electrical battery is cited that covers the general evolvement in medicine. Since the collector of medical electrical batteries is concerned about the characteristics of the collected artifacts, some information about the construction and operation of the early batteries is provided. Selected pulse forms, and characteristics of electrical components are given that may enhance the collector's background for understanding the function of the devices. An abbreviated table of patent numbers and dates is provided that may help to date the devices.

This book in Parts 1 through 4 will review briefly the histories of some of the most notable American manufacturers and retailers of electrical machines and supplies during the late nineteenth and early twentieth centuries. Several companies represented essentially physician interests, while several companies directed their business to the public and home use market. Some companies covered all business fronts by making or selling or both electrical apparatuses to physicians and public consumers. Many medical electrical batteries of these American companies are described and illustrated. This book is not inclusive of all medical electrical battery businesses and their manufacturers.

In this book medical electrical apparatuses are presented. These devices throughout time have been called by different names. They have been named medical electrical batteries, medical electrical apparatus or machines, electrical stimulators, and recently on the internet auctions as quack boxes, shock machines or devices, as well as electrical batteries. Other names may have been associated with the apparatuses from time to time. These medical electrical apparatuses evolved over time according to their type of electrical outputs.

CHAPTER 1. INTRODUCTION

Instrument making (eg, medical electrical machines; viz, surgical instruments) in the first half of the nineteenth century in the United States was a skilled craft by an elite small group of men who lived mostly in the Middle Atlantic and New England States. Their workmanship was excellent and could generally match the English quality in their trades. Instrument making was thus a slow labor intensive process that kept up, however, with the demands of scientists and of educational institutions early in the century. American instrument makers prided themselves for the accuracy, precision, and quality of their products. Quality instruments of various kinds and uses were also imported from England and other countries, but often these were very costly to the American consumers of education and science.

The Civil War, beginning in 1861, made immediate demands on manufacturers to produce accurate, precise, quality, and reliable instruments at a fast rate and affordable prices. The elite small group of instrument makers had to take on more employees to meet the demands. These owners of the instrument shops also had to find other ways to meet the demands for instruments, keep the costs down, and yet make the instruments accurate and reliable. The medical electrical battery was not yet a featured item.

The first factory to manufacture instruments of science was opened in 1855 in England. Manufacturing in the factory setting had been introduced in the United States before the Civil War so this approach was the solution to meeting demands for quantity during the war years[1] for some medical instrumentation, but not yet for medical electrical batteries.

A few American instrument makers engaged in the construction of medical electrical batteries in the 1850s. Medical electrical machines (viz, galvanic) were used in the Civil War in cases where respiratory obstruction occurred with anesthesia.[2] After the Civil War physicians demanded electrical machines for use in their offices and to some extent in hospitals. The popularity of the medical electrical battery in medicine was spreading from England and Europe. The demand for medical electrical machines (galvanic, faradic, magneto electrical) was sufficient by 1870 that small factories or manufacturing shops appeared. Compared, with today's factories the manufacturers of 1870 to 1900 were small employing a few to perhaps 75 individuals. The manufacturers of the 1870s often were extensions of the instrument making shops, but soon effectively replaced the instrument makers of pre Civil War times in the United States. Various types of factories and plentiful in numbers were existing in the United States to serve as roles for small manufacturers of medical electrical machines and for which to learn existing technology for fast and mass production.

Factory made instruments were reduced in quality of workmanship compared with those made previously by the elite small group of instrument makers (eg, Daniel Davis, Thomas Hall). Reduced quality of medical electrical batteries by mass production generally did not occur in the United States because manufacturers of these apparatuses remained small in scope. These small operations were just one step removed from the elite skilled craftsmen only because some machines were now used to replace the craftsman to increase production. The wooden box was used to house or encase the electrical machine, but generally of equality to those previously made manually by instrument makers. Quality was reflected by costs, however, and quality did change. Wooden boxes of mahogany and cherry were top of the line and of better quality than oak or pine. Those having comers dovetailed, grooved, and glued were better than those whose comers were squared and nailed together. Later in the nineteenth and early in the twentieth centuries metal and cheap wooden boxes covered, with buckram (leatherette like) replaced the solid wooden boxes of cherry, mahogany, or oak. The transition from quality wooden cases to buckram covered and metal cases occurred roughly from 1912 to 1925. The demands of fast production through the manufacturing or factory process sacrificed the nonessentials of decoration and ornamentation.[1] The medical electrical apparatus of the twentieth century that were factory made erased the character of those constructed by the skilled craftsmen. Apparatus of the twentieth century, although superior with advanced technology and in function, were not always as attractive as the units of the eighteenth and nineteenth centuries; or at least to the collector. Present day manufacturers do, however, make great efforts to make their products attractive by color, adding fabrics, and simulated materials. In the late twentieth and early twenty-first centuries, metals have often been replaced by plastics that again are changing the quality and appearance of the devices. Electrical apparatus demand accuracy, precision, reliability, and sophistication, which necessarily requires metal and mathematical input.[1] Superior technology of the twentieth and twenty-first centuries has in most cases reduced the weight and size enormously of the medical electrical apparatuses compared with those of the eighteenth and nineteenth centuries.

As the manufacture of medical electrical machines progressed after 1870, the issuance of trade catalogs, at least by the giants (leaders of the industry), also progressed. The introduction of trade catalogs in the United States began with Benjamin Franklin who printed catalogs of his books for sale. He suggested that people living in rural areas should have similar benefits of book sales as those living in the cities. His catalog of 1750 even listed fireplaces. He, however, indicated that this would work only if the rural resident sent cash first. Catalogs were used for the mail order business in the United States that began in 1872. Montgomery

Ward and Co distributed circulars in 1872 (ca 1894 for medical electrical batteries), while Sears, Roebuck and Co made 10,000 catalogs available to the public in 1880 (ca 1896 for medical electrical batteries).[3] These retail companies used the best printers after often securing quality writers to author particulars about the listed items and even about the companies. Catalogs were often enriched with lithographs and woodcuts by quality artists and engravers even though the volumes were considered lowly giveaways.[3] The outdated catalogs were often found in rural outhouses.

Catalogs of medical electrical batteries probably existed prior to 1848 when Daniel Davis, Jr, published his Manual of Magnetism. His manual was both a text and a catalog for listing and describing his products for sale. His manual was a hard cover publication rather than the throwaway paperback type of catalog associated with the later mail order business.

SHORT HISTORY OF MEDICAL ELECTRICAL BATTERIES

From the first man made electrical machine in 1675 by Otto Van Guericke (1602-1686) of Germany to 1800 the only output was static electricity or static charge. The first recorded electrical treatment of patients was in 1745 by Christian G Kratzenstein of Germany. In 1800, Alessandro Volta (1745-1827) of Italy built the first battery or pile as it was called. A pile or series of metal discs (eg: zinc, copper) alternating with a brine soaked substance (paper, cloth, cardboard, and then in order repeated) was developed by Volta to produce the first source of constant or direct current. The pile became known as a battery when cells or discs (zinc, copper, soaked substance repeated to increase effectiveness) were repeated in or piled in a series, and named in honor of Luigi Galvani (1737-1798) who experimented with electricity (animals and lightning). In the year 1800, two sources of electricity on demand were known and apparatuses were built to produce either static or constant (direct, galvanic) electricity. In 1831, Michael Faraday (1791-1867) of England and Joseph Henry (1797-1878) of the United States invented the induction coil and soon afterwards from 1831 to 1834 several apparatuses to produce magnetoelectrical currents were built by Hippolyte Pixii (1808-1835) of France, Edward Clarke (1804-1846) of England, and Joseph Saxton (1799-1873) of the United States. The magnetoelectrical devices produced a crude alternating current and were named in honor of Faraday (Faradic, faradic currents). The name most commonly given these magnetoelectrical devices was faradic electrical machines or apparatuses. Thereafter, magnetoelectrical apparatuses were constructed as another source of artificial or man made electricity. After the discovery of the induction principle three forms of electricity (static, direct current, and alternating current) were available. In 1836, Nicholas J Callan (1799-1864) of Ireland invented the style of induction coil used commonly in subsequent faradic batteries[4] constructed in the United States between the 1870s into the 1930s. His style of coil was powered by a wet cell (direct current) rather than being magnetoelectrically produced.

The construction or engineering of electrical apparatuses improved with demand. The demand for electricity in medicine really took off in the United States after the Civil War or around 1871 when manufacturers improved the medical electrical battery to become more efficient, more powerful, more affordable, reliable, and manageable apparatus for physicians than apparatus of the early nineteenth century. From the 1870s into the 1920s the medical electrical battery had its "heyday" in medicine.

In the 1870s to World War I electrical treatments were administered by physicians who were known as electricians, electrotherapeutists, electrotherapists, and physical therapists. In the 1920s, a large proportion of medical electrical treatments were administered by nonphysician physical therapists. Physicians in the 1920s had stopped calling themselves physical therapists, and later were named physiatrists. Early (1745-1845) electrical treatments for patients were administered by lay people knowledgeable of electricity, and then later by physicians of physical medicine and rehabilitation and physiatrists.

During the peak period of time (1890s) for the medical electrical battery in medicine, medical practitioners theorized that external healing powers (eg, electrotherapeutics) could be transferred to a patient's body to energize it for improving health. Electrical belts, medical electrical batteries, electrical batteries for prostrate massage, and other devices or nostrums (medallions, rings) were modalities of choice in the 1890s to transfer energy to the ailing body. Because of electricity's association with the nervous system and sexual performance, not only medical electrical batteries by physicians but by home consumers increased in popularity. The developments in electricity during this era were most promising, the public was fascinated and gullible by promises read in magazine and newspaper advertisements.

Electricity was thought by many, especially the electrotherapeutist (physician promoting electricity in treatments), to be the force of life (Dr Scott's hair and flesh brushes, Pulvermakers' belts) or the source of the body's energy. Electrotherapeutists promoted the idea that electricity worked similarly to the electrical phenomena of electrical lights, motors, telegraphs, and telephones. While promoting electrical force for life, the electrotherapeutist faulted others as quacks for using electrotherapeutics, like them, as a real dangerous problem.[5,6]

Even the leading electrotherapeutists of the 1870s and 1880s (eg, Drs Beard and Rockwell) theorized that modern man was stressed and was in need of added electrical energies. These men even blamed

Thomas A Edison for speeding up life with his electrical lights and telegraph, yet developing their renown treatment of general faradism. Beard and Rockwell generated a large following in medicine for treating neurasthenia (nervous debility and exhaustion) with medical electrical batteries.[6]

From the 1870s to about 1905, the boxed faradic or galvanic or both (combined) battery was very popular among those physicians using electricity in their medical treatments of patients. The boxed battery was an apparatus well constructed and encased in wooden boxes that were designed for office or portability uses. Among the faradic type apparatuses were the conventional induction coil and the sledge inductorium style batteries of DuBois-Reymond of Germany. The conventional induction coil (after NJ Callan) used a fixed primary and secondary coil or helix arrangement, and then having a sliding metal tube between the two coils to control current. This arrangement of coil and sliding tube was a technological advancement over the magnetoelectrical apparatus to produce and control the amplitude of alternating current. The sledge inductorium unit on the other hand, used the principle of moving the secondary coil over the primary coil to control current amplitude. Moving the secondary coil over the primary coil to control small increments of current amplitude was still another technological advancement in the history of the medical electrical battery. A portable boxed unit would generally be small enough to be carried by physicians in their buggies on their travels to patients' homes. During this same period of time (1870s to 1930s), the influence or static electrical machine was reintroduced and used in medicine. The influence machine was larger and superior in function to the previous static electrical models of the eighteenth century (eg, Ben Franklin's era).

In 1883, Dr JH Kellogg of Battle Creek (MI) Sanitarium and cornflakes fame introduced sinusoidal current. The name "sinusoidal" was coined by Jacques A d' Arsonval of France in the early twentieth century for high frequency current that described the same waveform as that of Kellogg. After 1900, manufacturers began offering the sinusoidal current in medicine. Sinusoidal current was similar in physiological effects to that of faradic current but the sine wave offered less discomfort during machine controlled muscle contractions of patients. Sinusoidal current is a smoother and more symmetrical form of alternating current than that of faradic current. Medical electrical apparatus producing sinusoidal currents required the use of a motor and used commercial electricity or power grid to operate it. In early 1900, power grids were replacing the wet and dry cell as the major power source of the medical electrical battery. By 1910, fewer and fewer medical electrical batteries that were powered by dry cells were being sold. Manufacturers were now making medical electrical apparatuses that were powered by grids or sources of commercial electricity; first, the commercial power was by direct current (Edison type), and then alternating current was introduced by Nikola Tesla. After World War I the medical electrical apparatuses that delivered galvanic and sinusoidal currents used by physicians were mostly powered by commercial (power grids) electricity.

The influence or static machine was used in the United States mostly in the 1880s through the 1920s, and then faded in use. The machine was very large (cumbersome), expensive, and physiologically did not prove to be more effective than the combination of faradic and galvanic currents so had a limited market. In the 1900s commercial power and engineering of the medical electrical apparatus provided small portable compact units that could deliver all forms of electricity which then replaced the influence machine. The static current of the influence machine of the 1880s to the 1920s was also known as frictional, Franklinic, and static electrical current. Although static electricity was considered a form at rest, it was produced under tension. These machines separated the positive and negative forms of electricity by first generating it and then accumulating it. Since static electricity was a form at rest, for a long time clinicians thought that it did not penetrate the skin. Dr William J Morton of New York City demonstrated it otherwise.[7]

Morton brought the influence machine with him in 1880 after some training in Europe, and showed that it did penetrate skin with its very high tension (10,000 to 500,000 volts) and very low amperage (0.2 to 3mA). He even modified the influence machine, and his modified model produced electricity in a form known as the Morton current. He showed that 100,000 volts was safe to treat patients yet could power the x-ray.

As stated, up to the 1870s, medical electrical batteries were sold mostly to institutions of learning, researchers, and some physicians. The medical electrical batteries were mostly customized for the customer by individual instrument makers. In the 1870s manufacturers began to mass produce medical electrical batteries that had the effect of replacing the individual instrument maker in the United States. Manufacturers advertised their products and marketed them with the physician in mind yet made quality items at reasonable costs. As a product the medical electrical battery became very competitive with modest profits for the manufacturer.

Early instrument makers in the United States were concentrated in Boston, Philadelphia, and New York. In the 1870s, New York began to pull away from manufactures of other cities as the dominant location for the production of the medical electrical battery. Chicago came into the picture of the medical electrical battery when manufacturers there became well known and started to erode business from New York in the 1890s. Boston and Philadelphia never reached the height in the medical electrical battery business as did Chicago and New York. Boston and Philadelphia were better known for their manufacture of medical and surgical instruments.[7]

Some manufacturers of medical electrical batteries prospered between 1870s and 1920s during which time the business was unstable. These companies endured the problems of the market over time and remained in business during the early to middle of the twentieth century (eg, Betz, Bunnell, McIntosh, Pilling, Waite & Bartlett). Some manufacturers endured while many did not. Manufactures started and ended business after several years (eg, Signal Electric, Van Houten & Ten Broeck, Voltamp Electric), often changed partners, and frequently moved their business location.

Competition certainly was responsible for changes within the industry, but profit margins were never great. The advancement of commercial electricity replaced the use of the wet and dry cell as a primary source of power. Physician interest and acceptance of the medical electrical battery dropped appreciably after 1896 when the x -ray became the "fair haired" apparatus in medicine. After World War I, the non-physician physical therapist (then an agent of the physician) became the prime caregiver rather than the physician of medical electrical treatments. Engineering of the products changed frequently with clinical research to support the changes and uses. The period of time from the 1870s to the 1920s was the golden years of the medical electrical battery in medicine. Thereafter the medical electrical battery, more or less, became the tool of the physical therapist when the physician abandoned it to engage in other areas and specialties of medicine. The medical electrical apparatus and its principles endure to this day in the medical field under the direction of medically educated caregivers (eg, physical therapists).

The medical electrical apparatuses presented herein are dominantly of the direct current (galvanic) and alternating current (faradic, sinusoidal). Since the popularity of the static current (through the influence machines of the 1880s) returned, some of these machines are also included, but their marketed volume was never great in the United States.

Direct current was used medically for electrolysis (iontophoresis) to introduce selected chemical (ions) through the skin and hopefully for local and systemic physiological effects. This approach of introducing ions or chemicals into the body preceded the now commonplace injectables (chemcial solutions). The use of injectable medicines mostly replaced the use of galvanic currents in medicine. Faradic current was used for local muscle contractions, and systemic physiological effects. Sinusoidal current replaced faradic current in the United States for medical use, although the British medical literature continues to use the term faradism for most types of alternating currents. Both galvanic (unipolar or positive or negative currents) and alternating current (faradic and sinusoidal) can be pulsed to form muscle contractions with proper and specific current characteristics (rapid rate of change, amplitude, duration, and frequency).

The medical electrical apparatuses or batteries, as they were often called, presented in this book represent the state-of-the-art for the dates cited for each. Apparatus design changed with time to improve their operation and the sensory perception of the patient. The reader is advised to consult textbooks on medical electrical therapeutics for detailed information about the design and operation of medical electrical batteries, and the physiological effects produced by current variations. This book is aimed at helping collectors to date and identify their medical electrical batteries that were once used by physicians to treat patients, and used by public consumers for treatments at home. The quality of apparatus is reflected according to its intended use (physician vs home). Today, electrical therapy treatments are given by physical therapists in the clinic, home, office, and hospital. Battery powered electrical apparatus (stimulators) are available for home use when recommended or prescribed by the physical therapist or physician. These home units (TENS, transcutaneous electrical nerve stimulators) are mostly used for treating pain, while others of different designs are used for treating some prescribed muscle and neural conditions.

The latter part of the nineteenth century and early twentieth century were periods of time when medical electrical batteries were used extensively and intensively to assist medical care. Therapeutic treatments using medical electrical batteries were given by a variety of people in early times (1745-1830), but mainly by physicians from 1870 to and for several years after World War I. Just prior to World War I and thereafter electrical treatments were mainly given by physical therapists. Medical electrical apparatus continue in use by physical therapists to treat patients having a variety of muscle, joint, neural, and vascular conditions. Medical electrical batteries (now called muscle and nerve stimulators) are also used today in medicine as heart pacemakers, incontinence control, respiration assistance, and muscular paralysis assistance.

References

1. Pearsall R. Collecting and Restoring Scientific Instruments. New York, NY, Arco Pub, 1974

2. Wilbur CK. Civil War Medicine 1861-1865. Old Saybrook, CT, Globe Pequot Press, 1998, pp 43-45

3. Romaine LB. A Guide to American Trade Catalogs 1744-1900. New York, NY, RR Bowker, 1996, pp 235-241

4. (www.corrosion-doctors.org/Biographies/CallanBio.htm)

5. Ives J. Electricity as Medicine. New York, NY, JT Ives, 1879

6. de la Pena CT. Powering the body. Favourite Edition (of NY Acad Med). Feb 2000, pp 8-9

7. Malone D (ed). Dictionary of American Biography. New York, NY, Charles Scribner's Sons, 1964, pp 267-268

CHAPTER 2. CHARACTERISTICS OF APPARATUS

Chapter 2 deals with construction characteristics of the artifacts, dating artifacts, and grading them. General information about faradic coils, interrupters or rheotomes, and current regulators or rheostats is discussed. Some selected examples of currents discussed within the book conclude this chapter.

1. Information for Collecting

While attempting to identify and date the various artifacts, the collector is aided by knowing the construction aspects of medical electrical batteries. These several tips may be helpful in learning about specific artifacts in a collection.

Handles. Prior to 1880, handles for cranking of electrical batteries (eg, Davis-Kidder magnetoelectrical apparatus) were often bone, or ebony. After 1880, handles were made of hard rubber, wood, or metal. Leather straps were used to carry some models. After 1900, some models with wooden boxes had the combination metal and leather for carrying handles.

Metal: Between 1871 and about 1920, metal on the medical electrical batteries of quality was nickel plated. Since some surgical instrument manufacturers also produced medical electrical batteries, nickel plating began on their devices in 1870.[1] Nickel plating on surgical instruments started for the purpose of resisting corrosion on metal instruments while providing an attractive coating; a nice silvery white color of the metal. Quality of plating varied on the batteries. Various forms of nickel compounds were used to plate metals because of its hardness and resistance to oxygen and rust. Nickel plate was started in the 1860s and continued on medical electrical batteries into the twentieth century. Items such as coils, switches, binding posts, and interrupters of faradic and galvanic electrical apparatuses were nickel plated to give a nice appearance yet not rust after a short time like unplated steel or tin. Nickel plate was the most commonly used metal on medical electrical batteries from the 1870s to the 1920s when chrome began to replace nickel plate.

The quality medical electrical units of the 1850s to about 1880 also used brass (alloy of copper and zinc) at times for components mounted on the face panel. When polished to remove effects of oxygen the metal was attractive to the consumer while hard and workable to the manufacturer. Brass was used early in history, and is seen on the earliest dated medical electrical batteries (eg, 1850s to 1875).

Chrome provided the brightness that manufacturers liked to have displayed for components mounted on the face panels of their electrical apparatuses. Chrome is a shortened term for chromium plate that provides a bright finish for metal electrical components, but it was not used prior to the 1920s (ca 1923).

Like chrome plate, stainless steel was used for its resistance to chemicals and rust. Stainless steel is an alloy of iron, carbon, and four percent chromium, and is hard yet workable. Available in the 1920s, stainless steel was used on some medical electrical apparatuses sparingly until after World War II when it replaced chrome plate. Unplated metal, particularly steel and tin, was used prior to 1900, but both rusted easily and did not offer an impressive appearance. Tin and unplated steel were used on some of the cheaper home units. Unplated metal was used occasionally for minor parts on quality medical electrical batteries, but its use was very limited and usually to that of the low cost units. Unplated steel parts on medical electrical batteries, as seen today, are most often rusted and unattractive.

Enameled porcelained steel was used in the 1920s to form the face plate and encasement of some medical electrical batteries. This metal seemed to be used with the availability of the direct current (Edison's current), later alternating current as a commercial (wall or power grid) source of electricity. The so called polysine models exemplify the porcelained apparatuses.

Cases: Most faradic and galvanic medical electrical batteries were housed in wooden boxes from 1871 to the 1920s. The construction of the wooden boxes varied in quality. Quality boxes had dove tailed corners that were glued. Boxes having tongue and groove corners were also well constructed and these were mostly glued joints. Boxes that were nailed together and having straight or mitered corners were usually associated with cheap apparatus intended for home use. Quality boxes were made of cherry, mahogany, or walnut. As the supply of these woods in the United States decreased the quality wooden boxes were made of oak. Often golden oak was preferred. Oak cases are found on both physician type units and those for home use, quality wooden boxes made for physician use were still available with cherry, mahogany, and walnut with early twentieth century quality electrical apparatuses. Many boxes were polished (smooth and semiglossed) by the manufacturers.

Quality wooden cases had heavy metal (brass, nickel plate) latches to secure lids of the boxes, and heavy metal carrying handles on the lids. Wooden boxes of cheaper quality (eg, home use) often are found having nickel plated metal, or unplated steel for latches and carrying handles which often are rusted. Earlier boxes sometimes had ornate metal latches and handles. Most manufacturers of wooden boxes used ordinary type hinges that sometimes matched the metal of devices on the face plate or panel, but more often were made of unplated steel. These hinges are now showing rust. After 1900, wooden boxes or cases were being replaced by cheaper wood (eg, pine) that was covered by black buckram (a leatherette like fabric) and in some leatherette. Measurements cited in the text for the cases listed are length (front facing) x width (depth or side) x height in inches.

Directions: Some of the physician quality electrical batteries had directions printed on labels that were glued to the inside lid of the box. Many batteries did not display directions, since physicians were supposed to be knowledgeable in operating the machines. Electrical batteries intended for home use often had similar displays of directions, but some manufacturers had booklets published that instructed the consumers about various conditions and diseases for treatment. These booklets often contained basic information about electricity and about the electrical battery, care of the unit, how to prepare and handle wet cells, and occasionally some advertisements about product lines (eg, Bunnell, Pilling, Sears, Voltamp, PG Williams). The trade catalogs of some manufacturers (usually large companies) offered instruction about electricity and the operation of various electrical units to physicians in lieu of directions on individual models.

Since the subject of medical electrical batteries was not included in medical curricula, physicians using electrical treatments could learn from manufacturer catalogs, textbooks, correspondent courses, graduate program lectures, and perhaps from the manufacturers' representatives.

Face Plate or Face Panel: This is the plate or panel used as a foundation for mounting and supporting the electrical components (coil, switches, interrupter, outlet posts, input binding posts from battery (s), rheostat when available), and insulating the electrical components from the wiring of the circuitry. In early quality medical electrical batteries the face plate might be matching wood of the box. Some quality units of the twentieth century had marble, metal, porcelain, or slate while those of the nineteenth century also had gutta percha, hard rubber, or wood.

Gutta percha was introduced to the Royal Society of Arts, London, England in 1842 or 1843 by Dr William Montgomerie, an army surgeon in Singapore. It was the first natural plastic material, but by 1851 the International Exhibit showed that it could be used for many commercial applications (golf balls, cable and wire insulation, medical and surgical uses). Michael Faraday of England used gutta percha to insulate electrical components in his many experiments. Face plates of medical electrical batteries were often made of this material from 1870 in the United States. Gutta percha is extracted from tropical evergreen trees (Isonandra, Palaquium, Payena, sapodilla) in countries of the Malayan Archipelgo. It is a concrete milky sap that dries to become dark brown. After being collected from the tree it is coagulated, washed, purified, and molded for shipping and manufacturing. Often the gutta percha is mixed with powdered glass, silica, or zinc oxide to make it harder than the natural drying. Between 1858 and 1866, the milky juice of Malaysian trees was molded in hot water to soften, but then hardened after cooling. The substance was mostly black colored by processing.

Gutta percha was used mostly in the 1880s and 1890s, and into the early twentieth century, but was replaced by the plastics or synthetic materials of the twentieth century. This material was called hard rubber.

Bakelite was developed by LH Baekeland of the United States in 1907 and patented in 1909 as a phenol formaldehyde resin that provided a hard polished, shiny surface that would withstand heat and moisture. Bakelite was a good nonconductor of electricity. It was produced in a variety of colors but black was the most common color on medical electrical apparatuses. Bakelite became one of the most versatile materials and was used into the 1940s.

Bakelite is always solid, never hollow. When two pieces of bakelite are banged together a clunk sound is heard that typifies the material. Also, when heated in hot water or hot water is dropped onto a piece a distinctive smell is detected. Many other materials have been substituted for bakelite because of their reduced costs of manufacture, and these substitutes are sometimes presented as being bakelite.[2] Bakelite was not commonly used with medical electrical batteries of the faradic and galvanic types because of its timing in the history of the battery (eg. 1870-1930).

Manufacturers: Some medical electrical batteries had metal signature plates that cited the name and city of the maker. Some of the metal signature plates had patent dates of the device or components of the device. Paper labels glued inside of the lid of the box might have the maker's name and address, but often this means of identification only cited the name and city of the manufacturer. Manufacturers seldom provided the exact date of construction. Manufacture dates are usually associated with patent dates. Often manufacturers made and retailed a particular medical electrical battery for 20 years without significant design changes. Occasionally, a manufacturer made only subtle changes in a particular model within a 20 years period of time. Examination of the metal components may yield a name, or date. Occasionally, the case was made by a company other than that of the manufacturer of the medical electrical battery, but most often the wooden case was made in the same factory as the battery (eg, The Chloride of Silver Dry Cell Battery Co, the Signal Electric Co). GP Pilling manufactured both the medical electrical battery and the box, like most, and he may have his name on both or just one of the items.

Unfortunately, some manufacturers of medical electrical batteries did not cite the name, address, or date of their items. In such cases the collector must consult trade catalogs of manufacturers and hunt for a particular item by description. Confusion occurs when manufacturers produced the medical electrical battery for a particular seller (a second party). For example, a medical electrical battery manufactured by JH Bunnell, GP Pilling, The Voltamp Electric Co, and Signal Electric Co may not bear their names but may have a paper label or signature plate on their items with the name of the seller (eg, EH Mahady Co; Max Wocher & Son Co; George Frye Co; Montgomery Ward & Co; Sears, Roebuck and Co, or the name of other regional sellers from various sections of the United States). This guide will help identify and date specific artifacts.

Familiarity of medical electrical batteries will assist collectors in identifying features or trade characteristics of a particular manufacturer. Knowing a manufacturer's product characteristics will help the collector when a particular item is labeled with a name other than that of the maker. Close examination of your artifacts or those of a friend or of a museum will teach familiarity. Study of a manufacturer's trade catalogs or bulletins for various years will also teach familiarity. Trade catalogs are usually obtained only in certain centers like medical libraries, museum libraries, or university libraries associated with a medical school. The many references cited in this book will be helpful to those who are serious collectors.

Dating Medical Electrical Batteries by Numbers: Batteries can be identified by their patent, design, or design patent numbers if and when these are available on a specific artifact. Occasionally, a medical electrical battery will have a patent date on it so the collector will be able to identify the date that the model was patented. Patent dates do not, however, provide information about the date the particular battery was manufactured. The patent date might agree with the date or year that the item was first manufactured, but it does not provide any other date that the battery was made. Many medical electrical batteries were manufactured over a life that ranges for 20 years, not all in a single year when patented. Most often, however, the battery does not contain any information about its date of manufacture, and the collector must turn to other methods for dating a model. Models of medical electrical batteries are identified by descriptions of listings from a company's trade catalog. The small companies often did not issue such trade catalogs. Advertisements in magazines and journals will also provide clues to the date of a particular battery as well as the owner's manual of a specific unit.

Ideally, if and when medical electrical batteries have patent, design, or design patent numbers the collector only has to match the particular number with a date. In the event that a medical electrical battery has one of the numbers a crude table of corresponding dates is provided to help in dating your medical electrical battery. In the table the numbers are cited for six years spans of time (range). The average numbers for a year within the span are approximate and are cited in parentheses below the average number. For a more exacting date of your medical electrical battery with a patent number the reader is referred to Digger Odell's patent numbers listing on the internet to date your artifacts.[3]

Patent numbers increase for most years after 1870, while those for design numbers often varied from year to year. Design patent numbers varied from year to year but between 1924 and 1929 the

PATENT NUMBERS TO DATE MEDICAL ELECTRICAL BATTERIES[3]

Dates	Patent #	Design #	Design Patent #
1870-1875	98,460- (16,522/yr)	3,810-7,969 (830/yr)	1-2,150 (430/yr)
1876-1881	171,641- (12,900/yr)	8,884-12,082 (640/yr)	3,288-8,139 (970/yr)
1882-1887	251,685- (20,721/yr)	12,647-17,046 (880/yr)	8,973-13,939 (793/yr)
1888-1893	375,720- (22,651/yr)	17,995-22,092 (819/yr)	15,072-22,272 (1440/yr)
1894-1899	511,744- (21,025/yr)	22,994-29,916 (1,384/yr)	23,956-32,308 (1,670/yr)
1900-1905	640,167- (27,733/yr)	32,055-37,280 (1,045/yr)	33,957-43,932 (1,995/yr)
1906-1911	808,618- (34,312/yr)	37,766-41,063 (659/yr)	48,446-80,506 (6,412/yr)
1912-1917	1,013,095- (39,458/yr)	42,073-50,117 (1,609/yr)	84,711-114,666 (5,991/yr)
1918-1923	1,251,458- (37,781/yr)	51,629-61,748 (2,024/yr)	120,005-163,215 (8,642/yr)
1924-1929	1,478,996- (43,580/yr)	63,675-77,347 (2,734/yr)	177,785-251,129 (14,669/yr)
1930-1935	1,742,181 -1,985,878 (48,739/yr)	80,254-94,179 (2,785/yr)	265,655-320,441 (10,957/yr)

numbers increased greatly. The table allows you to roughly estimate the year of your medical electrical battery between 1870 and 1935 if any number from one of the three categories is cited on a particular model. By subtracting or adding the average number/yr to the numbers above it you will approximate the year that a particular number falls in for the specific medical electrical battery.

Grading Batteries for Value: The value or worth of a medical electrical battery is not necessarily based on a commercial price. It is first based on your appreciation of the artifact, and secondly, value is the price it would bring on the antique market. Both appreciation and commercial values are based on certain grading factors or standards that hold with time. Some of these grading bases are considered.

Condition. The condition is paramount unless the item is of significant historical worth or rare then less than a mint state is acceptable. Medical electrical batteries, even if cabinets, are not dated furniture, and therefore restoration is acceptable. So called "museum quality" is often associated with a seller's description of an artifact. Restoration is frequently necessary to bring an unit to "museum quality" which is desirable.

Case. The wooden box should be quality constructed and without defects (chips, cracks, water marks). Dove tailed corners and enforced brass are usually considered first rate. If the box is covered with buckram then the material should be unmarred (not cut, torn, faded). Modern apparatuses are often metal encased. The metal cases should be unmarred (without scratches, dents, paint touch ups). Missing or broken hinges, locks, keys reduce the value of a battery.

Face Plate or Panel. The wood, hard rubber, or marble (or slate) should not be cracked or otherwise marred (scratched, chips, water marks).

Induction Coils. The coils are often covered with a fabric that should be intact and unmarred (without tears, rips, scratches). Coils that are labeled by a signature (trade mark, logo) are of more value than unmarked coils unless they are of superior construction. For example, some manufacturers made coils having nickel plated caps, sleeves, or bands that offset a dull fabric finish. These latter coils offer a pleasing appearance that make the units more valuable.

Metal. Earlier units offered brass or steel metal components. The stainless steel components replaced the brass and steel components and improved the appearance of the batteries. The nickel plate also varies in quality. The better batteries have heavier nickel plated components than batteries made for home use. The better batteries are mostly those made for physicians while cheaper units were usually made for home use.

Completeness. The age of medical electrical batteries often reduce the completeness of the unit. Accessories and wet cells are frequently missing on units found in antique shops and on eBay. The battery is more valuable if there are no missing or broken parts.

Named Batteries. Certain units of manufacturers are more valuable than others. Some models by certain manufacturers command worth because of reputed quality. Models that are labeled with the manufacturer's name or signature are more valuable than those unnamed. The engraved plates or embossed units are more valuable than those unnamed (identity is harder without names or labels). Labels add to the value of a battery. Rarity of the model contributes value, and rarity could be the size or a unit as well as the number manufactured. One of a kind is more valuable than one that is commonplace. Influence machines are more valuable than the common faradic and galvanic batteries because of their size and reduced numbers available. Cabinet and table models are more valuable than the box units for reason of numbers and size. Early (1830s-1860s) batteries or coils are more valuable than mass produced units after 1870.

Grading Scale. A simple method of assessing the value or worth of medical electrical batteries is to assign a scale that summarizes the above criteria. A suggested scale to help collectors might be:

Mint. Like new, unmarred, no missing or broken parts, museum quality, rare;

Excellent. Museum quality but with a few small marks, no missing parts, no rust;

Good. Some marks, no rust, dirty, missing cells; and

Fair to Poor. Scratched, marred, some rust, dirty, missing or broken parts.

2. Faradic Coils

The manufacturers of medical electrical batteries in the United States mass produced versions of models using the induction coil to deliver faradic currents starting in 1871. These models became known as faradic batteries (after Michael Faraday of England who invented the induction coil principle in 1831, making the model possible by Nicholas J Callan of Ireland in 1836). The faradic electrical battery or medical induction apparatus was a type of electrical motor that produced current of make and break or alternating current (AC). Alternating current offered an improved current for contracting muscles compared with galvanic current that had to be interrupted manually each time. Although crude, faradic or the first AC current could be pulsed by making (On) and breaking (Off) its flow at various rates by automatic interrupters.

The induction coil was the basic component for producing faradic current required two coils: a primary and secondary coil. Manufacturers marketed their batteries to accommodate practitioners, but promoted the use of currents produced by both the primary and secondary coils. In reality after many years of clinical use, current from the primary coil was found to add nothing to the physiological effects of body tissue. The currents produced by the primary coil were not used much clinically after about 1897. Practitioners concentrated the use of the faradic battery for the alternatives offered by the secondary coil. The induction coils were manufactured in varies diameters, lengths, and windings for specific uses.

The primary coil often consisted of a cylindrical soft iron core that was wound by a few layers of thick copper wire. The secondary coil consisted of several layers of thin insulated copper wire wound over the primary coil. An electrical cell served as a power source to the primary coil but when the current to the coil was interrupted (Off/On) another current (induced) is created in the secondary coil. This induction process changed the voltage from the source current (electrical cell) into a higher voltage to deliver the interrupted or alternating electricity. See Fig I for diagrams.

Some induction coils were wound by different sized wires that were then spliced together to form continuous winding. By changing the size (diameter and length) of the windings in the secondary coil, the coil could serve functionally as two to six or more coils. The Dr Jerome Kidder Co was best known for this practice, although others followed the practice sparingly (as a fad). This practice never really captivated the market on faradic batteries nor did it offer any practical advantages physiologically. This practice of multiple induction coil windings was a gimmick from a historical perspective.

The medical electrical batteries using the faradic currents with their induction coils were classified as: 1) pocket batteries, 2) portable or box batteries (varying greatly in size and construction), and 3) stationary or sledge inductorium (for fine work in research and treatment).[4]

3. The Interrupter

Once the electrical effects and operation of the primary and secondary induction coils were recognized in medicine, manual interruptions became a real burden to the operator of a faradic battery. Mechanical devices to control the interruptions (On/Off) of the current from the power source (electrical cell) to the primary coil soon appeared.

As early as 1836, automatic interrupters were devised to break (interrupt) and make (close) the circuit of the induction coils. By automatic regulating the interruptions, rates, or frequency of the faradic current the pulses can be controlled by increasing or decreasing the rates. Pulse rates are used to alter the effects of electrical current on biological tissues. The automatic interrupter freed the operator of the medical electrical battery from manually regulating the pulse rates, thus offering a smoother and more reliable operation.

Numerous attempts were made to regulate faradic current pulses automatically after 1836, but in 1839 Neef of Frankfort-am-Main, Germany, presented his device to a meeting of the Freiburg Scientific Society. Need then published the descriptions of his device in Annales edited by Poggendorff. Neef's device used a hammer that was moved from its contact (the anvil) to the core of the primary coil when magnetized by the primary current. The hammer fell back into the anvil when the magnetic attraction was completed by breaking the circuit.

Neef's early device used the principle of a mercury contact cup. He later

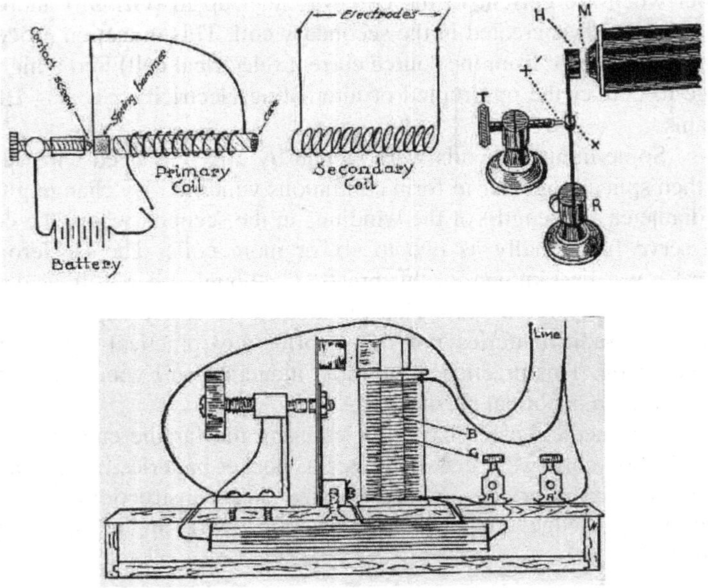

Fig 1. Mechanical Vibrating Interrupters (Top, Circuit and Primitive Type; Bottom, Auxiliary Twin Coils type)

replaced the mercury contact cup with platinum contacts and binding screws when Johann Wagner (1799-1879), also of Germany, gave him the idea.[5]

Several years later (ca 1850), Alexander Kemp of Edinburg and William Neeves of London developed the hammer break of the interrupter. A small device or keeper of soft iron was attached to a leaf spring that was attached to a plate on the base of the device. The device was connected to the poles of the circuit that would open the contact with the platinum contact.

This spring lever, hammer adjustable screw contact vibrated at various rates determined by the adjustable screw. The operator could set the adjustable screw to deliver slow or rapid pulses, but precise rates were not generally possible. The vibration caused a humming sound that was commonly referred to as the "musical note." This hammer type of vibrating interrupter remained in common use on faradic current medical batteries until replaced by thermal glass tube switches in the twentieth century.[4]

A few faradic electrical batteries use two interrupters on a single model. One interrupter of the conventionally designed spring hammer and vibrator is used to regulate fast interruptions (rapid pulses). The second interrupter, sometimes of conical shape design or pendular operation, moves like a pendulum to regulate slow interruptions. Examples of these dual interrupters on faradic machines are seen on a few models by Hall of Boston; Flemming of Philadelphia; and Kidder of New York.

Operation of the interrupter: The vibrating interrupters were mechanical type interrupters powered by the one or more cells (wet or dry) operating the electrical battery. The earliest form was a primitive vibrating interrupter that used two small disc surfaces (contacts) of platinum or soft iron for the point of make and break (upper left, Fig1). Later models offered the choice of the earlier type or the type that used an auxiliary make and break feature (upper right, Fig1). The auxiliary type of mechanical vibrating interrupter had its own twin inductive coils separate from the major induction coil of the faradic electrical battery. These coils were small and operated as a separate device. Each type of interrupter required little attention, no recharging, and did not overheat.

The simple and early design (upper right, Fig1) operates by having the lever (RH) pulled back which allows (x) to contact the circuit for current to flow through the primary circuit. The flowing current magnetizes the iron core (M) of the induction coil which then pulls the lever (RH) so that the soft iron or platinum disc (H) touches the iron core (M). When the small iron or platinum disc makes contact with the iron core of the induction coil the other end (x) of the lever loses contact (break) so current stops its flow, the core loses its magnetism, and the lever (armature) is pulled back by the spring action of the material of the lever (RH). The action at (x) is repeated. The adjustable screw (T) is connected to the circuit (left). The screw contact is adjusted manually to set the rate or degree of rapidity desired by the operator to change the period (timing) of the moving spring lever. The twin coil vibrating interrupter used on faradic electrical batteries were placed on some batteries by Otto Flemming, and by Thomas Hall.

4. Rheostats

An important aspect in operating a medical electrical battery is the control of current amplitude. Several approaches to solving this problem occurred ever since artificial electricity was used in medicine. One of the easiest and most economical (from a cost basis) methods for control of faradic current was the sliding metal tube current controller or rheostat. This approach was used commonly by American manufacturers from 1871 through the 1920s. The metal tube was moved out (away) from the coils to increase current amplitude, and then pushed in (closes) to decrease the current amplitude. Current amplitude was maximum when the sliding metal tube controller was pulled away from the coils which allowed the two coils (primary and secondary) to be fully exposed to each other. In other words, movement of the sliding metal tube interfered with the magnetic field or flux of the primary coil to control the current amplitudes.

Another method used to control current amplitude was to introduce gradated resistances into the circuit by means of fluids. Columns of water or salt solutions (eg, sulfate of zinc) were used in fluid rheostats. Fluid rheostats are unreliable with continued use because electrolysis and polarization occurs from the electricity.

In 1843, Sir Charles Wheatstone (1802-1875) of England invented the bridge or a method of varying manually the amount of resistance in an electrical circuit. He assigned the word rheostat to describe his electrical bridge device. In 1849, DuBois-Reymond of Germany described in the second volume of his works a method of sliding the secondary coil manually over the primary induction coil to finely control faradic current amplitude for clinical and research work. He called his device a sledge inductorium. Between 1871 and 1885 American manufacturers of faradic batteries used either the sliding metal tube controller or the sledge inductorium style to manually control current amplitude. Some Kidder faradic current models exemplify the inductorium style for control of current amplitude.

In 1885, Charles Willms of the Charles Willms and Co of Baltimore, MD, invented a new disc style rheostat to control both faradic and galvanic current on medical electrical batteries (Fig 2A). In 1886, The Chloride of Silver Dry Cell Battery Co of Baltimore (Willms also worked for this company) began marketing some of its units with the new Willms Current Controller. The Willms Current Controller is seen only on the Chloride of Silver Dry Cell units that were quality products for physicians. In 1887, Dr GB Massey, renown electrotherapeutist of Philadelphia, designed a disc rheostat along the basic design of Willms. Otto Flemming, a manufacturer of quality medical electrical batteries in Philadelphia, made and marketed the Massey style rheostat on his models (Fig 2B).[5]

Soon after the new disc style, Dr AH Goelet of New York City designed a smaller disc style rheostat that could operate effectively on portable medical electrical batteries (Fig 2C). The Waite & Bartlett Manufacturing Co of New York City made and marketed the Goelet disc rheostat.[5] In 1899, Manes Fuld of both The Chloride of Silver Dry Cell Battery Co and the Voltamp Electric Co of Baltimore developed a disc style rheostat that was then used on several models of the Voltamp family batteries (Fig 2D).

The disc style rheostat designed by Massey and representing that of others was made of slate with a cone shaped roughened surface for adhesion of a graphite coating. A spring nickel plated rotating lever with a brush like attachment was manually moved over the graphite of varying thickness to regulate current amplitude through the graduated resistances offered by the graphite. Slate was used as a material because of its enduring and pleasing appearance. The graphite offered resistance

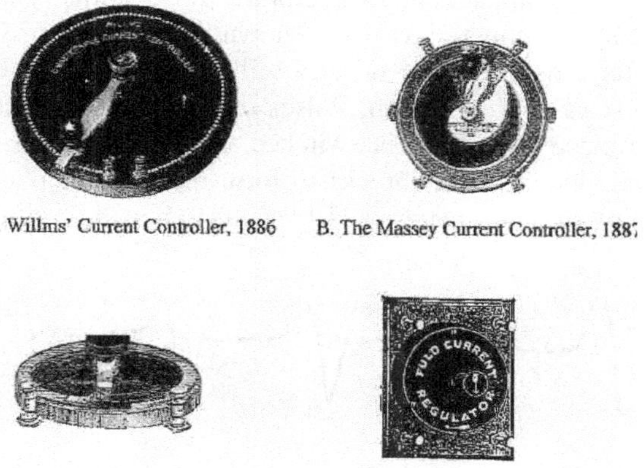

A. Willms' Current Controller, 1886 B. The Massey Current Controller, 188

C. Goelet's Pocket Rheostat D. Fuld Current Regulator, 1899

Fig 2. Disc Current Controllers of Willms, Massey, Goelet, Fuld

to the passage of current so it made a good nonconductor for regulating current amplitude.[5]

The Willms disc rheostat used glue, graphite, and brass fillings to resist current. These combinations of materials are mounted on the under side of the disc. The rotating lever made contact with the circuit and resisting graphite to control current amplitude.

5. Types of Currents and Their Waveforms

The types of waveforms delivered from a medical electrical battery are based on the direction of flow of current. In galvanic or direct current units the flow is unidirectional. That is, the current direction is either negative or positive because of its direction or polarity; the current can flow negatively or be reversed to flow positively at a given pole or in a given electrode. Galvanic current is continuous if it flows in one direction for one or more seconds up to several minutes (Fig 13). Monophasic pulses are formed when the galvanic current is modulated or interrupted for short periods of time (eg, less than 1 second, Fig 14).

Alternating current is current that is bidirectional or biphasic. As alternating current flows its direction is constantly reversed (eg, 2 directions). Thus, unidirectional, continuous, or monophasic pulsed currents are usually considered direct current or galvanic source. Bidirectional and biphasic currents that alter directions continuously are alternating, faradic, and sinusoidal currents. Pulsed currents are monophasic or bi-directional currents of very short durations (less than 1 msec) and separated by an even shorter period of time.

The characteristic waveforms for faradic current that are produced by an induction coil are shown in Figures 3-5. Waveforms are drawn after those depicted on an oscilloscope. The waveforms are not drawn to scale in this section. Pulses (or faradic or induction) are made when the electrical circuit is switched On (make) to form the negative phase, and switched Off (break) to form the positive phase. The pulses delivered by the early batteries (19th century) may be controlled manually

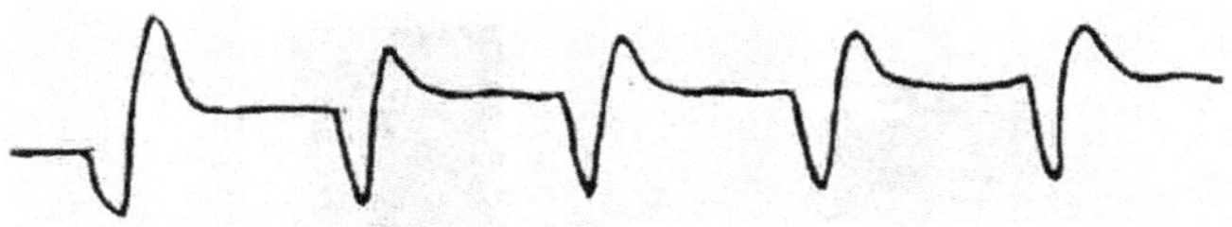

Fig 3. Waveform from Common Induction Coil

or by a mechanical interruptor. The advantage of pulsed current is the contractile effect on muscle. Different models of faradic electrical batteries may provide slight modifications in the biphasic waveform, but

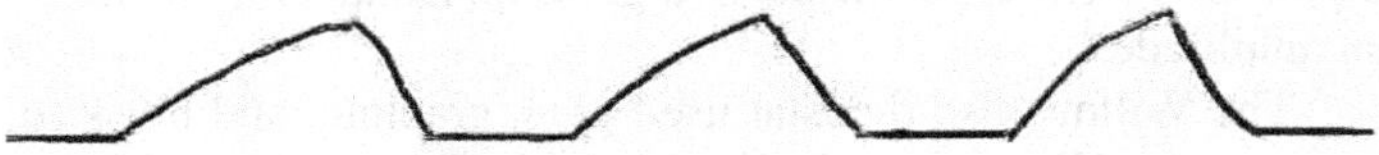

Fig 4. Waveform from Primary Coil

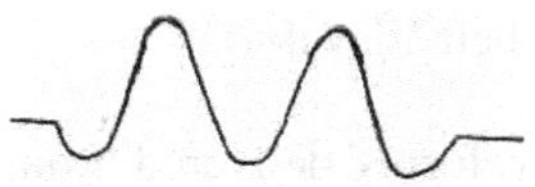

Fig 5. Waveform from Secondary Coil

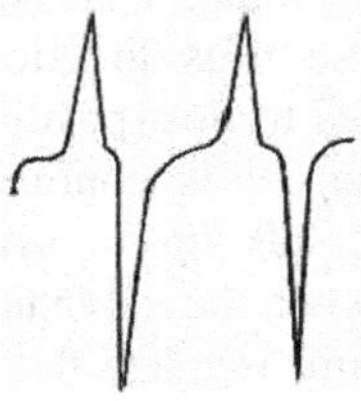

Fig 6. Symmetrical Biphasic Waveform

all faradic pulses give contractile effects of muscle. The following figures show waveforms of some medical electrical batteries discussed herein. These waveforms were obtained when the particular medical electrical batteries were powered by four D-sized dry cells (ca 6 volts), and recorded by an oscilloscope. A typical recording represents the waveform produced from the combined primary and secondary induction coils receiving a mean 5.8 volts direct current input and a mean 2.6 volts alternating output (35 to 40 % of input); 18 millivolts peak to peak pulse; and two milliseconds pulse duration (Figs 6-12).

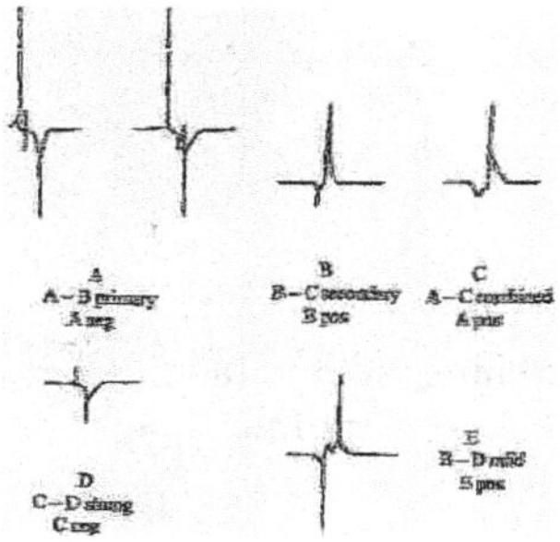

Fig 7. Williams' Dial Electro-Magnetic Machine, Posts A to E

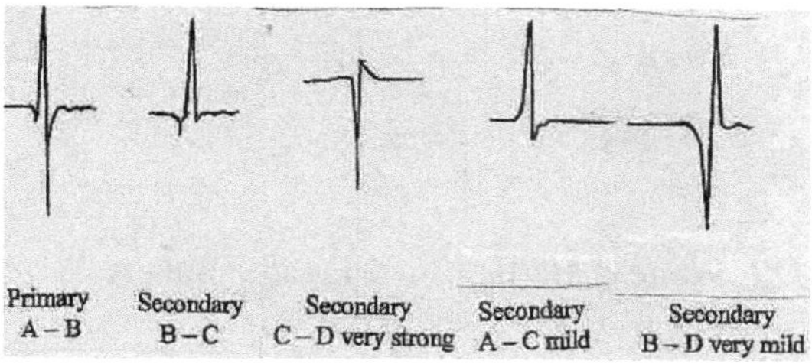

Fig 8. PG Williams' Perfection Electro-Magnetic Battery

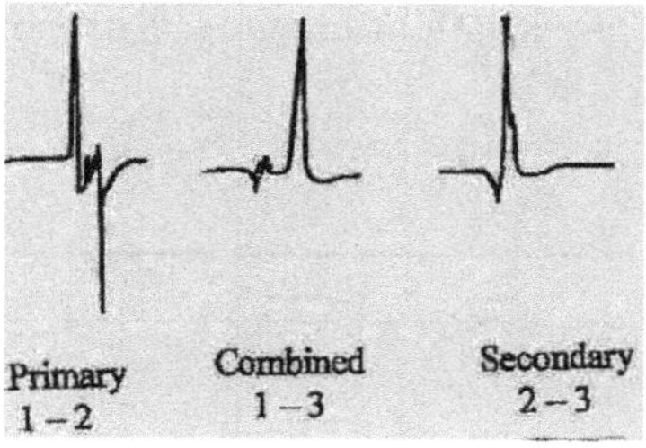

Fig 9. Voltamp No.2 Faradic Battery

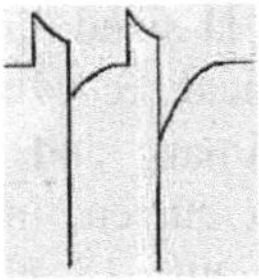

Fig 10. Voltamp No.3 Faradic Battery

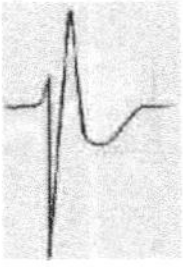

Fig 11. Flemming No.3 Faradic Battery
with Rocking Arm Interrupter

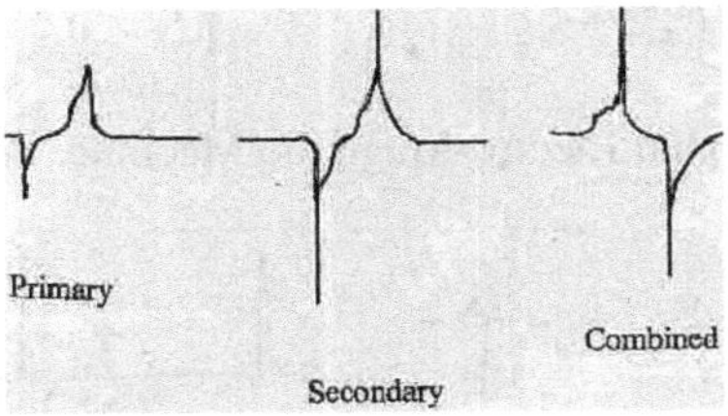

Fig 12. Waite & Bartlett No.2 Faradic Battery

The monophasic current of galvanic or direct current is unidirectional, but can be changed with a pole changer to provide either positive or negative current at the active or designated electrode. Galvanic current basically provides chemical changes to the skin if allowed to flow for any length of time (eg, 1 or more seconds to several minutes).

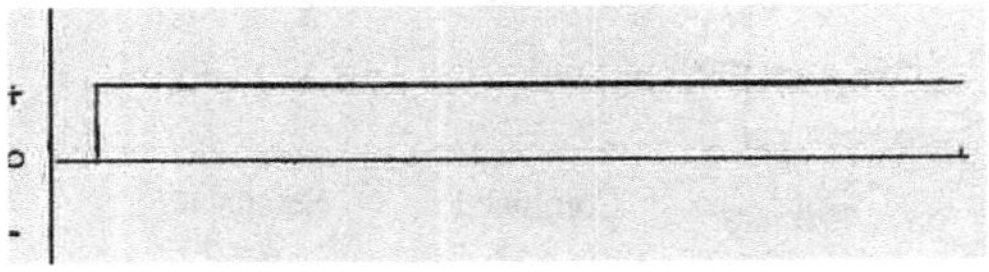

Fig 13. Positive Galvanic Current

Galvanic current may be pulsed manually or automatically to provide a monophasic pulse for contracting muscle. If the galvanic current flow is modulated by interrupting it at a fixed or unfixed rate a pulse (monophasic) is formed. Galvanic current can be reversed by switches or manually so that negative or positive monophasic pulses are produced.

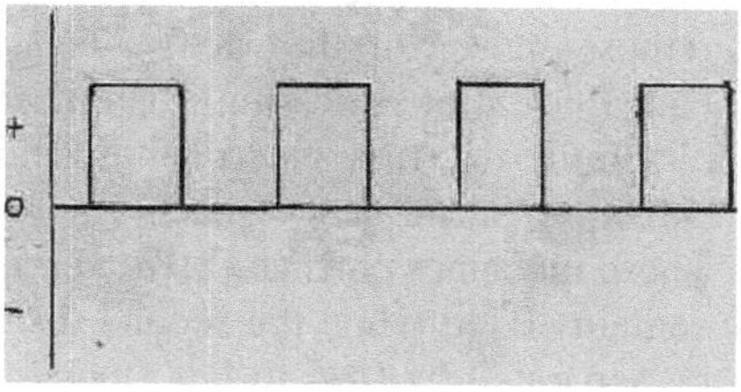

Fig 14. Monophasic or Galvanic Pulses

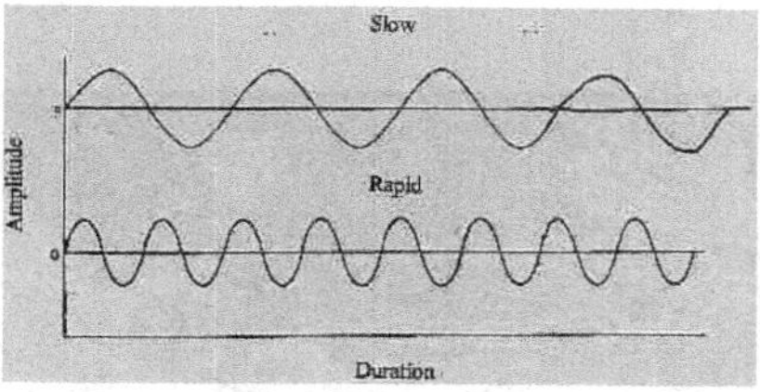

Fig 15. Slow and Rapid Sinusoidal Current

The sinusoidal current has some similarity to the faradic current because it is alternating waves and causes muscle contractions. The sinusoidal wave form is smooth and balanced biphasic pulses, and less painful to the sensory nerves than faradic current that is unbalanced biphasic pulses.

Dr JH Kellogg of the Battle Creek (MI) Sanitarium in the 1880s discovered sinusoidal current, made apparatuses to produce it, recorded its wave form by an electrograph, and studied its effects on muscles. Years later d'Arsonval of France experimented with high frequency currents and coined the named "sinusoidal" after their wave form, however, the high frequency current effected tissue as heat unlike the slower frequencies used by Kellogg to contract muscles. Around 1900, sinusoidal currents became accepted and fashionable among those physicians using electrical batteries.

The waveforms of pulsed current vary (mono-, bi- phasic), but it is the interaction of charge, current, energy, and voltage that excites peripheral nerves to cause muscle contractions. The interaction of the current characteristics rely on the area under the curves that depend on time and peak current amplitude. Shape of the waveforms is just a twist to the area under the curve and relates to angular velocity and pulse rates. Today, the waveforms of pulsed currents may be somewhat different than those shown in this section; however, the differences relate to the interactions of the characteristics above and to the electrical engineering of apparatuses. The pulse times are generally shorter now than in the 1880s and the current shapes are smoother and more accurate. The area under the curves (pulses) may be smaller today that in affect offers more subject comfort than those pulses of the 1880s. Today's apparatuses permit greater control and current modifications than those of the 1880s.

In 1865, Holtz built the first electrical machine that was to become a class of induction or influence machines to produce static sparks or electricity. These machines consist of two varnished glass discs or plates. One disc remains fixed while the second disc revolves on its axis. The two discs are separated by 0.25 to 0.50 inches. The fixed disc has two holes or openings oppositely located from the axis. A strip of paper with one end pointed extends from each opening and is called an inductor. Opposite the inductors on the other side of the revolving disc is

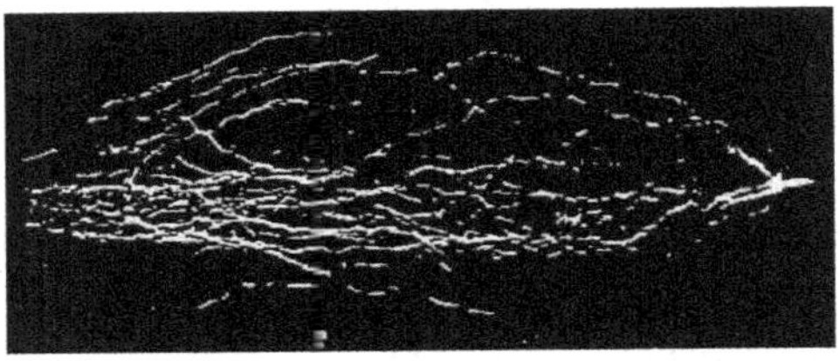

Fig 16. Sparks from Influence Static Machine with Leyden Jars

a pair of metal combs connected by wires to the poles of the machine.

When the inductors are charged positively and electrodes are brought into contact, the comb opposite the inductor is charged negatively by induction. A positive charge occurs at the comb and since the combs are connected through joined electrodes the positive electrode is repelled from the inductor.

The negative electricity on one comb begins to discharge itself through the point on the comb to the glass disc or plate in front of it to form a brush. The negative charge is then carried around the disc in a direction toward the other inductor and comb. Positive electricity is then discharged onto the disc to the comb on one side and inductor on the other side of the disc while the inductor receives negative charge. The discs become strongly electrified (high voltage, low amplitudes) positively and sparks pass between the electrodes. In some cases Leyden jars (capacitors) are attached to the electrodes to increase energy of the sparks that were used in treatments.

References

1. Edmonson JM. American Surgical Instruments. San Francisco, CA, Norman Pub, 1997, pp 86, 90

2. Shatx SC. Bringing home the bakelite. Antiq Trader's Collect. Nov 2000, pp 7-9, 14-15

3. Digger Odell's web page,www.google.com; (http:www.bottlebooks.com/patenteddates.htm)

4. Hackmann WD. The Induction Coil in Medicine and Physics 1835-1877. In Blondel C, Parot F, Turner A, Williams M (eds). Studies in the History of Scientific Instruments. London, Rogers Turner, 1989, pp 235-250

5. Englemann GJ. The Faradic or Induced Current; Electromagnetism; Electro-massage, and Instruments. In Bigelow HR (ed). An International System of Electro-Therapeutics. Philadelphia, PA. FA Davis, 1894, pp A117-A177

PART 2. MANUFACTURERS OF PHYSICIAN USE OF APPARATUS (PHYSICIAN SHOCK MAKERS)

Electrical batteries and apparatuses and supplies in the United States were first made for and sold to scientists of educational institutions and to physicians. Until the invention and commercial production of the telegraph and then the telephone almost all advances in the knowledge, theory, design, and manufacture of electrical devices were for medicine and science. Until the telegraph and telephone there really were no other commercial demands for use of electricity. Medicine and science were the major consumers and developers of electrical devices for centuries. The commercialism in the 1870s of the telegraph, telephone, dynamo, and lighting placed medicine as a sharer rather than a creator and innovator of electrical advances. Science on the other hand continued to be a reactor and innovator, but additionally became a partner with commercial developments to continue thereafter as a major contributor to advances in electricity. In Part 2 several major manufacturers and their electrical medical apparatuses for physicians will be discussed along with discussions of some of the smaller or lesser known companies. These discussions are limited by the availability of resources, and which necessitated exclusion of such companies as Fischer, Myers, Myrowitch, and Vetter.

CHAPTER 3. EARLIEST BATTERY MAKERS

Prior to the Civil War very few medical electrical batteries were made in the United States. Those batteries made were constructed manually by a few instrument makers who probably made most of them on request. Educational institutions that used electrical batteries, electrical philosophical instruments, and induction coils for laboratory demonstrations were the major consumers. No doubt some physicians were requesting the American made electrical batteries, but both educational institutions and physicians were buying electrical batteries and their accessories from European sources. The Civil War became a stimulus for faster, durable, and cheaper production for all products that included medical electrical batteries.

Although the Davis-Kidder magnetoelectrical unit was patented in 1854, it really was not put into mass production until about the 1860s and 1870s. Also, in the 1860s, especially the mid 1860s, a few instrument makers were converting their shops into capabilities for mass production. Europe was influencial in the American movement for medical electrical batteries. Medical electrical batteries were expensive, slow in delivery, and unseen products before purchase. Physician and public consumer demand for these electrical and mysterious devices increased after the

Civil War (viz, 1870s). Electricity was anticipated to offer improvements in medical treatments and could be applied without the physicians' intervention.

Prior to and immediately after the Civil War (ca 1848-1870) a few American instrument makers were involved in constructing and retailing medical electrical batteries. Most notable of these early makers of batteries was Daniel Davis, Jr, of Boston, MA, whose main emphasis was making medical electrical batteries and philosophic instruments. His successor, Palmer and Hall and in particularly Thomas Hall of Boston, after 1857, included an emphasis in making medical electrical batteries in addition to optical and surgical instruments. The other early makers of medical electrical batteries did so as a diversional or side line product. These latter makers (Pike, Jr; Ritchie) were best known for their medical instruments other than medical electrical batteries. In the case of the Ritchies, their efforts were accessories used with medical electrical batteries rather than their actual construction.

This chapter reviews four instrument makers that in reality were pioneers in the manufacture of American medical electrical batteries. Emphasis is placed on Benjamin Pike, Jr, Daniel Davis, Jr, Thomas Hall, and Edward S Ritchie.

THE PIKE FAMILY

Members of the Pike family were noted instrument makers of New York, NY, from 1841 to 1916. Benjamin Pike was born in England, but lived in the United States from 1777 to 1863 when he died. Benjamin Pike made and sold mathematical, nautical, optical, philosophical, and survey instruments. Benjamin Pike, Jr (1809-1864), the eldest son, joined his father in 1831 as a partner, and worked with him until 1843. The firm was known as Benjamin Pike and Son, and was located at 12 Wall Street, Boston, from 1831 to 1832. The address changed to 14 Wall Street in 1832 to 1833, and to 166 Broadway from 1833 to 1843. The second son Daniel (1815-1893) joined his father and brother in 1841 as a partner. The firm continued to make instrument categories as listed above (barometers, gunner's calipers, protractors, surveyor's compasses, transits) during this period of time. In 1843, Benjamin Pike, Jr, left Benjamin Pike and Son to work alone at 294 Broadway. In 1850, another son Gardiner (1824-1893) joined his father and brother Daniel. Benjamin Pike and Sons were located at 518 Broadway from 1850 to 1867.[1]

BENJAMIN PIKE, JR

Attention shifts to Benjamin Pike, Jr, since he is the only member of the Pike family to manufacture a medical electrical battery. He may also be the best known instrument maker of all of the Pikes.

Benjamin Pike, Jr, was born as the eldest son of Benjamin, Sr,[2] in New York City in 1809. Benjamin Pike, Sr, was an optician, and between 1831 and 1841 the Directory of New York City lists the Benjamin Pike & Son company as opticians. The company then was located at 12 Wall and 166 Broadway. The Directory listed the company as B Pike & Sons (Sr, Jr, Daniel) for 1841 to 1843 on 166 Broadway. Then in 1843 and 1844, Benjamin Pike, Jr, was listed alone as an optician on 294 Broadway. Benjamin Pike, Jr, continued to be listed in the Directory from 1845 to 1846, but now he was involved in the business of manufacturing varieties of magnets and electrical apparatuses for medical use, microscopes, philosophical and optical instruments, and telescopes. In 1846 through 1847 his optical business shop was at 294 Broadway.[2] He continued to be listed as an optical company from 1846 through 1864 at 294 Broadway. Benjamin Pike, Jr, died on 1 May,1864 near his home in Astoria, Long Island,[2] but the company with his name continued until at least 1881. In 1881, the company was a wholesale merchant for imported instruments from Europe. Like many American companies of the nineteenth century the Benjamin Pike, Jr, business imported the instruments unsigned and then attached its name by adding engraved plates to the instruments.

Locations for the Pike business were assigned to Benjamin, Sr, at 518 Broadway, and by Benjamin Pike, Jr, at 291 Broadway. Benjamin, Jr, made and sold early dial telegraph sending and receiving sets while at 291 Broadway. These locations are in addition to those cited above. Small manufacturers changed locations frequently in the nineteenth century to improve, downsize, and economize the business with changing times (similar to that today). The Pikes were early manufacturers of telegraph sending and receiving sets. Since the father and sons were master opticians, they easily got involved in making instruments that required similar skills and components. Their involvement in telegraph and medical electrical batteries was a natural involvement with market demands and savings.[2]

Davis and Dreyfus list Benjamin Pike, Jr's, address as 294 Broadway in 1848. The 1848 catalog listed and priced products as chemical, mathematical, optical, and philosophical instruments.[4]

Electro-Magnetic Machine. The Faradic Battery by Benjamin Pike, Jr, in 1848 had a logo that read "Electro-Magnetic Machine" and bore a golden eagle on the red Morocco leather cover of the induction coil. The eagle on the logo also has "E Pluribus Unum" impressed on the shield. The boxed case (6.25 x 6.25 x 4 inches) is walnut, and houses the induction coil that has a sliding metal current controller. The coil is contacted by an adjustable spaced contact screw to control vibrations of the interrupter. Metal binding posts are lacquered brass. The unit is powered by a single trough wet cell (similar to those made later by Thomas Hall of Boston) of copper and zinc components.[3]

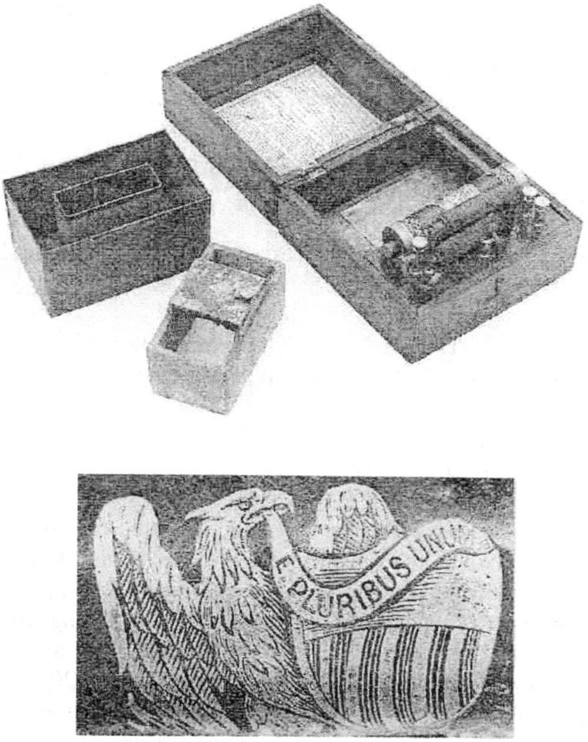

Fig P1. Electro-Magnetic Machine (Courtesy of Tesseract-Early Scientific Instruments)

Benjamin Pike, Jr, published trade catalogs of his products (viz, 1848 and 1856) that included another electrical faradic battery, the New Portable Magneto-Electrical Machine. Pike's faradic batteries were designed for physician use. The catalog for 1856, displayed an electrical egg (device that was a cross of the vacuum tube and high voltage technology of the time) that cost $6.00. The electrical egg was probably imported. The same catalog illustrated and described mathematical, optical, and philosophical instruments.

Summary

Benjamin Pike, Jr, was an early maker of medical electrical batteries (1848) in the United States. His proficiency resided in his making of optical products. Only one medical electrical battery (Electro-Magnetic Machine) has been identified with his signature. He perhaps custom made other models that would indeed be rare artifacts.

References

1…Websters Instrument Makers Database.(www. adlerplantarius (www.adlerplantarius.org/histoy/websters/p.htm)

2. Smart CE. The Makers of Surveying Instruments in America Since 1700. Troy, NY, Regal Art, 1962

3. Cofeen D, Coffeen Y (eds). Tesseract, ed 74 catalogue. Hastings-on-Hudson, NY, 2003, no 41

4. Davis AB, Dreyfus MS. The Finest Instruments Ever Made. Arlington, MA, Medical History Pub Assocs, 1986, p 258

DANIEL DAVIS, JR, OF BOSTON

Daniel Davis, Jr, may not have been the first instrument maker in the United States to concentrate a portion of his business to making and retailing medical electrical batteries, but he was among, if not, the most prominent of the early individuals (Pike, Jr; Pilling; Ritchie; Saxon) in the field. He was born (1813) and raised in Princeton, MA. Seeking a career trade, he went to Boston in 1833 when he was 20 years of age. He got a job with William King who made electrical machines and lightning rods. Davis, Jr, was apparently both quick to learn and to acquire skill of a credible craftsman.

He may have worked with his brother Ari around 1835 to 1837 at 11 Cornhill.[1] Ari Davis (1811-1885) worked as an instrument maker in Washington, DC, in 1834, but returned to Boston in 1835. Ari Davis was a maker of mathematical, nautical, philosophical, and survey instruments. He also was an inventor and a watchmaker. His shops were located at 11 Cornhill, 19 Court Square, and from 1839 to 1845 at 75 Court Square, Boston. In 1845 to 1885, Ari Davis worked in Lowell, MA. Ari died in 1885. From 1837 to 1844 Elias Howe was an apprentice under Ari Davis.[1]

Daniel Davis, Jr, left his association with brother Ari when he entered his own business of making electrical machines around 1837 in addition to making mathematical, nautical, and philosophical instruments. He located his business at 428 Washington Street, Boston, MA. At that period of time the greatest outlet for marketing electrical machines and medical electrical batteries was educational institutions that used the machines for lectures and laboratory demonstrations, and some physicians. Davis was able to form the association with educational institutions to make and sell them instruments. Even though the medical electrical battery had limited use in the United States in this period of time, Davis apparently was fortunate enough to forge ahead and make a comfortable living. He sold his magnetoelectrical machines for $25.00 to $35.00 that was considerable costs for medical electrical batteries that in the 1870s would sell for much less with mass production manufacturing.

Around 1836, a local physician, Dr Charles Grafton Page (1812-1868) had designed an improved version of the induction coil. By that year Dr Page was well known in electrical science after having a dozen of his research papers published in the Annals of Electricity, Magnetism, and Chemistry, a journal edited and owned by William Sturgeon of England.[2(1-36)] Sturgeon was renown for his work with electrical magnets.

Dr Page apparently went to Daniel Davis, Jr, in 1837 because of his reputation from making electrical machines. Dr Page probably used electrical batteries in his practice, but more importantly he had an advanced knowledge of physics that provided him the ability to invent, improve electrical machines, and to investigate. A relation of business, interaction of science, and mutual admiration began between Dr Page and Davis, Jr, in 1837 and lasted until 1852. During this period of time, Dr Page probably shared his knowledge of electricity and magnetism with Davis who increased his understanding about the phenomena. Davis is not known to have had formal education in electricity, magnetism, mathematics, or physics.

By 1838, Davis Jr, began to illustrate Page's instruments in his trade catalog. Davis made instruments that Dr Page designed and then retailed them through his catalog. Mutual interests and shared benefits encouraged the relation between the two individuals. Davis constructed many units of Page's electrical machines and was able to sell them at considerable profit; Page, however, did not benefit financially from these sales.[3] Page's current breaker was the first magnetic driven interrupter for the induction coil. Earlier (1837) Sturgeon found that a bundle of iron wires used as the core for his electromagnets was most effective. He was working with various metals for use as cores. His work involved studying bundles of iron tubes, bundles of iron wires, gun barrels, iron bars, and rolled iron foils to improve the electromagnets.[4] The improved coil of Sturgeon was then introduced into Page's medical electrical machines.

After leaving Salem, MA, in 1838 and moving to Washington, DC, area Page searched the area to find a suitable instrument maker to help him. He apparently worked with Ari Davis, brother of Daniel Davis, Jr, for awhile. Through the years Daniel and Ari Davis were Page's only association with instrument makers, but Daniel Davis, Jr, was in contact with many notable scientists of that period of time. Notable scientists frequented the Davis shop in Boston where he demonstrated both experiments and instruments to his visitors. The visiting scientists may have reciprocated by showing Davis various experiments using his shop and instruments.[5] Davis conducted his own experiments in his shop similarly to Francis Hauksbee (d 1713)[6] of England using the various instruments that he made.

Ari Davis, brother of Daniel, who was an experienced machinist in making philosophical instruments came to Page's aid. Ari Davis patented the earliest compact electromagnetic machine for use in medicine in 1854. He sold the patent to Walter Kidder, an investor of New York City, for $4000.00 (ca 1855). After awhile Kidder sold the patent to Walter Burnley for $6000.00 profit. Burnley eventually (ca 1856) developed, manufactured, and marketed the Davis/Kidder electromagnetic machine.[7] The first units used a bone handled crank to operate a gear & pulley drive that turned twin coils at high speeds to generate current. Ari Davis placed the magneto-electrical components into an attractive wooden box. This particular medical magnetoelectrical machine was very popular for home use during the years between 1856 and 1900 so that the unit is commonly found in antique shops and on eBay auctions.

Daniel Davis, Jr, continued to gain a credible reputation for his craftsmanship and knowledge of electricity. He became the first instrument maker in the United States to design and produce machines that generated constant electrical current mechanically for use in electrochemical experiments. At the 1839 exposition of the Massachusetts Charitable Mechanics Association he won a gold medal for his workmanship and display of a variety of magnetoelectrical instruments and engines. He even received a commendation for understanding the rationale of the instruments that he displayed and produced.[5]

During their relation Page would mention Davis' work in his published papers, and Davis listed Page's instruments in his various catalogs. Of 21 instruments shown in Davis' first catalog, Page had invented 14 of them. Davis' first catalog Descriptive Catalogue of Apparatus and Experiments, To illustrate the following Branches of Science, Namely: Galvanism, Electro-Dynamics, Magnestism, Electro-Magnetism, Magneto-Electricity, Thermo-Electricity in 1838. Sixty-eight instruments were described in this 72 paged catalog. In 1839, he had improved or introduced 41 of the instruments described in the 1838 catalog.[5] Only five of Page's instruments were cited in Davis' catalog of 1839, but 18 are listed in the catalog of 1848.

In 1842, D Davis, Jr, now with several years of experience and much knowledge about electricity and magnetism published his Manual of Magnetism. Including also Electro-Magnetism, Magneto-Electricity, and Thermo-Electricity. With Description of the Electrotype Process. For the Use of Student and Literary Institutions, Boston.[5] The second edition of the manual was released in 1848 as an enlarged and extensively written book. The manual not only contained descriptions and prices of instruments that Davis was selling (5 pp), but its contents included:

definitions and explanations, details of electrical current (frictional, galvanic, thermal, and animal electricity), magnetism, induction of magnetism, and induction of electricity. The manual was really a textbook of 322 pages. He intended college and high school students to use his manual; it was adopted as a textbook for the cadets at the United States Military Academy. A section of the manual stressed and detailed the use of one of his machines for electroplating and other electrolytic experiments. Electroplating was new at the time, and his manual never became well known. The next year, however, a Frenchman presented electroplating to the French Academy that became the standard for the new industry.

Daniel Davis, Jr, did however put his new found process to work for his own use. He began to gild (place a thin layer of gold) or silver plate on medical instruments such as: canulas, forceps, knives, lancets, and needles. His process enabled him to gild very economically to make his instruments most attractive, and prevent their rusting. His electroplating method preceded the nickel plating that became so popular and commonplace on medical electrical batteries in the late 1860s or early 1870s. The George Tiemann Co of New York City followed the practice of electroplating in 1843, and then others in Boston and Philadelphia.[8]

The fourth edition of the Manual of Magnetism was published in 1852, although entered in Congress in 1847. The fourth edition contained 322 pages of text and an additional 46 pages as a catalog of products. The manual basically was about magnetism and its relation to electricity. Each edition was intended as a practical rather than theoretical approach to the subject. His manual was mainly under the direction of Drs John Bacon, Jr, and William F Channing. New articles of the apparatuses presented were credited to EB Horn. His Manual of Magnetism endured 13 editions until 1872. The 13th edition was similar to the second,[5] except for the catalog section. Professor Silliman of Yale College and editor of the American Journal of Science once lauded Davis for his Manual of Magnetism.

In 1846, Daniel Davis, Jr, published his The Medical Application of Electricity, Boston.[8] In this pamphlet Davis, Jr, alluded to a form of quackery that included galvanic belts and rings. He described the belts as being made of two different metals that when activated with the skin might deliver a small amount of galvanic electricity. He doubted the ability of the current amplitude from these devices to pass through organs of the body.[9]

In the meanwhile, Daniel Davis, Jr, severed any relation with Dr Page in 1852. Daniel Davis, Jr's business in Boston was so successful that after just 15 years (age 39 years) he sold it in 1854 and retired to his farm.[5] The business was bought by Palmer & Hall of Boston in 1854, and in 1857 Thomas Hall became the sole owner of the instrument company.

Thomas Hall probably contributed to Davis' revisions of the Manual of Magnetism in 1852 to 1872; especially with price setting and the deletion and addition of apparatuses that he was making and marketing. The 4th edition of Davis, Jr's, Manual of Magnetism contained 322 pages of machine descriptions and figures. Pages 35 to 46 lists medical electrical batteries, and 46 pages served as a "Catalogue of Appraratus" with prices. The business was still located at 428 Washington Street, Boston, in 1854 when Davis retired and sold it. Although published in 1852, the 4th edition was entered in Congress in 1847 (title page). Like earlier editions Davis, Jr, credited Drs John Bacon, Jr, and William F Channing as principals in the books' preparation. EB Horn contributed the new articles cited in the manual.

In 1867, Page published his book History of Induction in which he credited Davis several times for illustrations and catalog descriptions. Daniel Davis, Jr, died on 22 March 1887 (age 64 years; 1813-1877). Rowbottom and Susskind cited Daniel Davis, Jr's, birth as 1777 and his death as 1841.[9]

Double Helix and Electrotome. This double helix is mounted by three brass bands onto a wooden base with knob legs. The central helix is wound with several strands of large insulated copper wire. Wires at one end of the central helix are connected to a screw post on the wooden base at the same end of the helix wire. The other ends of the helix wires are soldered to the middle brass band. On the middle band is a brass cup that holds mercury. From this cup holding mercury is a wire secured to a clockwork above. On each side of the middle brass band is the clockwork from which extends a wire to each glass cup mounted on a brass band at each end of the helices. The spring controlled clockwork dips the wire ends into the glass cups that also contain mercury. This

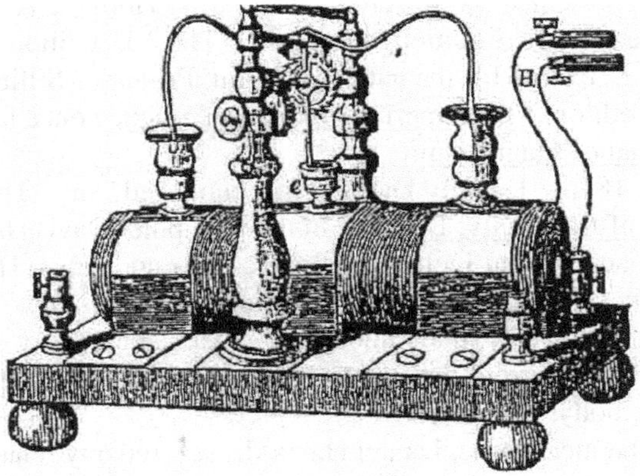

Fig D1. Double Helix and Electrotome

action of the clockwork and wires make circuit connections.

The outer helix (coil) is wound by 2000 feet of fine wire. One end of the helix are two screw connecting posts to join the power cell(s). The unit is activated when one end of the wire dips into one mercury cup. The spring clockwork is released to start a vibration for flow of pulsed current. When either end of the wire leaves the mercury (a spark occurs in the cup) the current is interrupted.

An electrical shock occurs in the electrodes (connected to a person's hands) when a spark shows. The unit was used for educational demonstrations, but could also be used medically. It is believed to have been one of Dr Charles G Page's designs, and it cost $20.00 between 1848 and 1852.

Double Helix and Vibrating Electrotome. This unit is simpler than that of Fig D1 because its rheotome is not a clockwork, thus the reduced cost. The unit has the electrical components of the circuit mounted on top of a wooden base or face plate. No box encases the unit. The interrupter or vibrating electrotome (later rheotome) is self acting by

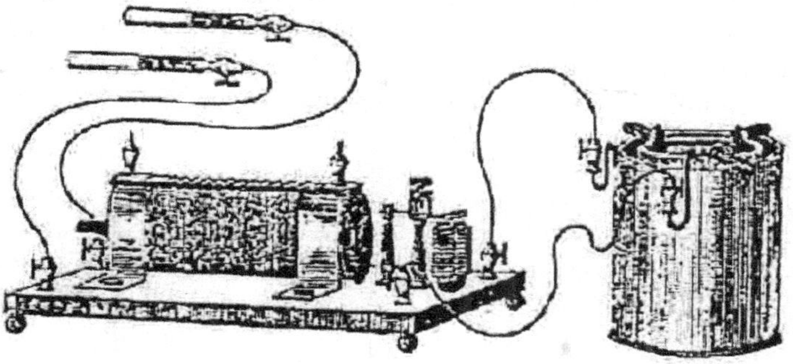

Fig D2. Double Helix and Vibrating Electrotome

which faradic pulses can be varied in rate. It is fixed to the base. The helix or induction coil is mounted horizontally on the base. The helices are not separable but are insulated from each other. The inner helix is a bundle of wires that are moved at will to regulate current amplitude. The number of wires in this small movable helix will also control amplitude. Two screw posts or cups near the electrotome are used to connect to a Grove wet cell. At the other end of the base are two more posts that connect to electrodes and patient. In 1848 to 1852, the unit sold for $12.00 complete, but without the vibrating electrotome it sold for $10.00.

Compound Magnet and Electrotome. A double helix or induction coil is mounted on the wooden base in a horizontal position. The smaller of the two helices is fixed within the larger helix. At one end of the wooden base are two posts or screw cups for connection to a wet

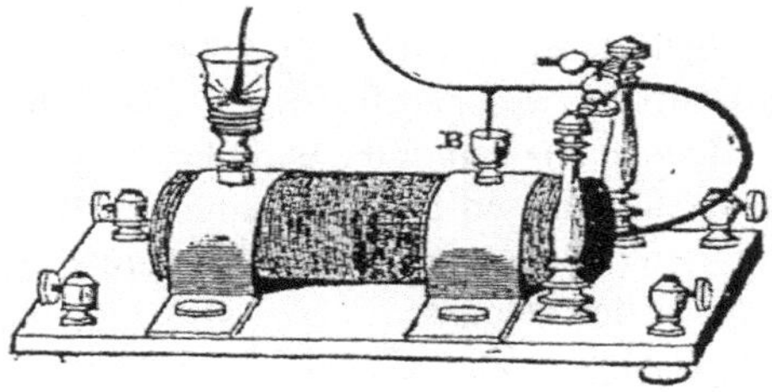

Fig D3. Compound Magnet and Electrotome

cell. One of these two posts is connected with a band that holds a glass cup of mercury. The second post is joined to the coarse wired coil while the other end of the wire connects to the band that holds the brass cup. A formed wire moves on a horizontal axis, and dips its ends into the two mercury cups. A curved iron rod is attached to the side of the axis at one end and approaches the fixed wire helix at its other end.

When the wet cell is connected and the circuit is activated the formed wire and the iron wires of the small helix is magnetized causing the motion of the iron rod to rise out of the mercury cup to break the circuit. From 1848 to 1852, this compound magnet sold for $8.00 to $10.00.

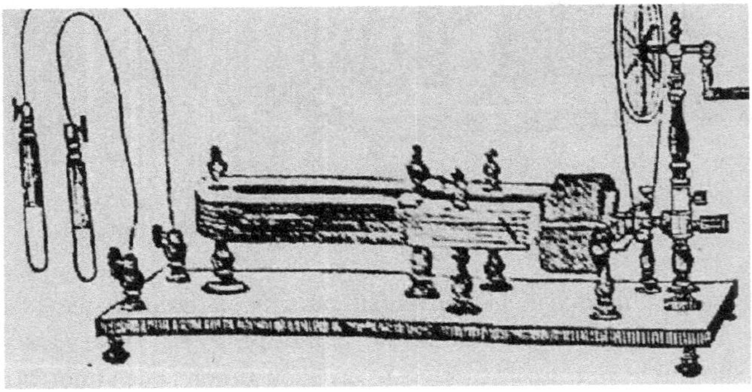

Fig D4. Magneto-Electric Machine

***Magneto-Electric Machine*.** This magnetoelectrical machine uses an armature mounted on an axis. The armature revolves at right angles to a compound horseshoe (U-shaped) steel magnet. The rapidity of the armature (double coils) is determined by a multiplying wheel, manually turned, that is connected by a belt with a small wheel on an axis. The double coil armature is designed to open and close the circuit alternately as it revolves near the magnet. This design and revolving action alternately changes the direction (north to south) of the pulsed current.

The operating components of this machine in Fig D4 are mounted on a wooden base having four knob legs. The motion of the wheels and armature excites electrical currents in the helices. This current amplitude is determined by the rapidity of the turning wheels. The ends of the coil are soldered to a pole changer fixed to the axis. Two silver springs press against these segments and send electricity to the two screw cups (posts). The currents in the helices are reversed twice with each revolution of the armature but changes into one direction by a pole changer. The position of the armature determines the amplitude of current in the various parts of the revolution.

The primary current is not of amplitude sufficient to deliver strong shocks, but when the secondary currents are interrupted with the primary circuit strong electrical shocks are obtained. The shocks are regulated by varying the rate of the revolving armature. This unit cost $30.00 to $35.00 between 1848 and 1852. The mechanism for achieving magnetoelectrical pulses is similar to that used in Ari Davis' design used later in the popular Davis-Kidder magnetoelectrical machine (patented 1854, manufactured after 1856).

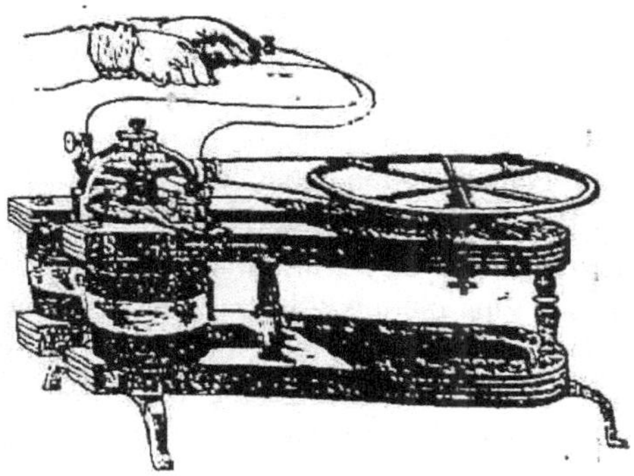

Fig D5. Improved Magneto-Electric Machine

Improved Magneto-Electric Machine. In this model two straight armatures have insulated copper wire that revolve between two U shaped magnets. This model was designed by Dr CG Page with modified (shorter) armatures by Davis, Jr. The permanent magnets are fixed horizontally with mounted legs on the bottom of the lower magnet. Like the unit of Fig D4 this model has a multiplying wheel that can revolve the armature rapidly. A pole changer is present that conveys the alternating currents in a constant direction. Brilliant sparks are emitted as the wire of the helices pass over the pins. The Improved Magneto-Electric Machine offers more power than the previous unit (Fig D4). This model sold for $40.00 to $50.00 in 1848 through 1852.

Magneto-Electric Machine with Vibrating Electrotome. The model is similar to that of Fig D5 except it has a vibrating electrotome

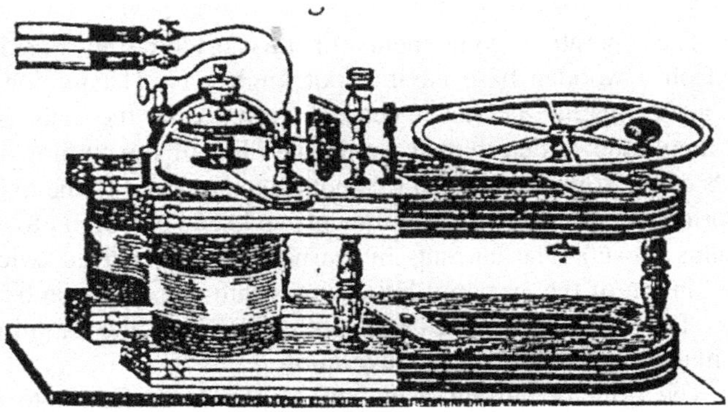

Fig D6. Magneto-Electric Machine with Vibrating Electrotome

that interrupts the electrical circuit to provide pulses. The interrupter device provides more uniform pulses than the previous units of Figs D4 and D5. By turning the screw the platinum point from the attached spring to the armature is raised to permit sparks and primary current use without passing through the coil of the electrotome.

The vibrating electrotome is an electromagnet enclosed in a helix consisting of several layers of coils. It has an armature (device moved by magnet) fixed to a spring supported by the pole. Screw cups or posts are available to connect to the patient and to the machine.

When the machine is put into motion, the electromaget is immediately charged and moves the armature. The motion depresses the spring and separates the the platinum disc. On interruption of the circuit, the armature is raised by force of the spring. The force retention is prevented by a slip of brass brazed to the face of the armature. The current amplitudes are varied by turning the screw. The cost of this unit was $45.00 in 1848 through 1852.

Box Apparatus for Medical Use (Fig D7). Davis offered his double helix and vibrating rheotome in a wooden box for convenience of the physician. Davis simply called this unit the Box Apparatus for Medical Use. This unit is very similar to that cited in Fig D2 except it does not have the spikes on the brass bands as does the model in Fig D2. The wooden box contains all electrical components including a single wet cell to power the unit. The box is hinged and fastened in front by a lock with key. The double helix or induction coil is mounted horizontally to the base of a wooden face plate by two brass bands.

The helices are insulated from each other with the inner helix as an iron rod wound by heavy iron wire, and is moved in and out to control current amplitude. The outer or secondary helix is wound by fine wire. The unit has a self acting interrupter that controls rapidity of current pulses. The interrupter is a vibrating rheotome fixed at one end of the double helix. It forms an electromagnet; the unit's rate is controlled by an

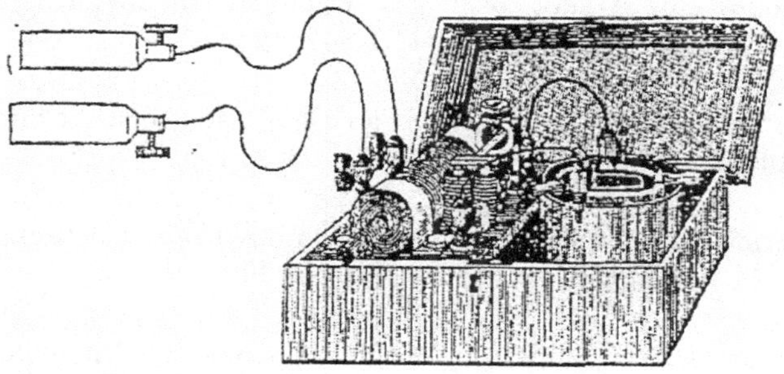

Fig D7. Box Apparatus for Medical Use

adjustable screw. Two adjustable screw posts are located near the interrupter for connection with the wet cell, while two adjustable screw posts at the other end of the helices connect with the patient. Depending on elective features and qualities the unit cost $1.00, $12.00, or $14.00 between 1848 and 1852. The design of the unit is very similar to the faradic units made by Thomas Hall of Boston (eg, Deming, Prof Wells' batteries). Palmer and Hall (Thomas) of Boston bought Davis' business in 1852 so no doubt continued manufacturing Davis' products until such time that Hall came out with the French faradic battery series.

Summary

Daniel Davis, Jr, is credited with making custom medical electrical batteries as early as 1837 in the United States. His association with Dr Charles G Page led to his involvement with medical electrical batteries, and he custom made medical electrical batteries until he sold his business in 1852 to Hall and Palmer. Daniel Davis, Jr, is best known as a master craftsman of mathematical and philosophical instruments. His name is also well known in the medical electrical battery field as a pioneer.

References

1. Websters Instrument Makers Database. (www.adleerplantarius.org/history/webster/p.htm)

2. Post RC: Physics, Patents, and Politics: A Biography of Charles Grafton Page. New York, NY, Science History Pub, 1976, pp 1-36

3. Malone D (ed): Dictionary of American Biography, vol 7. New York, NY, Charles Scribner's Sons, 1934, pp 136-137

4. Geddes LA: A short history of electrical stimulation of excitable tissues. The Physiologist 27 Suppl S1-S47, 1984

5. Sherman R: Charles Page, Daniel Davis, and their electromagnetic apparatus. Rittenhouse 2:34-37, 1989

6. Sherman R: Joseph Henry's contributions to the electromagnet and the electric motor. Rittenhouse 12:97-106, 1999

7. Warner D. Everything from Watch to Locomotive. Rittenhouse, 5:81-93, 1992

8. Edmonson JM: American Surgical Instruments. San Francisco, CA, Norman Pub, 1997, pp 281-282

9. Licht S (ed): Therapeutic Electricity and Ultraviolet Radiation. New Haven, CT, Elizabeth Licht Pub, 1959, p 48

10. Rowbottom M, Susskind E: Electricity and Medicine: History of Their Interaction. San Francisco, CA, San Francisco Press, 1984,pp57-64

THOMAS HALL OF BOSTON

Thomas Hall of Boston, MA, although best known as a manufacturer of electrotherapeutic apparatuses, was not always in that business field. Thomas Hall began his career as a silversmith in Boston (1852-1885;[1] 1849-1878[2]) located at 22 Reade Street.

He was a partner in Palmer and Hall from 1849 to 1857 while making philosophical instruments.[2] During this period of time, Hall was a minor manufacturer of telegraph instruments (eg, the camelback key) which was a natural sideline for him since experience in making various instruments provided the necessary skills. The manufacture of telegraph instruments was in demand then, and additional revenue could be earned through its manufactory. Telegraph instruments shared similar induction coils and contact spacing screws (interrupters) with medical electrical batteries. Hall was listed as an instrument maker of Boston from 1854 to 1872 while operating from a shop at West Broadway (1853-1878).[1]

In 1852, they located their business at 78 West Broadway until 1854 when 72 West Broadway became the center of the business. Palmer and Hall bought the medical electrical business from Daniel Davis, Jr, of Boston in 1854 when Davis retired. In 1857, Palmer and Hall separated when Hall went into the medical electrical business for himself. Hall apparently continued to operate his business in 1857 from 72 West Broadway. His residence was next door (73 West Broadway) to his business in 1862 (1855-1865),[1] but he relocated the business two times between 1862 and 1855 before finally moving to 18 North William Street (1866-1885[1]). The two intermittent locations of his business were 153 Washington, and 19 Bromfield Streets. The Washington Street address was just three blocks from the former business location (430 Washington St) of Daniel Davis. These latter two addresses are inscribed on two of the faradic batteries (Prof Wells, and Hall) presented in this section. He was still involved as a silversmith in 1866 and in the surgical instrument making business in 1884,[1] but was out of the manufacturing business of medical electrical batteries after 1885. Thomas Hall then sold his medical electrical battery business to Otto Flemming of Philadelphia, PA, in 1886. Flemming continued to manufacture and retail the French Battery series of Hall after buying the business from Thomas Hall.

Thomas Hall designed his early faradic battery model to accommodate the galvanic trough wet cell within the accompanying wooden box after he and Palmer bought the business from Daniel Davis, Jr, in 1854. Two of the three medical electrical batteries displayed in this section with the galvanic trough wet cell are similar in design to that by Dr Charles G Page and to that made and retailed by Daniel Davis, Jr. Daniel Davis, Jr, made and retailed the medical electrical batteries designed by Dr Charles G Page (Washington, DC). The three faradic batteries in this section could possibly date between 1854 and 1870. All three faradic batteries displayed in this section have coils secured by brass bands, have vibrators that use an armature device to control pulse rates similar to Page's design (continued by Hall and later by Flemming), and use similar brass fixtures. Brass electrical components or fixtures mostly precede the 1880s in medical electrical battery construction.

Daniel Davis, Jr, was a well known maker of custom electrotherapeutic apparatuses, although featuring the designs of Dr Charles G Page (later of the US Patent Office), never constructed any trough wet cells with his coils or batteries. Davis, Jr, did, however, describe a trough wet cell in his catalogs of 1848 and 1852. Thomas Hall was the manufacturer of the Hall, Prof WR Wells, and the Deming (Demming) faradic batteries featured in this section. Thomas Hall did manufacture a galvanic trough wet cell for a faradic battery that displayed his signature on the induction coil similarly to the Prof Wells, and the Deming (Demming) units. These three particular faradic batteries share the open copper trough-molded zinc insert type of wet cell (Fig H1). This particular design of the galvanic trough wet cell and faradic battery style are not common among the models sold in the United States and appear to have been manufactured by only one manufacturer, Thomas Hall of Boston. Since Hall's manufactory between 1854 and the 1870s was still manually constructing each battery, the numbers of faradic batteries using the open style galvanic trough wet cell are limited.

Collectors may have difficulty in locating an open galvanic trough wet cell.

The Galvanic Trough Cell. The trough cell (Fig H1,upper left) was invented in 1802 by Dr William Cruickshanks of Woolwich, England. His trough cell at that time was an improvement over the pile and couronne de tasses (crown of cups) invented by Alessandro Volta of Italy in 1800. The galvanic trough wet cell by its design offered the first electrical battery (group of cells) that could be produced in quantity. Cruickshanks constructed his galvanic trough cell by soldering together rectangular plates of zinc and copper at their ends. The plates were arranged horizontally in grooves in a box of baked wood that was insulated and held a solution of brine or diluted acid.[3]

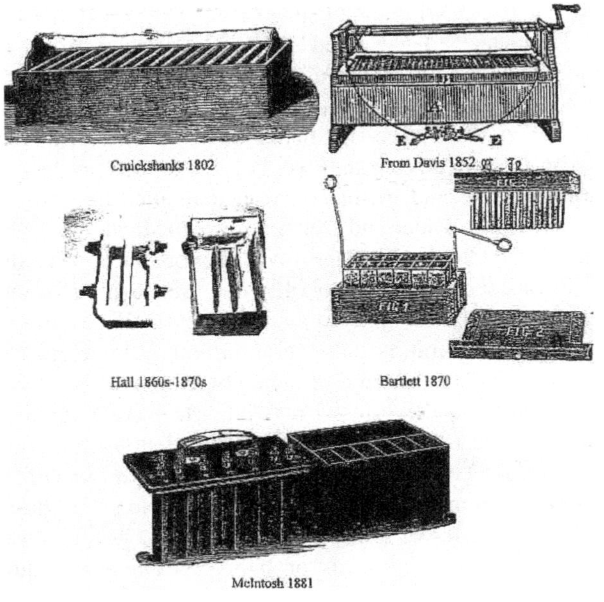

Fig H1. Galvanic Trough Cells

The galvanic trough cell with design changes from that of Cruickshanks was used by Nicholas Callan of Ireland around 1836. Callan's galvanic trough consisted of a ceramic trough divided into 10 cells. He devised zinc and copper (bent around the zinc) elements that could be lowered into the trough with solution to activate the cells. Callan's arrangement allowed for several cells to be connected in series.[4] The galvanic tough battery became popular in the United States to power both faradic and galvanic medical electrical batteries. Davis, Jr, stated that in the galvanic trough battery the zinc plates are flat and placed between copper cases that are open both at the top and bottom. (Fig H1,upper right). The plates are contained in a wooden case that is inserted into the trough. Nitric acid was added to the sulfuric acid when more cell power was desired.[5] Thomas Hall no doubt redesigned the trough wet cell from Davis, Jr's, catalog description, and then constructed them for use with the Prof WR Wells, Deming, and Demming trough wet cell style faradic batteries after 1854 (Fig H1,center left).

This Figure features examples of the trough cell historically with Cruikshanks 1802, Davis, Jr's, example of 1852, Hall's open galvanic trough cell of 1860s, Bartlett's hard rubber trough of 1870 (Fig H1-center right), and McIntosh's hard rubber cells of 1881 (Fig H1,bottom). Hall used a rectangular copper tray as the trough to replace the earlier wooden cases. The open rectangular zinc base (open at top and bottom) was inserted (not touching) into the copper trough. The galvanic trough cells of the 1870s and 1880s were similar in design to that of Callan but a hydrastat was used to cover the trough and separate the zinc and carbon elements from the solution when not in operation. The trough was divided into cells and was made of hard rubber (gutta percha). The carbon and zinc elements were placed into the hard rubber trough. Examples of companies using this style of galvanic trough cells to power their faradic and galvanic electrical batteries were: the Galvano-Faradic Mfg Co of New York, the McIntosh Battery & Optical Co of Chicago, and the J Kidder Mfg Co of New York. The galvanic wet cell played a role in the succession and advancement of the electrical cell in the late nineteenth century. The sealed or capped wet cell became an alternative to the galvanic trough cell in the 1890s as an improvement to avoid spillage and emission of unpleasant odors.

The galvanic trough cell featured in this section was designed by Thomas Hall that differs from that designed by Cruikshanks and that by Callan, and those later used by some American companies. Hall designed and used the rectangular zinc element as an insert (On/Off switch) placed into the copper trough. When the zinc element was lowered into the solution in the copper trough the cell was activated or turned On to operate the faradic battery. Raising the zinc element from the solution turned Off the power to the battery and operations ceased. The galvanic trough cell of Thomas Hall was open to the environment at all times, and when activated an unpleasant odor was emitted and the likelihood of spillage was greatly increased. The galvanic trough cell of Hall was cruder than that of competitor companies that used the design of Cruickshanks. Technology for the use of the hydrastat with the trough cell was available to Hall in the 1870s, but he did not elect to use it. The question then is why not use the improved design? Why did Hall use a technology that could then be labeled as outdated?

Perhaps the answer lies in the personality of the manufacturer Hall who was a silversmith and instrument maker from earlier days when items were custom and constructed manually. He was no doubt nearing the end of a successful career when mass manufactured products were being introduced and becoming commonplace in the United States. He may have elected to continue with custom and manually construct batteries rather than convert his shop into a factory for making medical electrical batteries. He operated his battery business from 1854 to 1886. Thomas Hall did not mass produce batteries using the galvanic trough cells, but did sometime in the 1880s mass produce the French series of faradic medical electrical batteries.

Hall Faradic Battery with Trough Cell. This faradic battery was probably manufactured by Hall prior to that of Prof Wells' model and that of the Deming-Demming models. Hall placed his customary logo on the induction coil that is covered by reddish fabric, and enclosed at each end by a circular hard rubber disc. This unit dates between 1864

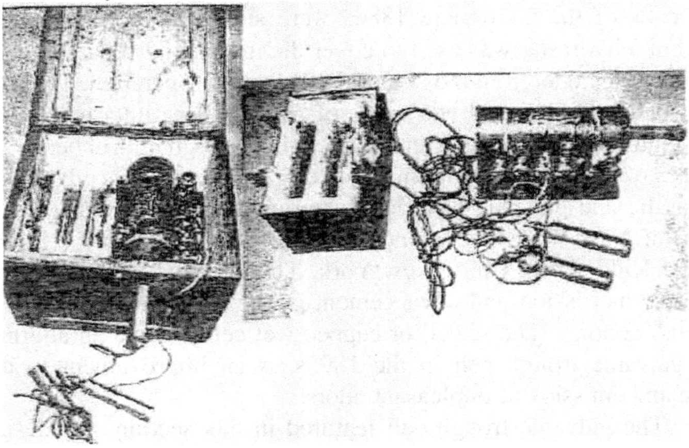

Fig H2. Hall Faradic Battery with Trough Cell

and 1870 with Hall's address on the logo being 153 Washington Street. The unit is enclosed in a walnut stained box (9.25 x 8 x 6.12 inches) that has recessed panels on each side of the box. The box lid is hinged and secured by a lock and key. A metal carrying handle is located on top of the lid. Other than the lock, hinges, and handle all metal is brass. The induction coil (6 x 2 inches) is covered by reddish fabric, and contains the Hall logo (shape) that reads "Dr A Paige's Electropathic Instrument," it resembles the design of those faradic models manufactured and retailed by Daniel Davis, Jr. That is, identical electrical components of the Davis' faradic batteries of 1848 to 1852 are seen as early as Hall's faradic batteries. These particular styled faradic batteries of Page, Davis, Jr, and Hall were also similar to those in use in England in 1849.[7] Dr A Paige was the designer and retailer of the "Perpetual Electromotors and Galvanic Supporter" that were labeled as forms of quackery by Rowbottom and Suskind.[8] Oddly, Daniel Davis, Jr, made reference to this form of quackery as early as 1846 in his first edition of The Medical Application of Electricity with Descriptions of Apparatus and Instructions for Its Use, Boston, MA, Daniel Davis, Jr, 1846. Davis, Jr, was referring to galvanic belts and rings of metal. Thomas Hall must have been aware of the contemporary concern about devices of medical quackery yet he manufactured and retailed a faradic battery (identical to that of Daniel Davis, Jr's) with Dr A Paige's name on its logo.

This unit also has the T-shaped spring leaf vibrator with adjustable screw and the wound U-bolt type of magnet. The current controller is pulled out and pushed in the coil through the front of the box. The four brass connecting posts are labeled "N, P, C, and Z." The unit has a galvanic trough wet cell composed of a copper tray and zinc rectangular insert.

Daniel Davis, Jr, illustrated a similar faradic battery with and without a wooden box. It is possible that Thomas Hall continued to make the Davis, Jr, Page style faradic battery also with and without the wooden box. The wooden box in the unit displayed seems to have been an after thought because its quality does not match those constructed by competitors of the 1870s. Thus, the wooden face plate with the coil, interrupter, and connecting posts may have been the original faradic battery of Hall, and without a wooden box like Davis, Jr, illustrated in his Catalogue of Apparatus, 1852.[4]

Prof WR Wells' Current Electropathic Instrument. The trough wet cell was made by Thomas Hall, electrician of 19 Bromfield Street, Boston, who produced the "French Battery" series. In the late 1860s to the early 1870s (possibly in 1868 or 1869), Hall produced a faradic battery using a trough type wet cell exactly like that accompanying the

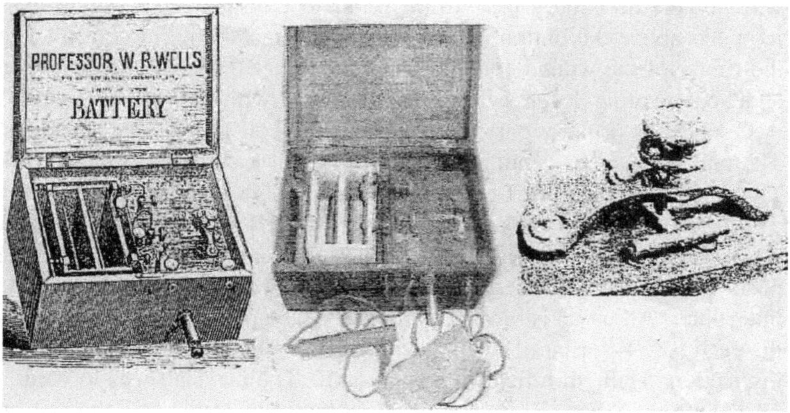

Fig H3. Prof WR Wells' Current Electropathic Instrument

Deming, Demming units (Fig H4). Hall was a manufacturer while Deming and Demming were consumers. Hall's faradic battery with the trough wet cell was labeled the "Prof WR Wells' Current Electropathic Instrument." The earliest picture of this electrical battery was located in SM Well's Electropathic Guide, edition 1, 1867, p 13. The unit was labeled "Prof Wells' Battery" and resembles that depicted in Fig H4 (left). In his book SM Wells discussed and listed Hall's glass castors for insulating bedsteads which indicates that he had association with Hall (a clue to identifying the manufacturer of Wells' Battery). WR Wells sold his battery in 1867 for $26.00 with full case of accessories), and $16.00 without the case of treatment accessories. The recommended solution for use with this battery was two ounces of sulfate of copper (blue vitriol) mixed in one quart of water.[9]

This unit by Hall is encased in a walnut box (9.5 x 7 x 6 inches) that is slightly larger than the later batteries labeled Deming and Demming. The wooden case is well constructed with its grooved cut corners that are sealed tightly by glue. Directions for operations are glued inside of the hinged lid. This case was carried by a leather strap mounted on each side by two screws. Each battery was accompanied by a copy of SM Wells' Electropathic Guide. According to the label with directions an additional copy of the Guide cost $1.00.

The vibrating interrupter is comprised of an adjustable screw that controls a vibrating T-shaped spring metal armature. The cross bar on the T-shaped spring makes contact at two points with a U-shaped bolt wound on each leg by heavy insulated copper wire. The U-shaped bolt (adjustable) attached to the wet cell and served as a magnet to operate the vibrator. Another binding pole on the walnut face plate connects with the wet cell and the induction coil winding. Connecting wires from patient to two connecting posts (adjustable) join the induction coil. The connecting wires enter the battery case from the patient through two button eyes mounted above the button eye for the sliding metal current controller to the center of the wound coil. One post is marked "P" and along with an attached pivoting lever switch then connects with "S" or "P" buttons (secondary or primary currents) that join the coil at different locations. The coil appears as a multi-wired unit without a soft iron primary coil. This type of coil was used on batteries of the 1860s and earlier.

The trough wet cell is exposed on the left side to the operator while the right side is a wooden face plate containing only the connecting posts (2 for the cell, 2 for the patient), and On/Off lever, and the interrupter. All metal is brass which places the date of the manufacture in the early 1870s (or late 1860s). Also, the brass On/Off lever contains the inscription "Hall Bromfield Boston Patent." Thomas Hall was located at 19 Bromfield Street, Boston, for awhile between 1864 (or before as an optician) and 1886. Hall was a manufacturing electrician and optician. The Hall unit for the Prof WR Wells Battery, unlike the Deming, Demming units located the induction coil (4.75 x 1.75 inches) underneath the face plate. The coil is uncovered and open at the ends. The sliding metal controller is moved in an out of the coil by the operator through an opening in front of the box. Also, underneath the face plate is the dual coils (formed from wound U bolt) serving the interrupter. The Deming, Demming faradic batteries were also among the few American models that used the dual or double coils type of interrupter (Flemming used this on some models of the 1880s after buying Hall's business). Directions for the unit are glued inside of the lid. WR Wells claimed that his battery had the advantage over those with a single current, since his has primary and secondary currents combined into one battery that can be chosen by a switch rather than changing wires in connector button holes on the face plate.

The Prof WR Wells' faradic battery was probably designed by SM Wells for WR Wells, but manufactured by Thomas Hall. In 1862 and in 1869, WR Wells published books about his theory of disease based on man being a compound electrical magnet. He stated that cures for diseases could be obtained through various qualities of electricity. WR Wells did not picture any electrical battery in either of his books.

WR Wells, MD, of Mount Morris, NY, published his 144 paged book A New Theory of Disease Based Upon the Principle of the Various Qualities of Electricity in 1862. He revised and enlarged his book to 178 pages in 1869.[10] HE Waite, MD, of 108 East 23rd Street, New York City, wrote an inscription in the second book by WR Wells. Dr Waite later founded the Waite & Bartlett Co of New York City; manufacturer of quality electrotherapeutic apparatuses and later of quality x-rays.

Dr WR Wells was a practicing physician in Mount Morris, NY, and used electricity to treat his patients. He needed an apparatus to provide the electricity proposed by his theory, and may have suggested a design for a faradic battery that was a precursor to the Deming and Demming faradic batteries. He may have had the design concept in his mind that would serve his theory about electrical magnets, although the Hall faradic battery (Fig H2) using the open galvanic trough wet cell was produced earlier and the Prof Wells' unit resembles it.

SM Wells, medical electrician, of Beaver Dam, WI, wrote The Electropathic Guide: Prepared with Particular Reference to Home Practice; containing hints on the care of the sick, the treatment of disease, and the use of electricity sometime in the late 1860s. The third edition of his book was published in 1872 and featured the Prof Wells' Current Instrument in his, rather than WR Wells' book. The two individuals are conjectured as either brothers or close relatives. SM Wells listed himself, in his book, as the seller of the Professor WR Wells unit, and used his Beaver Dam, WI, address as the source for those ordering the apparatus. SM Wells used an accessory electrode designed and made by Thomas Hall, instrument maker of Boston, with the Prof WR Wells Battery.[10]

The Electropathic Guide...... by SM Wells was later adopted (early 1890s) by the JH Bunnell & Co of New York to accompany each of its New No.4 D.D. Home Medical Battery. Bunnell batteries from about 1892 to at least 1915 were accompanied by an updated edition of The Electropathic Guide. The ninth edition (98 pages) was authored by SM Wells in 1888 and published in Chicago, IL.

Deming Faradic Battery. The unit is housed in a rather well constructed walnut box (9.25 x 7 x 5.25 inches) that has tongue and groove joints that are glued. The lid is secured by a lock and key on its front. The box is divided into two compartments. The compartment to the left houses the open copper trough wet cell that is composed of a copper container or trough (6 x 3.75 x 3.5 inches) that has two dividers or walls partially divide the container into three sections. Accumulator plates

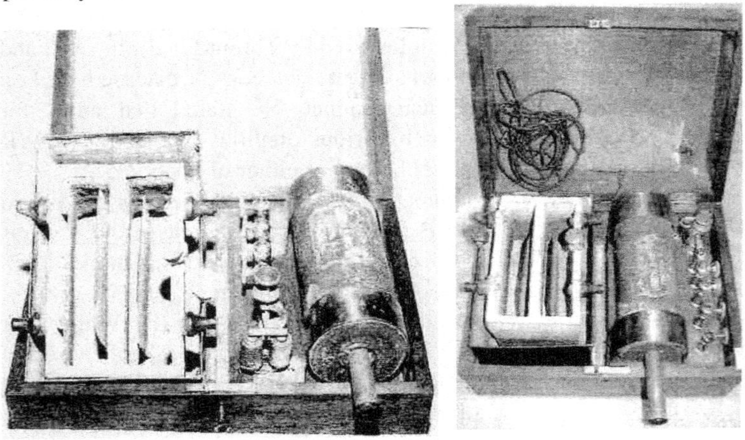

Fig H4. Deming Faradic Battery

were formed by soldering the two copper dividers to the bottom of the copper container. The copper container has a brass adjustable screw binding post soldered to the top of one side, and serves as the positive wet cell post. The copper container or trough holds the acid solution. A twin chamber cast zinc insert with a divider plate that forms two divisions is placed into the copper trough. The cast zinc insert has four wooden supports welded at each upper corner. These supports keep the zinc insert from touching the copper trough when immersed into the container. A brass adjustable screw binding post is soldered to one side, and serves as the negative post of the wet cell. The insert with a two sections is bottomless, and measures 5 x 3 x 3 inches. A mixture of nitric and sulfuric acids after the Grove design of a porous iron pot held zinc and copper plates was used for the cell. The nitric acid was added to the sulfuric acid only when needed to boost the power of the cell.

The cast zinc insert is lifted from the copper trough and acid solution when not in use. The matching wood face panel is flush to the bottom of the box, and contains a large induction coil (5.13 x 2.13

inches) that has a hollow metal tube current controller that is surged (pulled/pushed) to regulate current amplitude. The coil is covered with a reddish fabric that contains a logo with the Deming inscription, and is secured near each end by a one inch brass band. The ends of the induction coil are exposed. The face panel also contains an adjustable screw T-shaped (armature) spring type interrupter that approximates a horseshoe shaped magnet wound on each leg rather than commonly approximating the core of the coil through a hammer, vibrator type interrupter. The cast zinc insert has two connector posts to connect with two of four screw posts on the face panel to select the type of current. Most metal on the apparatus is brass except the surging tube in the coil and the spring coils of the interrupter.

Searches in directories of businesses, advertisement, or name sections of any directories[11] or other source[12] of cities of Providence, RI, and Portland, ME, did not reveal any listing of a manufacturer or retailer of electrical apparatuses and supplies between 1879 and 1918. The word "battery" and category first appeared in the directory of Portland, ME, in 1891,[13] but never for Deming Brothers or William N Deming or William N Demming. Thomas Hall manufactured the faradic battery with the open copper trough wet cell for both Deming and Demming.

William N Deming was a physician in Providence, RI, and listed in the city directory of 1879. His office was located at 214 Broad Street at the junction of Praire Avenue. Dr Deming was not listed in the 1887 directory, but reappeared in the directory of 1891 with his office located at 420 Praire Avenue. This second location was a short distance from his location in 1879.[14] He was not practicing medicine in 1904.

WN Demming, MD, is the name shown on the brass bracket securing the induction coil of the unit for Portland, ME, and sold on eBay. A difference in the spelling of his last name was made between the units of Providence, RI, and of Portland, ME. The initials are the same in both cases, however. The question can be asked whether WN Deming, MD, of Providence, RI, and WN Demming, MD, of Portland, ME, are one and the same person? Could Dr Deming (Demming) have lived in Portland between 1887 and 1891 when his name was not listed in the directory of the city of Providence, RI? Each medical electrical battery has the same identical features except the names and addresses. Neither Dr WN Deming, nor Dr WN Demming is listed in the city directory for Portland, ME, between 1884 and 1890. A Wm N Demings, machinist, 224 Newbury appeared in the directory of Portland, ME, from 1884 through 1886. In 1888, William W Deming, hammersman, 222 Newbury, appeared in the directories, and in 1890 his business was located at 291 Commercial Street. Dr Demming apparently did not sell batteries nor practice medicine in Portland between 1884 and 1891.[11,12]

Only on four occasions has the author seen this particular style of faradic battery using a galvanic trough wet cell. Two units of note,

Deming and Demming, are identical in design and appearance, however, there is a difference between the units that raises an unresolved question. The two units are owned by different individuals, and the difference between the two units is that one (sold on eBay) is labeled "Electro-Magnetic Battery, W. N. Demming, M.D., Portland, Maine" on the induction coil, and the other is labeled "Deming Brothers, Providence, R.I." on its induction coil. The manufacture dates were first estimated independently as 1870 to 1875, and 1875, respectively. The uniqueness of these two units is that they are powered by an open copper trough type wet cell, and each unit was designed with the cell style in mind. These two similar units are unlike any other wet cells made and sold in the United States between 1867 and 1900.

French Battery. Sometime between 1875 and 1885, Hall manufactured and sold his French Battery. The French Battery developed into a series of models that even continued with Otto Flemming Co of Philadelphia that bought the electrotherapeutic battery business of Thomas Hall in 1886. Hall invited both physicians and families to use his French Battery. The first batteries in this series were mass produced, and

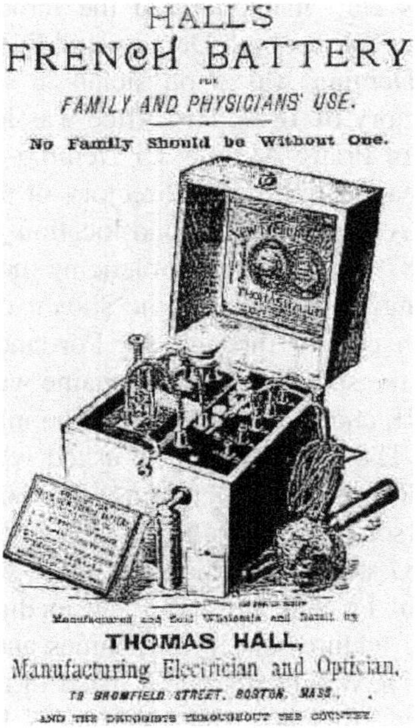

Fig H5. French Battery

may have been produced as successor to the Hall, Prof Wells, and Deming batteries. The fifth edition of Hall's catalog illustrated and described Hall's French Battery. This catalog may have been issued in 1864 but this author believes that it was issued between 1875 and 1885. The address on the catalog, however, is 19 Bromfield Street, Boston,

MA. Hall cited himself as a "manufacturing electrician and optician." This battery has nickel plated handles for hand held electrodes. The induction coil is underneath the face plate, but Hall used a silver plated armature with its interrupter. The wooden case is French polished black walnut, has a metal carrying handle, is secured by a lock and hooks, and weighs four pounds. This battery originally came with a Grove type wet cell that differed from Hall's earlier open galvanic trough wet cell. This battery complete originally sold for $15.00. Other French Batteries are covered under the section on Otto Flemming.

Hall also manufactured Hall's Body Battery that was an electrical belt. This belt has conducting wires that are attached to the arms of the wearer, and lead to India rubber gloves. The wearer controlled the power of the electrical belt through controls in the gloves. The price for this belt was $25.00 between 1875 and 1885.

Summary

The three faradic batteries (Hall, Prof Wells, Deming) displayed within this section were definitely manufactured by Thomas Hall, but their design is that of Dr Charles Page (see J Kidder). Daniel Davis, Jr, first manufactured the medical electrical batteries designed by Dr Page, Washington, DC. Daniel Davis, Jr, illustrated the "Box Apparatus for Medical use" in Davis' catalogue of apparatus Manual of Magnetism, ed 2, 1848, and in edition 4 of 1852. Davis, Jr, did not use the galvanic trough wet cell for his electrical devices, but Thomas Hall did after Palmer and Hall bought the business from Davis, Jr, in 1854.

The Deming and Demming names are believed to be assigned signatures to the respective medical electrical batteries that Thomas Hall manufactured and sold to individuals. Apparently the batteries with their galvanic trough cells were not as popular with consumers as other wet cells of the 1870 to 1885 period of time. The galvanic trough wet cells are open compared with other wet cells that are covered. The open galvanic trough cells are more likely to spill and give off unpleasant odors than the closed or capped wet cells. Why Thomas Hall made these particular faradic batteries using crude galvanic trough wet cells when other improved types of wet cells were available is unclear. Perhaps the Demings ordered such batteries that Thomas Hall then customized. The Wells may have influenced this type of cell by their books and booklets, but most likely the style was borrowed from Davis, Jr, along with his business after 1854.

These types of cells are not often encountered in antique shops or on eBay auctions. The galvanic trough wet cells made by Thomas Hall of Boston to power faradic batteries are considered rare to the collector. Galvanic trough wet cells with covers became popular with units built by other companies in the 1870s to 1900.

References

1. Edmonson JM. American Surgical Instruments. San Francisco, Norman Pub, 1997

2. Websters Instrument Makers Database. (www.adlerplanetarius.org/history/websters/p.htm)

3. Mottellay PF. Bibliographical History of Electricity and Magnetism, reprint. New York, NY Maurizio Martino Pub, 1984

4. Mollan C, Upton J. The Scientific Apparatus of Nicholas Callan and Other Historic Instruments. Dublin, Samton Otd, 1994, p 57

5. Davis D, Jr. Catalogue of Apparatus, ed 4. Boston, MA, Daniel Davis, Jr, 1852, p 30

6. Davis D, Jr. Manual of Magnetism, ed 4. Boston, MA, Daniel Davis, Jr, 1852, pp 280, 301

7. Bird G. Lectures on Electricity and Galvanism. London, 1849

8. Rowbottom M, Suskind C. Electricity and Medicine: History of Their Interaction. San Francisco, CA, San Francisco Press, 1984, p 64

9. Wells SM. The Electropathic Guide. Chicago, IL, Horton & Leonard, 1867, pp 13, 91

10. Wells WR. A New Theory of Disease; Based Upon the Principle That Man Is a Compound Magnet; also, A New Method of Cure. Rochester, NY, Printing House Tracy & Row, 1869

11. Portland City Directory. Portland, ME, 1884-1886, 1888, 1891

12. Board of Trade J. Portland, ME, 1888-1918

13. Bacon GF. Portland: Its Representative Business Men and Its Points of Interest. Portland, ME, Glenwood Pub, 1891, p 105

14. Correspondence, Public Library of Providence. Providence, RI, 2001

ES RITCHIE OF BOSTON

Edward S Ritchie (1814-1895) was a well known and an innovative American instrument maker of Boston in the nineteenth century. He was born in Dorchester, MA, to affluent parents John and Eliza (Eliot). Since he was the only surviving child of six, he enjoyed vantages. Although he attended the Friends Academy of New Bedford for one year (1827-1828), he had little additional formal education. His limited education was by choice; he preferred to stay home for several years conducting science experiments and sculpting. He even built a telescope that he later donated to the Friends Academy. During his years of self-tutoring, he developed both interest and talent for mechanics. He did work for awhile with a furniture maker.[1]

He moved to Boston by 1839, and became a partner with Ashur C Palmer in hardware. The business was known as Palmer and Ritchie, and they may have sold mathematical instruments as one of their products.[2] After three years of partnership, Ritchie decided to go into business for himself.

From 1842 to 1850, Ritchie's business was as a ship's chandler (supplier). The business was located in New Bedford. He played the organ for an Episcopal Church while there.[1]

In 1850, the Boston City Directory listed ES Ritchie as a merchant, married with four children, and holding property valued at $35,000.00.[1] He joined in partnership with Nathan B Chamberlain in 1850 to 1854, and their business was named Chamberlain and Ritchie. They made philosophical instruments. While repairing compasses for the United States Navy in Boston, he learned that he could improve upon the compass by eliminating the problems presented for repair. He developed the first marine compass manufactured in the United States that then eliminated foreign compasses that previously were requiring frequent repair for the Boston Naval Shipyard.[3] Ritchie paid Chamberlain $20,000.00 to associate with him while learning the trade as cited in a credit note of 1858.[1]

When the Chamberlain and Ritchie partnership dissolved in 1854 Ritchie again went into business for himself as Edward S Ritchie. Ritchie remained at the shop that he owned at 313 Washington Street, and worked alone until 1862. Chamberlain went across the street from Ritchie and established his own business. In 1861, Ritchie received a contract for making compasses for the United States Navy. He proceeded to build the first liquid filled compass,[3] and continued to build compasses for the United States Navy during the Civil War period. Also in 1861, Ritchie contributed toward the founding of the Massachusetts Institute of Technology as a reputable businessman.[1]

Induction coils up to 1857 did not deliver sparks over three inches between discharge points. Actually, coils at that time rarely delivered sparks over one inch between points because of problems with the insulation of the wire windings.[4] In 1855, Heinrich Ruhmkorff (1803-1920) of Germany opened up his electrical instrument shop in Paris, and exhibited his induction coil in Paris. His device became known as the Ruhmkorff coil and for awhile it served for the design and construction of the currents of the early faradic medical batteries.[5] In 1858, Ruhmkorff won first prize at the French Exhibition of Electrical Apparatus, and as a result was challenged (unsuccessfully) for invention credit by Dr Charles Grafton Page who invented a similar coil in the United States in 1836.[6] Although the Ruhmkorff coil was both efficient and reliable as a source of electricity, it could not deliver much tension (voltage). His induction coil could only deliver sparks one to three inches between discharge points.[1]

Induction Coil of 1869. In 1857, Ritchie modified the induction coil to make it an important science instrument. At this time he was making electrical instruments for educational institutions that were teaching courses in natural philosophy. In 1869, Ritchie made a small induction coil that produced a spark of six inches that was notable at the time. The coil sold for $337.00.[7]

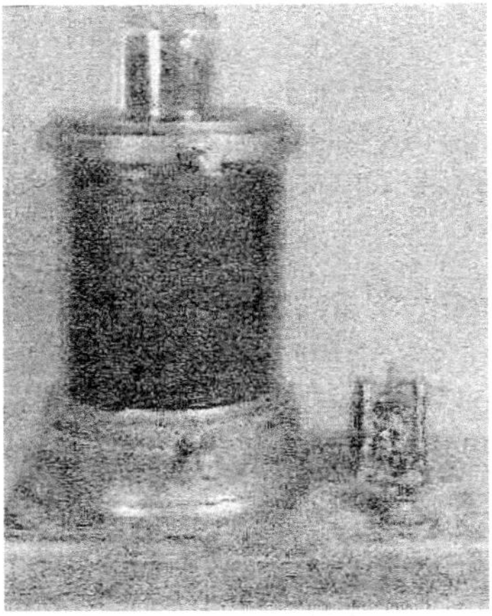

Fig R1. Induction Coil of 1869(Courtesy of
Dr T Greenslade Kenyon College, Gambier,OH)

Induction Coil of 1880s. According to the Ritchie trade catalog of 1890, he constructed his improved coil based on the principle of double helices of Henry, Page, Faraday, and Fizeau. Ritchie devised an improved manner that the secondary helix (coil) was wound. He wound the wires at right angles to the main axis that then permitted the use of only thin insulation.[4] Previously, the European manner of winding induction coils was parallel to each layer of thick insulated wire. Ritchie wound about 30,000 feet of thin insulated wire on his secondary coil that

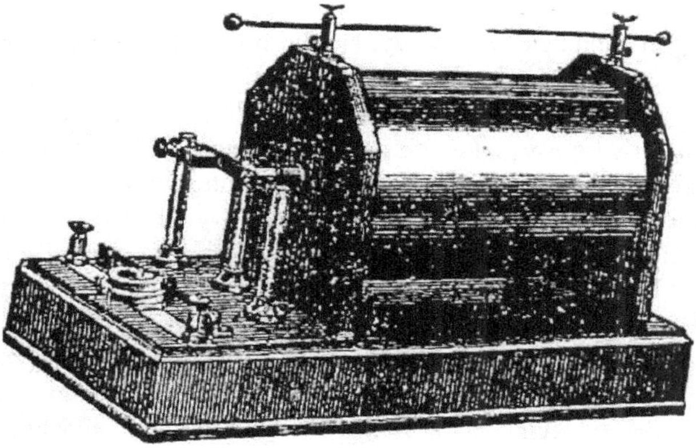

Fig R2. Induction Coil of 1880s

enabled his coils to deliver sparks six inches between discharge points. This manner of winding increased the tension (voltage) produced by the coil. Both Silliman's American Journal of Science and the Philosophical Magazine of London provided information about Ritchie's improved coil that gave him credible publicity. Ritchie presented a paper before the 1857 meeting of the American Association for the Advancement of Science.[1] Ritchie's manner of winding the secondary helix was also soon adopted by most manufacturers of induction coils. The 1890 catalog of Ritchie offered induction coils based on their ability to "throw" sparks. A coil delivering a spark of 0.5 inch cost $10.00. Sparks graduate in increments of one to two inches (3 to 4 to six to eight and 10 inches)

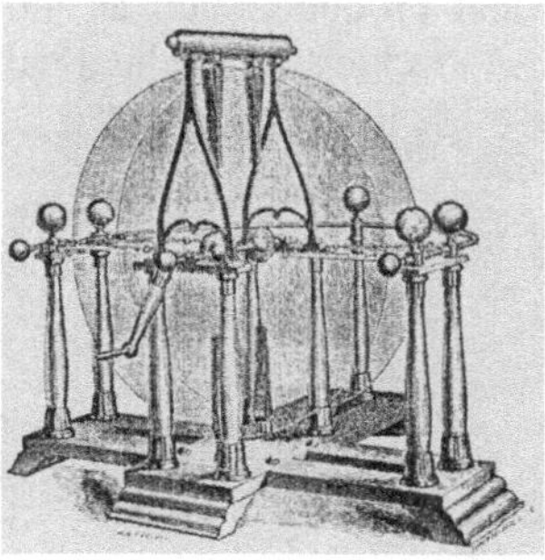

Fig R3. Static Machine for the University of Mississippi
(Courtesy of Dr T Greenslade, Kenyon, College, Gambier, OH)

were sold by Ritchie. At that time a coil delivering an one inch spark cost $28.00, and that of 10 inches cost $150.00.[4]

In 1857 and into the 1890s, Ritchie manufactured quality induction coils and electrical apparatuses. For unknown reasons he continued to manufacture his quality induction coils without introducing in their designs updated technology. He did not enter the popular market of faradic medical batteries. In 1857, Ritchie made a very large static electrical apparatus for the University of Mississippi. The static electrical apparatus had two glass plates of six feet diameter, and three cylinders as prime conductors. Most static influence apparatus of later design used two Leyden jars to store electrical charge, but Ritchie used 100 Leyden jars with his unit. Ritchie's large static apparatus seemed to under perform and became an item of curiosity.[1]

The Holtz influence (static) electrical apparatus was introduced by CF Varley (1832-1921) in 1860. He manufactured a static machine that soon was named the influence machine because it contained carriers mounted on the revolving plate. It was the first influence machine really constructed for electrotherapeutics. In 1867, Ritchie modified the Holtz apparatus that was unique enough to be patented. Ritchie's innovation proved to improve the electrical output of the Holtz apparatus more than designs of others at the time. Ritchie's static electrical apparatus at this time used a large thick glass plate, a thin revolving plate, and two or four sectors of glass. This particular static electrical apparatus of Ritchie's delivered sparks three feet between the contact points.[1] Ritchie's Patent Holtz Machine was an eight paged booklet that he had published.[8] In spite of Ritchie's improvement of the Holtz type influence machine his modification never achieved the level of notoriety of that of either August Toepler (1836-1912) or James Wimshurst (1832-1903).

Galvanic Batteries sold by Ritchie. Over the years ES Ritchie and Sons made physical products for high schools and colleges (anatomical models, calipers, gauges, lanterns and projectors, telescopes), and electrical products such as ammeters, galvanometers, and Wheatstone bridges. Ritchie sold medical galvanic batteries ranging

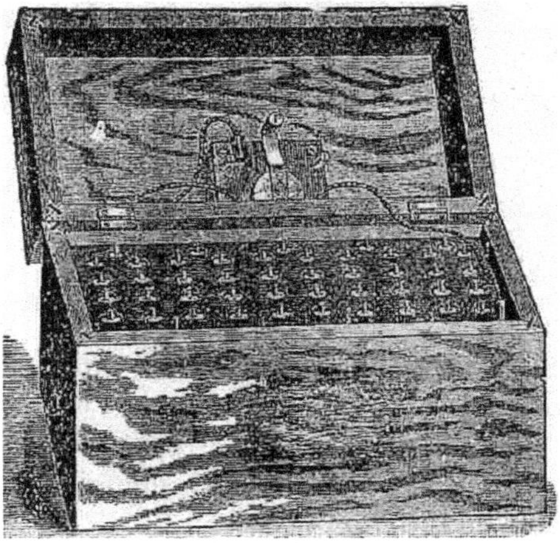

Fig R4. Galvanic Batteries sold by Ritchie

from six to 60 cells that were manufactured by the Silver Chloride and Dry Cell Battery Company of Baltimore, MD. Ritchie's prices in 1890 for these batteries were: six cells, $8.00; 12 cells, $13.00; 16 cells, $18.00, respectively; these models were encased in a plain oak case. The batteries for 24 cells ($38.00), 32 cells ($45.00), 50 cells ($65.00), and 60 cells ($75.00) were encased in a mahogany box with a current reverser.

From 1862 to 1864, Ritchie went into business with his friend John Kehew (1818-1889) who had worked at various Water Street locations in New Bedford, MA, (1841-1862).[2] The ES Ritchie and Company was formed in 1862 to make mathematical, navigational, and optical instruments. The marine compass became a major product of the company.

In 1866, ES Ritchie and Co was renamed ES Ritchie and Son when his oldest son, Thomas Pope (1842-1914), joined the firm. The company was now making mathematical, navigational, philosophical, and surveying instruments. The name was again changed in 1867 to Edward S Ritchie and Sons when the second son John (1844-1902) started work with his father and brother.[2] In 1868, the company moved from 313 Washington Street, Boston (1857-1867), to 149 Tremont Street, Boston.

The third son Andrew Montgomery (1849-1916) joined ES Ritchie and Sons in 1872, and continued to work for the company until his death in 1916. He became head of the company probably in 1895 when his father Edward S Ritchie died. Andrew M directed the company until 1916 when he died. Andrew M Ritchie's son Andrew Eliot (1878-1935) succeeded his father as head of ES Ritchie and Sons in 1916.[2]

In 1881, the company's address was 150 Tremont Street, Boston, and then the company relocated in 1886 to Brookline, MA,[2] where it located its factory and warehouse. After Edward S Ritchie's death in 1895, his three sons sold the philosophical instrument division of the business to LE Knott Apparatus Co of Boston, and then devoted their resources and efforts to the nautical division of ES Ritchie and Sons. ES Ritchie and Sons incorporated in 1935. In 1939, the Ritchies purchased the TS and JD Negus company that marketed chronometers.[1] In 1953 when Andrew Eliot Ritchie died the company was sold to Louis A Sherman who combined the Marine Compass Company with ES Ritchie and Sons. The company continues to operate today under Louis A Sherman's grandson Paul. In 1953 the company moved from Brookline to Pembroke, MA.[2]

While Edward S Ritchie lived trade catalogs were published periodically. He became a successor to Daniel Davis, Jr, in the instrument business by reputation, and like Davis he kept abreast of the latest trends in electricity. He was highly respected by scientists of the nineteenth century, and like Daniel Davis, Jr, would spend considerable time with scientists demonstrating his instruments and conducting experiments. ES Ritchie patented 28 devices during his career as an instrument maker.[1] ES Ritchie published trade catalogs of his products in 1857 and 1860 from 313 Washington St, Boston through his Illustrated Catalogue of Philosophical Instruments; in 1868 from 149 Tremont Street, Boston; in 1871, 1875, and 1877 through Illustrated Catalogue of Philosophical Instruments and School Apparatus, 1889, 1890, 1894, 1895, and in 1896 from 150 Tremont Street, Boston, through either Catalogue of Physical Instruments, or Laboratory and Experimental Apparatus for High Schools and Colleges.[1,8] Sometime in the mid 1890s Ritchie published his eight paged booklet Ritchie's Patent Holtz Machine.[8] These catalogs offered astronomical and optical instruments, but no ownership was mentioned. ES Ritchie and Sons manufactured most of their own instruments, but did list and show imported products as well. In 1880, the company employed 12 men, and advertised itself as the largest of its kind in the United States. The company grossed $ 40,000.00 with a net of $6,000.00 in the same year.[1]

Ritchie gained much acclaim for his instrument making by exhibiting instruments at the Massachusetts Charitable Mechanic Association in 1878[1] (winning a silver medal), the American Institute in New York (winning a medal), and the Franklin Institute in Philadelphia, and the Louisiana Purchase Exposition of St Louis. He also won awards at the Centennial Exhibition in Philadelphia in 1876,[1] and at several world expositions[3] (Paris 1901, Pan American 1904).[1] Ritchie was making quality products, and advertised his instruments at low prices.[1]

At one point in his life he formed the Ritchie Street Lighting Company of Allenstown, NH, that supplied lighting for the town's streets. He disseminated his electrical knowledge in many leading science journals in the United States and Europe during his career. He also used leading educational and science journals in the United States to advertise his electrical products.[1]

Summary

These makers of American medical electrical batteries evolved from their trade as instrument makers that constructed their products individually by skilled craftsmen. They made and sold most of their instruments to educational institutions and physicians. When the Civil War placed a demand for a larger quantity, cheaper, durable, and reliable instruments than previously many abandoned their custom making practice to mass produce.

These few American instrument makers remained as small businessmen after the Civil War and so continued to make and sell their products to educational institutions and physicians. These few individual craftsmen also entered the market of making medical electrical batteries prior to and after the Civil War. They did, however, open the market to public consumers who could buy directly from the makers after learning about them through catalogs, magazines, and newspapers. These small makers of the medical electrical battery were the pioneers of the American field that in 1870 developed into an expanding business.

References

1. Warner DJ. Compasses and coils. Rittenhouse 9:1-24, 1996

2. Websters Instrument Makers Database. (www.adlerplanetarius.org/history/webster/p.htm)

3. (www.ritchienaviagation.com/company/history.html)

4. Ritchie's Catalogue of Electrical Test Instruments. Brookline, MA, ES Ritchie and Sons, 1890, p 20

5. Maurer JF (ed). Concise Dictionary of Scientific Biography. New York, NY, Charles Scribner's Sons, 1981, p 595

6. Post RC. Physics, Patents, and Politics. A Biography of Charles Grafton Page. New York, NY, Science History Pub, 1976, pp 274-275

7. GreensladeTA. (http://physics.kenyon.esduc/EarlyApparatus/Electricity/Induction_Coil/ Induction_Coil.html)

8. Davis AB, Dreyfus MS. The Finest Instruments Ever Made. Arlington, MA, Medical History Pub Assocs, 1986, pp 274-275

CHAPTER 4. FRANK S BETZ COMPANY OF CHICAGO

This Chapter reviews Frank S Betz, his company, and his electrical batteries. Frank S Betz (1861-1940) founded his business of selling medical apparatuses and supplies in 1895. He used his name for the business (Frank S Betz Company) when he founded it. His name was still carried as the company title on its catalog (Supplies and Equipment for Physicians and Surgeons) of 1928, although Davis and Dreyfus,[1] and Grigg[2] referred to it as the "Frank S Betz and Company."

Frank Betz was born in 1861 (to George and Lomira; father was a Union officer in the Civil War), and attended rural schools while growing up on the family farm in Eau Claire, WI. He started work in a local sawmill around 1873, but realizing its limitations he soon changed jobs to learn the blacksmith trade. Next he worked as a blacksmith helper for the N Shaw Company that manufactured saw and gristmill equipment. He quickly transferred within the company to become an apprentice to learn the machinist trade. At the end of his apprenticeship in 1884 he moved to Minneapolis to work for the Union Iron Works that made flourmill machinery. Soon learning that salesmen of health insurance made much more money than him he entered that business (1884) by selling health insurance to men working in saw mills, lumber and logging camps in Michigan, Minnesota, and Wisconsin. In 1888, he married Alice May Roberston of Bay City, MI; he and wife had three sons; Irving, Frank R, and Lyman B. In 1889, Betz moved to Chicago where he worked in real estate. Anticipating a great number of visitors to Chicago for the 1893 Columbian Exposition (world's fair) he operated the Colonial Club hotel and speculated in real estate near the site of the Exposition.[3]

When the Exposition ended Betz was over extended with real estate and went broke. The ownership of the Colonial Club (on Oglesby Ave south of Sixty-Third St)[4] changed, but Betz continued as its operator on a commission basis. Within 60 days he had all rooms rented and was making money. During this period of time his former health insurance employer gave him the management of its hospital in Grand Rapids, MI, and of its district agents. While managing the hospital he learned that hospital and medical equipment and supplies could be sold at half the prevailing prices and still provide a profit.[3] At the end of his employment contract with the hospital in 1895 he founded the Frank S Betz Company of Chicago. The insurance company that he worked for went bankrupt so could not pay Betz owed money at the end of his contract. Betz then borrowed $25.00 and went into the hospital equipment and supply business.

In 1896, he invented and built as his first retail item a steel dry hot-air apparatus for patient care that he sold for $24.00 when his competition sold it for $350.00. His continued success was built on selling steel hospital furniture, x-ray machines, and surgical equipment and instruments directly to physicians to use in their offices at a price that was so affordable that they soon preferred to buy from Betz.[3,4] Also, Frank Betz used direct mail advertising, dealers, salesmen, and wholesalers, and operated his business from a building on 75th Street, Chicago. According to Davis and Dreyfus the first Frank S Betz Co was located at 35-37 Randolph Street, Chicago, IL.[1] (Note: Biographer Dunajeski had the first location of the company on 75th St, Chicago. Perhaps Davis & Dreyfus were referring to the location cited in the first trade catalog issued by the company.)

The Frank S Betz Co first issued a 16-paged illustrated catalog of surgical instruments and apparatuses in 1895. This source indicated that he had 20 years of experience which would put him in business in 1870 (a slight stretch). He released an illustrated special 30-day bulletin advertising medical instruments and furnishings in 1896.[6]

Shortly, he was successful enough to operate from five rented buildings. The Frank S Betz Co's selling of medical instruments and supplies at discount prices began a new trend in the United States in 1895. From the beginning in 1895, the Frank S Betz Co became the premier supplier of low cost medical equipment and accessories to physicians and hospitals in the United States.

In 1900, the Frank S Betz Co built its first true factory on the southeast of Chicago, at 1760 East Ravenswood Park.[3] (Hammond, IN, adjoins Chicago at Summerdale near Ravenswood.) The new building had 100 feet frontage and was two stories high. Each year he built an addition to the factory until it was one block long. His Chicago factory, however, lacked easy railway access so he began looking for a new location.

In 1900, the company published its 96 paged Manual of Physiological Therapeutics that covered the sale of invalid chairs. In 1901, Betz's Manual of Physiological Therapeutics with Special Reference to the Treatment of Acute & Chronic Diseases advertised electrotherapy, hydrotherapy, massage, and thermotherapy equipment with an appendix on orthopedic appliances, supporters, and trusses. The manual was authored by more than 50 individuals. This particular 96 paged manual contained prices of illustrated items, photographs and descriptions of their uses. The Frank S Betz Co published a Bargain Bulletin in April and September of 1902; another issue in 1903; and an addition to a catalog of its product line.

In 1903, Frank S Betz started a mail order business that became an immediate success. At this time the company was operating from 41 Randolph St, Chicago, IL. The company also in the same year introduced its static electrical machine and x-ray apparatus. The catalog that year listed 5000 electrical and related items which gives an indication of the size of the company's operations and product lines. The company had its salesroom located at 88-90 Wabash Ave and its factory at 1760 E Ravenswood Park, Chicago, IL, from 1900 to 1904.

In 1904, Betz accepted an earlier offer by the city of Hammond, IN, of 12 acres of land near a railroad north of the Grand Calumet River[4] (Hoffman Street and Sohl Avenue). The local newspaper announced the Betz pact on 10 November 1904,[4] and that the new company would hire 300 workers.[5] When his newly bricked factory was completed in Hammond in 1905 it was 536 by 100 feet in size. A rail spur was built along the factory.[5] Each year he added a wing to the building. Not wanting to be involved with the turmoil of business and moving, Mrs Betz and their three sons traveled Europe in 1904 until a new residence in Hammond could be completed. She and their three sons joined Frank in 1905.[4]

The factory in Hammond was the manufacturing base after 1904 with other locations (viz, Chicago) as a branch office.[2] He later named one of his medical electrical batteries (Fig B20) after the name of the river near the factory. The Frank S Betz Co was the name cited in 1895, and both Chicago, IL, and Hammond, IN, were often cited on the signature plates of its medical electrical batteries (these units are dated 1904 and later).

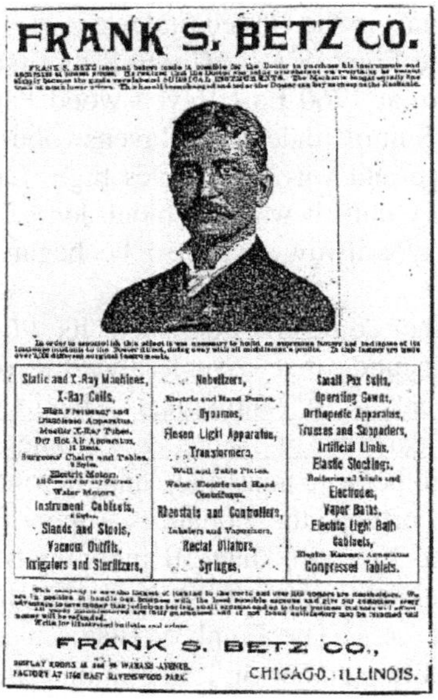

Fig B1. FS Betz, 1904

A 1904 advertisement stated that the Frank S Betz Co was the largest of its kind in the world, and that more than 1000 physicians were stockholders which if true did not hurt its business.[7] The FS Betz Co continued to publish bulletins or catalogs from two to four times a year through the years of 1907, 1910, 1912, 1913, 1915, 1916, 1917, 1918, and 1919.[1]

Offices of the company were subsequently located at several locations in Chicago, based on its various trade catalogs. For example, cited locations were: 35 & 37 Randolph St, 30 E Randolph St; 88-90 Wabash; 37,39,41 Randolph St; and 634 S Wabash Streets. Branch stores of the Frank S Betz Co were also located in other cities: 348-353 W 34th St and, 6-8 W 48th St in New York City; and the Santa Fe Building in Dallas, Texas.[1] The company branch in New York City only sold electrotherapeutic equipment.[2] The Frank S Betz Co sold electrotherapeutic equipment and accessories from the beginning of the company's founding in 1895. The company sold medical electrical batteries to both physicians and public consumers, although Betz is best known for its quality electrical machines for physicians. Betz went all out to sell his products to physicians. Besides discounts on purchases he provided published medical articles and history involving selected products for physicians.[1] He permitted physicians to use items on trial for 60 days while deciding to buy or not to buy the products from the Betz Co.[3]

In 1905, the Frank S Betz Co published the Journal of Physical Therapy that really was a pseudomedical periodical. The new journal was a commercial vehicle edited by GM Blech, but because of its nature it ended after two volumes in 1907.[3] Physicians rejected this approach to continuing education of electrotherapeutics because the journal was basically written by lay people or at least not by leading physicians in electrotherapeutics.

He traveled to Europe many times in the early twentieth century. On one occasion he attended the International Conference of Physical Therapeutics in Rome (1907), and while there he mailed postcards to his clients and friends (Fig 1A.)

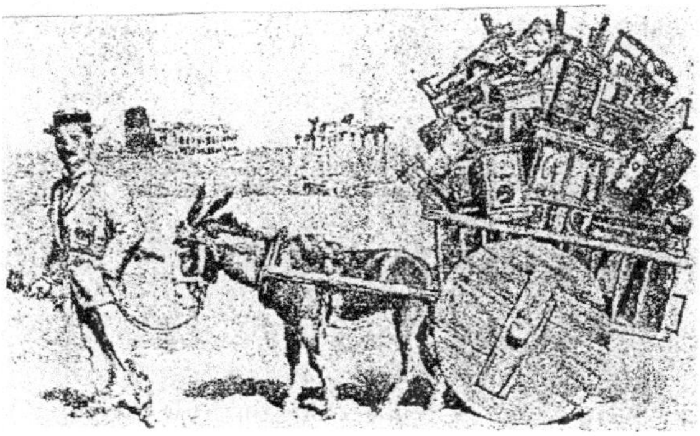

Fig B1A. Postcard from one of his travels

Betz's success in business is demonstrated by expansion of his factory at different times (eg, Fig B1B, ca 1910).

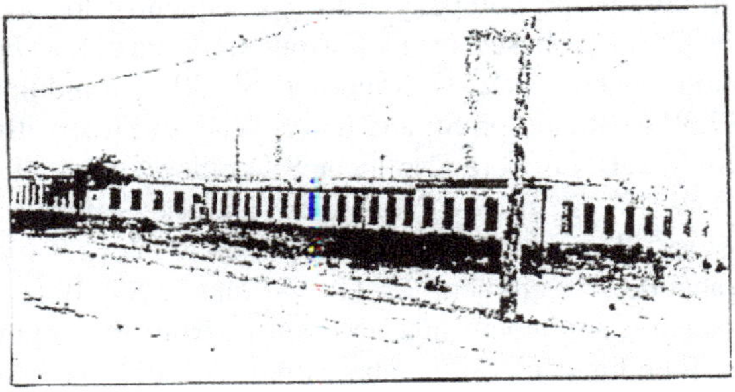

Fig B1B. The Frank S Betz Co of Hammond, IN, ca 1910
(Hammond Historical Society, 564 State St, Hammond, Indiana)

One son, Irving, designed the Betz 22 and 30 automobile models in 1911. The idea was to market the autos to the dentists and physicans who patronized the company's medical and dental business. Irving had worked in Detroit automobile plants where he apparently formed his ideas and plans to build his models in Chicago, and then later in Hammond, IN, if enough interest developed. By early 1911, considerable interest and demand for his autos developed, but since he did not have a factory to build the automobiles to meet demands the once interested parties and sale demands stopped when potential customers bought automobiles elsewhere.[8]

Frank S Betz decided to step down from the day-to-day operations of the company in 1914 (retired 1 Jan 15),[4] but remained in the capacity of president. He was listed in the 1914 Hammond City Directory as the president. Alvin F Rohrer was listed as the secretary-treasurer, and the company was cited as a physician supplier located at 274 Hoffman St. That 1914 Directory listed two of Frank S Betz's sons, F Herman and Irving as clerks in the company.[9(1914,p60)] The Directory in 1916 listed John E Murtaugh as the company's secretary and manager in addition to the positions of Betz and Rohrer.[9(1916,56)] In 1919, the company's officers remained intact except Charles A Taylor was its general manager. The Directory at that time listed Lyman Betz, the youngest son of Frank and Alice, as a student.[9(1919,,p65)]

Although Frank S Betz supposedly retired in 1914, he remained on the board of directors.[5] While still somewhat involved with the Betz Co, Frank S remained active in many activities. His other business associations were in auto manufacturing, an airline, a moving and storage company, a piano company, and a radiator cabinet company. He was also active in may civic organizations.[5]

By 1915, the company administrators were planning a second building (165 x 100 feet and three stories high). At that time the Frank S Betz Co was claimed as the largest and most modern business of its type in the world. The company manufactured and sold dental, embalming,

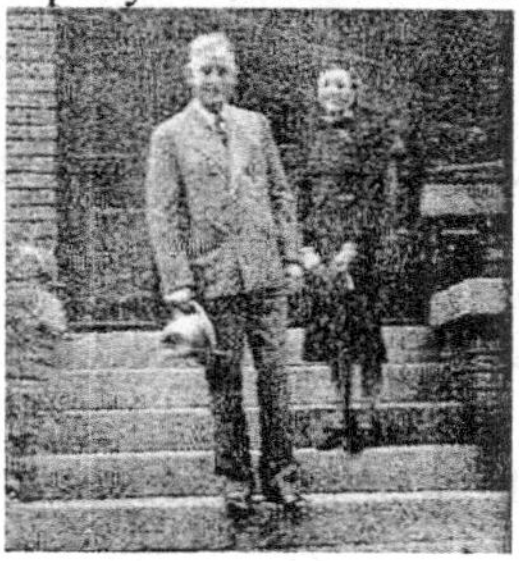

Fig B1C. FS Betz and Wife after 1915

surgical, and veterinary equipment; hospital and office furniture; drugs and pharmaceuticals; glassware; orthopedic appliances; and of course medical electrical apparatuses. The company's assests at that time were more than two million dollars, debt free.[3,4] Frank S Betz is believed to have turned the company over to one or three sons to operate when he retired. The company continued in business until about 1937 when it faced bankruptcy, and was sold to the AS Aloe Co of St Louis.[5] The catalog of The BETZCO line of 1928 did not display any evidence of a Betz family member in control. Others than Betz family members were listed as company administrators.

In 1920, the Frank S Betz Co (after Betz's retirement) was marketing physician and hospital supplies when they introduced the BETZCO electrical line of both dental and physician products, electrical cabinets, and electrical machines. This line of products continued through 1932. The company offered a "satisfaction or money back" policy in its catalog of 1925 (Montgomery Ward was first to offer such policy in 1904). In 1932, the company, in addition to selling x-rays, added a variety of x-ray supplies. The company continued to provide assistance to physicians buying its products by offering unassembled equipment that could easily be put together by the buyer with instructions that accompanied the product. This method was used to further reduce the costs of equipment to physicians.

The Frank S Betz Co also engaged in the manufacture of pharmaceuticals. The quality products under the BETZCO line included elixirs, medications, accessories such as medical bags, bottles, jars, needles, syringes, toothpaste, and narcotics. By July 1924, new Federal laws caused the Frank S Betz Co (as well as other similar companies) to discontinue the BETZCO line of pharmaceuticals.[8] One drug manufacturing building was destroyed by fire on 22 December 1913. The loss of the building amounted to $10,000.00 to $30,000.00 loss. The fire, however, did not curtail the drug operation for more than a day because the company had large amounts of stock maintained elsewhere.[5]

The company manufactured many instruments, and also imported additional medical items. By the middle of the 1920s the company served 100,000 physicians while it maintained items in stock valued at $200,000.00. Discounts to physicians on a direct purchase were offered with the BETZCO line. The company's catalog at this time was offering items like: anesthesia and anesthetic equipment; bath supplies; beauty parlor supplies; bed and bedding; blood pressure instruments; dental supplies; dental furniture; drugs; elastic stockings; hot air devices; medical cabinets; orthopedic devices; radiator covers; surgical instruments; equipment for urinalysis; pharmaceuticals (until 1924); hospital clothing; office furniture; and veterinary equipment. The company sold most items that were used in the medical field.[1]

The catalog of the Frank S Betz Co in 1922 listed parts for invalid chairs along with its prices; and in 1923 the BETZCO line of invalid chairs was introduced. By 1925, the Frank S Betz Co offered a

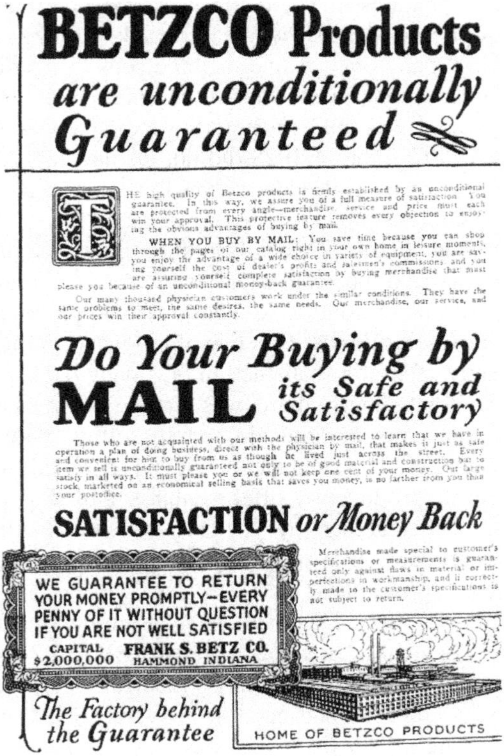

Fig B 2. Home of BETZCO Products

limited assortment of medical electrical apparatuses. The Betz name did not always appear on its medical electrical apparatuses at that time. By 1925, most electrical apparatuses were using alternating current (AC) for power source, however, direct current (DC) line power remained available for many of its apparatuses. Very few electrical apparatuses at this time were being powered by dry cells. Also, the faradic coil's dominance for producing alternating currents in medical electrical apparatus was disappearing.

The trade catalog of 1926 was the last year that electro-therapy apparatus was listed in the Davis & Dreyfus book for Betz.[1] Company catalogs of 1925 through 1932 offered BETZCO dental supplies and equipment. In 1936, the catalog was entitled Betz Book for Physicians and Hospitals.[1] Also, the Betz Co was still in the mail order business for medical, pharmaceutical, and surgical equipment and supplies. In 1925, the Betz Co contracted the manufacture of the Ultima line of electrical apparatus by another company of that name in Chicago.

Commonalties of Betz Electrical Apparatus

The Frank S Betz Co made a wide variety of medical electrical apparatuses. Other than a signature plate or trade name placed on the face plates or on the label of directions the company's product line is difficult to characterize with any commonalities.

Electrical Belts

The Frank S Betz Co never recommended nor vigorously promoted the use of electrical belts, but as a service to customers the belts were stocked and sold upon demand. Betz limited the line of belts to just two styles. Style A was a deluxe unit with spiral suspension for

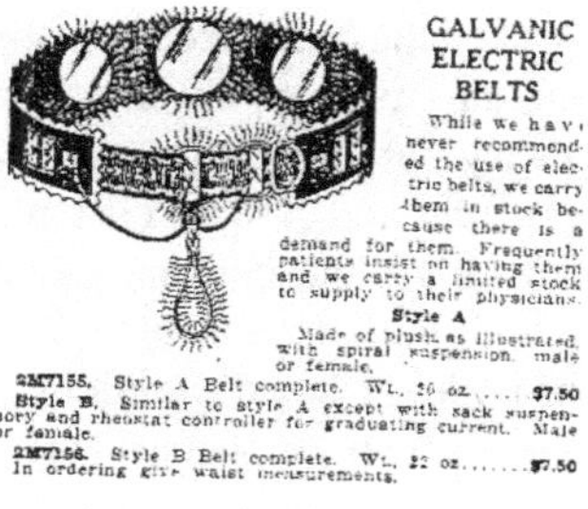

Fig B3. Betz Electrical Belts

both females and males at $7.50 each, and each weighed 20 ounces. Style B belts were also for females and males at the same price, but offered sack suspensory and rheostat control. These latter belts weighed 22 ounces, and came in various waist sizes to fit all customers.

Cabinet and Static Machines.

The Frank S Betz Co produced the Betz console plate that provided the combination of galvanic, faradic, cautery, and rapid sinusoidal currents. Parts of the console apparatus were patented in 1877 by others. The large marble face plate contained a rheostat, millammeter, automatic galvanic rheotome, faradic coil, cautery poles, sine transformer, dial selector, and a pole changer. These items were encased

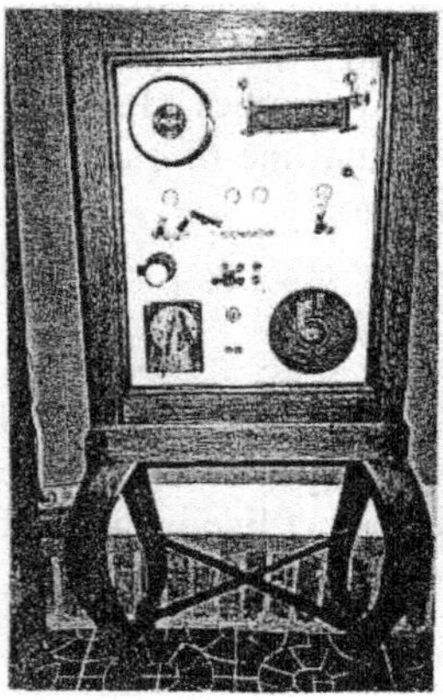

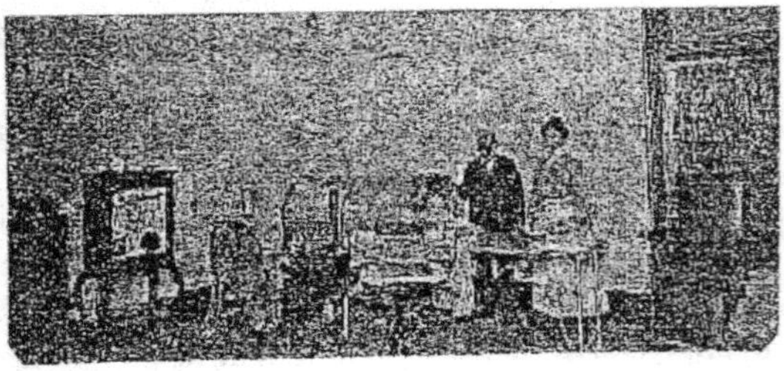

Fig B4. Cabinet Machine

in a quarter sawed golden oak cabinet with a plate glass door, and mounted on four wrought iron legs 26 inches high with cross braces. The dimensions of the oak cabinet are 19.5 x 31 x 15.5 inches. The overall height of the unit mounted on legs is 45.5 inches.

This Cabinet Model of medical electrical apparatus is capable of delivering galvanic current, fast primary faradic current, fast secondary faradic current, slow primary faradic current, slow secondary faradic current, combination of galvanic and faradic current, low potential rapid sine current, high potential rapid sine current, combination of galvanic and rapid sine current, and cautery current. The unit includes all accessories necessary to provide all listed functions. This Cabinet Model electrical apparatus is believed to be first marketed after being patented about 1900 to 1904, and continued for sale in 1918 and later. The unit could be operated by batteries or commercial direct current. This unit is drawn on the cover of this book.

In 1880, Dr William J Morton returned to New York City after studying for awhile in Europe. He brought and introduced the influence or static induced electrical current machine into the United States upon his return. The influence machine produced the first high frequency current used in medicine in this country. The Morton wave current was known also as indirect franklinization or static charge. The currents of d'Arsonval, Tesla, and Oudin were modifications of Morton's influence or static induced current.[10]

The influence machine differs from its forerunner static machines because a conductor gains an electrical charge when contacted whereas the older machines discharged when touched, and there is reciprocal accumulation of the electrical charges with the influence machine. The older static electrical machines did not accumulate charge until the Leyden jar was added as an accessory. The influence machine

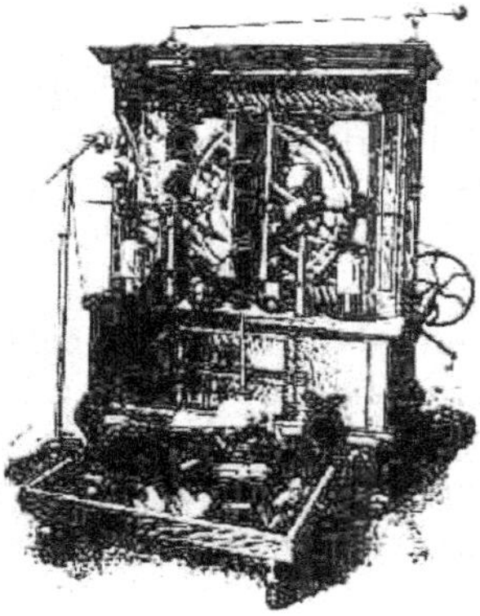

Fig B5. Static Machine by Betz

constantly builds up new charges that go from zero to very high frequencies. The voltage produced is the length (in inches) of the spark between or from conductors multiplied by 30,000. The number and speed of revolving plates determine the machine's amperage (the greater the number and faster the speed the greater the amperage). Voltage can be increased by increasing the size or diameter of the plates.[10]

This particular static machine in Fig B5 operates manually by cranking the two glass circular plates that are enclosed in a cabinet with glass windows. This particular cabinet design reduces atmospheric humidly from collecting on the plates so it is effective on damp days. The manual crank also started the machine so that a primary action made the unit immediately operational (earlier units required a separate starting action.)

The Betz influence machine of 1903 has two glass plates with fixed slots cut into the sides. One plate is fixed while the other revolves. The machine has the ability to separate positive from negative electricities and to accumulate them. The Betz machine like other modified Holtz machines produced unidirectional static current of high potential and very low amperage. The machine was used to generate power for use with x-ray tubes as well as use for therapeutics. The machine uses highly insulating materials (wood). Its poles are the prime conductors which have Leyden jars connected to accumulate charge. Like most influence machines Betz's unit was costly, large, heavy, and cumbersome.

Violet Ray Electrical Stimulators

High frequency electrical violet ray stimulators were first marketed around 1910 to 1915 and immediately became popular among public consumers and some physicians. The Frank S Betz Co was believed to have entered this market also around 1915 or 1916, and continuously sold the high frequency electrical violet ray stimulators at least through 1925, while offering five models.[11] Violet ray electrical stimulators were so named because of their use of glass tube electrodes that provide a violet glow when operating. No ultraviolet ray is emitted by these stimulators.

Electro-Therapeutic Cabinet. The deluxe model (Fig B6) was the Betzco Electro-Therapeutic Cabinet. This cabinet model was actually a portable unit that was housed in a wooden case (16.75 x 11 x 8.5 inches), dovetailed corners but covered by black buckram (leatherette like material). The corners of the case are protected by metal shields, and the case is carried by a leather ringed handle mounted on the front of the case. The front of the case also has two hinged snap latches. The double hinged lid of the case, lined with green velvet, contained all 15 accessories that were open for view of the operator. The face or panel plate of the unit is white marble that contains the controls and most

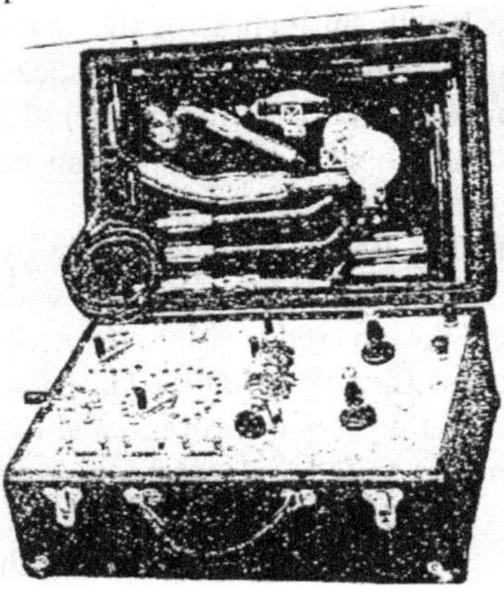

Fig B6..Electro-Therapeutic Cabinet (Lightning)

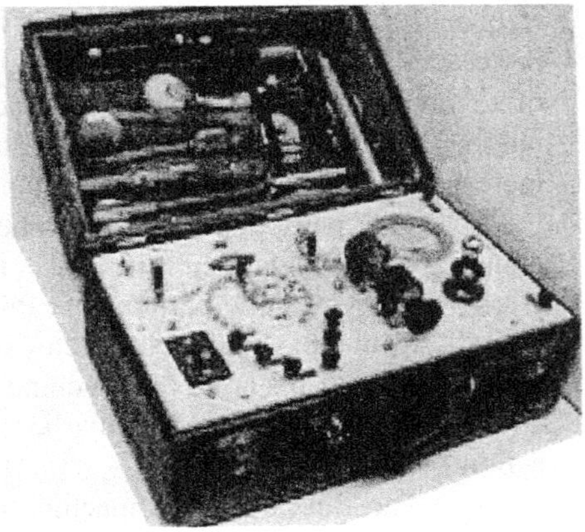

Fig B6A Electro-Therapeutic Cabinet

components of the electrical circuit. Underneath the face plate are three induction coils. One coil (5.5 x 1.75 inches) is for sine, primary, and secondary currents, while two coils (6 x 1.75 inches) are sealed at their ends with multilayered plate magnets to boost voltages sufficiently for cautery and x-ray functions. The unit delivers Tesla high frequency currents, fulguration (tissue destruction by electrical sparks), ozone, and has d'Arsonval and auto condensers (capacitors). The face plate contains two high frequency poles (center to center separation) that deliver sparks of 4.25 inches between them, and used to connect to a heavy glass x-ray tube; double throw On/Off switch; and 20 control studs or buttons with double lever controls (rheostat; selector for cautery, diagnosis, and sinusoidal). Three connector poles from the face plate to the patient are marked "sinusoidal, cautery, and diagnosis." The unit weighs about 50 pounds. The AS Aloe Co of St Louis sold the identical unit as the "Lightning" but Frank S Betz Co was the manufacturer of this popular unit around 1920, and those retailed directly by the Betz Co had no signature plate. Only the identical units sold through the retailer AS Aloe Co bears the tradename "Lightning." Lightning was coined for this series of electrical stimulators because of the violet colored sparks emitted from the conductor post(s). BETZCO models were 9M213 complete with accessories, and operated on 110 volts, 60 Hertz (cycles) alternating (AC) current for $115.00, and the 9M215 was sold without accessories for $85.00.

The Frank S Betz Co made variations of the Electro-Therapeutic Cabinet that were sold through the AS Aloe Co of St Louis. About 1925 or earlier a model of the Lightning (Fig B6A) included the addition of a "milliampere meter." The model was similar to that in Fig B6. The apparatus was housed in a pine box (17 x 11 x 8.5 inches) that was covered by black buckram. It had a leather carrying handle on top of the hinged lid. Inside of the lid held accessories. The face plate was marble and contained all of the features in Fig B6 including the capability of sinusoidal current, diagnosis, cautery, and high frequency current by a d'Arsonval condenser. The unit weighs about 35 pounds and operates on 110 volts, 60 hertz alternating current. The milliamperemeter was an option for some models of the "Lightning."

Thermode and Quatremod. Between 1925 and 1928 the Frank S Betz Co discontinued the Electro-Therapeutic Cabinet models (Fig B6 and B6A), and introduced the Thermode (Fig B6B) and the Quatremod (Fig B6C) Cabinets as shown in its catalog BETZCO Line for 1928. Like the previous models of the Electro-Therapeutic Cabinet series (B6 and B6A), these units were also portable. A Hand Book of Instructions and Suggestions for Operating The BETZCO THERMODE Portable Diathermy Apparatus and THE BETZCO QUATREMOD High Frequency Apparatus came with each unit. Although not stated, the booklet may have been written for the Betz company by Dr NM Eberhart who authored the book A Working Manual of High Frequency Currents, Chicago, 1920. His name is mentioned in different places within the booklet. The Thermode and Quatremod were second generation electrotherapeutic cabinets with some similarities of the "Lightning."

The Thermode is designed for automobile travel and bedside use by the physician; weighing 35 pounds and selling for $125.00 in 1928. The wooden case (17 x 11 x 8.5 inches) was covered exteriorly by black leatherette; bottom corners had protective metal cleats. A strong leather carrying handle is located on the front of the case along with two snap latches to secure the hinged lid. The inside of the lid stores many glass and metal electrodes The face plate contains dials, switches, a d'Arsonval and Tesla coil, milliamperemeter, and other controls to operate the unit's

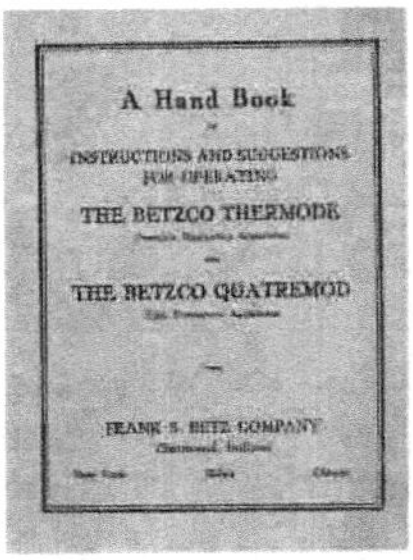
A Hand Book

INSTRUCTIONS AND SUGGESTIONS
FOR OPERATING

THE BETZCO THERMODE

THE BETZCO QUATREMOD

FRANK S. BETZ COMPANY

BETZCO Handbook

multiple functions of diathermy (direct and indirect), autocondensation with d'Arsonval pad electrodes and Telsa glass electrodes, sinusoidal current, cautery, and diagnostic illuminator. Diathermy or deep heat was

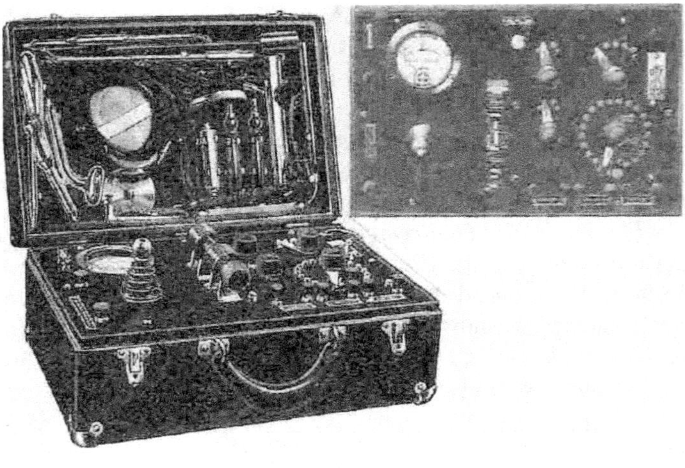

Fig B6B Thermode Cabinet, and Face Plate

becoming popular in physical therapy and rehabilitation medicine by 1928, and this unit served office and hospital applications.

The Thermode operates only on alternating current of 105 to 110 volts and frequencies of 50 to 60 hertz (cycles). A rotary converter was used with it when only a direct current source was available. The plug was screwed into a light socket of alternating current for operation. Lever switches on the face plate control currents for sinusoidal, modalities, condenser, and d'Arsonval and Telsa terminals. The meter ranges from 0 to 1200 milliamperes (mA), and a safety fuse is set for 1250 mA. The high frequencies range from hundreds of thousands to millions of alterations per second.

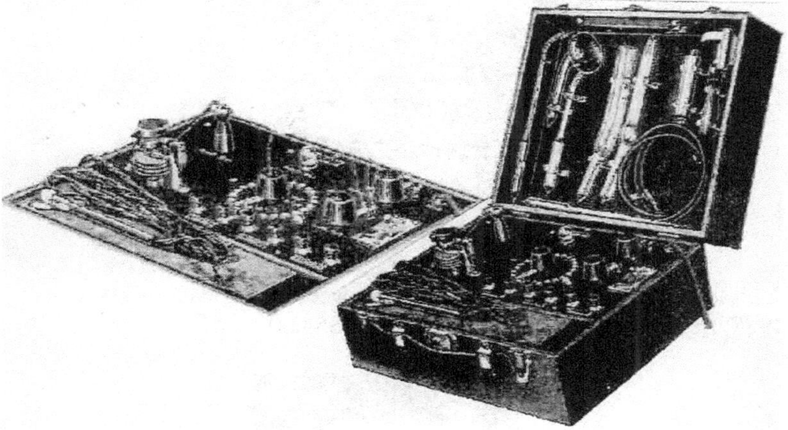

Fig B6C. Quatremod Cabinet

The Quatremod's wooden cabinet (12.75 x 10.75 x 6.75 inches) is covered exteriorly by black leatherette. The case has a hinged lid, and inside it is padded with a green felt lining. The inside of the lid stores the many glass electrodes. The front of the case has a strong leather carrying handle, and two snap latches that secure the lid. The unit weighs 13 pounds and sold for $51.00 in 1928. It was labeled a universal design because it operated either by 110 volts, 60 hertz (cycles) alternating or direct current source. It had only a Tesla coil for use with the glass vacuum tubes.

The unit was used for therapeutic high frequency treatments, for treating sensitive mucous membranes. It could also be used for light cautery (blemishes, boils, warts), and diagnostic and sinusoidal currents.

Universal High Frequency Apparatus. The model in Fig B7 was designed as a portable apparatus to function from 110 volts electrical power source. The unit has heavy induction coils and condensers (capacitors) to deliver a variety of currents that are well controlled. The unit provides for desired levels of violet ray glows, and sparks of varying degrees. The glass tube accessories are mounted on the inside of the hinged lid. The front of the black buckram covered case has a ringed, metal carrying handle, and two hinged snap latches. The unit operates

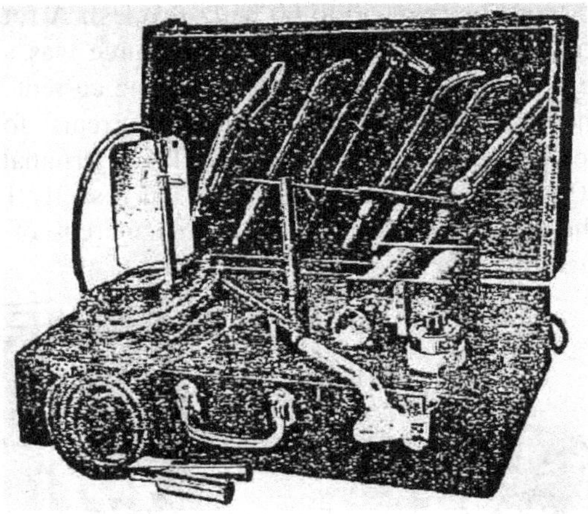

Fig B7. Universal High Frequency Apparatus

with either alternating or direct currents power sources having 110 volts. In 1925, Betz Co sold this unit (9M209) for $54.00.

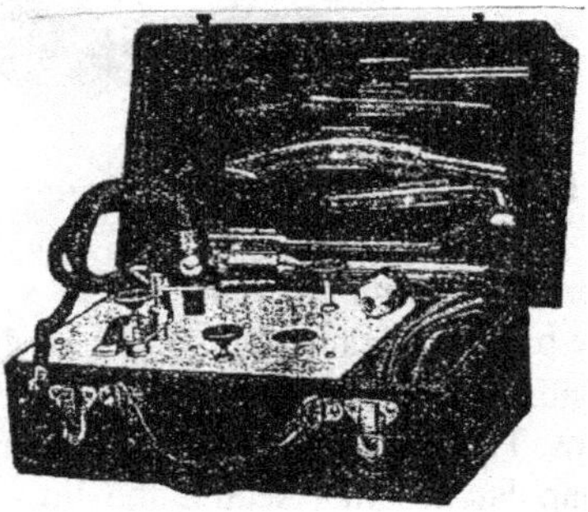

Fig B8. High Frequency and Violet Ray Generator

High Frequency and Violet Ray Generator. This portable unit (Fig B8) is housed in a wooden case covered by black buckram. Its front has a leather carrying handle that is attached by rings, and two snap latches. The unit operates with either alternating or direct current power sources. The voltage capacity (60,000 to 0 volts) varies from the highest amplitude currents for massage to the very high oscillations needed for fulguration (destroy tissue) or urethral treatment. The 9M204 model cost $32.50, while the 9M206 designed for cautery cost $43.50. Both models have a spring lever vibrator for setting frequencies.

Specialist's High Frequency Outfit. This model contains only the operator's handle and its two glass electrode attachments, a plain glass circular bulb tip, and a plain glass, general purpose electrode. This unit is a portable lightweight violet ray generator housed in a seal-grain carrying case. The 9M242 unit was designed for home use and operates

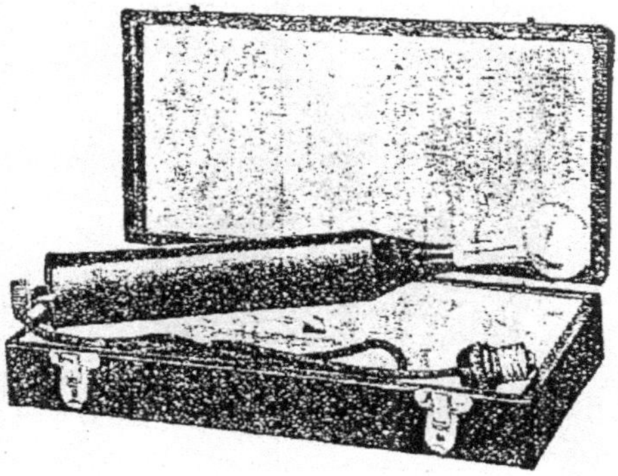

Fig B9. Specialist's High Frequency Outfit

on 110 volts alternating current source from a light socket. The original cost was $12.75 in the 1920s.

Violet Ray High Frequency Generator. The unit of Fig B10 is an efficient, compact, durable, and low cost generator for home use. Costing $9.95, the primary coil was installed in the case rather than the

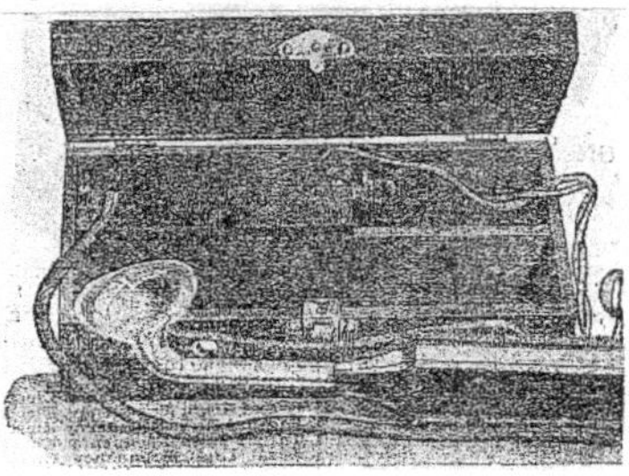

Fig B10. Violet Ray High Frequency Generator

operator's handle. The wooden case covered with black buckram (imitation leather) has a leather carrying handle mounted on the front of the case; nickel plated metal features, and one glass violet ray electrode. The power source (110 V, AC) connecting cord is for connection to a lamp socket that was still common method of obtaining source current in 1925. It cost $10.00 in 1928 and could operate on either 110 volts AC or DC. The unit converts the 110 volts source AC into higher voltages and higher oscillations.

Light Model High Frequency Set. The company increased its offering of high frequency units in 1928. The glass electrode type stimulators, introduced between 1910 and 1915, were still popular in 1928, at least by public consumers for home use. This unit is similar to the once popular High Frequency Generator of Fig B10, but additionally has three electrodes that fit all of the Betz glass electrodes. The Tesla coil

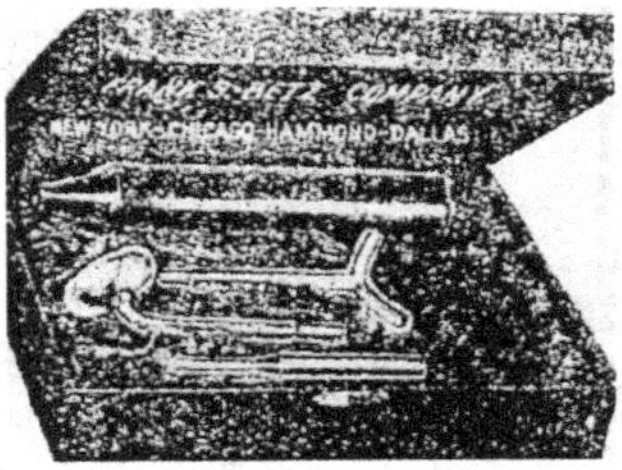

Fig B10A. Light Model High Frequency Set

is located in the operating handle. The inside of the case is silk lined, portable, and operates with 110 volts source AC. The unit cost $15.00 in 1928.

High Frequency Violet Ray and Ozone Set. The violet ray unit

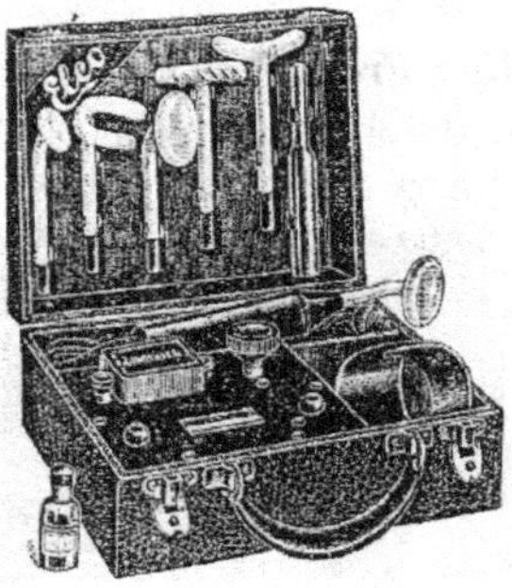

Fig B10B. High Frequency Violet Ray and Ozone Set

of Fig B10B is higher grade than those of Fig B10 and B10A. It provides high frequency current and fulguration (destroy abnormal tissue) treatment. Its 50,000 volts can be adjusted from zero to high potential in fine increments, and it operates with 110 volts source AC or DC.

The face plate (6.5 x 7.25 inches) is bakelite that contains the few needed controls for high frequency, and ozone treatments. The wooden portable case (11.5 x 8.75 x 5.38 inches) is covered exteriorly by black leatherette. All metal parts are nickel plated. The case has a hinged lid that is lined inside by satin, and serves to store accessories. The unit's logo is ELCO. The case has a leather carrying handle secured by strong rings, and two snap latches to secure the lid. It cost $25.00 in 1928, and was accompanied by instructions and charts. The ELCO violet ray electrical stimulator was manufactured by Lindstrom & Co, 2322 Indiana Avenue, Chicago, from 1924 to at least 1928 that again suggests that the Frank S Betz Co was not making all electrical generators that it sold.

Alternating and Galvanic Current Apparatuses

In addition to the line of violet ray generators Betz made and stocked several alternating and galvanic current generators. These 1925 generators are shown in Figs B11-B21.

Polysine. The top of the BETZCO line was the Polysine Generator with options. This generator provided a variety of glavanic and sinusoidal wave currents. The operator of this generator will find rapid

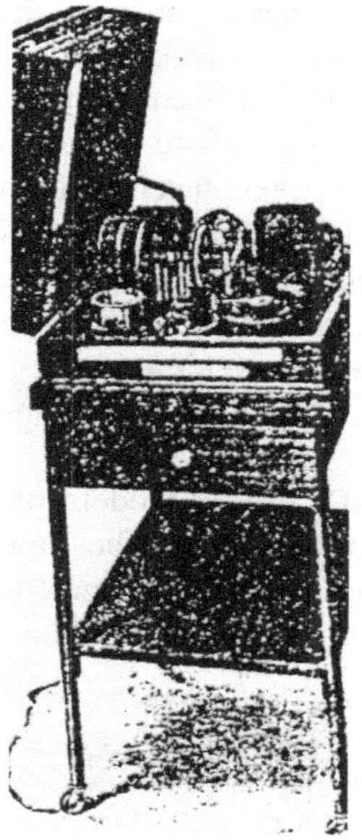

Fig B11. Polysine Generator

and slow sinusoidal pulse rates available. The generator functions when powered by a 110 volts alternating current source. The unit is enclosed in a wooden box that has a hinged lid. The face plate is black slate and contains a milliammeter, large horseshoe magnets, electrical motor, and current control dials. A sliding drawer is accessible from the left hand side of the case. The unit and wooden case is mounted on four metal legs with rollers (casters) on the bottom ends. A shelf is mounted between the rollers and the bottom of the wooden case. Two models were originally available: 9M1144 polysine with stand and 110 volts direct current power for $325.00; and 9M1145 polysine for 110 volts, 60 "cycle" (hertz) alternating current power source and without the stand for $400.00. Mahogany finished metal stand was $35.00 extra, and a mahogany wall bracket was $5.00 extra.

This polysine generator sold by the Frank S Betz Co in 1925 was in reality the McIntosh No.4 Polysine Generator that was manufactured and sold in 1918 for $130.00 without the metal stand. (Note: The Betz Co by 1925 had dropped the manufacture of most of its electrotherapeutic apparatus, but contracted other manufactures to supply them with units of its suggested design and signature. The Frank S Betz Co did not manufacture the polysine generator in 1925, but like others, contractred the manufacture of specific items for retail under the Betz name.) In 1918, the unit provided a full range of galvanic and sinusoidal currents. The No.4 unit was fitted with a universal motor and operated with either alternating or direct current. It has a dial current selector, and slow and rapid sinusoidal pulse frequencies. The face plate is a white enameled porcelained steel slab that is encased in a polished golden oak cabinet with a plate glass cover. The face plate also contained a sinusoidal device, rheostat, a milliammeter, and a pole changer. The unit sold for $175.00. The basic polysine generator design resembles that of Dr JH Kellogg's model of about 1893 except for the added meters.

Other units offering sine (sinusoidal) current were combination generators of both sine and galvanic currents. The BETZCO line included the Ultima Sinustat, two models of combined sine and galvanic currents.

Ultima Sinustat No.4. This model combines sinusoidal and galvanic currents into a portable unit. The unit was contained in a wooden case covered by black buckram (leatherette-like) with a carrying handle on top and two hinged snap latches on the front of the case. This

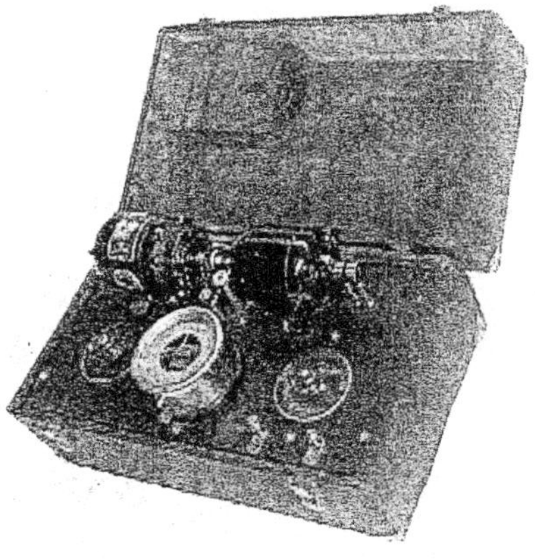

Fig B12. Ultima Sinustat No. 4

unit generates DC (direct current) by converting the AC (alternating current source). The unit operated from any lamp socket sources of AC or DC in 1925. The face plate has a milliammeter, rheostat, AC to DC convertor, selector dial, and connecting posts. Inside of the lid is a small box for storage of accessories. The 9M1166 Ultima Sinustat No.4 sold for $175.00 in 1925 through 1928, and was considered the deluxe combination generator of the BETZCO line. The Frank S Betz Co did not manufacture this unit or the Ultima line. By 1925, the Ultima line was made by the Ultima Physical Appliance Co, also of Chicago, and retailed by the Betz Co. The Ultima Physical Appliance Co was apparently a small manufacturer that received a contract from the Frank S Betz Co to make the Ultima line. This company has not been found in searches, and may have discontinued the Ultima line when the Betz Co stopped selling medical electrical stimulators in the 1930s. In 1928, the Ultima Sinustat No.4 was the only model of the Ultima series being sold, and it was then named The Sinustat Galvanic or Sinusoidal Generator.

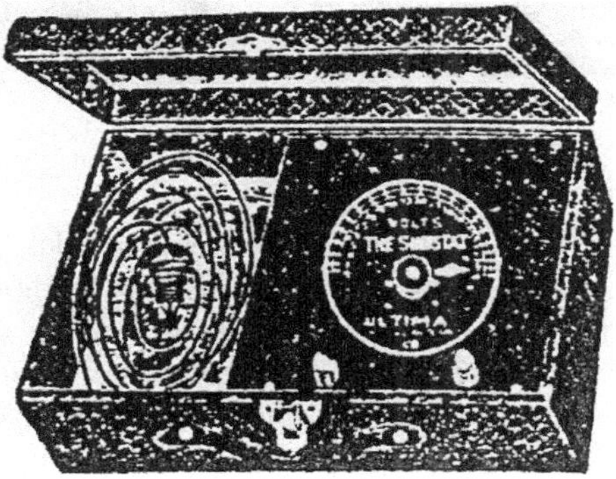

Fig B13. Galvanic and Sinusoidal Generator

Galvanic and Sinusoidal Generator. This unit (Fig B13) is a cheaper version of other BETZCO combination current generators, and the 9M1245 sold for $25.00. This unit was designed for home use. It operates on 110 volts DC for galvanic currents, and 110 volts AC for sinusoidal currents. The sinusoidal current is rapid pulses. The unit is enclosed in a portable wooden carrying case covered with black imitation leather. The hinged lid has a single snap latch on front and a carrying handle on top of the case. The face plate occupies about 75 percent of the box area with the remainder for accessories.

Ultima No.1 Sinustat. The Ultima series, although sold by the Frank S Betz Co, but was manufactured in Chicago by the Ultima Physical Appliance Company, 136 W Lake Street. In 1918, this company sold the No.1 and the No.3 models. Again, this is another example where the Frank S Betz Co was not manufacturing electrotherapeutic generators in 1925 or perhaps after 1918.

This unit (left) resembles the Galvanic and Sinusoidal Generator sold by the Frank S Betz Co in 1925 for $25.00. The Betz unit was labeled "The Ultima," that usually operated on either 110 volts alternating or direct currents. This No.1 Ultima Sinustat, however, operated only from 110 volts alternating current, and delivered only rapid

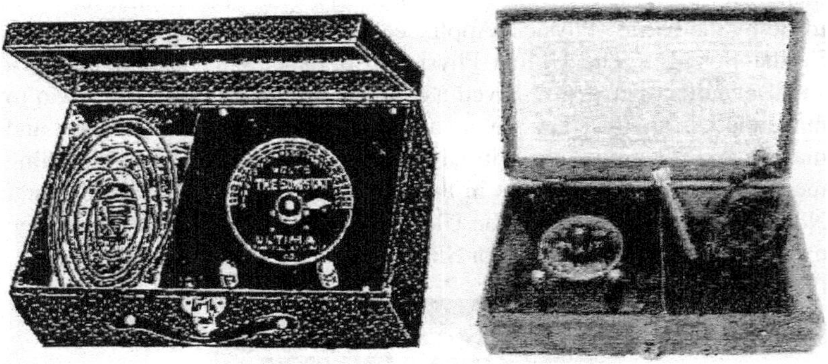

Fig B14. The Ultima No. 1 Sinustat

sinusoidal current. Since it was a portable model, the unit was recommended for house calls by physicians and for home use by the patient for neuritis, sciatica, lumbago, gastro-intestinal conditions, and uterine diseases. The No.1 was a shunt controller so provided perfect regulation of the voltage (via dial) without any surprise shock. The unit contained a special resistance in the circuit regulating from 0 to 100 volts. The metal is polished nickel plate; the face plate is black enameled metal; encased in a wooden box (12 x 7 x 3.5 inches) covered by leatherette. The front of the case has a leather carrying strap, and a hinged snap lock. A third of the case was open for storage of accessories. In 1918, the unit sold for $15.00 by competition of the Frank S Betz Co.

The Ultima No.1 Sinustat pictured on the right is the same design and function as that shown on the left, however, the casing of the model differs. The model on the right is also enclosed in buckram and measures 11.5 x 7 x 3.75 inches but the face plate is reversed from that on the left. The models are of the same date and cost.

Ultima No.3 Sinustat. Unlike the No.1 Ultima model, this No.3 provided slow and rapid sinusoidal currents (10 hertz or cycles per minute). The unit operates with 110 volts alternating or direct currents. The motor on the black enamel face plate adopts the operation to alternating or direct current. The slow sinusoidal current was used to stimulate the peristaltic action of the bowels and other gastro-intestinal conditions. The rheostat controls fine graduations of current amplitude.

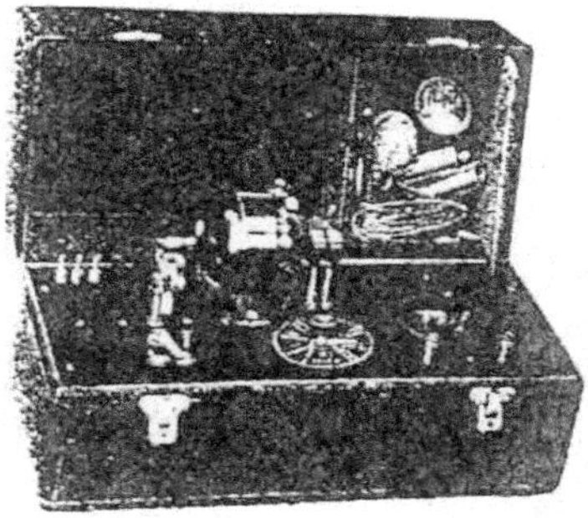

Fig B15. Ultima No. 3 Sinustat

The alternating current mode gives slow or rapid current pulses, while the direct current mode gives galvanic current or slow and rapid sinusoidal current amplitudes. The wooden case (7 x 16.5 x 8.5 inches) is covered by black leatherette and weighs 18 pounds. The unit sold for $60.00 in 1918.

Ultima Sinustat No.3. This No.3 Ultima (Fig B16) was also a portable unit with a wooden case covered by black imitation leather. The top of the case has a carrying handle, while the front has two hinged snap latches. The inside of the lid, right corner, has a storage box (about a

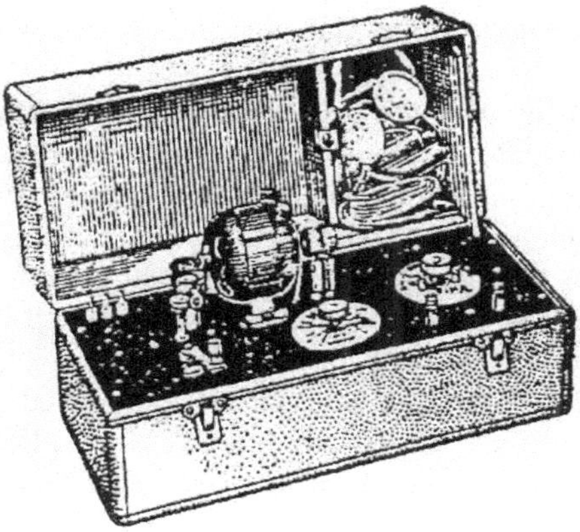

Fig B16. Ultima Sinustat No. 3

third of the lid area), and lid for accessories. The black face plate has a motor that helps to generate various rates and forms of sinusoidal pulses (eg, rapid and slow sine pulses; high voltage sine waves; and surging sinusoidal and galvanic currents). Surging pulsed currents are ramp modulations of cyclical increases in the phase charges of a pulse to change the amplitudes used in various therapeutic treatments.[12] The unit operates on AC and DC power sources. A current selector, and rheostat are also mounted on the face plate. An interrupter is adjacent to the motor to set pulse rates as well as an On/Off switch, and connecting posts. The 9M1165 No.3 Ultima Sinustat sold for $100.00 in 1925.

Century Model. This model of Fig B17 provides both faradic and galvanic currents, and was designed for exclusive use in sanitoriums. The electrical circuit and components are mounted on a white marble plate (18 x 24 inches). The model can be operated by electrical cells, AC

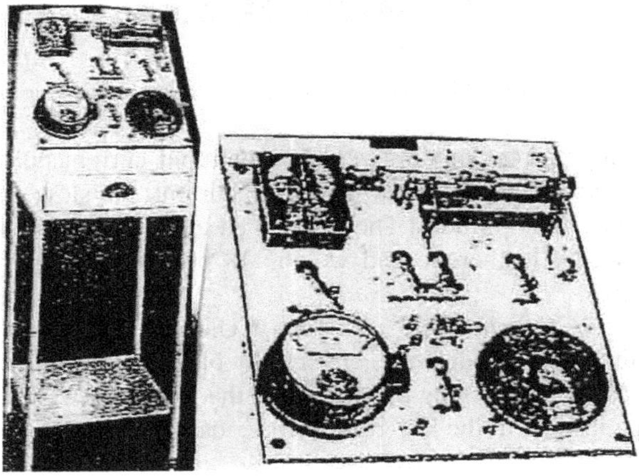

Fig B17. Century Model Galvanic and Faradic Wall Plate

with use of a rectifier or motor generating set, or DC power sources. The face plate contains: an automatic current rheostat for galvanic current, a "milliamperemeter," selector switch, On/Off switch; connecting posts, and a graphite circular type rheostat for faradic current control. An induction coil for faradic current is also mounted on the face plate. The 9M1117 face plate is mounted on a steel wall cabinet of white enamel. This unit sold for $125.00 in 1925.

The 9M1119 model was a table plate mounted on a tubular steel stand with an accessory drawer below the face plate. The metal is finished in white enamel, and the marble face plate (16 x 16 inches) with beveled edges contains the electrical components. It cost $115.00. A 9M1120 Century Model Table Plate without stand cost $75.00.

Dr Pope's Model Galvanic and Faradic Battery. Dr Pope's model is a wall mounted apparatus designed for offices with limited space. The cabinet is steel, white enamel. The cabinet has a glass door and a sliding drawer below the door. Components include: throw On/Off switch, graphite circular rheostat, induction coil, "milliamperemeter," automatic galvanic rheostat, and connecting posts. This 9M1124 unit cost $150.00 in 1925. This unit's operating components and face plate design resembles that of the Cabinet Model of Fig B2.

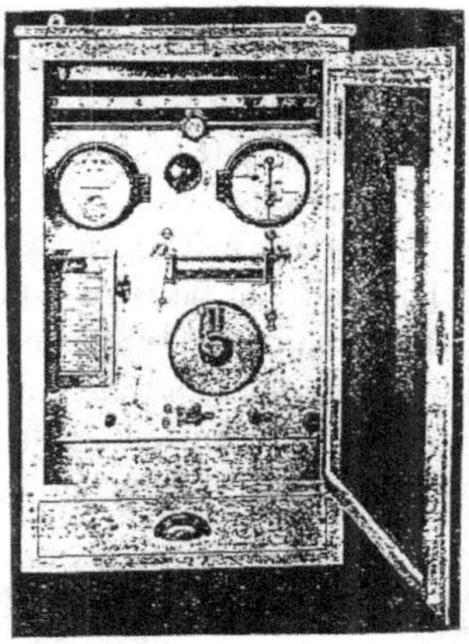

Fig B18. Dr Pope's Galvanic and Faradic Battery

The Granger Outfit. Granger's model is a portable combination faradic and galvanic generator that operates from a 110 volts AC power source. This unit is a mahogany case (12 x 16 x 10 inches) with hinged lid, carrying handle on top, and two snap latches on front. The face plate has a chemical rectifier, condenser (capacitor), graphite rheostat controller, pole changer, selector switch, switch for controlling input current, fuse holder, "milliamperemeter" with a double

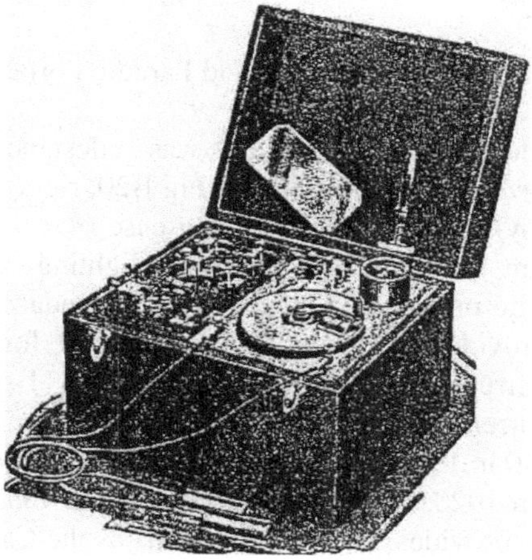

Fig B19. Granger Portable Outfit

scale, and a compartment for accessories. It sold for $72.50 in 1925. This unit may have been designed by Frank B Granger, MD, who was a Boston physician, and an US Army officer in World War I. He paved the way for physical therapists to practice professionally, was author of the book Granger FB. Physical Therapeutic Technic. Philadelphia, PA, WB

Saunders, 1929, and a leading electrotherapeutist in the United States between 1915 and 1930.

The Calumet. This model (Fig B20, left) is a lightweight, durable, portable battery that provides faradic and galvanic currents. The galvanic current is sufficient for use with reflexes and removal of hair and small skin growths. The unit can be used with lights of 1.5 to 15 volts in diagnostic work. The cost of 9M1285 was $29.50 ca 1925. The face plate contains the induction coil, a lever, button current controller for galvanic current and a sliding tube current controller in the coil, and a selector switch. It was named for the Calumet river near the company's plant in Hammond, IN.

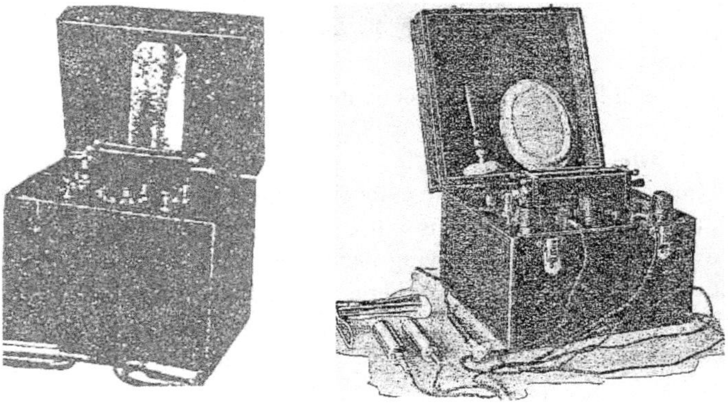

Fig B20. Calumet Galvanic and Faradic Portable Battery

The Calumet Portable Battery was redesigned, improved, and renamed the ***Galvanic-Faradic Battery*** (Fig B20, right) in 1928. The unit is housed in a "Whitekraft" steel carrying case (9 x 9 x 7 inches). This model offers an electric eye magnet, lighting diagnostic lamp, cystoscope, faradic or galvanic currents. Five standard (radio) dry cells were used to provide 22.5 volts that were used for electrolysis and massages. The current amplitude is controlled by a 11-point cell selector. An adjustable current interrupter is available with the faradic coil. The model cost $37.50 in 1928 (Fig B20, right). ***Portable Current Controller***. A new product in 1928, this combined current (galvanic and sinusoidal) unit in Fig B20A provides the same functions as the Calumet yet smaller and more convenient. It operated by commercial direct current or dry cells. It uses a circular dial type of current controller on the face plate while other circuit components are underneath. The wooden case is hinged, covered by black leatherette (12 x 7 x 3.5 inches), and has a leather carrying handle on the front with two snap latches. Accessories are carried in the left side of the case. The unit cost $17.50 in 1928.

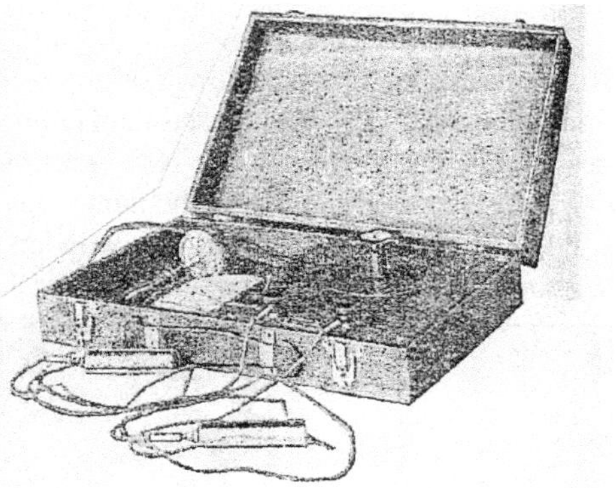

Fig B20A. Portable Current Controller[13]

Faradic Battery

Standard Faradic Battery (Cedergren, Home Faradic Battery). The Betz Co offered only one faradic model in 1925. The complete 9M1265 Standard Faradic Battery (Fig B21,upper right) sold for $10.75. The unit is powered by two dry cells but operates with one or both by means of a selector switch. A graduated scale with a pointer indicates an arbitrary value for current amplitude when the sliding metal tube is moved away or toward the induction coil. Accessories are stored in the lid of the wooden box that is hinged and has a self lock device on the front. Since the unit is portable, a carrying handle is mounted on top of the lid (box). A spring lever, hammer type vibrating interrupter is also mounted on the face plate.

This particular faradic battery resembles the Double-Cell Faradic Battery manufactured by Signal Electric Co of Menominee, MI, (Fig B21, bottom) and retailed through Montgomery Ward & Co and in 1908 by the Sears, Roebuck and Co of Chicago. The construction quality of the Betz unit is superior than those sold through the mail order catalogs.

Earlier, probably 1900 to 1910, Betz called this two cell powered boxed faradic model the ***Cedergren Family Battery*** (bottom picture). Perhaps the Cedergren was sold by other retailers, but it was made by Betz. The Cedergren has a glued dovetailed oak box (8.5 x 7 x 6 inches), and directions for operation on the inside of the lid (upper right).

Still another Betz unit labeled (Fig B21, left) was made and retailed by the company probably in 1904 when its New York office opened. This model is similar to both the Standard Faradic Battery and the Cedergren (upper right) with the exception that the hinged compartment of accessories on the inside of the lid is designed to allow the induction coil to occupy part of the lid's space. The accessory compartment in this unit occupies the front half of the lid. Like other Betz batteries a signature plate is attached on the face plate of the unit, and this model shows both Chicago and New York as well as Hammond locations for the company. Although Betz used the Hammond location in 1896 on signatures, it was not until 1904 that New York was added. (The company was not yet in Hammond, perhaps the name was used for tax or license purposes.-ed) The model was housed in a wooden case (9 x 6.5 x 6.5 inches) with a hinged lid. A metal carrying handle is located on top

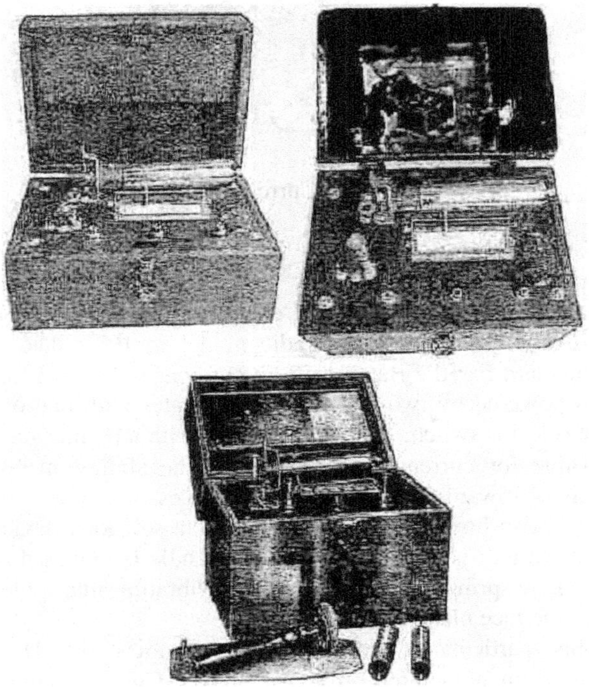

Fig B21. Standard Faradic Battery (Cedergren, Home Faradic Battery)

and a snap latch to secure the lid is on the front of the case.

In 1928, this model was renamed the Home Faradic Battery (ID #9DX1265) (Fig B21, upper right) and was similar to that shown on the left side of Fig B21. The unit sold for $13.50 in 1928, its steel case measures 9 x 6.5 x 8 inches, the lid has a compartment for accessories, and the top has a carrying handle. The coil provides primary (low amplitude) or secondary (high amplitude) currents, or combined primary and secondary currents. Two No.6 dry cells powered the unit, but could be operated by either or both.

BETZCO Line of Galvanic Batteries

The Frank S Betz Co was offering four galvanic battery models in 1925. Each unit used dry cells for its power source.

Wilson's Galvanic Battery. The 9M1283 Wilson Portable Battery sold for $26.00. The unit used nine standard dry cells for power source, and was contained in a carrying case (10 x 9 x 12 inches) with a handle on top and two snap latches on the front. The face plate has a 10-point selector switch, two primary binding posts, and a large accessory box to the rear of the plate. The unit was designed for light or small work such as facial blemishes; removal of hair, warts, and moles. The unit has

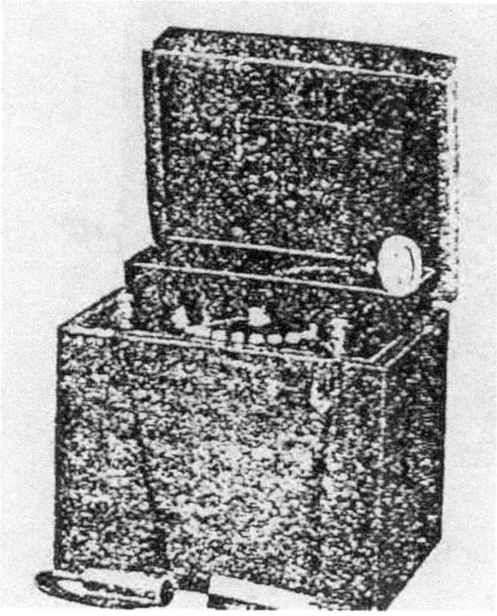

Fig B22..Wilson's Galvanic Battery

lights, controls for small eye magnets, a diagnostic lamp, and a cystoscope.

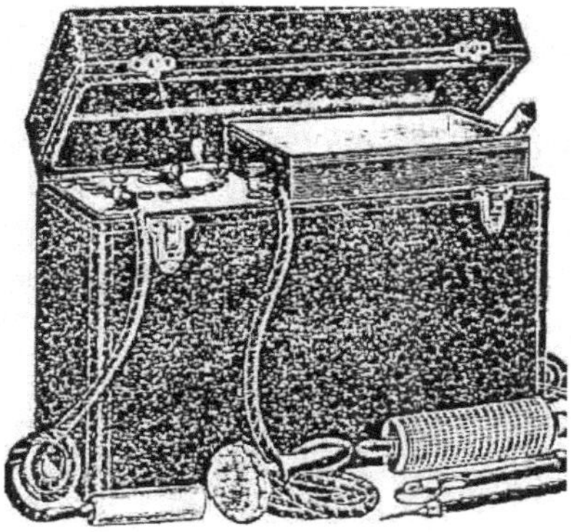

Fig B23. Portable Galvanic Battery

Portable Galvanic Battery. This model of Fig B23 operates from 12 dry cells that are controlled by a selector cell switch. The unit is housed in a carrying case (17 x 11 x 17 inches) with a top leather handle.The lid is hinged and has two snap latches on the front of the case. The face plate occupies about a third of the area with the remainder compartmentalized for accessories. Two connecting posts are located on the face plate. The complete 9M1282 unit cost $25.00 and weighs about 30 pounds.

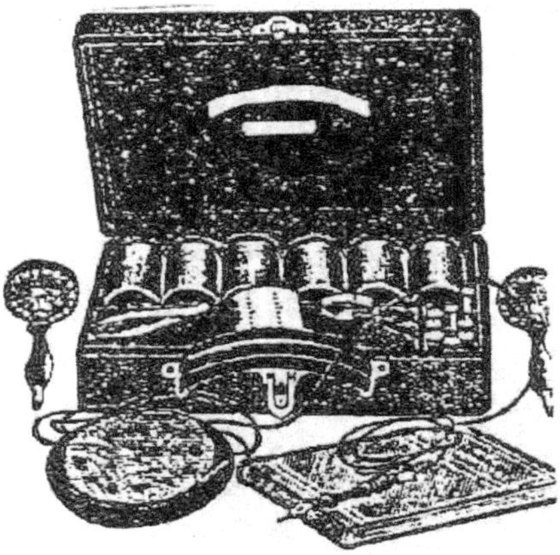

Fig B24. Electrolysis Battery

Electrolysis Battery. The small hand carried battery of Fig B24 was designed to be used for the removal of hair and facial blemishes. The unit is powered by six dry cells mounted to the rear of its small face plate, and has a compartment for accessories. The Betz Co recommended and provided a copy of the book Hayes PS. Electricity and the Methods of its Employment in Removing Superfluous Hair, ed 2. Chicago, IL, 1899. The complete 9M1222 Electrolysis Battery with a copy of Hayes' book sold for $20.00 in 1925.

Dermatologist's Galvanic Plate. The unit of Fig B25 is in plate form for use with a 110-volt DC power source, wall or dry cell). The operator used the galvanic plate in series with a 16 CP lamp.The white marble plate (12 x 15 inches) contains a "milliamperemeter" with ranges of 0 to 10 and 0 to 50 mA scales. The face plate also has a pole changer, a fire-burned rheostat, a double throw On/Off switch, two binding posts, and two connecting posts. The unit could be mounted on the wall or on top of a table by four screws. The 9M1189 Dermatologist's Galvanic Plate sold complete for $40.00. The unit could also be run on a 110-volt AC service with an electrolytic rectifier or motor generator set.

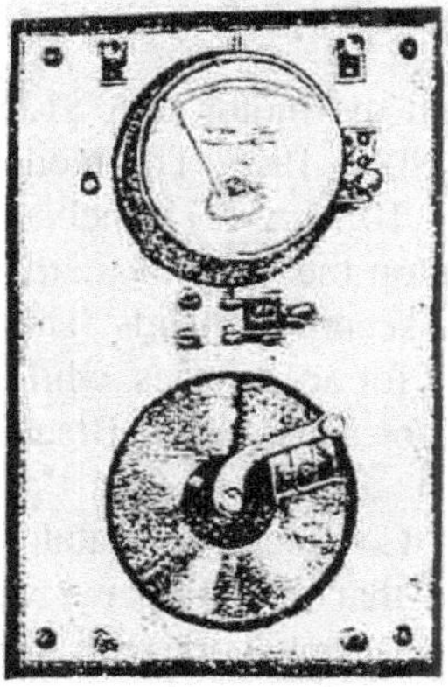

Fig B25. Dermatologist's Galvanic Plate

New Galvanic Set. Two models (Fig B26) were offered in 1928 for this galvanic set: with (left) or without (right) a motor generator, otherwise the models are near identical. The motor converts commercial or source AC to DC. These models provide galvanic treatments, and electrolysis; control diagnostic lamps, cystoscopes, lamps, and other devices.

On the left is the model with the motor. It is designed for the office use of a physician and its case measures 13 x 14 x 4.5 inches. The voltage and current of the model are controlled by a potentiometer (rheostat) that permits constant smooth increments of direct or galvanic current. The current amplitude is displayed by a "milliamperemeter." A control next to the meter permits adjustments for measurement ranges of 0 to 10, 0 to 100, or 0 to 500 milliamperes.

Both models have many electrodes, and a set of operating

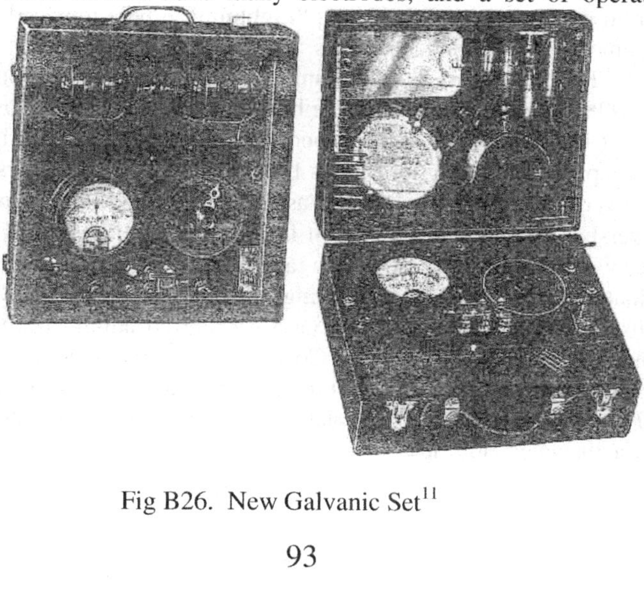

Fig B26. New Galvanic Set[11]

instructions. The model with the motor cost $125.00, while the model without the motor cost $75.00 in 1928. The model without motor has a case that measures 12.75 x 10.75 x 6.75 inches. Both models have a heavy leather carrying strap on the front of their cases, hinged lids, and two snap latches on front to secure their lids. The model with the motor has no separate compartment for accessories, while the model without the motor uses the extra space for accessories. Black leatherette covers the exterior of each case.

The Frank S Betz Co issued its catalog BETZCO LINE for 1928. The catalog indicated that the company was still operating from offices in Chicago, Dallas, and New York with the factory in Hammond, IN, and a sizable warehouse in Dallas. The president and director was John E Murtaugh, secretary and treasurer was Robin E Amoss, while managers of the Chicago and New York Offices were OK Mitchell and JA Padden, respectively. In 1928, the company manufactured steel furniture, electrotherapeutic apparatus, orthopedic appliances, sterilizers, soft metal instruments, and certain specialities. Other products listed in that catalog were imported and purchased direct from makers. The company still claimed a capital of two million dollars in 1928.

Many of the electrotherapeutic apparatuses listed and described in the 1925 catalog were no longer available through the catalog of 1928. The Ultima series that had been around since 1918 was discontinued, but the Sinustat Galvanic or Faradic Battery was a replacement. The New Galvanic Set with two models was introduced, while the Improved Calumet and the Portable Current Controller offered both faradic (sinusoidal) and galvanic currents. The Standard Faradic Battery was renamed the Home Faradic Battery. The most noticeable product omission was the series of electrotherapeutic cabinets and high frequency apparatuses that resembled the "Lightning," but replaced by the Quatremod and Thermode Cabinets.

Busines affairs of the Frank S Betz Co began to soon change after 1928, and into the 1930s. The business volume dropped, as well as financial losses because of the economic depression in the early 1930s. The company was losing money by 1934, and local stockholders went to court over the liquidation of some assests that forced the company into receivership. The AS Aloe Co of St Louis acquired the Frank S Betz Co in early 1937. The AS Aloe Co apparently was most interested in eliminating competition and acquiring remaining stock from the Betz Co because it immediately upon purchase transferred administrative, sales, and marketing aspects of the Betz Co away from Hammond, IN. AS Aloe was not a manufacturer nor was it interested in maintaining that aspect of the Frank S Betz Co so by late 1936 or early 1937 shut down manufacturing capabilities.[5]

The former Betz property on Hoffman St was sold to a candy company by 1939[5] to end an era of the once world's most successful physician supplier and maker of electrical medical batteries.

Summary

The Frank S Betz Co grew from a shed in 1895 to become one of the largest companies of its kind. The company was both a manufactory and a retailer. It accommodated local and regional retailers

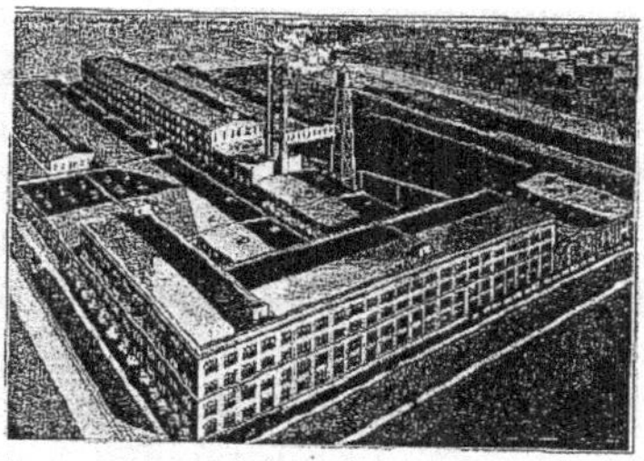

Hammond, IN, Factory

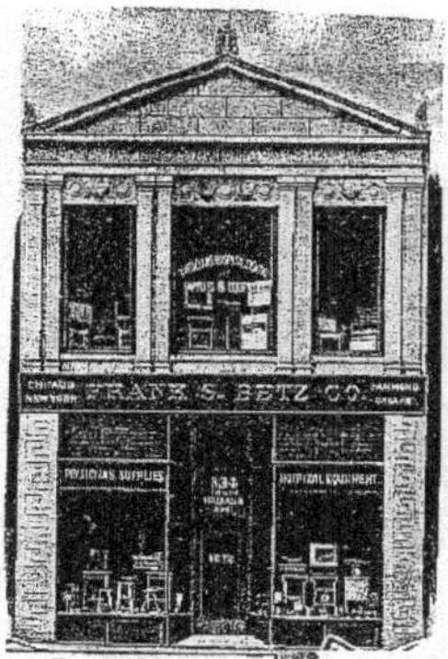

THE BETZ BUILDING
At 654 So. Wabash Ave.,
Chicago, Illinois

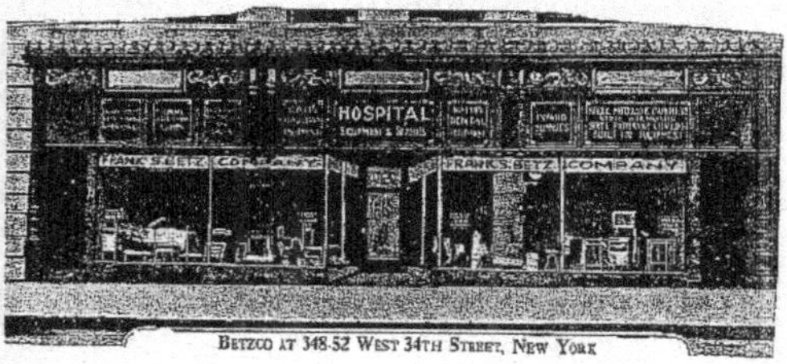

BETZCO AT 348-52 WEST 34TH STREET, NEW YORK

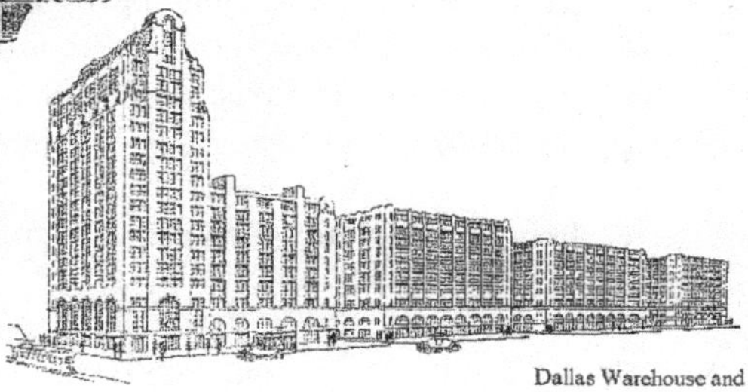

Dallas Warehouse and Office

Fig B27. BETZCO Offices of Chicago, Dallas, and New York, 1928[11]

Although the Betz Co manufactured quality items, the company was by manufacturing specific items for them (eg, medical electrical batteries) and placing various signatures on the contracted products committed to providing physicians with very reasonable costs for satisfactory products. The company stood behind its products.

Following the retirement of Frank S Betz in 1915, the company changed directions somewhat, at least in some product lines. The manufacturing aspects were reduced to fit the demands of the times which saw decreased volumes of medical electrical batteries, particularly those supplied by electrical cells. The company offered batteries powered by commercial electrical power, and even went into the violet ray stimuator business that became more oriented to sales for home use. By 1925, however, the company was contracting the manufacturing of most of its line of medical electrical batteries. The Frank S Betz Co was sold to the AS Aloe Co of St Louis in 1937.

Frank S Betz was a conservationist, inventor, manufacturer, and philanthropist. A newspaper in 1915 described him as fiery, energetic, dominating personality, while other descriptions have included eccentric millionaire, globe trotter, and philanthropist. At times he was a member of the directory board of several banks and other prominent local businesses. He was a member of several civic organizations. He enjoyed travel and is known to have crossed the Atlantic Ocean 41 times and the Pacific Ocean five times. Betz promoted conservation and natural resources (viz, trees); worked with school children, and was active in the Boy Scouts.[3] He donated a water front property in Berrien Springs, MI, for Boy Scout activities. The camp is used year round, and is named Camp Frank S Betz.[5] He also created a home for working women of Hammond, and aided in the development of a city park. After several strokes he died at the age of 78 years on 28 February 1940.[4]

References

1. Davis AB, Dreyfus MS. The Finest Instruments Ever Made. Arlington, MA, Med Hist Pub Assocs, 1989, pp 15-16, 63-68, 370

2. Grigg ERN. The Trail of the Invisible Light. Springfield, IL, CC Thomas, 1965, pp 52, 64-65

3. Dunajeski JG. Frank S Betz Biographical. Hammond, IN, Hammond Hist Preserv Comm, 1994, pp 1-8

4. Long S. Calumet Room, Hammond Public Library. Hammond, IN, 2002

5. Lytle RM, Personal Correspondence.Hammond Public Library, Hammond, IN, May 2004

6. Romaine LB. A Guide to American Trade Catalogs 1744-1900. New York, NY, RR Bowker, 1966, pp 235-241

7. Advertisement. In Polk's Medical Register and Directory of North America. Baltimore, MD, RL Polk, 1904, pp 1669, 3055

8. Twentieth Century Time Capsule. , and capsule 68, 1999-2000, (http://www.hammondindiana.com/20thcentruy/time_capsule62.htm)

9. Smith's Hammond City Directory, Hammond, IN

10. Dugan WJ. Hand-Book of Electro-Therapeutics. Philadelphia, PA, FA Davis, 1910, pp 42-45

11. The BETZCO Line 1925, Hammond, IN, FS Betz Co

12. Electrotherapeutic Terminology in Physical Therapy. Alexandria, VA, Am Phys Ther Assoc, 1990, pp 21-22

13. The BETZCO Line of 1928, Hammond, IN, FS Betz Co, pp 101-108

CHAPTER 5. THE CHLORIDE OF SILVER DRY CELL BATTERY COMPANY OF BALTIMORE

Chapter 5 reviews the company, personnel, and its battery products. The founding date for The Chloride of Silver Dry Cell Battery Co is conjectured to have begun on or before 23 February 1886 when the company's first of many patents were registered in the United States Patent Office, Washington, DC. The Chloride of Silver Dry Cell Battery Co was also an English firm located in London (Saracen Chambers, Snow Hill EC) about the same time. Patents for components of the company's faradic electrical aparatuses made in the United States show many patent dates between 1886 and 1910, while those same inventions were later patented in England between 1895 and 1900. One could speculate that The Chloride of Silver Dry Cell Battery Co originated in the United States and that the English firm was a branch. The patent date of 1886 was taken from one of the company's medical electrical batteries, yet the 1902 catalog lists 22 patents in the United States ranging from 7 May 1889 to 2 July 1901. Patents in England (7 patents) ranged from 18 June 1895 to 15 September 1900.

Review of company trade catalogs is often a good source for revealing the histories of manufacturers and retailers. Using this source of information for The Chloride of Silver Dry Cell Battery Co may be risky because the catalog would suggest that the company may have been founded in 1889, since the sixth edition of its trade catalog was dated 1895 with its 55 pages of items. However, the problem with assigning credit to this source is that catalogs were not issued on a strict annual basis by manufacturing companies. The catalog of The Chloride of Silver Dry Cell Battery Co of 1892 with its description of medical electrical batteries was edition four with 32 pages. The Baltimore based The Chloride of Silver Dry Cell Battery Co issued a catalog in 1898 as its eighth edition with 72 pages. The company also issued catalogs in 1900 (supplemental issue to catalog No.8 with 20 pp), and 1902 (63 pages) listing batteries, electrodes and accessories.[1] The catalog of 1900 (supplement No.8) illustrated the company's combination medical electrical batteries Nos.13, 17, 18, and 19.[2] These few trade catalogs of The Chloride of Silver Dry Cell Battery Co are the only known editions available (1890 to 1902) through library sources, and the specific edition and year are not often cited.

The Chloride of Silver Dry Cell Battery Co may possibly have been established in 1885 or earlier. The date of 1885 is attributed to the trade catalog of Leach & Greene of 165 Treamont St, Boston, MA. The Leach & Greene signature plates were placed on the lids of some boxes of the early portable units of The Chloride of Silver Dry Cell Battery Co units that Leach & Greene retailed. The Leach & Greene Co also issued a trade catalog in 1885 that illustrated surgical instruments, orthopedic appliances, trusses, microscopes, and medical electrical batteries (eg, The Chloride of Silver Dry Cell Battery Co).[1] The second edition of the Leach and Greene catalog was dated 1888, and it illustrated medical items in 126 pages. Leach & Greene also sold the medical electrical apparatuses of the Voltamp Electric Mfg Co of Baltimore, MD, as did other distributors (eg, GC Frye Co of Portland, ME, and Wocher & Sons Co, Cincinnati, OH).

The Chloride of Silver Dry Cell Battery Co apparently issued at lease three trade catalogs between 1886 and 1889. The fourth edition of their catalogs indicated that the company had just moved to larger and permanent facilities and were incorporated between issuance of the third and fourth catalog editions. The fourth edition of The Chloride of Silver Dry Cell Battery Co trade catalog was issued around 1890 to 1892, and shows that the president of the company was JA Pfarre; vice president was GA Liebig; secretary was Claude Van Bidder; consulting electrician was John A Barrett; and general manager was Charles Willms (from 1890 to 1897).[2] JA Pfarre (son of successor to G Tiemann in 1868) worked for the George Tiemann Company of New York City which was one of the largest and best known surgical instrument manufacturer and medical suppliers of the time. Working in New York would mean that Pfarre was not involved in 'hands on' operations of the company, but like many company presidents today he may have set policy and direction with help of the members of the board. Pfarre may also have been a major investor in the company. Perhaps as president he brought marketing expertise to the company. GA Liebig, Jr, held a doctorate degree (PhD) in electrical engineering, and besides being an officer of the company, vice president, he was the company's principal electrician. He no doubt set policy in design and construction of the electrical items manufactured and sold by The Chloride of Silver Dry Cell Battery Co. Dr Liebig coauthored with Dr CH Rohe their book Practical Electricity in Medicine and Surgery. Philadelphia, PA, FA Davis, 1890;[3] was an assistant in electricity at Johns Hopkins University; lecturer on medical electricity at the College of Physicians and Surgeons, Baltimore; and a member of the American Institute of Electrical Engineering. Dr Liebig discussed briefly and illustrated a 50-cell Chloride of Silver Co battery pack mounted in a wooden box in his book (p 103), and the same unit was featured on the title page of the company's trade catalog for around 1890 to 1891.

Dr Claude Van Bidder in addition to being the company's secretary around 1890 was a general practitioner of medicine in Baltimore. He graduated in medicine from the University of Maryland in 1877, and maintained his office for medical practice at 9 E Read St.[4] John A Barrett was living and working in New York City while serving as consulting electrician to The Chloride of Silver Dry Cell Battery Co around 1890, yet he was the owner of the John A Barrett Battery

Company of Baltimore. Barrett's company at the time was selling the Two-Cell Faradic Battery (until ca 1897). Charles Willms was managing the daily operations of the Chloride of Silver Co in 1890, yet a few blocks away he owned and managed the Charles Willms Surgical Supply Co. Willms designed and held the patent to the Willms' rheostat that was part of The Chloride of Silver Dry Cell Battery Co's faradic batteries numbers 6, 8, 9, and 14. The Chloride of Silver Dry Cell Battery Co was the first manufacturer to depart from the common sliding metal tube for regulating current amplitude and to use a circular resistance type rheostat on the face plate of its medical electrical batteries. The Willms rheostat allowed the induction coil to be hidden underneath the face panel rather on top as most models were previously designed. In other words, the Willms' rheostat or controller replaced the sliding metal tube current regulator on most of The Chloride of Silver Dry Cell Battery Co's faradic batteries for physician use, and served to advance technology in the developmnet of medical electrical batteries. The resistance of the Willms' rheostat ranged from 0 to 10,000 ohms.

The Chloride of Silver Dry Cell Battery Co of Baltimore under went a major administrative change in 1897. Manes E Fuld (1863-1956) took over The Chloride of Silver Dry Cell Battery Co as its general manager and ran the day to day operations of the company, while at the same time being the general manager and owner of the Voltamp Electric Manufacturing Co of Baltimore. Officers of the company in 1890 appeared to be gone or disassociated with The Chloride of Silver Dry Cell Battery Co after 1897. Frank B Cahn held the title of counsel or consultant to the company.

The Chloride of Silver Dry Cell Battery Co was located at 409 North Paca Street while the Voltamp Electric Mfg Co was nearby at 408 North Pace Street, Baltimore, MD. For some reason the medical electrical apparatus of either company did not provide the street address with signature labels or plates attached to the units. Booklets accompaning each unit sold by the two companies also did not give the street addresses. Most often the address was just cited as Baltimore, MD. Manes Fuld and his Voltamp Electric Mfg Co may have absorbed or purchased The Chloride of Silver Dry Cell Battery Co in 1897 or soon afterward when he became general manager of both companies. The Chloride of Silver Dry Cell Battery Co seemed to have faded sometime around 1920, perhaps its volume of sales began to wane as early as 1911 or 1912, while the Voltamp Electric Co continued to manufacture medical electrical batteries for family or home use, and sell chloride of silver dry cells for several years after World War I. The last trade catalog of The Chloride of Silver Dry Cell Battery Co cited by Davis & Dreyfus was for 1902, and was a 63-paged general catalog of product lines.[1] The Chloride of Silver Dry Cell Battery Co supplied its electrical apparatuses only with sliver of chloride dry cells only, and when commercial (AC)

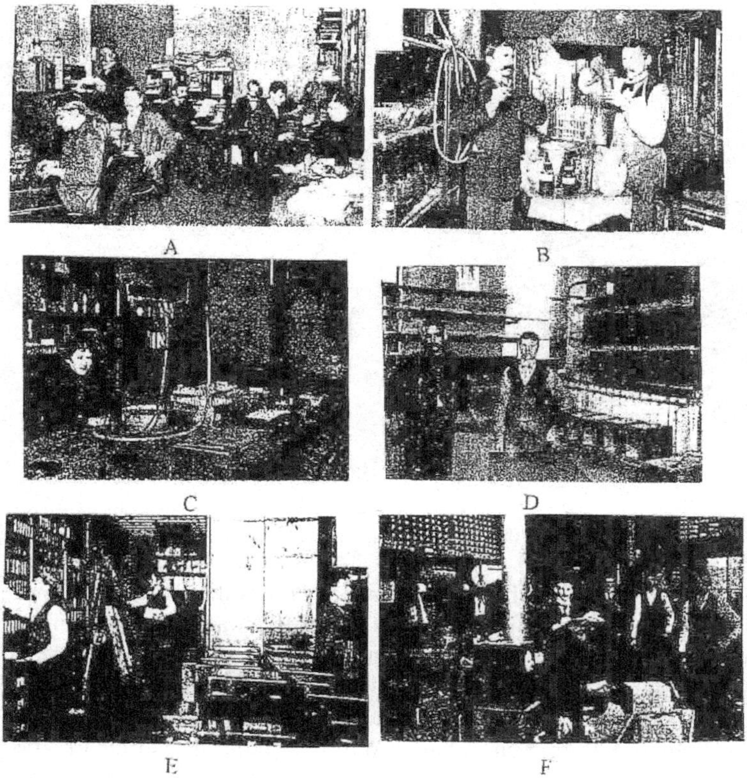

Fig C1. Factory and Offices, 1898. A. General Office, B. Chemistry Laboratory, C. Cell Room, D. Cabinet Room, E. Stock Room, and F. Shipping Room.

(alternating current) and DC (direct current) became the electricity sources or grids for powering medical electrical apparatuses the battery powered units in medicine became obsolete.

Commonalties of The Chloride of SilverDry Cell Battery Co Electrical Batteries

Features to be identified on the faradic medical electrical batteries of The Chloride of Silver Dry Cell Battery Co are: 1) labels on the inside lid of all models are black, mostly with yellow lettering; 2) some units contain a Willms' current regulator; 3) the hardware is heavy nickel plated; 4) units contain the silver of chloride cell packs; and 5) units other than portable contain hidden induction coils.

The galvanic batteries, like the faradic batteries, had signature labels on the inside of the lids, wedged and glued corners on the wooden boxes, some have the Willms rheostat and a milliammeter, the hardware is heavy nickel plated, and the units always use chloride of silver cell packs.

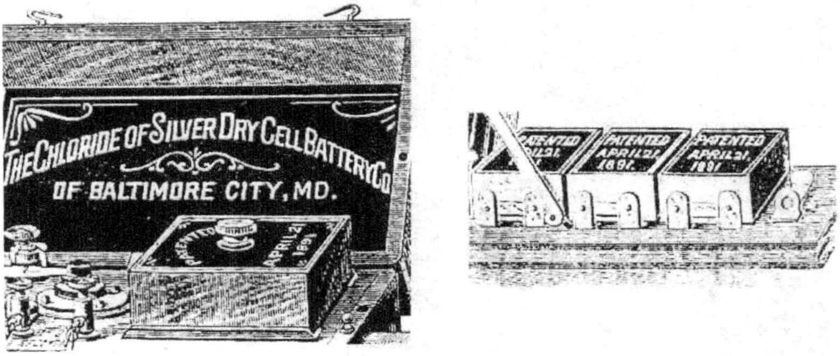

Fig C2. Chloride of Silver Battery Pack with Cells

Chloride of Silver Dry Cells

In 1860, Marie Davy of France advanced the idea that chloride of silver was a deep depolarizing agent. Soon afterward the noted English astronomer, chemist, physicist, and inventor, Warren de la Rue (1815-1889), demonstrated a constancy of electromotoforce or voltage when using chloride of silver as a crude electrical cell. Not until about 1884 when Dr John A Barrett and Charles Willms combined chloride of silver with an appropriate electrolyte did the chloride of silver dry cell become practical. De la Rue used a fine powdered form of chloride of silver in his crude cell, but Barrett and Willms solved the problem to sufficiently make the cell a useful source of galvanic current for powering medical electrical batteries.

Thus the company's name was formed and derived from the unique product that it produced around 1886; ie, the chloride of silver dry cell. This particular battery (resembles the AA battery of today) may have been the first really successful minature dry cell to bridge the gap between the inconvenient wet cell and the reliable and durable dry cell battery. The absence of liquid through the method of the hermetical sealing made the cell appealing to consumers. Each electrical apparatus (battery) of The Chloride and Silver Dry Cell Battery Co was equipped with a number of the dry cells, arranged in series (battery), and enclosed in a japanned (varnished) metallic box or pack. The boxes were secured in the apparatuses by a screw and nut.

The advantages of this unique battery were that: 1) no corrosive fluid leaked onto its outer cover, thus the cell did not destroy the clothing of its consumers, 2) no elements (metal plates) had to be removed from fluid like the wet cells, 3) it was ready for use upon wilful demand without any preparation, 4) it was constantly available for action and performed constantly when in action, thus durable without needed repairs, and 5) it was very portable, easily carried. The early batteries of chloride of silver type wore out when not in use because of their design. This type of battery was sold by the Chloride of Silver Co in 1886 and perhaps as early as 1882, and continued to be its franchise item into the early 1900s (ca 1910), and was available in the 1920s through the Voltamp Electric Mfg Co of Baltimore.

The chloride of silver dry cell battery lasted between three months to three years, depending upon its use. According to the AS Aloe catalog of 1895, the battery pack worked for 100 hours of continuous use that averaged in cost of $0.015 per hour to operate. In 1890, one cell cost $0.30 to replace. Since chloride of silver batteries do not have as much

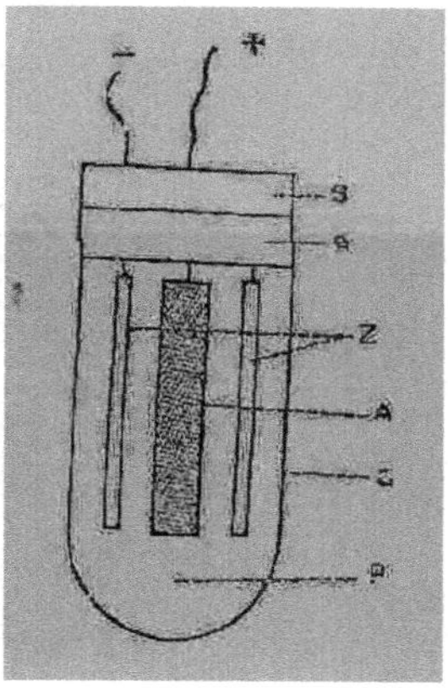

Fig C3. Cell and Its Cross Section: Connecting wires (copper wire from zinc -, silver wire from chloride of silver +); S – plaster of Paris stopper; O – resin and resin oil stopper; Z – zinc plates; A – chloride of silver plate; G – glass vessel; P – flour and sulfate of zinc paste.

electromotive force (EMF, ca 0.8 to 0.9 volt) as the carbon-zinc batteries, about one-third more cells than the standard available cells of the time were needed per application. When the first chloride of silver batteries were placed into use currents increased in amplitude for a time and then remained almost without variation until all silver chloride was converted into nonfunctional silver. The unique cell was considered expensive at the time because of its use of silver; the more silver that was used the higher the cost but the more voltage produced. Fortunately, silver could be recycled so dead cells could be traded with the purchase of new cells that kept the price down on trade-ins for new cells. The Chloride of Silver Co's chloride of silver dry cell batteries were unique at the time. Each cell's size varied in length according to demand (2 to 3 inches), measured 0.75 inch in diameter, weighed 1.5 ounces, and produced about 1 volt (50-cell battery is ~ 45 volts). Each battery consisted of four to six external dry cells that were patented in the United States from 1886 to 1892 and in England from 1895 to 1900. The cells did not contain any liquids or acids, and could be turned or stored in any direction without loss of performance. An average sized battery (with multiple cells) had a working life of 200 to 700 hours and cost $15.00 over its lifetime. The Chloride of Silver Dry Cell Battery Co stated that this duration amounted to more than two years with usual office use of a medical electrical apparatus.

The cells for the faradic batteries were generally grouped in a series of four and constituted a pack or case. Each cell was attached by a contact screw to a replaceable individual cell on the plate could be easily removed and replaced when needed. Each wooden plate matching that of

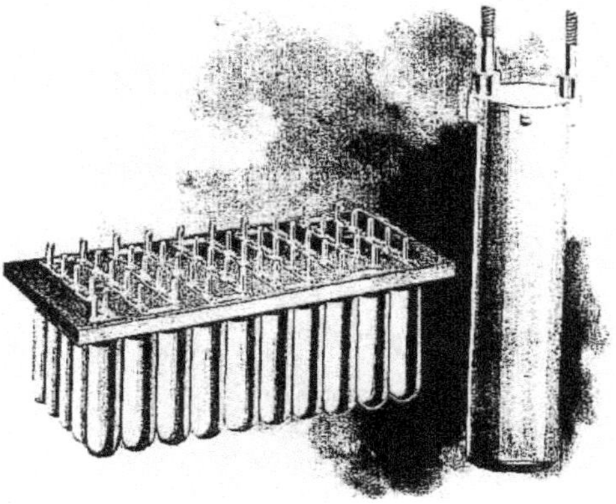

Fig C4. Chloride of Silver Cells used in Faradic Apparatus

the face plate of a given unit. The cell group or a pack was rectangular and each cell inside of a pack was cylindrical and oval in shape (pack size was about 2.75 x 1.63 x 0.88 inches).

The cells for the galvanic batteries were cylindrical in shape (2.75 x 0.75 inches) and weighing 1.5 ounces each. The chloride of silver dry cells for the galvanic apparatuses were replaced individually or the entire number could be replaced simultaneously.

The Chloride of Silver Dry Cell Battery Co seems to have been the first company in the United States to have marketed the cell. The Chloride of Silver Dry Cell Battery Co was, however, not the only company to market the cell. The McIntosh Battery & Optical Co of Chicago had its version of the chloride of silver dry cell. The eighteenth edition of the McIntosh Electro-Therapeutic Catalogue (1897, page 4) stated "An experience of many years in the manufacture and use of the chloride of silver cells, has convinced us of their entire unreliability; chemical action with the cells even when they are suppose to be at rest, continues uninterruptedly, and at the most critical moment when the

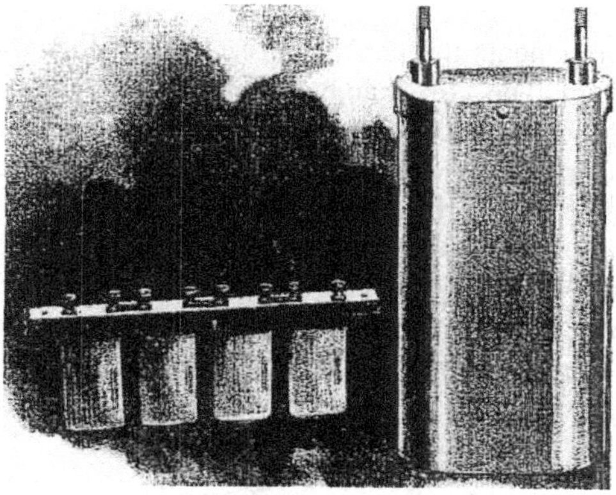

Fig C5. Chloride of Silver Dry Cells for Galvanic Apparatus

operator is most desirous of expected service, the cells are discovered to be exhausted and the battery 'dead'." McIntosh Battery & Optical Co of Chicago cornered a large proportion of the market for medical electrical batteries so therefore had considerable influence. Thus, if McIntosh was dissatisfied with the chloride of silver dry cell and promoted the MESCO (Manhattan Electrical Supply Co) dry cell the company's position may have had an affect on the dry cell battery market. The year 1896 or 1897 was when the reliable standard sized dry cell (6.25 x 2.5 inches) was marketed (eg, MESCO, Burnley cells; Eveready came later).

The Chloride of Silver Dry Cell Battery Co was mostly a medical firm that manufactured and sold to physicians from 1886 to at least 1910. The last faradic type of the medical electrical battery produced by The Chloride of Silver Dry Cell Battery Co held a patent date of 1910. The electrical batteries (apparatuses) manufactured by The Chloride of Silver Dry Cell Battery Co were considered high quality units and were well received by physicians that used them. By 1910, however, most manufacturers of medical electrical apparatuses were converting their units to alternating current power (grid) or direct current source but The Chloride of Silver Dry Cell Battery Co did not convert. Also, The Chloride of Silver Dry Cell Battery Co emphasized only the dry cell battery of its innovation and in time these factors rendered it obsolete which no doubt ended the marketability of The Chloride of Silver Dry Cell Battery Co's medical electrical batteries.

Faradic Batteries

Double Coil Faradic Battery. The unit of Fig C6 is a portable faradic battery designed for use by physicians, and is similar in design to the No.7 unit except it has induction coils built of the DuBois-Reymond sledge inductorium principle, and two cells packs. The unit is housed in a small hardwood box; when upright the hinged lid opens from the top to the electrical components that are comprised of: a DuBois-Reymond or sledge inductorium type coil that has interchangeable fine and course windings of wire for the secondary coil, while the primary coil is a wire horseshoe; two hermetically sealed chloride of silver dry cells each in a wooden pack (patented 13 December 1887); an adjustable screw spring lever, hammer vibrator type of interrupter that sets the current pulse frequencies; and connecting posts are attached to the coil. All metal are nickel plated. A manually interrupting handle electrode is furnished. The lid of the box has a self lock on front, and a metal carrying handle on top of the lid. This particular unit dates before or from 1890 to 1895, but was

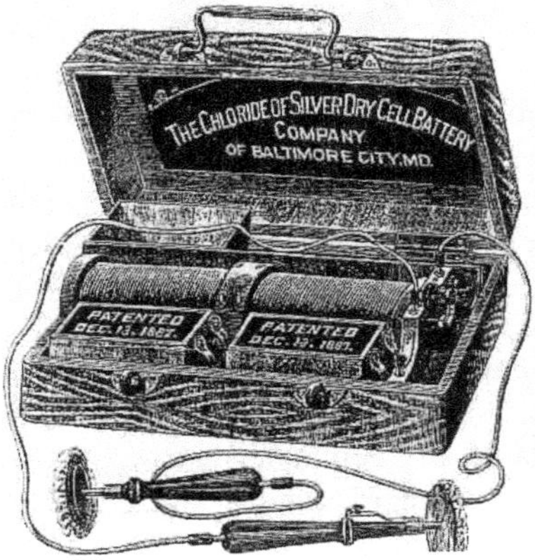

Fig C6. No. 5 Double Coil Faradic Battery

closed out between 1895 and 1898. The No.5 unit sold for $20.00 from 1890 to 1895. The two chloride of silver cell packs could be replaced for $1.50 in 1890 and 1895. The cells were claimed by The Chloride of Silver Dry Cell Battery Co to operate continuously for 100 hours at a cost of $0.015 per hour.

The Lord Baltimore Family Battery or No.7A. This unit was a quality product designed for home and travel use. The unit is small and portable because of its size (4 x 5 x 2 inches) and purpose, and could be carried around easily by a metal carrying handle.

The unit provides primary, secondary, and combined currents. The faradic coil uses the DuBois-Reymond principle where the secondary coil slides over the wound primary coil to control current amplitudes. This unit has an adjustable screw spring lever, hammer type of interrupter that vibrates to set the pulse frequencies. A wooden cell pack that contained four chloride of silver dry cells powered the unit. No conventional face plate is used. All components are mounted to a bottom panel of the inside of the box (circuitry is underneath). The wires connecting the patient to the apparatus leave two posts from the right end

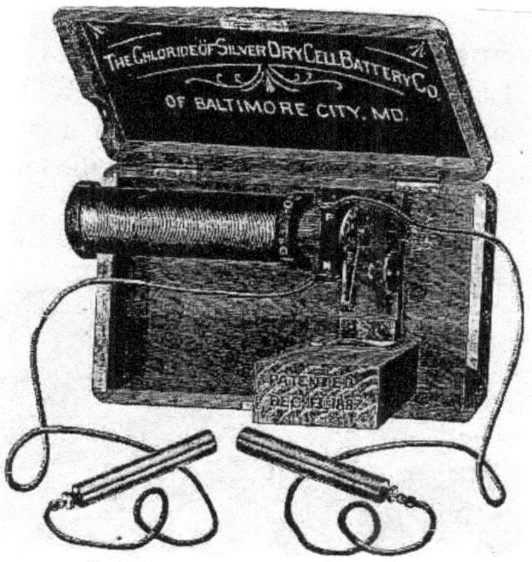

Fig C7. No. 7A, The Lord Baltimore Family Battery

cap of the coil. This particular unit is one of only two faradic medical electrical batteries that The Chloride of Silver Dry Cell Battery Co designed for home use and its cell pack bears the patent date of 13 Dec 1887. Accessories were placed between electrical components in the box. The unit was listed for sale at $6.50 in the 1892 through 1902 catalogs of The Chloride of Silver Dry Cell Battery Co.

Physicians' Pocket Faradic Battery No.7. One of the faradic batteries of The Chloride of Silver Dry Cell Battery Co was a compact, durable, easy to operate, and a small portable unit (Fig C8) much like the popular device designed and sold by Gaiffe of France. A similar portable unit was also sold by Montgomery Ward & Co (the 1894-1895 catalog), and Sears, Roebuck and Co (1897 catalog). This particular portable battery was encased in a cherry box (8.75 x 4.5 x 2.25 inches) with a hinged lid that has two silver plated sliding clasp locks on the front part of the lid. Inside of the lid are directions, cautions, chloride of silver dry cell information and the patent dates 23 Feb 1886 through 26 July 1892, "The Chloride of Silver Dry Cell Battery Co, of Balt City, MD, sole mfg–galvanic, faradic, and combin batts, mil-am-meters, electrodes." The unit does not have the conventional face plate or panel as electrical components are mounted to the inside bottom of the box that matches the wood of the box, and the dry cells are enclosed in a separate pack (4 cells). The battery pack pictured above from the 1893 AS Aloe catalog shows a patent date of 21 April 1891, and is a finished and polished outer wooden box secured by a single nickel plated screw. The battery pack is mounted to the right and held by a brass screw. The induction coil (4.25 x 1.25 inches) on the left is a sledge inductorium type, after the DuBois-Reymond principle, where the secondary coil slides over the primary wound coil to control current amplitude. The induction coil delivers primary, secondary, and combined currents. An adjustable screw spring lever, hammer interrupter or rheotome on the right of the coil controls the pulse frequency. The connecting cords insert into a "Fone Plug-EZ" that also inserts into a single connector pole with a monurial type plug. Accessories are kept in another compartment on the left side of the case.

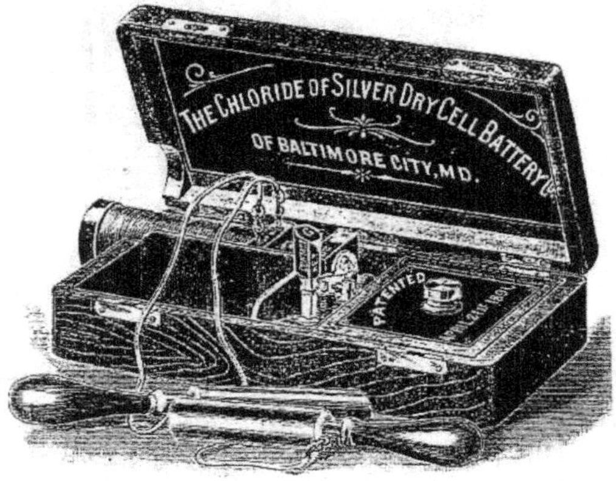

Fig C8. Physician's Pocket Faradic Battery No. 7[5]

The unit in Fig C8 above dates before or from 1890 through 1902 or later. This unit is small and portable so that it could be transported easily in a doctor's bag. The battery contained in the wooden case held four chloride of silver dry cells, and could produce slightly less than four volts. The exhausted battery would be replaced by the company when returned for a smaller price than when new. Unlike most faradic apparatuses with connecting posts from the face plate to the patient, this unit connects the patient by wires directly from two metal posts on the inside of one end cap of the coil. This portable unit sold for $10.00 in 1892 through 1902.

Split Top Faradic Battery. This model (Fig C9) was described in the catalog of 1892 only. The unit was contained in an upright hardwooden box (5 x 5 x 6 inches). The lid opens and splits into two halves. One half has the metal carrying handle, while the other half locks the lids when closed. This is perhaps the only American medical electrical battery that opens in this manner. The electrical components consist of: a powerful induction coil that provides a constant uniform current of primary, secondary, or combined currents; a spring lever, hammer vibrator type interrupter; and a lever control that turns the current On and Off. One section of the lid shuts off current when closed to protect the four-cell pack. The face plate is only 2.5 x 5 inches; the open area of the box is for accessories; and the cell pack is underneath the coil with the circuitry. This unit sold for $15.00 in 1892.

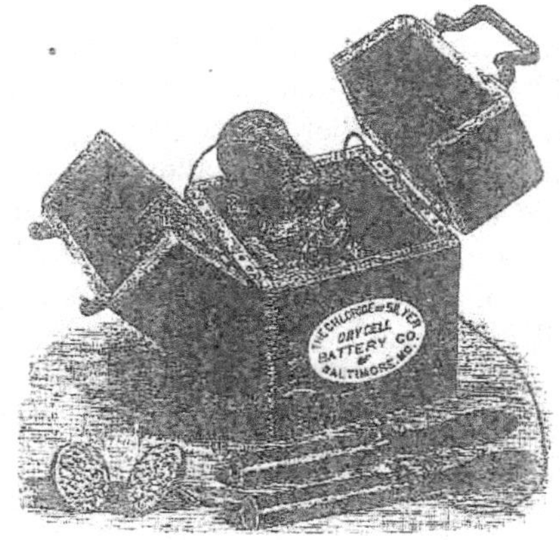

Fig C9. No. 6 Split Top Faradic Battery[2]

Upright Faradic Battery. The No. 6 Split Top Faradic Battery of 1892 was redesigned and in 1895 was presented as the No. 6A "Upright" Faradic Battery. The battery was designed for use by physicians who wanted an apparatus to take to the patient on home visits.

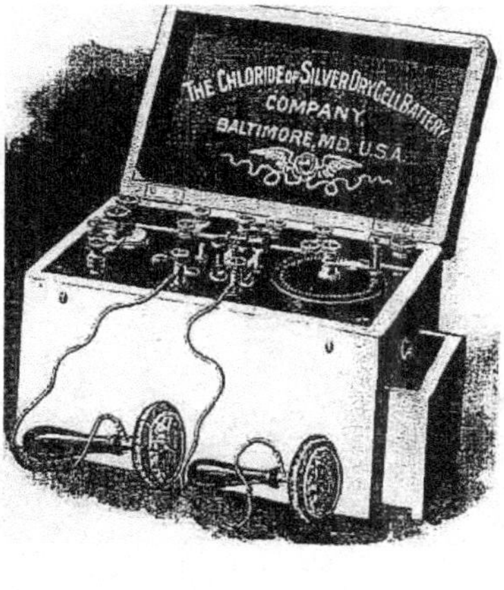

Fig C10. "Upright" Faradic Battery No. 6A

The mahogany box is upright as were most conventional electrical apparatuses of that time. The wooden box measures 7.5 x 7 x 5 inches, and has a metal carrying handle on top, and two lever hook eye latches on front to secure the lid. A drawer slides in and out from the bottom right side of the box. The four-inch secondary coil slides over the primary coil through the right side of the box (sledge inductorium), and is located underneath the face plate that is flush with the opened lower section of the box. The coils provide primary, secondary, and combined currents. The coils (4 inches in length) are located underneath the face plate. The face plate contains the four-cell pack (patented 21 April 1891);

four adjustable screw connecting posts that supply the primary, secondary, and combined currents; and an adjustable screw spring lever vibrating interrupter that is parallel to the face plate and indirectly contacts the coil. A metal key is inserted to allow the circuit to be closed and opened. All metal are nickel plated, and a metal disc secures the drawer. The unit sold for $15.00 in the 1893 AS Aloe trade catalog.[5] Unit 6A was the first model of this company's faradic battery product line to have its induction coil concealed.

The No.6 Upright Faradic Battery of 1898 (Fig C11) is a redesign of the No.6A of 1895. The No.6 of 1898 was designed after the No.8 that was very successful and well received by physicians. The redesign was aimed for the family or the consumer for home use so is less powerful than the No. 8 for physicians. The faradic battery delivers primary, secondary, and combined currents. The cell packs are underneath the face plate and concealed from view at the rear of the top panel. This unit has the Willms current regulator; a contact key for turning current On/Off and selects the current type; and the parallel interrupter on the face plate. The electrical components are housed in an up right mahogany box (9.38 x 5.88 x 5 inches) with a hinged lid that is

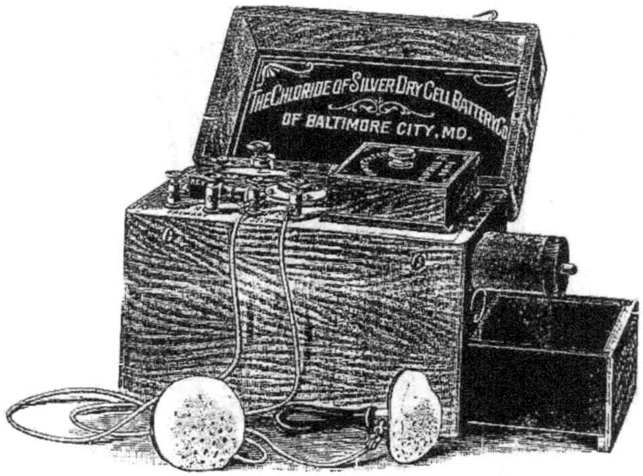

Fig C11. "Upright" Faradic Battery No. 6

secured by two hook latches on front, and weighing 6.75 pounds. A sliding drawer for accessories is located on the bottom right side of the box. In 1898, this unit sold for $15.00.[2] This unit was continued with the same design and components for $15.00 in 1902. The box size of 1902 differed very slightly from that of 1898 (9.25 x 5.75 x 7 inches).

Physicians' Faradic Battery No.8. This particular faradic battery is only the second portable unit of this company to have the coil or coils located underneath the face plate. Portable medical electrical batteries No.6 and 7 by Chloride of Silver Dry Cell Battery Co were the customary designs where the coil or coils were exposed to view so that

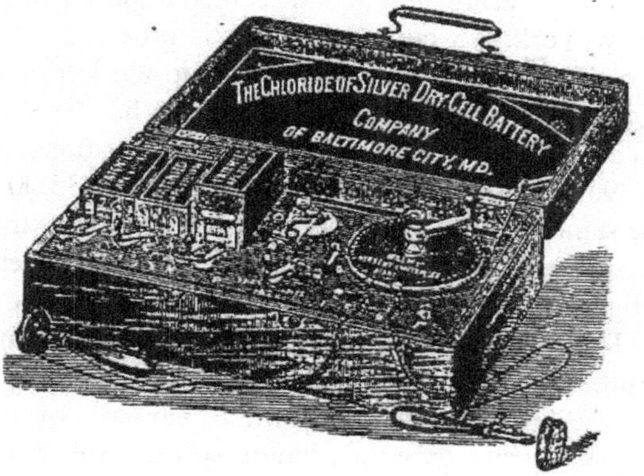

Fig C12. Chloride of Silver Physicians' Faradic Battery No. 8

the DuBois-Reymond principle (1849) could be incorporated. The state-of-the-art design of medical electrical faradic batteries in the 1880s and 1890s used the DuBois-Reymond principle where the secondary coil could slide over the primary coil to finely control current amplitude. The No. 8 model used the Willms' current controller that was considered so fine or precise that this design was used for electrodiagnosis and physiological research. The Willms current controller was first used on this model in perhaps 1889, and thought to be infinitely superior to the older customary designs of controlling current amplitude. The Willms current controller used graphite of different sizes to alter resistance to passing current, thus changing the amplitude. This new method of using a lever to move a metal pointer over the graphite allowed for the finest increments of current that improved patient comfort as well as laboratory and diagnostic work. Current controllers, like that of Willms design, soon replaced the sledge inductorim design in the United States in the 1890s. The No.8 battery was housed in a polished mahogany box (15.25 x 9.5 x 6 inches) with a metal carrying handle on top of the hinged lid. The lid had a self lock device on the front of the box to secure the lid. This unit used three battery packs for power that were mounted to the face plate along with the Willms controller, horizontal, parallel spring type vibrating interrupter, cell selector switches, lever On/Off control, and four metal connecting posts.

The No.8 model has a primary and four secondary coils with switches for controlling each. The design allows combining the primary coil with each secondary coil to provide nine different currents. (Note: The primary and secondary coils provide different faradic waves, but all others have no difference on physiological effects. The tapping of the coil windings with different lengths and diameters of wire to deliver currents of slight variations seemed to be a fad between 1875 and 1890. The idea is an engineering delight and seemed to have originated by Dr J Kidder of New York.). A current reverser is provided by the switch in front of the right cell pack; the ivory button to the left of the connector posts is the manual current breaker. This model has three cell packs for power that can be used individually or in combinations. The unit cost $35.00 in 1893, $30.00 in 1895 but increased to $35.00 in 1898 and remained the same for 1902. The model of 1898 has an extra high tension (voltage) secondary coil wound by No.36 wire 5000 feet long that is capable of lighting an eight-inch Geissler tube. This unit also has two interrupters. The slow or pendulum interrupter works by withdrawing the vibrator spring away from the magnet; the stroke of the pendulum is controlled by a lever at the rear of the vibrator spring. The rapid interrupter works by swinging the vibrator spring away from the operator so that the hammer rests over the magnet, and the spring is under the adjustable screw (platinum) point mounted on the post. The size of the wooden boxes change with the year; ie, 1895 (15.25 x 9.5 x 6 inches); 1898 (14.13 x 10 x 8.25 inches); and in 1902 (13.13 x 9.25 x 7.75 inches).

No.9 Faradic Battery. This unit by the Chloride of Silver Dry Cell Battery Co (Fig C13) is encased in a cherry box (11.75 x 7.5 x 7 inches) with the inside lid (double hinged) having a signature label giving all of its patents ranging from 26 July 1892 to 31 May 1910, and a trade mark registered 29 January 1907. The right side of the case has a drawer (5.13 x 3.25 x 8 inches) containing directions and accessories for its operation. A circular brass latch secures the drawer.

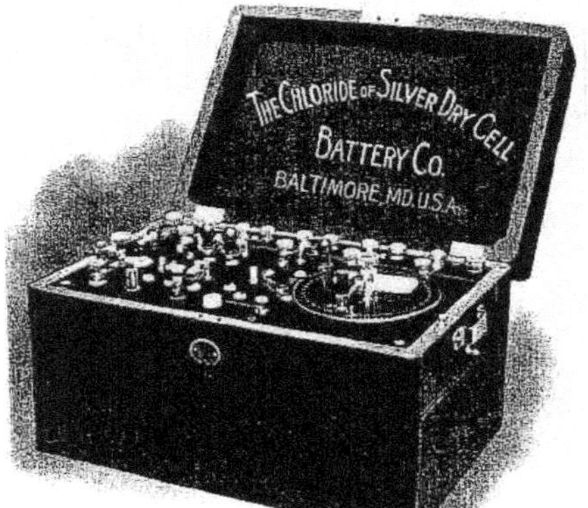

Fig C13. No. 9 Faradic Battery

The face panel is hard rubber with all metal heavy nickel plated, two adjustable screw poles that connect with the patient, a pole or current changer (P), a lever control with four buttons (0-3) for secondary coil control, two lever controls (A, B) with three buttons (In, 0, Out), and a lever control with four buttons (5 positions; Off, Cell 1 + 3, Cell 3, Cell 4, D) to switch to the number of batteries. The No. 9 Faradic Battery has a high tension (voltage) secondary coil that is wound and tapped to provide four coils (a primary and three secondary coils). The secondary coil is wound by No.22, No.32 and by No.36 wire. The arrangement of the coils provides seven different currents, and the primary and secondary coils can be used independently of each other or in combination. The rear of the face panel is separated by a wood strip to off set the binding posts to the batteries. Between the two connecting poles in the front part of the panel is a small circular ivory button to manually make and break the current. The four-inch circular black disc on the right of the face panel is the Willms rheostat that he invented around 1894. The Willms rheostat or current controller of this No.9 model has extra contact points. This rheostat used the principle of a large number of contact points underneath to vary resistance for controlling the current amplitude. The lever control marked with "D" near the rear controls the cells; center button brings cells 1, 2, and 3 into the circuit, left button brings cells 1 and 2 into the circuit, and when positioned to the right all cells 1 to 4 are in the circuit. Four chloride of silver dry cells are attached underneath the face plate. This model was probably made from 1900 to 1920. In 1900, it sold for $25.00, and weighed nine pounds. The No.14 Faradic Battery was an updated version of No.9, but did not offer all features of the No.9 (eg, coil of as high voltage).

The Chloride of Silver Dry Cell Battery Co offered four faradic coil type medical electrical batteries for physician use; numbers 6, 8, 9, and 14 in 1910 and perhaps later. The machines generally varied by the number of cells powering a particular unit, the tension (voltage) delivered, and the varied pulse frequency rates per apparatus.

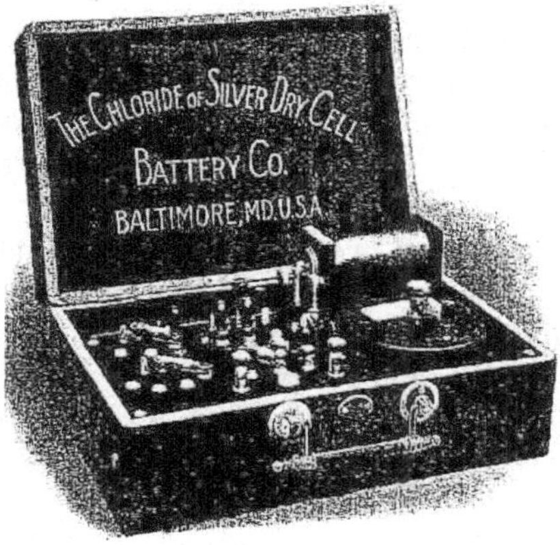

Fig C13A. "Satchel" Faradic Battery No. 4

"Satchel" Faradic Battery No.4. In 1902, The Chloride of Silver Dry Cell Battery Co produced this portable unit for physicians who went to the bedside of their patients. The No.4 unit, operationally, is the same as the company's No.9, but No.4 has the coil in view mounted on the face plate rather than hidden beneath it as in the No.9. The No.4 was packaged in a polished mahogany case (11.75 x 8 x 5.38 inches), hinged top, and with a swivel metal carrying handle and a lock on the front. The unit weighs 7.25 pounds, and in 1902 it cost $25.00.[2]

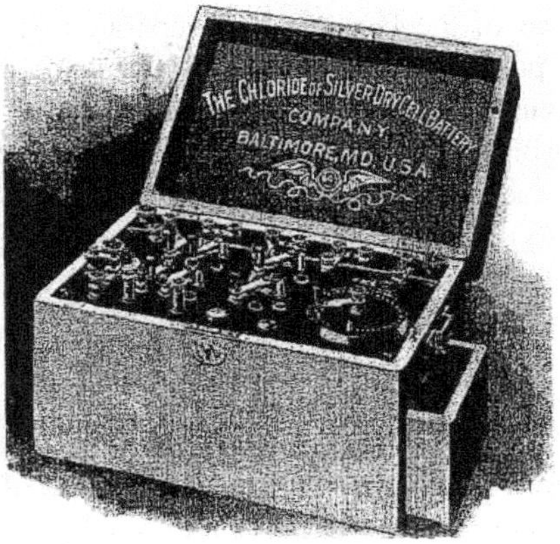

Fig C14. Faradic Battery No.14[2]

Faradic Battery No.14. The Chloride of Silver Dry Cell Battery Co added the No.14 to its product line between 1895 and 1898, and designed it for physician use. The Chloride of Silver Dry Cell Battery Co considered this as a deluxe unit. Underneath the hard rubber face plate was mounted four chloride of silver dry cell packs that could be replaced easily. Also hidden are three induction coils (a primary coil wound with No.26 wire, the secondary coil to serve as two coils; wound with No.22 and 32 wire, respectively). The three coils can be used independently or in combinations. The face plate contains: a Willms current controller; a cell selector switch to control one to four cell packs; a current reverser; and a manually operated contact or circuit breaker. A conventional interrupter, and two adjustable screw, connecting posts are mounted parallel on the face plate. The rear of the face plate contains screws for securing the battery packs and for contacts between cells and circuitry. The unit is housed in an upright mahogany box (10.75 x 7.5 x 7 inches) with a hinged lid, and sliding drawer at the bottom of the right side of the box. The lid is secured in front by a lock and key, and is carried by a leather strap mounted on each side of the box. The unit weighs about 8.5 pounds and cost $20.00 from 1898 through 1902.

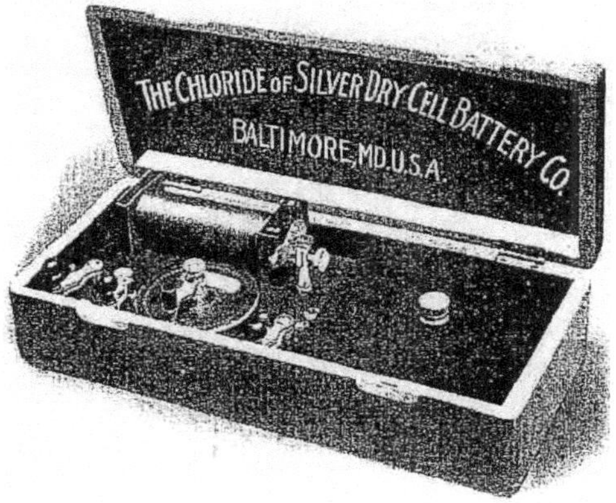

Fig C15. Faradic Battery No. 20

Faradic Battery No.20. This portable faradic battery was introduced in 1902. The unit was designed after the suggestion of a leading electrotherapist of the time, and has the advantage over the previous The Chloride of Silver Dry Cell Battery Co's pocket models by doubling the available current amplitude. The No.20 battery has a Willms current controller; a conventional induction coil rather than a sledge inductorium; a conventional spring lever, hammer vibrating interrupter; two metal buttons for connecting with the subject; and three control levers. The metal is nickel plated. The unit is contained in a wooden box (11 x 5.13 x 3.13 inches) that has a hinged lid with two self locks on front, and a battery pack of four chloride of silver dry cells. The unit weighs four pounds and cost $18.00 in 1902.[2]

Galvanic Batteries

Chloride of Silver Dry Cell Battery Co also manufactured galvanic electrical batteries in addition to faradic batteries. The company manufactured basically two galvanic batteries between 1892 and 1895. One small galvanic battery was designed for family or home use in treating small growths (warts, moles) and superfluous hair by electrolysis. Galvanic currents for family use were of low amplitude while using different numbers of cells (6, 12, or 16 cells). The second galvanic battery was designed for physicians, and it offered models with 24, 32, 50, 60, and 84 cells in 1892 to 1895, but also 100 cells in the 1898 to 1902 models. These galvanic batteries did not change much in design between 1892 and 1902. The costs of these units also remained constant over those 10 years.

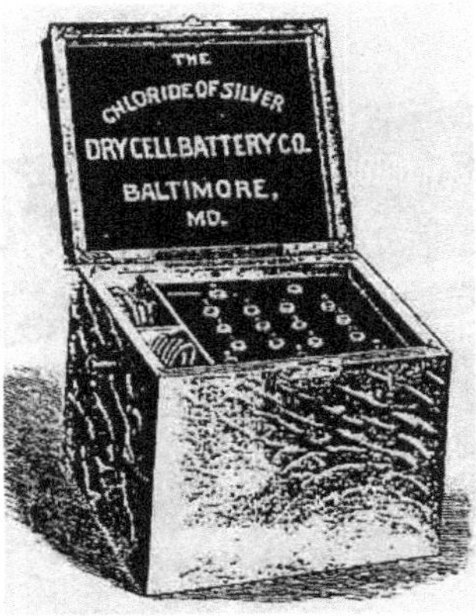

Fig C16. No. 3 Family Galvanic Battery

No.3 Family Galvanic Battery. This series of small galvanic batteries were contained in walnut boxes varying in size over the years, each having a hinged lid with self lock on the front, and carried by a leather strap mounted on each side of the box. The current amplitude was controlled by selecting the appropriate metal button for connecting with the subject, without a current reverser. The face plate is of hard rubber, covering most of the box area but leaving an open area on the left side for accessories. The chloride of silver cell packs were located underneath the face plate. The cells averaged 120 hours of use when current was applied over about 3000 ohms of body resistance. The estimated cost of operating this battery was $0.0025 per hour. The costs for the battery remained constant between 1892 and 1902; 6 cells cost $10.00; 12 cells cost $15.00; and the cost for 16 cells was $20.00. The box size in 1892 and 1895 were: 6 cells (4.5 x 4.5 x 5 inches), 12 cells (5.5 x 5.5 x 5 inches), and 16 cells (5.5 x 5.5 x 5 inches). The box size and weight for 1898 were: 6 cells (4.38 x 4.5 x 5.5 inches and 2.25 pounds), 12 cells (5.75 x 5.5 x 5.5 inches and 3.5 pounds), and 16 cells (6.63 x 5.63 x 5.5 inches and 4 pounds). The box size and weight for 1902 were: 6 cells (4.5 x 4.5 x 5.5 inches and 2.25 pounds), 12 cells (5.5 x 5.5 x 5.5 inches and 3.5 pounds), and 16 cells (6.63 x 5.5 x 5.5 inches and 4 pounds). Electrode needles used for the removal of superfluous hair were 32 gauged steel or iridio-platinum.

No.1 Galvanic Battery. Designed for physician use this galvanic battery came with a variety of cells (24, 32, 50, 60, and 84 in 1892 to 1895 then increased to 100 cells in 1898 to 1902). The costs remained rather stable over the 10-year period of time. The 24-cell unit cost $38.00 in 1892 to 1895, but decreased to $27.00 in 1898 to 1902. Likewise, the other sizes also changed in cost (1892 to 1895, 32 cells were $45.00; 50 cells were $65.00; 60 cells were $75.00; and 84 cells were \$95.00), and (1898 to 1902, 32 cells were \$35.00; 50 cells were \$50.00; 60 cells were \$60.00; 84 cells were \$82.00; and 100 cells were

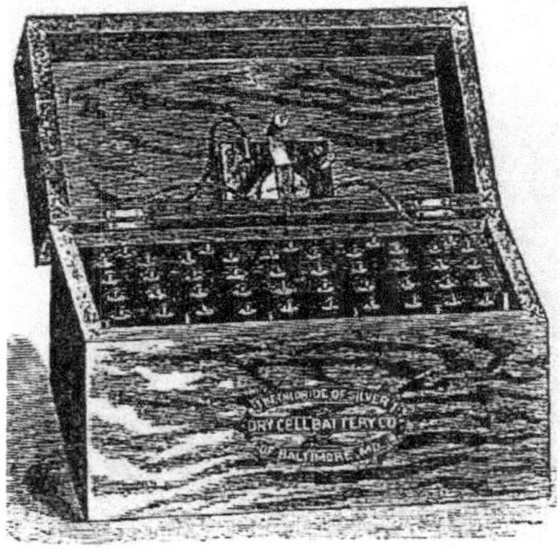

Fig C17. No.1 Galvanic Battery[2]

\$95.00). The units were housed in light (cherry), boxes (10 x 6 x 7 inches) in 1892, but changed in 1898 to mahogany and varied in sizes in 1898 and 1902. In 1898, the box sizes were: 24 and 32 cells (10.33 x 5.75 x 7.25 inches and 8 and 8.75 pounds, respectively); 50 cells (11.33 x 6.25 x 7.25 inches and 12 pounds); 60 cells (13 x 6.25 x 7.38 inches and 14 pounds); and 84 and 100 cells (11.25 x 11.25 x 7.5 inches and 12.5 and 19.5 pounds, respectively). The face plate was of hard rubber and contained a metal button for each number of cells it contained. The box lid was hinged and contained a small hard rubber base for a current reverser and switch for On/Off. The face plate contained two connecting posts while underneath the unit has a water rheostat, and tray for accessories. This unit was available in 1890.

Constant Current Galvanic Battery No.10. This galvanic battery (Fig C18) for physicians was introduced in 1898 and was still available in 1902 and perhaps later. The chloride of silver dry cells are arranged in series, and attached to an insulated supporting panel. The hard rubber face plate covers the tops of cells. The 25-cell unit is arranged for the operator to select cells in groups of five; the 35-cell unit is selected in groups of seven; and in the 50-cell unit the cells are selected in groups of 10. The face plate contains the binding posts, current reverser, cell selector, and the Willms current controller. The units are housed in mahogany upright boxes with a front lock, hinged lid, a drawer for accessories located on the bottom of the right side of the box. All of the constant current galvanic batteries of 1898 had the same box size (12 x 7.25 x 11.25 inches), and all of those of 1902 also had the same size box but differed slightly from those of 1898 by being 0.25 inches higher. The batteries each remained the same weight and cost from 1898 through 1902. The 25-cell unit weighed 13.5 pounds and cost $43.00; the 35-cell unit weighed 14.5 pounds and cost $52.00, and the 50

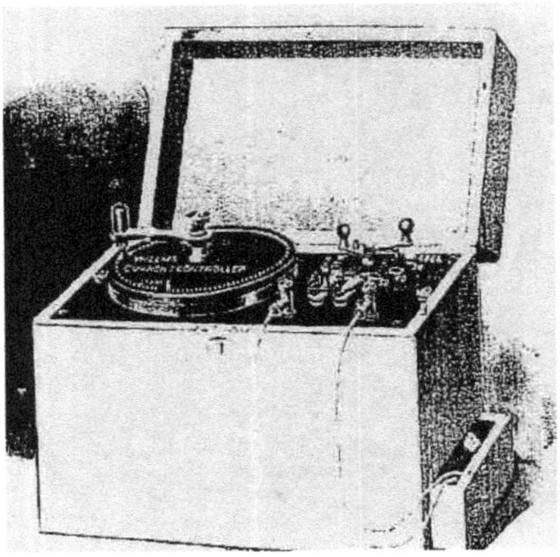

Fig C18. Constant Current Galvanic Battery No.10[2]

cells unit weighed 16 pounds and cost $65.00 in 1898 to 1902. The chloride of silver dry cell changed in design between 1898 and 1902.

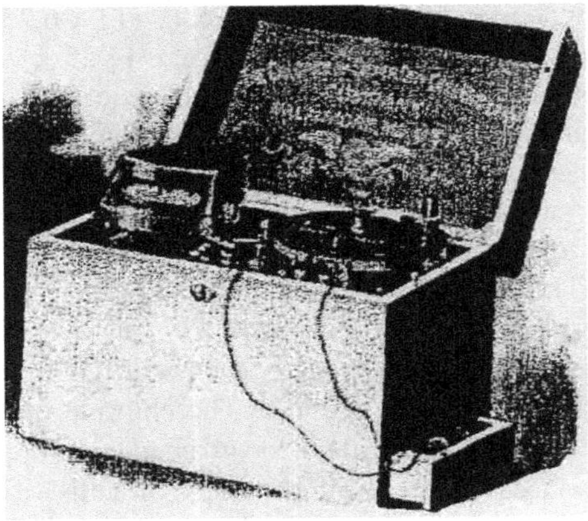

Fig C19. Constant Current Galvanic Battery No.11

Constant Current Galvanic Battery No.11. The No.11 galvanic current battery of The Chloride of Silver Dry Cell Battery Co was designed for physician use in the treatment of sensitive cases where knowledge of the amount of current was essential. For this reason the unit has a milliammeter on the face plate and built into the electrical circuit. (Note: Meters for measuring current quantities were perfected enough by 1898 to become standard equipment on deluxe models.) The unit also has a Willms current controller, a current reverser, a cell selector for 25, 35, or 50 dry cells, and two connecting posts. The electrical components are contained in an upright polished mahogany box with a hinged lid that locks in front, and has a sliding drawer on the bottom right side of the box for accessories. The box sizes and the weight of the unit differed slightly between 1898 and 1902. The 25-cell unit was 13.13 x 8.75 x 11.25 inches, 16.75 pounds and $63.00 in 1898, but was 13 x 8.5 x 11.25 inches, 17 pounds and $63.00 in 1902. The 35-cell unit was the same size as the 25 and 50 cells units but weighed 18 pounds and sold for $72.00 in 1898; in 1902 the price and weight were the same, but the box was the same as the 25 and 50 cells apparatus of 1902. The 50-cell unit was 19.5 pounds and priced at $85.00 in 1989 through 1902.

An earlier version of the No.11 galvanic battery varied only from the wooden box and the number of cells. The 1894 version of the No.11 battery used 50 chloride of silver dry cells to give it an electromotive force of just less than 50 volts. The apparatus was cased

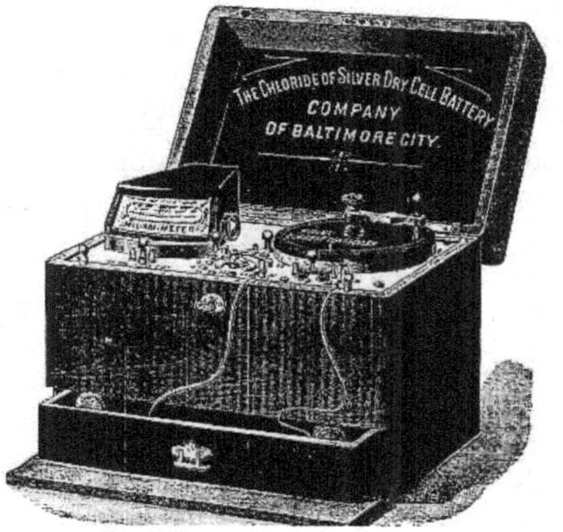

Fig C19A. Constant Current Galvanic Battery No.11 (1894)[6]

in a mahogany box (10 x 7 x 6 inches) and the complete unit weighed 11 pounds. This version had the drawer for accessories open from the front, and a metal carrying handle on top. This unit is shown in Fig C19A.

The galvanic batteries offered units of 25, 35, or 50 cells capacity. Options also included each unit with a Willms dry current controller, but with or without a "milammeter." The galvanic battery in Fig C19A represents a 50 cells unit with both a "milammeter" and a Willms' dry current controller. Both components are placed permanently. The unit has a black hard rubber face plate that holds the meter, controller, binding posts, selector switch, and On/Off switch. The wooden case is hinged at the top and locked in front with a key. A sliding drawer is located at the bottom front and holds the accessories.

In 1893, Charles Truax & Greene Co of Chicago retailed the galvanic unit with the Willms' dry current controller for $45.00 (25 cells), $57.00 (35 cells), and $69.00 (50 cells). With both the Willms'controller and the "milammeter" the units sold for $65.00 (25 cells), $82.00 (35 cells), and $95.00 (50 cells). This galvanic unit combined with the faradic components of No.8 Faradic Battery served as a combined battery and was also available in 1893.

Constant Current Galvanic Battery. This model of Fig C20 was introduced in 1898 and continued through at least to 1902. The model varied with 25, 35, and 50 cells. Unlike the galvanic battery models 10 and 11 this unit has an automatic rheotome (6 to 900 pulses per minute) in additional to the customary Willms current controller, a current reverser, a cell selector, and two connecting posts. The unit is enclosed in an upright polished mahogany box with a hinged lid that locks in front. A sliding drawer is located at the bottom right side of the box. This battery is carried by a leather strap that is mounted on each side of the box. All No.15 units of 1898 were contained in a box (13.13 x 8.75 x 11.25 inches), while those built in 1902 were in a different sized case than that of 1898 (13 x 8.75 x 11.25 inches). The 25-cell unit weighed 16.25 pounds and sold for $53.00 in 1898 to 1902. The 35-cell unit weighed 17.5 pounds and sold for $62.00 in 1898 through 1902. The 50-cell unit

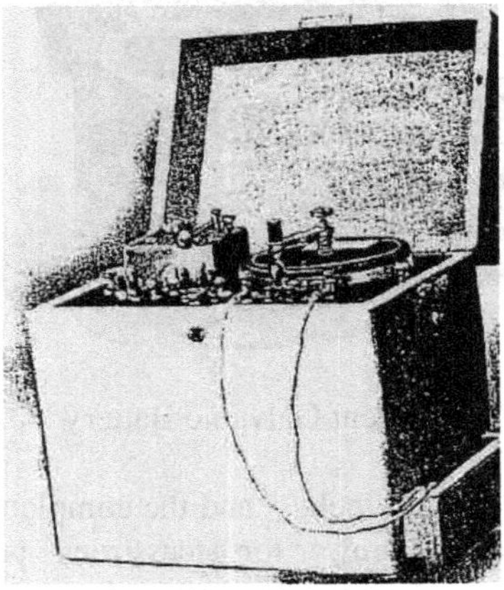

Fig C20. Constant Current GalvanicBattery No.15

sold for $75.00 in 1898 to 1902, but weighed 19 pounds in 1898 and 18.75 pounds in 1902.[2]

Constant Current Galvanic Battery No.16. The No.16 unit differed from the components of No.11 and No.15 by having both an automatic rheotome and a milliammeter in addition to the customary current reverser, cell selector, Willms current controller, and two connecting posts. This was the first model that offered so many updated electrical components to the physician. All units came in a mahogany

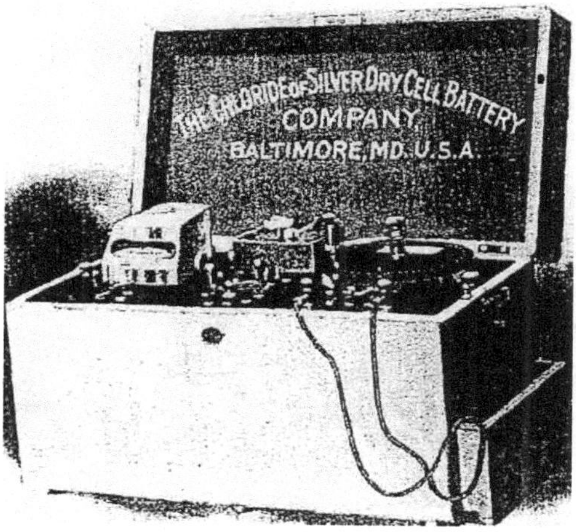

Fig C21. Constant Current Galvanic Battery No.16

upright box with a hinged lid that locks in front, a hard rubber face plate, and a sliding drawer at the bottom right side of the box for accessories. Each unit was carried by a leather strap mounted on each side of the box. This model was offered with 25 cells ($73.00, 20.25 pounds in 1898 and 20.5 pounds in 1902), 35 cells ($82.00, 21.5 pounds), and 50 cells ($95.00, 23 pounds) in 1898 to 1902. The box sizes were all the same for 1898, but slightly different for 1902 for all units. In 1898, the box size was 18 x 9.5 x 10.38 inches, and in 1902 it was 18 x 9.5 x 10.5 inches.[2]

Combination Faradic and Galvanic Batteries

Combination Battery No.2..This combination battery was available in 1895. These units (Fig C22) were constructed for 24, 32, and 50 cells, and varied in prices of $47.00, $55.00, and $70.00, respectively. The faradic electrical system of the battery was powered independently with three battery packs (12 cells) that could be used singularly or in combinations. The faradic device has a current reverser; current breaker; and delivers primary, secondary, and combined currents. The coil is underneath the hard rubber face plate. Current amplitude was controlled by the sliding secondary coil.

Combination Galvanic and Faradic Battery No.2. This No.2 combination battery of Fig C23 changed designs drastically from 1893 to 1898, and then was dropped from the product line in 1900. The design of 1898 was the same as that of No.1 for the galvanic section, and No.14 of 1898 for the faradic part. This unit came in 24 cells (16.25 x 7.88 x 7.63 inches, 15.75 pounds), 32 cells (17.88 x 7.88 x 7.63 inches, 17 pounds), or 50 cells (20.63 x 7.88 x 7.63 inches, 20.5 pounds), and costing $47.00, $55.00, and $70.00, respectively. For the faradic part the face plate is

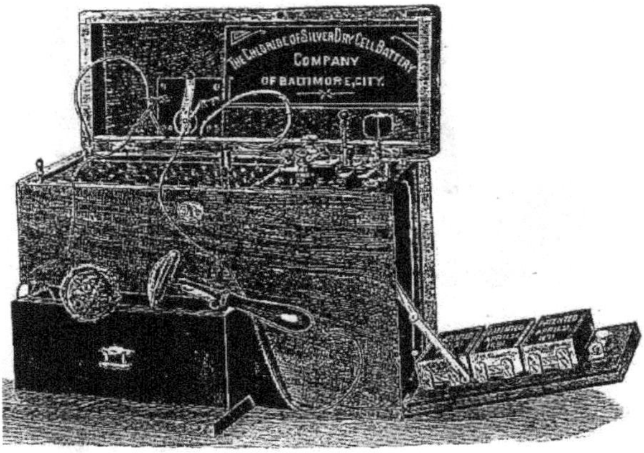

Fig C22. Combination Battery No.2[5]

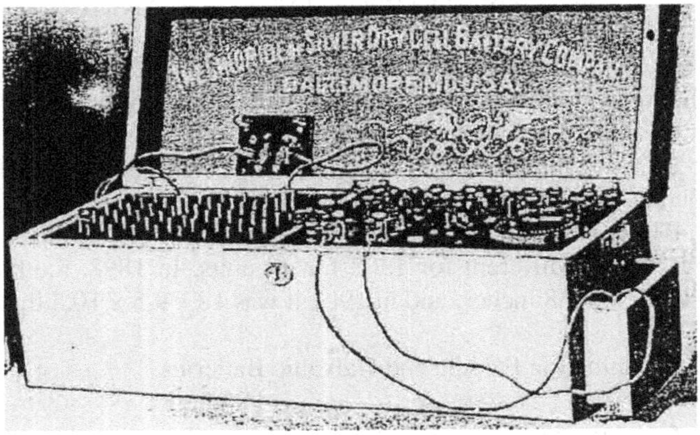

Fig C23. Combination Galvanic and Faradic Battery No.2

hard rubber that has a Willms current regulator, cell selector switch, a current reverser, a manual contact breaker, and a conventional type interrupter that is parallel to the plate. Underneath the face plate are three coils; a primary and two secondary coils made by different wire sizes and lengths (Nos.22, 26, and 32 wire) that can be used independently or in combination. For the galvanic section a current reverser is available along with a raised button for each cell. All units are housed in mahogany wooden boxes, hinged lids, and a key lock in front. The boxes are carried by a leather strap mounted on each side of the box. A sliding drawer is on the bottom right side of the box for accessories.

Combination Galvanic and Faradic Battery No.19. This combination battery was introduced by The Chloride of Silver Dry Cell Battery Co about 1898 as a low priced portable apparatus for general practitioners to carry to the bedside of their patients. This model varied in

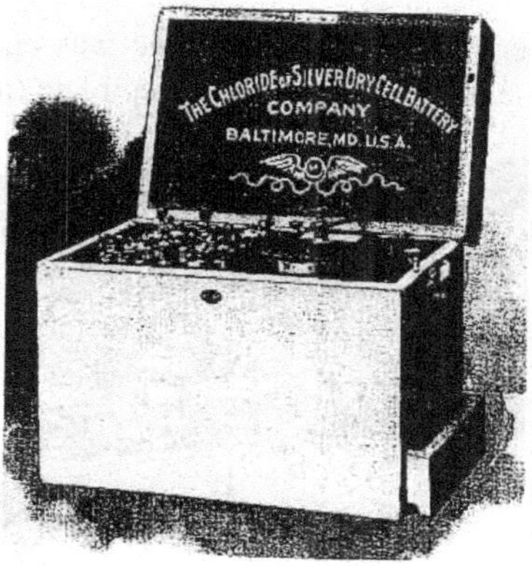

Fig C24. Combination Galvanic and Faradic Battery No.19

size from 25 to 50 dry cells. The chloride of silver dry cells are concealed from view (mounted underneath the face plate) along with cell posts and their connections. The coils are also mounted underneath the face plate as a primary and two secondary coils (wired differently by size and length), and coil outputs can be manually selected. The face plate has a cell selector switch for both galvanic and faradic currents; a current reverser to change polarity of electrodes; a switch that combines faradic and galvanic currents; a manually control contact breaker for electrodiagnostic work; and a contact key for starting faradic current. The unit is contained in an upright polished mahogany box varying in size according to the number of cells. The 25-cell unit (15.13 x 9.63 x 11.38 inches) weighs 23.75 pounds and cost $55.00 in 1898 through 1902. The box size changed in 1902 from that of 1898 (15 x 9.5 x 11.5 inches) and weighed less, 20.5 pounds. The 35-cell unit in 1898 through 1902 cost $65.00, and weighed 25 pounds. The 50-cell unit cost $80.00 in 1898 through 1902. All units of 1898 (25, 35, and 50 cells) had the same sized box, while all units of 1902 had a smaller sized box (same as the 25-cell unit) but their weights varied by the number of cells contained (25 cells = 20.5 pounds; 35 cells = 21.5 pounds; and 50 cells = 23 pounds, respectively). This No.19 combination battery of The Chloride of Silver Dry Cell Battery Co is exactly like the No.17 battery except that it does not have a milliammeter.[2]

Combination Galvanic and Faradic Battery No.18. Model No.18 (Fig C25) was offered by The Chloride of Silver Dry Cell Battery Co for the first time in 1898 and continued in the catalog of 1902.[2] The advantage of this particular combination unit was obtaining various functions for electrodiagnoses. The Chloride of Silver Co had just invented an automatic rheotome that it offered for the first time through this unit. The rheotome produced pulses automatically ranging from six to one hundred per minute. The rheotome was enclosed in hard rubber and mounted on the left rear side of the face plate (also hard rubber).

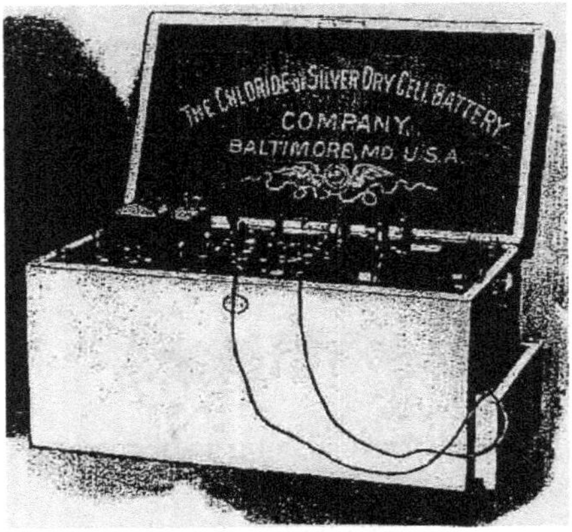

Fig C25. Combination Galvanic and Faradic Battery No.18

Underneath the face plate were four interchangeable dry cell packs with cell post and connections, and the induction coils. The coils were primary, and two secondary units that provide a variety of current combinations that can be preset. The face plate also contains: a cell selector for both faradic and galvanic currents; a current reverser for changing electrode polarity; a control switch for changing faradic and galvanic currents; a current breaker used in diagnostic work; and a contact key for starting the faradic current. The No.18 came in three different numbers of batteries, but in the same sized upright polished mahogany box (18 x 9.5 x 10.25 inches). The number of cells, weights, and costs were: 25 cells, 21.75 pounds, and $65.00; 35 cells, 23 pounds, and $75.00; and 50 cells, 24.5 pounds and $90.00, respectively. The No.18 combination battery combines the faradic battery No.9 and the galvanic battery No.15 of The Chloride of Silver Dry Cell Battery Co.[2]

Combination Galvanic and Faradic Battery No.17. This battery of Fig C26 was manufactured to meet the needs of the general practitioner and the specialist. This battery as one of the higher priced medical electrical batteries of the company and was offered in units by the number of cells. All No.17 units came in polished mahogany upright boxes of the same size (18 x 9.5 x 10.25 inches) with a hinged lid that has a lock and key on the front, and sliding drawer at the bottom of the right side of the box for accessories. The 25-cell unit weighs 22.25 pounds and cost $75.00; the 35-cell unit weighs 23.25 pounds and cost $85.00; and the 50-cell unit weighs 25 pounds and sold for $100.00. The No.17 combination battery was introduced in 1898 and was selling yet in 1902. Both size of the mahogany box and weight of the No.17 battery differed in 1902 from that of 1898. The box size was 18 x 9.5 x 10.5

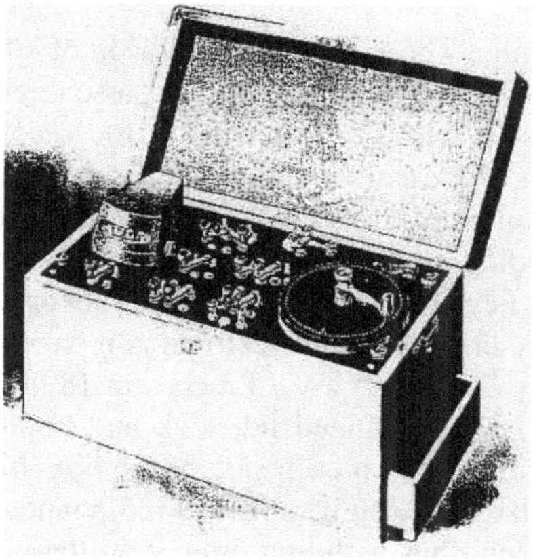

Fig C26. Combination Galvanic and Faradic Battery No.17

inches each, while the 25 cells unit weighed 22 pounds, the 35 cells unit weighed 23 pounds, and the 50 cells unit weighed 24.5 pounds in 1902. This unit features the Willms current controller, and the three-scale direct reading milliammeter for measuring galvanic current otherwise this combination battery is the same as the No.9 faradic unit and the No.11 galvanic unit of The Chloride of Silver Dry Cell Battery Co. The box is carried by a leather strap mounted on each side of the box.

Combination Galvanic and Faradic Battery No.13. This particular combination faradic and galvanic Battery (Fig C27) was the most costly deluxe model of The Chloride of Silver Dry Cell Battery Co product line. It cost $115.00 in 1898 and 1902, and came only in the 50

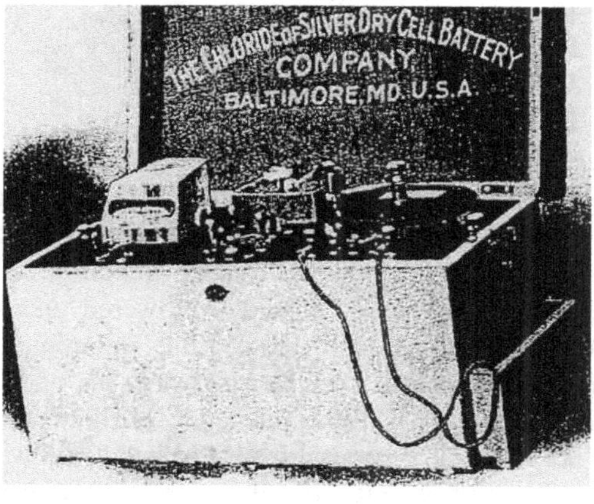

Fig C27. Combined Galvanic and Faradic Battery No.13

cells size. The Chloride of Silver Co considered this unit as the most perfect medical electrical battery of its time, and combines No.8 faradic and No.15 galvanic units. The unit has 50 chloride of silver dry cells; a Willms current controller; the best coils serving as one primary and four secondaries by means of wiring differences in the secondaries (No.30, No.26, No.24, and No.22 wires); an automatic rheotome for both faradic and galvanic current pulses (6 to 900 pulses per minute); a cell selector; a three-scale direct reading milliammeter; a current reverser; a current breaker; and a contact key. The face plate is hard rubber, and the metal is nickel plated. The case enclosing the electrical components is a polished mahogany upright box (21 x 10.5 x 9.75 inches in 1898 and 21 x 10.5 x 10.25 inches in 1902) with a hinged lid, lock and key on front, and a leather carrying strap mounted on each side of the box. In addition to the slight change in box sizes the weights differed (33 pounds in 1898 and 27 pounds in 1902). The unit has a sliding drawer on the bottom right side of the box for accessories.

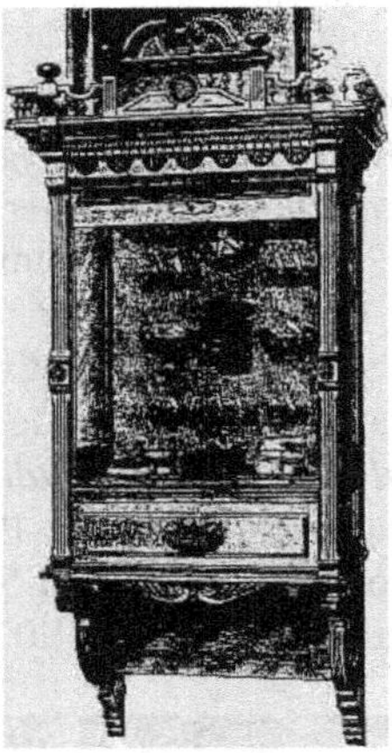

Fig C28. Wall Cabinet

Wall Cabinet. This combination faradic and galvanic battery of Fig C28 was designed in 1896, and is somewhat out of character with the previous product lines by its design. It has a mahogany cabinet (49 x 23 x 15 inches) with glass sides and its front is French bevelled glass plate. The front door is made to be raised or lowered and is balanced by weights. The unit is powered by 50 Willms' interchangeable galvanic cells. The faradic induction coil has one primary and four secondary windings, mil-am-meter, Willms' current controller, and an automatic rheotome. The unit has a series of switches that allow connections to combine primary current with any of the four secondary currents, and permit faradic and galvanic currents simultaneously. In 1896, this unit sold for $150.00 (via Wocher & Son Co[7]).

Electrical Cabinet. Sometime between 1890 and 1893, The Chloride of Silver Dry Cell Battery Co seemed to be competing with

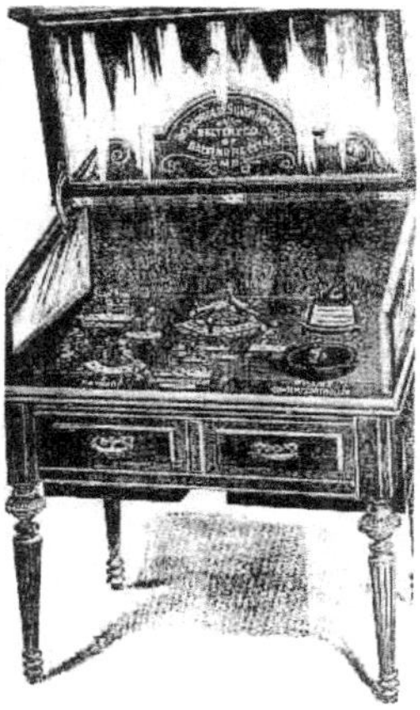

Fig C29. Electrical Cabinet[6]

companies like Flemming of Philadelphia and the Waite & Bartlett Co of New York for elaborate office model batteries. This desk style cabinet was a combination battery that delivered faradic and galvanic currents. The induction coils for the faradic currents were located underneath the wooden face plate that contained switches for selecting and controlling the operation of the primary and secondary coils. A current reverser is present, as is a galvanic cell selector control, and a switch for galvanic currents. The Willms' current controller regulated the current amplitudes. A millammeter is available, and has scales of 0 to 5, 0 to 25, and 0 to 250 milliamperes.

Sliding drawers on both sides of the cabinet hold cells to power the unit. The model used 100 chloride of silver cells connected in a series of blocks to a switch, 10 sets of 10 cells each. The switch operated any set of 10 cells. When the switch is thrown current passes to the reversing switch, then to a water rheostat, then through the mil-am-meter, and finally to the connecting posts to the patient. Drawers in front of the cabinet hold accessories. Access to the electrical components is from the rear of the cabinet. The cabinet has a lid containing glass and a view of the face plate when closed.

Summary

The Chloride of Silver Dry Cell Battery Co of Baltimore, MD, was a company that manufactured medical electrical batteries and retailed them directly and through medical supply stores around the country. The company is not known for manufacturing units for retailers who then sold the units using different trade names for their models. The company appears to have been founded by a group of professional and business personnel who ran the business for a little more than a decade before selling it to the new owner, Manes Fuld, who was a home use medical electrical battery manufacturer. Under the second owner the business lasted for another 12 years. The company's life was based on its innovative and patented cell for power source, but when the company did not change and up date its product line by converting the power source of its batteries to commercial electricity the business ended. The medical electrical batteries having the logo of The Chloride of Silver Dry Cell Battery Co were quality units, and the company offered a wide variety of units. This company held many patents for an American manufactory of medical electrical batteries.

References

1. Davis AB, Dreyfus MS. The Finest Instruments Ever Made. Arlington, MA, Med Hist Pub Assoc, 1986, pp 93, 185

2. Catalogs of the Chloride of Silver Dry Cell Battery Co, 1892, 1898, 1900, 1902

3. Liebig GA, Rohe GH. Practical Electricity in Medicine and Surgery. Philadelphia, PA, FA Davis, 1890, p 102

4. Polk's Medical Register and Directory of North America. Chicago, IL, RL Polk, 1904

5. Catalog of AS Aloe. St Louis, MO, AS Aloe, 1893

6. Catalog of Charles Truax & Greene of Chicago, IL, 1893

7. Catalog of Max Wocher & Son, Cincinnati, OH, 1896

CHAPTER 6. OTTO FLEMMING OF PHILADELPHIA

Otto Flemming was an instrument maker in Philadelphia who also engaged in the medical electrical battery business. This Chapter provides a brief story of Flemming and describes his batteries.

The City Directory of Philadelphia for 1877 (p 507)[1] listed the company as Otto Flemming & Talbot, electricians, on 814 Filbert Street. Otto Flemming of 729 Arch Street, Philadelphia, PA, was successor to Flemming & Talbot after 1877.

One of the first trade catalogs issued after 1877 listed Flemming as an electromedical instrument manufactory. This catalog listed a cabinet battery; combination battery; portable constant galvanic current battery; the 0 faradic battery; a keyboard for a galvanic battery; the number 1, 2, and 3 faradic batteries; a faradic apparatus for office table; the Drescher's Patent Electromagnetic Pocket Battery; an imported Gaiffe battery of France; rheostats; and electrical bells.[2]

The Illustrated Catalogue of Flemming's of 1886[3] indicated that the business was then located at 1009 Arch Street, Philadelphia, PA, and that it was formerly Flemming & Talbot. So between 1877 and 1886 the company changed ownership from Flemming & Talbot to Otto Flemming and relocated. Since the 1886 Catalogue was copyrighted in 1883, it is suggested that was the year in which Flemming & Talbot became the company of Otto Flemming. In 1886, he offered the sale of electrotherapeutic apparatuses, electrosurgical apparatuses, and electrodes. In a brief message to the reader (medical profession) the company's name was cited as The Flemming Electro-Medical Instrument Manufactory, however; the literature refers to the company as simply Otto Flemming.[2]

The company was then known as an electrical medical instrument manufacturer of cabinet batteries, faradic batteries, keyboard for galvanic batteries, faradic apparatuses for office tables, Drescher's patent electromagnetic batteries, imported French Gaiffe battery, water rheostats, and electrical cells. The company was selling the Queen's New Toepler-Holtz Electrical Machine, rheotomes, Grenet cells, and electrodes in the 1890s.[2] In 1896, the Flemming Electromedical Instrument Manufactory had an illustrated catalog (42 pp) of faradic and electrotherapeutic apparatus, electrical surgical apparatus, and electrodes.[2]

In 1904, Otto Flemming was located further down the street at 1025 Arch Street.[4] He was still selling electrotherapeutic items in 1904 by advertising faradic batteries with rapid and slow interrupted induction currents, galvanic cell batteries combining with faradic and galvanic currents, cautery batteries, and stationary and cabinet office batteries. The Flemming business was directed to that of physicians, although a few of his electrical batteries were marketed for home or family use.

Commonalties of the Flemming Batteries

The induction coils of the faradic batteries of Flemming were hidden from view (ie, mounted underneath the face plate). All models have quality workmanship, and brass metal components were used unless the buyer paid extra for nickel plated components which then were offered. The Flemming batteries are embossed or have an etched signature somewhere on the battery (wooden face plate or edge of the wooden box). The boxes had a metal lock and key on the front. Flemming manufactured at least five medical electrical batteries for home use, but, as stated, the major business efforts were aimed toward the physician consumer.

The more elaborate or deluxe models of Otto Flemming for physician use contained the unique rheotome (interrupter) devices. These particular units had separate devices for rapid and slow pulse frequencies, and communicated indirectly with the coil. The rocking arm lever for slow pulse frequencies was first devised as early as 1837 in England yet in 1886 was still being used in quality physician faradic batteries. Other manufacturers in the United States of faradic medical electrical batteries did not use the rocking arm style of interrupter.

Faradic Batteries

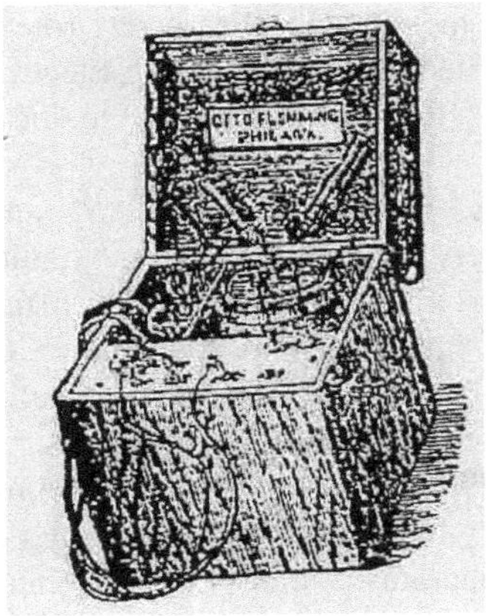

Fig Fl. No. 00 and No. 0 Faradic Battery

No.00 and 0 Faradic Battery. In his trade catalog of 1886, Flemming illustrated and described briefly five medical electrical batteries for family or home use. The No.00 and No.0 were the lowest priced faradic batteries of the Flemming line for the public consumer who had a choice of metal components. The $10.00 unit had brass metal, while the $12.00 unit had nickel plated metal components. The face plate is about half of the box's area, and contains four metal receptacles for connection with the subject to provide three different currents (primary, secondary, and combined). Two binding posts at the rear of the face plate join with the power source of the single wet cell. Since the coils are mounted underneath the face plate, the current amplitude is regulated manually by sliding the metal tube out or into the right side of the box. The pulse interrupter is the spring lever vibrator type that communicated indirectly with the coil.

No.1 Faradic Battery. This unit (Fig F2) was a low cost electrical apparatus designed for physician use on home visits, and specially adapted for treating muscular paralysis. The unit was powered by a single wet cell that connected to two binding posts on the face plate. The face plate is matching wood with the box. The No. 1 is upgraded

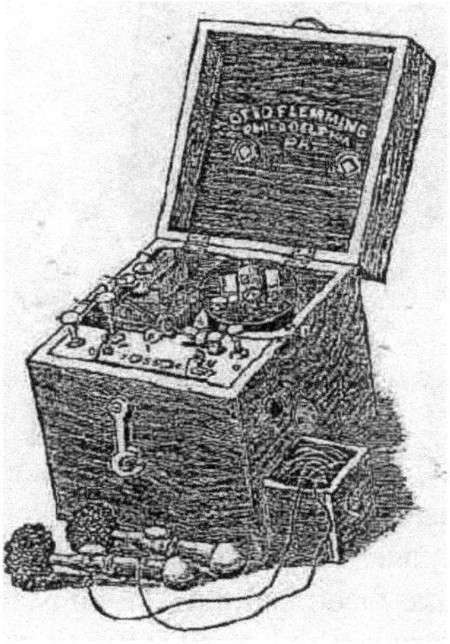

Fig F2. No.1 Faradic Battery of Flemming

from 0 and 00 by having manually adjustable vibrating interrupter to crudely control pulse rates. It also contains a manually adjusting lever control for slow frequencies. The unit contains the conventional induction coils underneath the face plate with the sliding metal tube current regulator operated from the right side of the box. The interrupter communicates indirectly with the induction coil. The unit came in either a polished black walnut or morocco style wooden box (6 x 6 x 7.5 inches). The box is hinged and fastened in front by a hinged twist type latch or lock and key. The lower right side of the box has a sliding drawer for accessories. The five-pound unit cost $22.50 complete in 1886 through 1896. Without the rapid and slow rheotomes its price was $15.00.

Another Flemming Faradic Battery No.1 (Fig F3) is believed to predate the above No.1 unit and to be made between 1877 and 1880. It also used a single wet cell for power. The unit was encased in a walnut box (6.25 x 6.5 x 7.5 inches), or slightly larger than that above No.1 unit of 1886. The box has a hinged lid that has the Flemming signature embossed as "The Flemming Electro Med Apps Manfty Otto Flemming Philadelphia." The wooden box has a brass lever lock on its front, and an engraved metal carrying handle on top. On the right side of the box is a

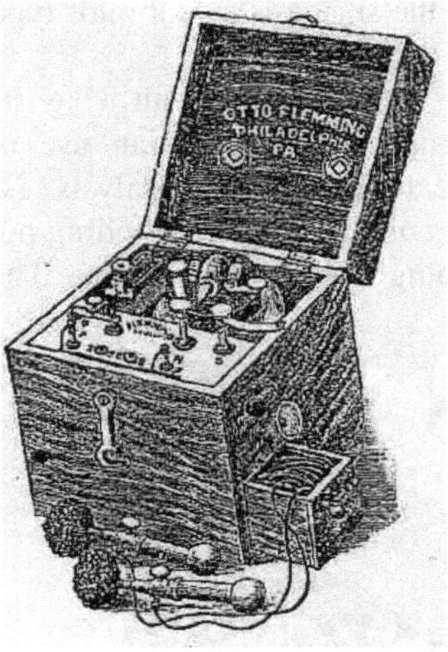

Fig F3. No.1 Flemming Faradic Battery

drawer (2 x 2.5 x 5.75 inches) used to hold accessories, and it is secured by a brass disc (0.88 inch). The corners of the box are glued with tongue and grooves. The face panel is wood matching the box. All hardware is brass. The left side of the face panel has an adjustable screw leaf spring lever, hammer type interrupter embossed "Otto Flemming, maker, Phila." The hammer of the interrupter contacts the coil (underneath the face plate) indirectly by striking a button that connects the coil by a bar attachment. Four connecting receptacles "1, 2-5, 3-6, 4-7" are recessed in the wood along the front of the face plate. The right side has two brass binding posts for joining the wet cell. The face panel lifts from the case with removal of the hollow surging tube that slides over the core of the induction coil. The induction coil is hidden underneath the face panel and occupies one third of the area of two compartments. The other compartment is open and houses the wet cell. A metal nickel plated tube (4.25 x 0.88 inches) serves as the current regulator, and is scored into 10 units and arbitrarily marked from 1 to 5. A thin brass latch secures the current regulator when not being used.

This No.1 Faradic Battery of Flemming (Fig F3) was still being sold in 1896 for $15.00. Although nearly the same as the earlier No.1, this No.1 changed slightly in 1896. It was advertised for family use and physicians making their daily visits, and came in only a polished walnut case of same size (6 x 6 x 7.5 inches) as No.1 of Fig F2. The cell was then a patented sealed unit. The unit also came only with a rapid interrupter, and weighed six pounds.

No.2 Faradic Battery. Flemming like other manufacturers gradated the quality or operations of his faradic apparatuses by either increasing current output or by adding electrical components. With the No. 2 (Fig F4) the power of the two coils is increased over that of No. 1.

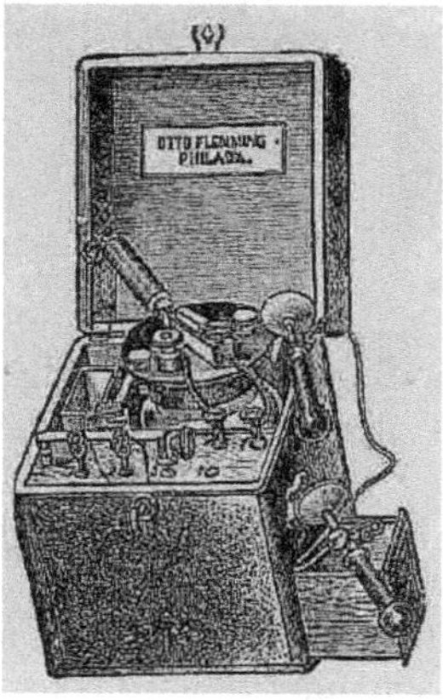

Fig F4. No.2 Faradic Battery

The coil in No.2 is one inch longer than that of No.1. This battery (7 inches sq) in a polished walnut box is hinged with a lock and key in front. An indirect connection with the induction coil is through an adjustable lever interrupter (horizontal to the face plate), and is located on the face plate. Like other Flemming faradic units the sliding tube current controller is manually adjusted from the right side of the box. Below the sliding tube is a sliding drawer for accessories. Two high adjustable binding posts connect with the single wet cell by lever type connecters. The unit is provided with a commutator (pole changer). All metal is nickel plated. This unit cost $20.00 in 1886 through 1896.

No.3 Faradic Battery. This No.3 unit of Fig F5 is similar to the No.3 unit of Fig F6 of 1877, and was sold by the National Commercial Co of Cincinnati, OH. This particular unit in Fig F5 was made by Flemming & Talbot, a company that ended in 1877 to become the Flemming Electro-Medical Instrument Manufactory.

This No.3 unit is similar to the No.3 unit of 1877 (Fig F6), and was sold by the National Commercial Co of Cincinnati, OH. This particular unit above was made by Flemming & Talbot, a company that ended in 1877 to become the Flemming Electro-Medical Instrument Manufactory. This unit above dates about 1873 to 1876. The Flemming

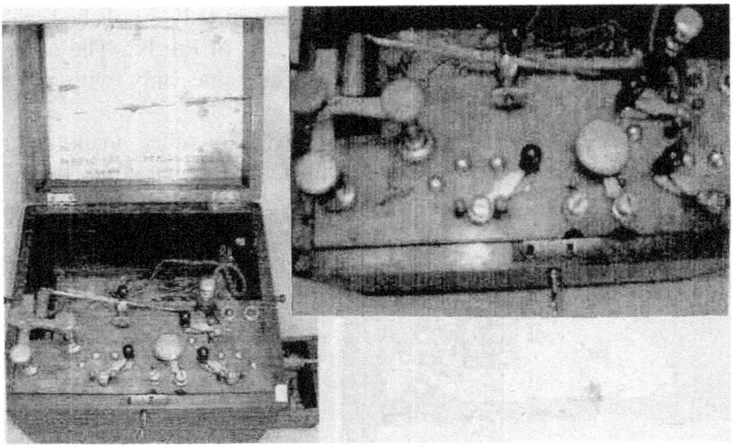

Fig F5. No.3 Faradic Battery of Flemming & Talbot
(No.9 National, Commercial Co of Cincinnati)

wet cells for this unit were a hard rubber container that has 10 sections, each section serving as an independent wet cell. The container of cells was placed in the open compartment (3/5 of area). Carbon and zinc plates were lowered into the cells containing fluid to activate the battery. After connecting cells 1 and 3 the battery would deliver galvanic current only, and then when rearranged according to directions the battery operated as a faradic apparatus. This particular No.3 unit is really a combination battery. Two minor differences existed between the two No.3 apparatuses pictured here. The unit of the National Commercial Co had a lever On/Off switch rather than a double throw switch, and it has a drawer (glued dovetailed) for accessories located on the bottom right side of its wooden case. It was carried by a leather strap secured to the sides of the box by metal eye holders. This battery is of the same basic design as the Flemming rocking arm interrupter unit of Fig F6 that was sold directly by Flemming. The National Commercial Co is believed to have been a retailer of medical equipment and supplies. The Cincinnati, OH, company had electrical apparatuses made for them by Otto Flemming who obliged the company by printing a paper label of directions and the Commercial Co's signature for the inside lid. Manufacturers always welcome retail outlets that promote their products. The nickel plated metal is thinner than that of the 1877 unit, also. This unit is housed in a walnut case (7.25 x 7.5 x 8.5 inches), and was the No.2 Faradic Battery of Flemming & Talbot in 1873 to 1876 period of time, but then became the No.3 unit of Otto Flemming after 1877. This unit cost $30.00 in 1873 to 1876 and weighed 10 pounds with cells. The Flemming medical

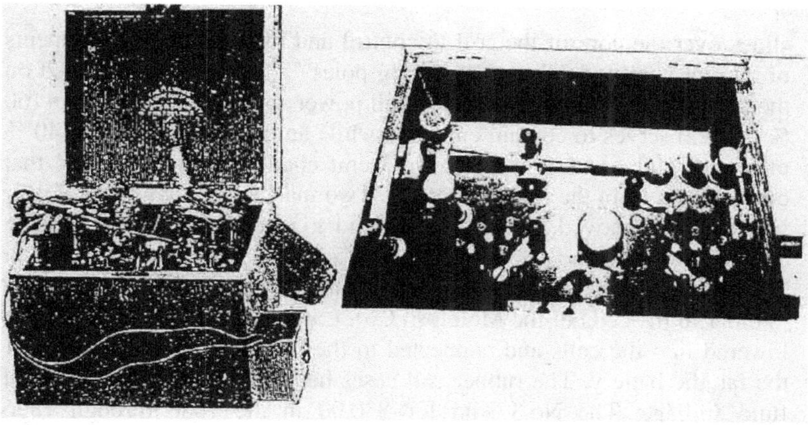

Fig F6. No.3 Faradic Battery (Flemming Rocking Arm Interrupter)

electrical batteries were of quality construction. The Otto Flemming No.3 Faradic Battery was probably first built in 1885 or 1887. Rather than a signature plate the unit has the identity of the company recessed on the polished black walnut face plate that reads "The Flemming Battery, Phila, Pat June 23.85." This particular faradic battery was encased in a wooden box (ca 8.75 x 6.75 x 8 inches) with glued tongue and groove corners. The lid has a folding onyx carrying handle, and is secured by a rotating type latch in front. Attached underneath and horizontal to the face plate is an induction coil (5.38 x 1.5 inches) covered with paper, and enclosed in a walnut box. On the left side and horizontal to the face plate is an adjustable screw spring lever, hammer that vibrates (rapid pulses) against two separate and heavy wired coils (armature, 2 inches long) having soft iron cores vertically mounted (to the face plate). The slow pulse controller is a long lever (ca 6 inches), right end has a ball, the center is the axis with a ring mount and a movable ring lock (when not in use), and the left end has a roller that is near the two vertical coils. The lever rocks when activated as slow as one per second. This arrangement was first designed and used by McGauley of England in 1837. The rocking arm interrupter seems to be characteristic of units in the United States by the, Otto Flemming Co of Philadelphia and the Galvano-Faradic Manufacturing Co of New York. All hardware are nickel plated.

On the left side of the face panel are 0, 1, 2, 3, 4 buttons with a control lever connected to the primary coil, "P;" on screw "N" for two connecting poles, the secondary coil is connected to 0, 1, 2, 3, 4 buttons with lever control, "S," on the right side, between the two controls is a lever switch "S/P", and to the rear on the right side is a vertical throw switch for On/Off On the right side of the box is a nickel plated surging tube (7 x 0.38 inches, 13 half-inch sections scaled with 1 to 6 marks) that slides over the core of the coil to control and offer crude measurements of current amplitude. Two connecting poles "Z" and "C" are located on the panel and connect with the wet cell power source. The face panel (60 % of area) serves to contain circuitry, while an open compartment (40 % of area) is for accessories. The No.3 unit changed in 1877 to one that opened both from the top and bottom. Two machine screws on the lower front, when removed, allow a hinged lid to open the area for housing cells. This bottom lid is beveled (9.38 x 7.13 x 0.5 inches). The cells in 1877 were of hard rubber and continuous as a pack for 10 wet cells (similar to the cells of the McIntosh Co). Carbon and zinc elements were lowered into the cells and connected to the two binding posts to power the faradic battery. The rubber cell cases had a hydrastat that prevented fluid spillage. The No.3 sold for $30.00 in the 1886 through 1896 Flemming trade catalogs, and was described as having a slightly different sized walnut case (7.5 x 7.5 x 8.5 inches) than that described herein (weighed 10 pounds). The No.3 Faradic Battery originated about 1876 or 1877 and was then the No.2 Faradic Battery of Flemming & Talbot. The unit was carried by a leather strap prior to 1877, but with the 1877 model the nickel plated handle was used. The metal is nickel plated and the unit weighs 10 pounds.

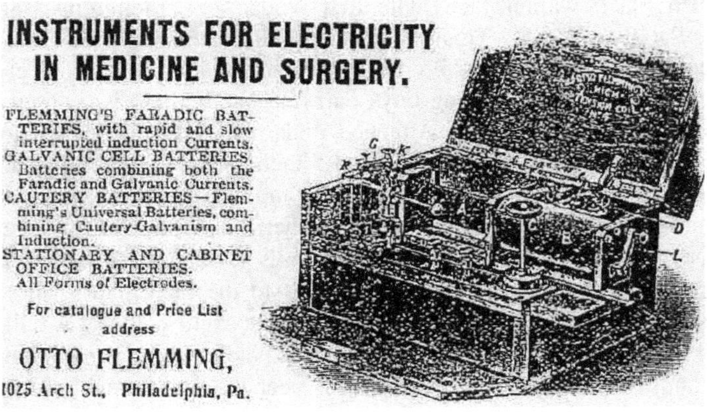

Fig F7. No. 4 Faradic Battery

No.4 Faradic Battery. In 1904 or before, Otto Flemming made the No.4 Faradic Battery from its earlier DuBois-Reymond sledge inductorium type coil. The No.4 battery was the DuBois-Reymond coil enclosed in a walnut box. The box was designed with a full (area) sized hinged lid that had a self lock and key in front. The front of the box was also hinged to drop the front side to allow a drawer to be pulled out for accessories. When the lid of the box was open the secondary coil could be moved over the primary coil because a hinged section of the right side of the case dropped to allow movement. Because of the sledge unlike other Flemming batteries, this unit has both the rapid and slow rocking lever interrupter. To the rear of the coil is an open compartment to contain the wet cells.[4]

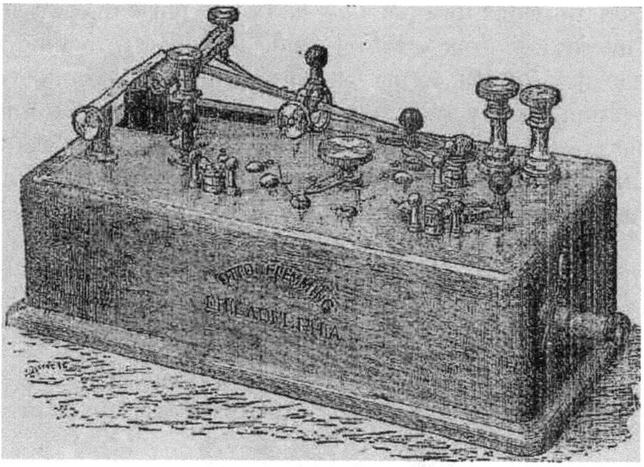

Fig F8. Faradic Apparatus for Office Table

Faradic Apparatus for Office Table. Like the No.3 Faradic Battery of Flemming, this model (Fig F8) also has the rocking arm lever type interrupter for slow pulse rates. The model is an alternative to the box type No.3 for consumers not wishing to have a complete case. The face plate and bottom portions are wood, but this unit is without a lid. The face plate has all of the features of a No.3 faradic battery, and can be connected with an external wet cell for power source. In 1886, the unit sold for $25.00.

DuBois-Reymond Coil. Otto Flemming made one of the best American representations of the DuBois-Reymond battery, most often called the sledge inductorium (Fig F9). The secondary coil of the faradic electrical battery is supplied with rails so that it slides over the primary

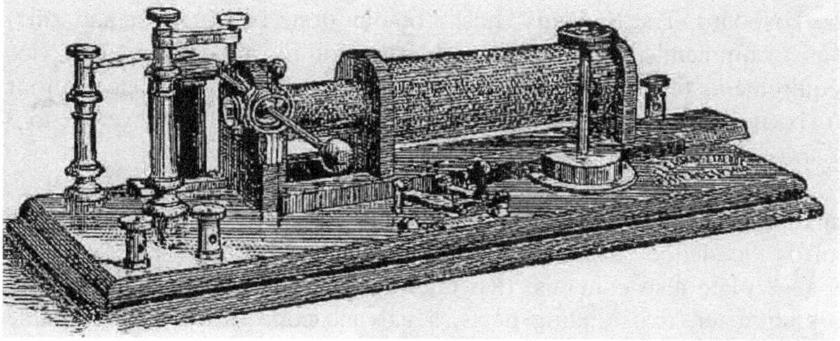

Fig F9. DuBois-Reymond Coil

coil. The unit has a double scale and pendulum that provides a slowly interrupted current. The unit made by Flemming was not portable, but suitable only for the physician's office and for hospital work.[5] The unit pictured here provides for both slow and rapid pulse rates by having two different interrupters (one a vibrator and the other a rocking arm). The unit has a switch for connecting with the primary and secondary currents, and a governing screw for controlling the voltage of the current. The power source is external to the coil and requires a single wet cell (eg, a Grenet cell). The wooden base is polished walnut, and the metal parts are nickel plated. Without the power source the unit cost $30.00 in 1886.

Combination Batteries

Permanent Office Table. The office table (Fig F10) is a keyboard containing the electrical components and a full sized drawer. The unit uses 60 to 100 cells that are kept externally (cellar or closet) to

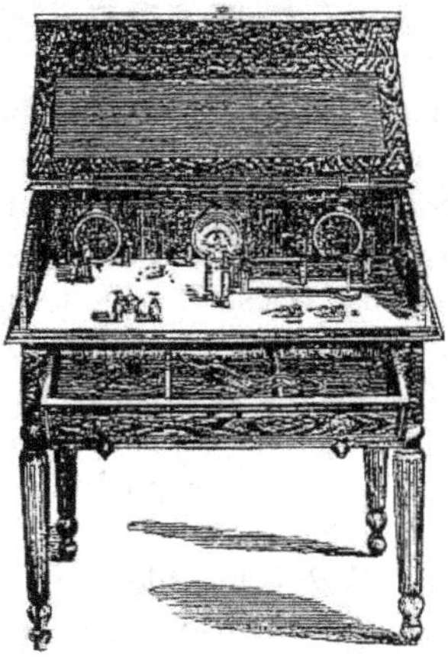

Fig F10. Flemming's Permanent Office Table

the keyboard. The Seimens Halske or bluestone cell (copper and zinc) was recommended by Flemming because of its minimal maintenance requirements (eg, a little water and a few chemical crystals once in four to six months were added, and zinc elements were replaced every 2 to 3 years).

The table and cabinet are black walnut (35 x 20 x 40 inches), carved legs, and an elegant piece of furniture for a physician's office. The coil is the sledge inductorium of DuBois-Reymond type. The keyboard or face plate also contains: two interrupters (slow and rapid pulses), a milliammeter, two binding posts, a galvanoscope to indicate available voltage, two current selectors to activate the desired number of cells, a pole changer (commutator), a water rheostat for faradic and galvanic use, switches to manually pulse galvanic current (monophasic pulses) at slow to rapid rates, and terminal posts for connecting faradic and galvanic currents to the patient. The unit without cells sold for $140.00 in 1886, and with 60 cells-it cost $200.00 or 100 cells for $250.00.

Cabinet Battery. This model of 1886 (F10A) has the same electrical components and functions as the Permanent Office Table, but offers a different style of case. The lid is basically designed like the unit

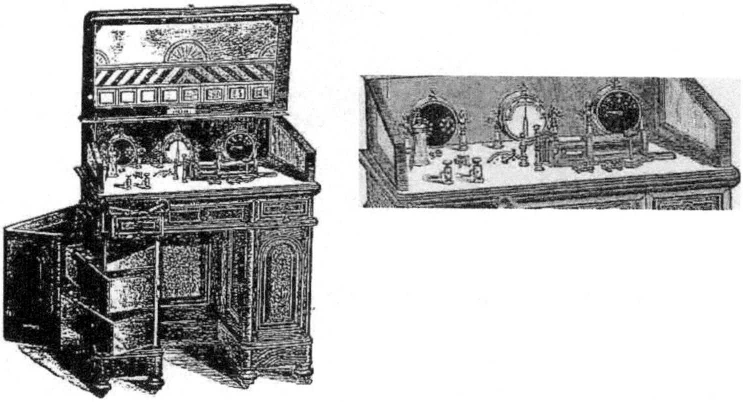

Fig Fl0A. Flemming's Cabinet Battery

of Fig F10, but is more elaborate with carvings. The signature plate is mounted on the inside of the lid. Two sliding drawers for accessories are located in front just beneath the inlaid face plate. Each side of the desk style cabinet is a folding type of door that opens in two hinged parts. The doors hide three pivoting drawers that hold and store up to 100 cells. The center portion of the cabinet is open like a desk for the operator's feet when seated. The size of the desk type cabinet measures 35 x 20 x 40 inches.

Wall Cabinet. This unit has the same electrical components as the office table of Fig F10 but was designed to save space, and to be located on a wall of the office. The cabinet is black walnut and has two hinged glass plated doors. Underneath the door are two drawers for accessories. The overall size of the cabinet is 25 x 7 x 40 inches. The 40 or 60 cells are located externally to the cabinet (eg, cellar or closet). Flemming recommended either Grenet or Siemens-Halske cells to power the unit. The wall cabinet's face plate contains: a galvanoscope (indicates EMF); two current selectors (controls set number of cells in use); a pole changer (commutator); a water rheostat for faradic and galvanic currents; a DuBois-Reymond induction coil; a slow and a rapid interrupter; switches to control the type of current at the connecting posts; and two binding posts to join the cells. Without any cells the cabinet model sold for $85.00 in 1886, while with 40 or 60 cells the cost was $135.00 and

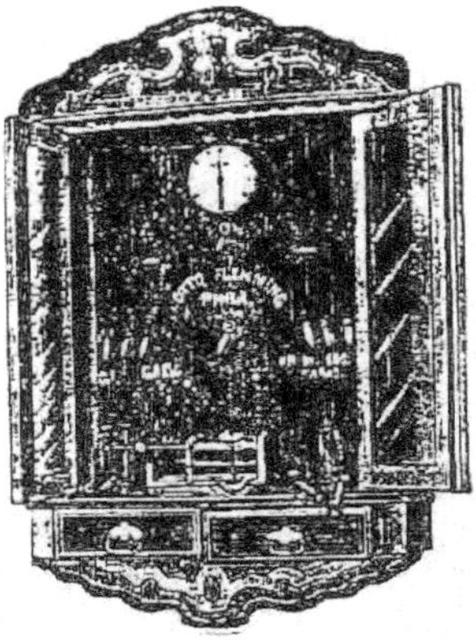

Fig F11. Flemming Wall Cabinet

$160.00, respectively.

Portable Combination and Galvanic Battery. This is a rather large boxed unit in Fig F12 (18 x 7 x 15 inches) is made with polished walnut weighing about 30 pounds. The lid is hinged and two hook type latches secure it in front. A leather carrying strap is mounted on each side of the box. The faradic portion of the unit is the same as that of the No. 3

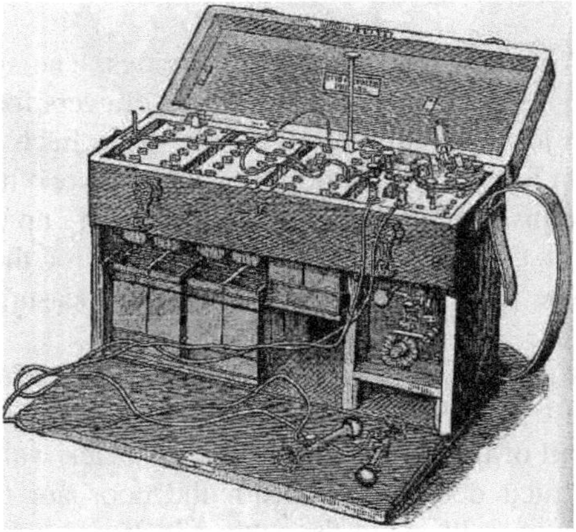

Fig F12. Portable Combination Batteries
(10, 20 & 30 cells)

Faradic Battery. The slow or the rapid functioning interrupters can be changed by a switch. The number of cells range from 10 to 30 dependent on the consumer who also chooses the rheotome (rapid faradic or slow and rapid). The prices of the unit in 1886 varied accordingly: with only the rapid faradic rheotome (10 cells cost $35.00; 16 cells were $45.00; 20 cells were $55.00; and 30 cells cost $75.00), and with slow and rapid faradic rheotomes (10 cells cost $50.00; 16 cells were $60.00; 20 cells cost $70.00; and 30 cells cost $90.00). The Flemming signature is embossed on the inside of the lid. The unit was designed for physician use.

Twenty-cell Combination Battery. Flemming also made a smaller unit than the 30-cell combination battery for physicians. This smaller model is the 20-Cell Combination Battery (Fig F13) that uses the same electrical components as his No.1 Faradic Battery. The No.1 Faradic Battery has the rapid interrupter (rheotome), but Flemming offered the slow as well as the rapid rheotome for an extra $15.00. The basic unit with only the rapid rheotome sold for $55.00 in 1886.[3] The

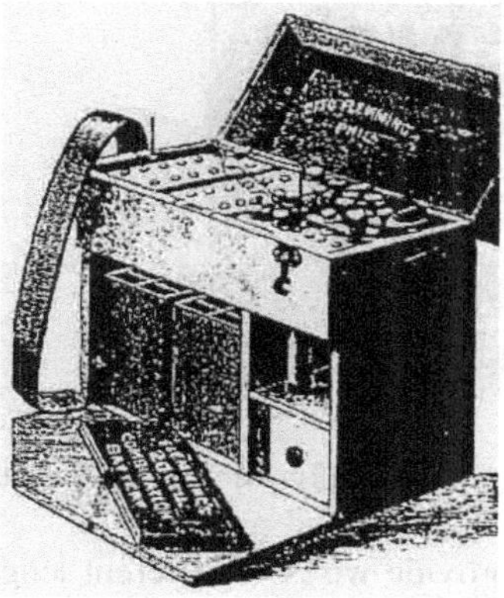

Fig F13. Flemming's 20-Cell Combination Battery

black walnut box has a hinged lid, a lock and key, and two hook latches on the front. The box is carried by a leather strap mounted by a clasp type holder. In addition to a top lid, part of the front of the box opened as another lid to form a desk like base. This latter lid opened to allow access to the two wet cells for recharging or replacing. Flemming wet cells for this unit were a hard rubber container that has 10 sections, each serving as an independent wet cell. The cell elements are carbon and zinc. Flemming in 1886 recommended bichromate of potassium as the cell fluid. The cells were raised for activation by metal rods at the back of the box. The rods are part of a spring system that allows the depth of the elements to control the amount of current. The cells are covered by a hydrastat when not activated. The hydrastat is controlled by two rods. The unit has a commutator for reversing polarity. The induction coils on Flemming's faradic batteries are hidden since being mounted underneath the face plates. This particular model has a small drawer located under the small face plate and access is from the front when the front lid is open. The size of the box is 14 x 7 x 12 inches, and weighs about 20 pounds.

Electro-Therapeutic Gynecological Cabinet. Flemming introduced this cabinet battery around 1887 or 1888 with its new Massey disc style rheostat. This is an exquisite wooden cabinet desk style (30 x 45 x 15 inches) with a hinged lid that closes diagonally over the face plate. The face plate contains a sledge inductorium style faradic coil. The coil could be varied as one compound helix or with several separate

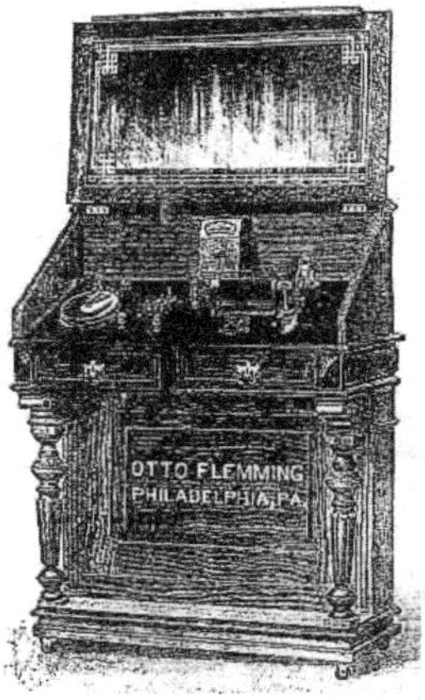

Fig F14. Electro-Therapeutic Gynecological Cabinet, 1887

interchangeable coils to provide wires of different lengths and diameters to vary currents. The interrupters provide for rapid and slow pulse frequencies. The apparatus delivers faradic and galvanic currents, separately or combined. The electrical components include a water rheostat, a Flemming milliammeter for measuring 0.5 to 1,000 milliamperes, and a current controller. Three Leclanche cells power the unit. Max Wocher & Son Co sold this unit in 1905 for $200.00.

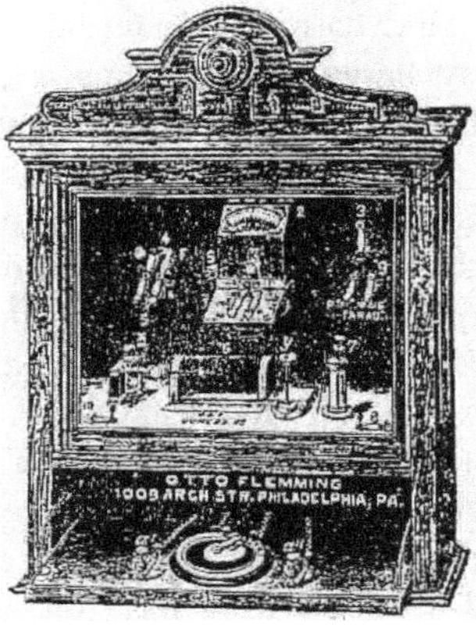

Fig F15. Electro-Gynecological Wall Cabinet

Electro-Gynecological Wall Cabinet. In 1890 to 1893, Flemming made an electrotherapeutic electrical battery (Fig F15) that works similarly in respect to the Flemming Wall Cabinet of 1886. This unit was designed for gynecological use; it has a Massey-Flemming current controller that varies the galvanic current; a DeWatteville current combiner is available for selecting either faradic or galvanic currents or both combined; current passing into the subject is measured by a Flemming milliammeter; a commutator (pole changer) is present; a DuBois-Reymond type of induction coil is available that has devices for rapid and slow current interruptions; varying and softening faradic currents can be done with the liquid rheostat with a switch; a double switch controls primary or secondary faradic currents; and a single switch starts or stops faradic currents on the coil and the two terminal posts. This unit sold for $123.00 in 1893, and $125.00 in 1896.

The Massey rheostat (see Rheostats, Part I) is featured in models of Fig F14 and F15. This unique current controller was the idea of Dr Massey of Philadelphia, a leading electrotherapist in the United States specializing in gynecological treatments by electricity.

Movable Table Battery. Around 1888 or 1889, Dr GB Massey, a gynecologist and inventor of the Massey disc rheostat, designed a combination battery (Fig F15A) in which most electrical components were placed underneath the face plate. The table has a hinged lid that holds the Flemming milliameter and when closed hides all components. The Massey disc rheostat controls both faradic and galvanic current amplitudes, and various switches on the face plate control the electrical operations. Binding posts are also located on the face plate. This model was powered from the wall source (power grid) of the new Edison direct current.

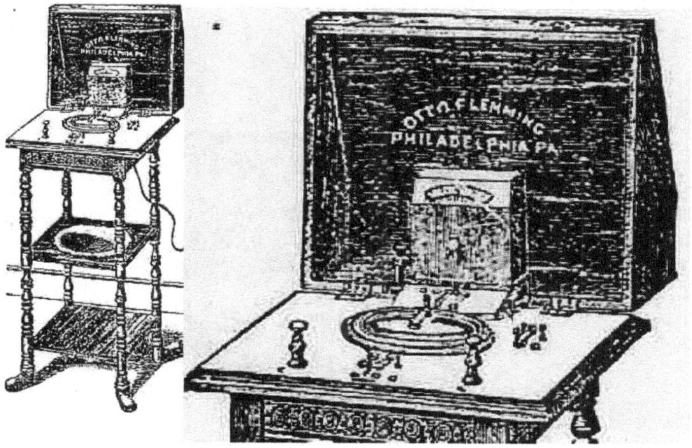

Fig F15A. Massey's Movable Table[7]

Table Plate. This model (Fig F16) is a combination battery with the same electrical components and operational features as the Gynecological Cabinet of Fig F14 except for a water rheostat. The wooden face or table plate has a Massey-Flemming current controller, a milliammeter, a DeWatteville current combiner, commutator (pole changer), a DuBois-Reymond induction coil, two current interrupters (rapid, slow), and binding (connecting) posts. The buyer had the option of a walnut cover for $85.00 to match the wooden base or a unit without

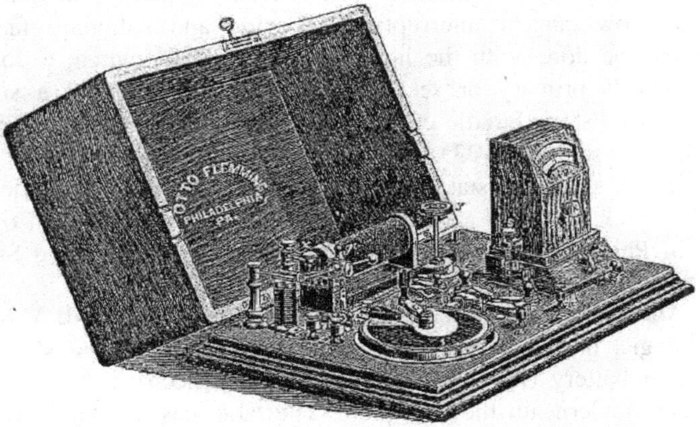

Fig F16. Electro-Therapeutic Table Plate

a cover for $80.00 in 1905 through Max Wocher & Son of Cincinnati.[6] Along with the wood cover was a self locking device and key on the front, and a metal carrying handle on the top. This unit was introduced about 1888 or 1890 by Flemming. The price in 1893 was the same as that in 1905.

Galvanic Batteries

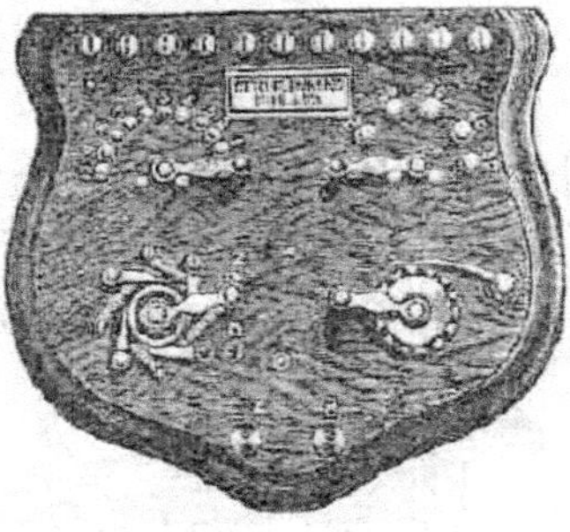

Fig F17. Key-Board for Galvanic Battery

Keyboard for Galvanic Battery. For the consumer who did not want an office table or wall cabinet medical electrical battery the keyboard was available for $25.00 in 1886. Although designed for electrical batteries and wall mounting, the keyboard can be used in the general office of a physician. The unit is essentially a large face plate for mounting on a wall. The face contains: a current selector for engaging the desired number of cells, and a polarity reverser (pole changer or commutator). The keyboard can be used independently for galvanic current or in conjunction with an office table model. The cells of 19 to 100 are externally located.

Portable Constant Galvanic Current Battery. Flemming advertised this model (Fig F18) as the most perfect ever available to physicians. It came in sizes ranging from 10 cells to 60 cells. The 10-sectioned cell unit is lighter in weight and considered more durable than glass cells. A rod on each side of the box raises and lowers the cells for activation or deactivation. When not in use the cells are covered and protected by the hydrastat (rubber cushioned sliding board). The cells are

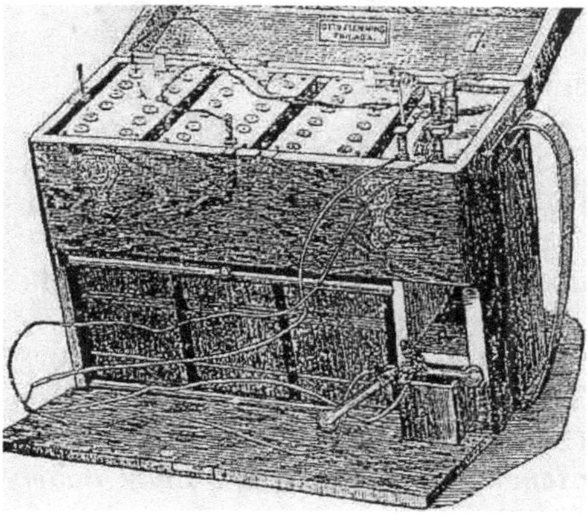

Fig F18. Portable Constant Galvanic Current Battery

removed through an opened front, hinged lid. The unit has a commutator, and binding posts for joining the cells to the circuitry. A galvanoscope, and an automatic rheotome (adjusts galvanic or monophasic pulses 2 to 8 per second) were available.

All of the black walnut boxes to house the electrical system were made by Flemming's firm, the boxes are polished, and the nickel plating was also done by Flemming. The unit is easily transportable, and ranged in price in 1886 with the size of the unit. The sizes and costs were: 1) 10-cell battery (14 x 12 x 6 inches), 10 pounds cost $25.00; and 2) 16-cell battery (14 x 10.5 x 6.5 inches), 15 pounds cost $35.00.

In 1896, this unit could be bought as a galvanic unit with 10 cells ($25.00), 20 cells ($45.00), or 30 cells ($65.00 basic or with slow interrupter for $90.00). A combined faradic and galvanic unit of 10 cells was $35.00, 20 cells was $55.00, and of 30 cells was $75.00.

Portable Galvanic Physicians' Battery. Around 1888 or 1890 Flemming improved on his Portable Constant Galvanic Current Battery of Fig F18 by adding the Massey disc rheostat, the Flemming milliammeter, and a current controller. This series of batteries like earlier galvanic batteries were made for 6, 12, 18, 24, 30, and 36 wet cells. The

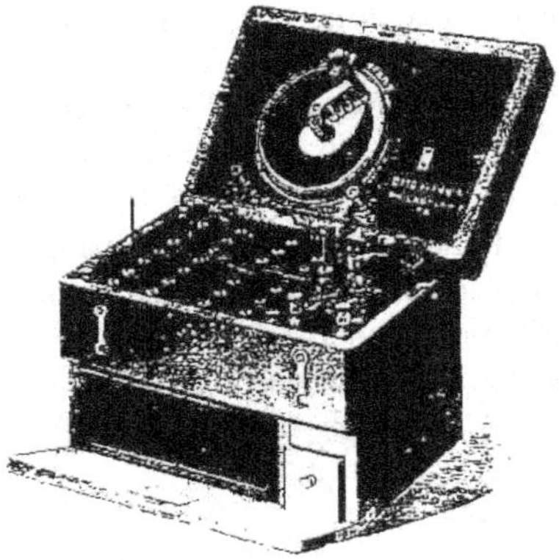

Fig F19. Improved Portable Galvanic Physicians' Batteries

wet cells came in sections of six or 12. The price of this unit in 1905 by Max Wocher & Son Co varied from $20.00 to $95.00 as a basic unit but the meter and current controller additionally cost $20.00 and $10.00, respectively.[6] This improved model has all of the features of the previous model except the additions noted.

Constant Galvanic Current Family Battery. Occasionally

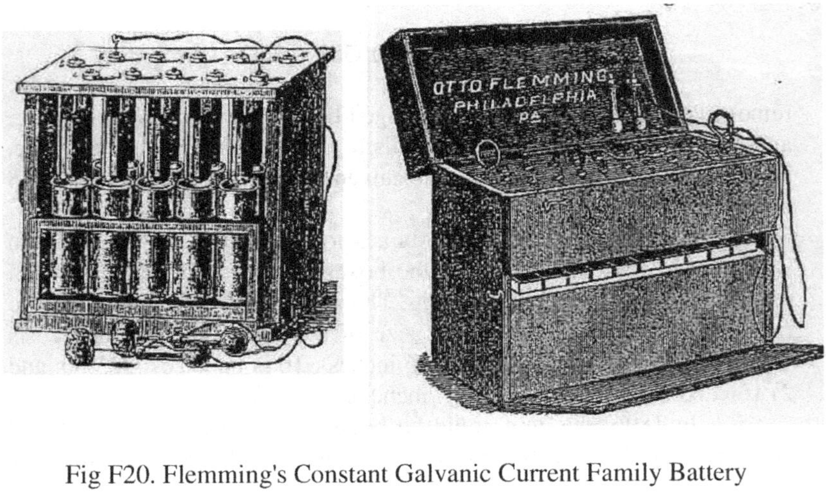

Fig F20. Flemming's Constant Galvanic Current Family Battery

physicians wanted a cheap galvanic battery to recommend to their patients for home use. Flemming came up with the Constant Galvanic Current Family Battery to meet this need. This galvanic unit accommodates 6 to 50 cells according to the need. The circular glass cells are on a tray inside a wooden box that moves as a frame by two screws on knobs to raise or lower the tray. The unit was simple in design and to operate. It could be activated and deactivated with two rotating screw knobs. The proper two metal receptacles for selecting the number of cells can be manually controlled when connecting the patient to the circuit. The galvanic battery (Fig F20, left) in 1886 was sold as a basic unit without a box or with a box case for 6 cells ($6.00 or $7.00); 8 cells ($8.00 or $9.00); 10 cells ($10.00 or $11.50); 16 cells ($16.00 or $17.50); 20 cells ($20.00 or $22.00); 30 cells ($30.00 or $32.00); 40 cells ($40.00 or $42.00); and 50 cell: ($50.00 or $52.50).

By 1896, the Constant Galvanic Current Family Battery (Fig F20, right) was redesigned slightly. The cells are closed glass tubes set in a movable frame that is raised or lowered by two set screws. The elements are carbon and zinc. This unit was offered with wooden case, hinged lid with two latches; drop drawer in front to expose sliding container holding the cells. Two latches on sides secured the lower drawer. The unit came with six cells ($7.00), eight cells ($9.00), 10 cells ($11.50), 16 cells ($17.50), 20 cells ($22.00), and 30 cells ($32.00) in 1896.

Flemming Cell. Flemming made an improvement on existing glass jar cells with a cap or top that allowed the jar to be filled with fluid rather than half full like others (Fig F21). The special cap allowed the zinc element to be pulled out after each use and a hydrastat to seal the vacated space in the cap to prevent spillage. This method of removing and saving the zinc element enabled the zinc to last a long time and be

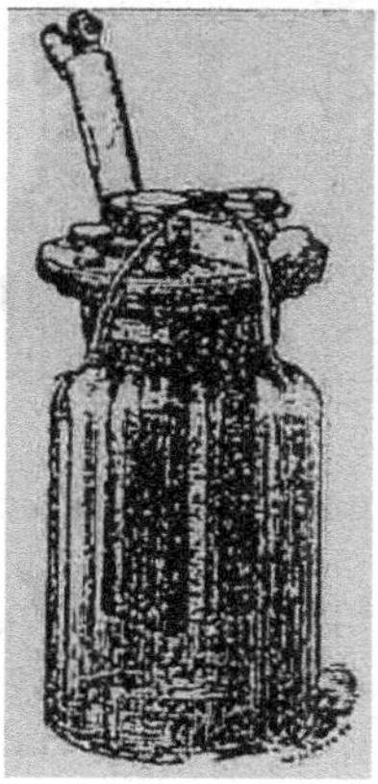

Fig F21. Flemming Cell for Faradic Battery
Miscellaneous Units

nearly the length of the jar. A long zinc element meant more voltage. The patent was pending in 1886 and the unit sold for $3.00.[3]

Miscellaneous Units

Dr French Batteries. Daniel Davis, Jr, the noted instrument maker of Boston, retired in 1854 and Thomas Hall, manufacturer of electrical and optical equipment, took over Davis' operation in Boston (Ari Davis, brother of Daniel, Jr, was instrument maker in Boston and Washington, DC). Hall's shop was located at 19 Bromfield Street, Boston, MA, for 34 years. In 1886, Otto Flemming acquired the Thomas Hall business. Thirty- four years is often enough for the lifespan of an individual to run a business; particularly if the individual was engaged in similar work prior to assuming ownership of the firm. Hall was probably pleased to sell his business before retiring (or dying) around 1886. The Hall line then was moved from Boston to Philadelphia where Flemming was in business. Although the French Battery series helped to keep Hall

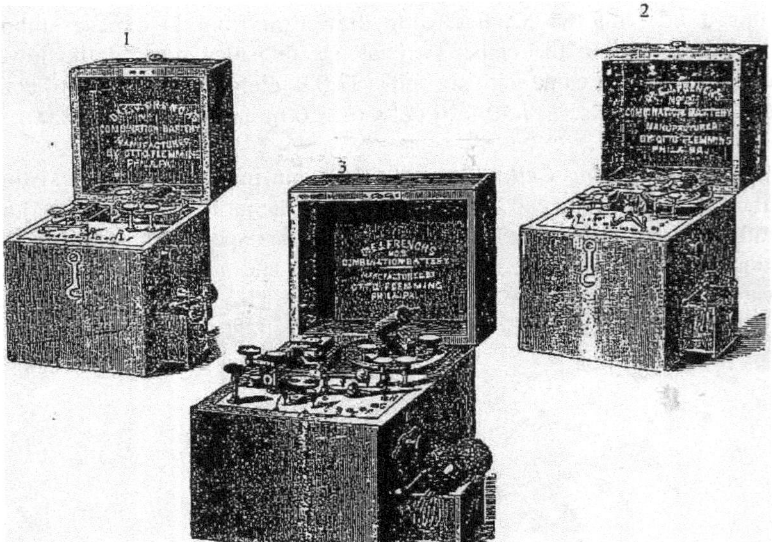

Fig F22. Dr EJ French Combination Batteries

in business locally (published few catalogs), the line was apparently not a nationally popular battery based on the paucity of artifacts found today.

Flemming took over the Thomas Hall line of three batteries of Dr EJ French around 1886. The French batteries are known for delivering many variations of currents. The No.1 Combination Battery delivered 15 different variations of current, and sold for $25.00. The No.2

Combination Battery sold for $30.00 and had 23 current variations. The No.3 Combination Battery of French furnished 28 grades of current. These variations of current were produced by wiring the induction coils with different lengths, metals, and sizes that, in turn, produce different thermal outcomes. In 1886, the different current variations were believed to produce different therapeutic effects, but sometime later this belief was dropped as false and the change is reflected in the design of the medical electrical batteries. The No.1 and No.2 batteries have vibrating rheotomes for rapid pulse rates, but the No.3 has both slow and rapid interrupters. Additionally, the No.3 battery has a pole changer (commutator) along with the conventional electrical components for $35.00 in 1886. Dr EJ French published two books of note, on electricity. In 1863, Medical Electricity Chicago, IL, was published, while editions of his A New Path in Electrical Therapeutics were published in 1873, 1875, and 1876 in Philadelphia, PA. This latter book and edition was selling for $2.00 in 1886, and was a popular book on anatomy, hygiene, physiology, and the value of electricity for curing disease.

The French batteries were quality units housed in French polished black walnut with a carrying handle on top, and a hook latch on

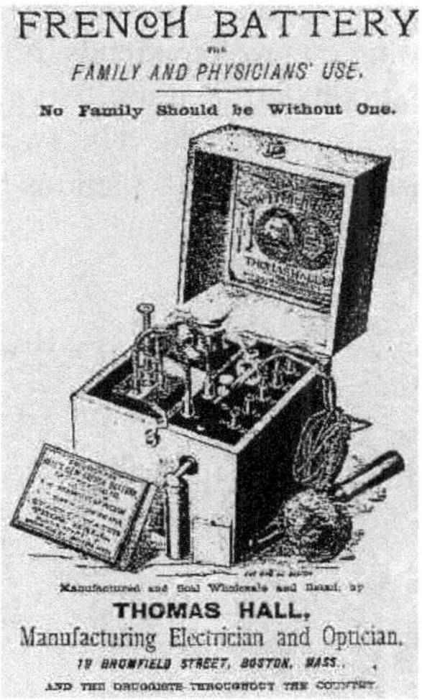

Fig F23. Hall's French Battery for Family and Physicians

the front. With cell, its fluid, box, and electrical components the weight is only about four pounds.

This faradic battery (Fig F23) was designed for travel and to operate for six months before renewing the wet cell. Unlike other French batteries this particular unit made by Hall, and then made and sold by Otto Flemming Co offered three different currents (primary, secondary, combination).This unit has an armature that vibrates on an elastic like substance to control the vibrations. The current amplitude was controlled by a regulating rod of immersion of the zinc element in the battery fluid. Five metal receptacles line the right side of the face plate and are marked "N, P, N, PN, and P," respectively. The faradic battery pictured here dates around 1877, and is unlike No.1 through No.3 offered in 1886 by Flemming.[3]

Universal Battery. This was a newly marketed combination model and first listed in the 1886 catalog, although its patent was filed in March 1883 and issued in June 1885. It served as a double-cell cautery (20 to 40 cells), a 20-cell continuous galvanic current battery, and a faradic battery with slow and rapid interruptions. The model cost $120.00 complete, but without the faradic function it cost $95.00. The wooden case (29 x 11.5 x 18 inches) is designed to permit convenience and efficiency for the operator.

Two systems of 10 zinc and carbon plates were suspended from two hard rubber platforms, adjacent to each other on the face plate. A brass connector joins the packs of two cells. Two binding posts are connected to each cell so in combination one or two cells can be used (10 to 20 plates can function). The face plate has a polarity changer, a two point switch to interrupt the current, and on the right side is the faradic section. The current's sliding controller extends through the case.

In the lower front compartment are two movable platforms that can be lowered and raised by a treadle. The two hard rubber cups (6 inches sq x 8 inches); partitioned into 10 sections each that hold the wet

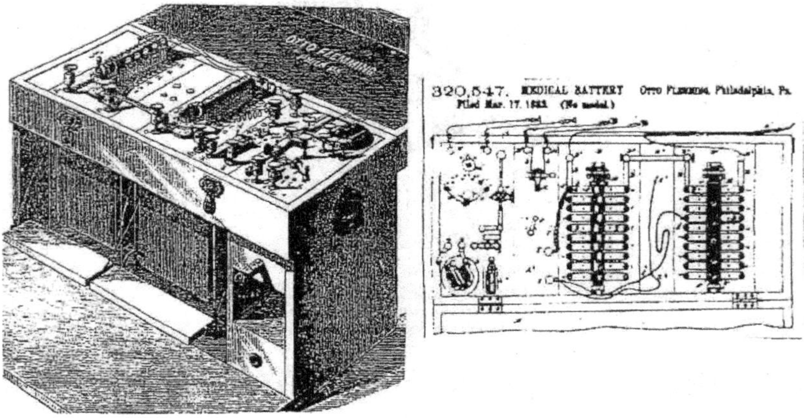

Fig F24. Flemming's Universal Battery

solutions. A ratchet hook at the bottom of the case allows for desired heights. Accessories are stored on the bottom right side of the case. A crude circuitry diagram is shown.

Dental Helix. This small faradic coil was designed by Dr Flagg for relief of pain while extracting teeth. The coil is mounted on a

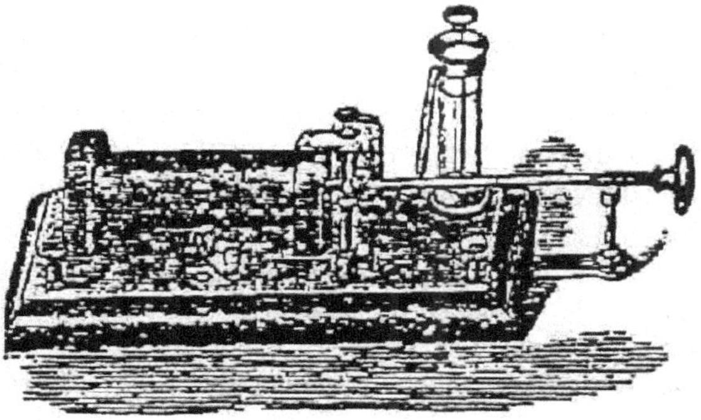

Fig F25. Dental Helix

wooden base as is the adjustable vibrating interrupter, and a water rheostat. The water rheostat has a central brass rod that controls the volume of water in the glass tube offering resistance to the current. The unit sold for $18.00 in 1886.

Galvano-Cautery Batteries

Otto Flemming offered physicians an electrical source to destroy tissue beneath specialized electrodes (eg: for nasopharyngeal operations, skin problems, warts), and to provide galvanic current. These particular batteries used wet cells in 1886, and Flemming provided directions for making fluid just for these cautery batteries. His recommendation was to dissolve one pound of bichromate of potash in

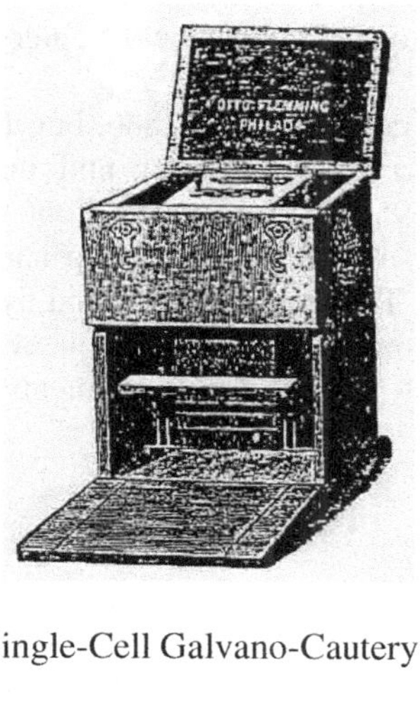

Fig F26. Single-Cell Galvano-Cautery Battery

one gallon of boiling water. Twenty-four fluid ounces of commercial sulfuric acid was added when the solution was cold. Then eight fluid ounces of nitrate of ammonium (saturated sol), and one and a half ounces of bisulfate of mercury was mixed with one pint of cold water before being added to the solution. Since the cell (s) of the galvano-cautery batteries were quite large, three quarts of solution were required for one cell.

Double-Cell Galvano-Cautery Battery. The unit of Fig F27 has a commutator (pole changer) for switching the cautery into a 10-cell galvanic battery. The wooden case (13.25 x 11.5 x 18 inches) was hinged at the top for reaching the electrical components, and hinged in front of the case (0.5 of area). This simple designed battery cost $30.00 in 1886. The open ends of the face plate are used for accessories.

This cautery model was housed in a wooden case (23.5 x 11.5 x 18 inches) with the case designed similarly to that of the Single-Cell unit.

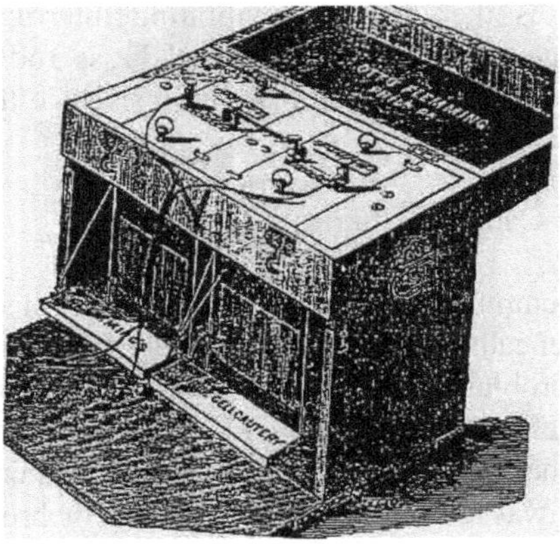

Fig F27. Double-Cell Galvano-Cautery Battery

The basic unit cost $50.00 in 1886, but if the consumer wanted the capability of converting the cautery unit into a 20 cell galvanic battery the cost was $95.00. The hinged front of the case permitted access to the cells. The top lid has a carrying handle and is secured by two latches in the front. The front lid is secured by a pivot hook latch on each side of the case. Connecting cords were heavy and doubled (split at each end). The face plate has small compartments with lids on each end for accessories.

Summary

The last trace of Otto Flemming found in the literature was in 1904. The company was a small manufactory that produced fine medical electrical batteries for over 27 years. Otto Flemming was best known on the east coast so he probably never had a sales force other than his few catalogs and perhaps sellers of medical supplies in cities of the east. His batteries are not equipped for commercial power sources of alternating or direct current that became standardized between 1900 and 1915. Otto Flemming like several other small manufactures of medical electrical batteries of the same period of time disappeared when their product lines failed to convert to the commercial power sources or the company did not enter the x-ray business.

Of course Otto Flemming may have closed his business because of age and retirement after many years in business with Talbot and for himself. Technical advances were taking place in his field that he did not care to confront.

References

1. The City Directory. Philadelphia, PA, 1877, p 507

2. Davis AB, Dreyfus MS. The Finest Instruments Ever Made. Arlington, MA, Med Hist Pub Assocs, 1986, pp 34, 134

3. Illustrated Catalogue of Flemmings. Philadelphia, PA, 1886

4. Polk's Medical Register and Directory of North America. Chicago, IL, RL Polk Pub,1904, p 2561

5. Stewart DD, Lawrance ES. Essentials of Medical Electricity. Philadelphia, PA, WB Saunders, 1892, pp 55-59

6. Catalog of Max Wocher & Son Co. Cincinnati, OR, 1905

7. Liebig GA, Rohe GH. Practical Electricity in Medicine and Surgery. Philadelphia, PA, FA Davis, 1890, p 223

CHAPTER 7. GALVANO-FARADIC MANUFACTURING COMPANY OF NEW YORK CITY

Chapter 7 reviews the role of Frederick Bartlett of the Galvano-Faradic company, and electrical batteries that the company produced. Frederick Bartlett along with SA Banks founded the Galvano-Faradic Manufacturing Company of New York City in 1870. This company became one of the earliest firms in the United States after the Civil War to manufacture (mass produce) medical electrical batteries and their accessories. After the war a market developed with physicians in the United States demanding quality electrotherapeutic apparatuses with the latest technology. Electrotherapeutics, while popular in England and Europe was gaining popularity in the United States. Technology of electricity was also advancing, although there was still limited commercial use for it in 1870. Thus, the source of electrical power for medical batteries was the cell (wet or dry).

SA Banks was the president while F Bartlett was the secretary of the new company located at 167 East 34th Street. The new company did not waste anytime before going into production (maybe as early as 1870) with several models of electrical batteries. The company issued a trade catalog (27 pp) as early as 1871 for portable electrical magnetism, galvanic batteries, and apparatuses.[1] Many of its products were patented in 1870 prior to publication of the catalog. The company issued its fourth edition trade catalog in 1874 (56 pp with additional 3 pages of testimonials by satisfied physician customers). This catalog in addition to promoting product lines served to instruct and make physicians more knowledgeable in medical electricity. The approach of placing instructional material in advertisement and product catalogs was a good business practice to keep those already using medical electrical batteries informed while recruiting new customers by educating them about the use of manufactured products. The editor of this catalog in 1874 classified medical electrical apparatuses into electromagnetic devices and the galvanic battery. Differences between the apparatuses were the type of currents delivered: one was pulsed (electromagnetic for muscle contractions) and one was unidirectional (galvanic for chemical effects).

In 1877, the company was located at 288 Fourth Avenue, and was advertised as a manufactory of various types of medical electrical apparatuses. It remained at this location through 1881.[2]

The use of medical electrical batteries was growing in popularity in medicine in the 1870s. Since electrotherapeutics was not a traditional or even an accepted subject taught in the medical curricula, the manufacturers moved to close the knowledge gap. Success in the endeavor of educating physicians about electrical treatments was somewhat based on getting physicians to write the information for the catalogs. Bartlett gathered his writers from the Graduate

Electrotherapeutic School of New York, a post graduate program to educate practicing physicians in electrotherapeutics. This practice of using a company's trade catalog as an educational tool was followed by others (eg: McIntosh; Traux, Greene & Co). Noted electrotherapeutists were also commissioned by some firms to write books featuring the company's batteries.

The trade catalog of 1881 (107 pages) illustrated products that the company both manufactured and retailed, and its size reflects company growth since 1870. The catalog entitled <u>Electricity and Illustrated Catalog of Standard Electrical Apparatus for Medical Uses</u> was both a manual of basic information about medical electricity, its uses, and listing of products. Additional trade catalogs were published by this company in 1874, 1887, 1890, 1891 (ed 26), 1895, 1905, and its 45th edition in 1911. During these times, the company moved. In 1882, the company was operating from 335 4th Avenue, and in 1883 through 1895 the company was located at 300 4th Avenue and 314 East 22nd Avenue. The location of 300 4th Avenue remained stable through its acquistion in 1905 and until closure around 1914. The company produced quality electrical apparatuses for physicians that were powered by batteries (wet and dry cells), but like most other companies in this field the x-ray soon became a dominant product after 1896. The Galvano-Faradic Mfg Co is well known for its static electrical machine, The Morton-Wimshurst Influence Machine, in the 1890s. The influence machines powered the first x-ray tubes because of their high frequency and low amplitude current.

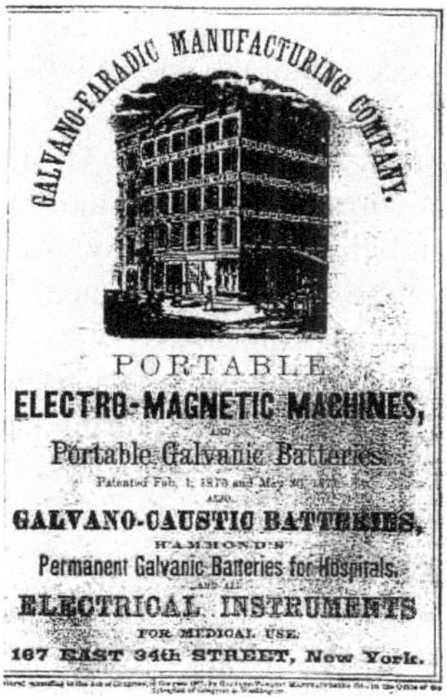

Fig G1. The Galvano-Faradic Manufacturing Company, 1871

A relation developed between the Galvano-Faradic Manufacturing Co and the Van Houten & Ten Broeck Company of New

York City that also formed in 1870. The relation is cloudy but either Galvano-Faradic Manufacturing Co was sold in 1879 to Van Houten & Ten Broeck when F Bartlett and Dr Henry E Waite founded The Waite & Bartlett Manufacturing Company of New York, or it was acquired by Van Houten in 1905 when F Bartlett died.

If sold in 1879, F Bartlett then concentrated all of his energies and innovations with The Waite & Bartlett Manufacturing Co until his death in 1905. Another version is that the Waite & Bartlett Manufacturing Co supposedly absorbed The Galvano-Faradic Manufacturing Co with Bartlett's death according to Grigg,[3] and probably sold the company to The Van Houten & Ten Broeck Co in 1905. Because of duplicated facilities and products the company was perhaps sold to Van Houten & Ten Broeck Co which then continued to market medical electrical products with The Galvano-Faradic Mfg Co trade name, but used both their own address (214-216 East 23rd St) and that of 300 Fourth Ave in 1911.

The products of The Van Houten & Ten Broeck Co were advertised and sold using those of The Galvano-Faradic Manufacturing Co through the 1893 catalog of AS Aloe, a retailing company in St Louis (see Sellers of Home & Physician Shock Machines). The Galvanic Battery was a series of galvanic apparatuses. The apparatuses were designed with selective battery power of 10, 12, 16, 20, 24, 30, 32, or 36 wet cells in 1911. Van Houten & Ten Broeck published the last catalog of The Galvano-Faradic Mfg Co's products about 1911, and soon afterwards developed financial problems. The company went into receivership in 1914 and by 1916 their stock was worthless.[1] Ironically, Van Houten & Ten Broeck catalogs once advised readers to "look before you leap."[3]

The Van Houten & Ten Broeck Co trade catalog for the 28th edition showed an assortment of Galvano-Faradic Mfg Co medical electrical batteries, and that the company was located at 300 Fourth Avenue. Up to this time The Van Houten & Ten Broeck Co was manufacturing influence machines and x-ray units, but retailing the product line of The Galvano-Faradic Mfg Co. Purchase of The Galvano-Faradic Mfg Co gave them the manufacturing capabilities for what was a new product line for them, the conventional faradic and galvanic medical electrical batteries. By 1905, however, the peak markets for these apparatuses had passed, although considerable volume of these apparatuses continued to sell. Section 1 of this catalog listed: faradic batteries, galvanic batteries, combined batteries, cautery batteries, milliampere meters, and electrodes.

Commonalties of Galvano-Faradic Mfg Co Electrical Apparatus

Major identifying features of the Galvano - Faradic's faradic apparatuses (batteries) are: 1) the induction coils have adjacent metal sleeves to the metal end caps that raise the coil above the face plate; 2) use metal signature plates on the inside lid of its apparatuses; 3) have vertical rather than horizontal (to face plate) spring lever, hammer vibrators, and 4) use heavy quality metal (nickel plated) fixtures. The galvanic units can be identified by: 1) use of metal signature plates on the inside of the lid of their apparatuses; 2) have a circular metal ring with metal buttons for each cell; 3) use heavy quality metal (nickel plate) fixtures; 4) use two hinged ring rods that lift the cell tray; 5) use a lever device on the wet cell to push down to elicit slow pulses and pull up to gain rapid pulse rates; and 6) the hydrastat is located on the front side of the wooden box.

Faradic Batteries

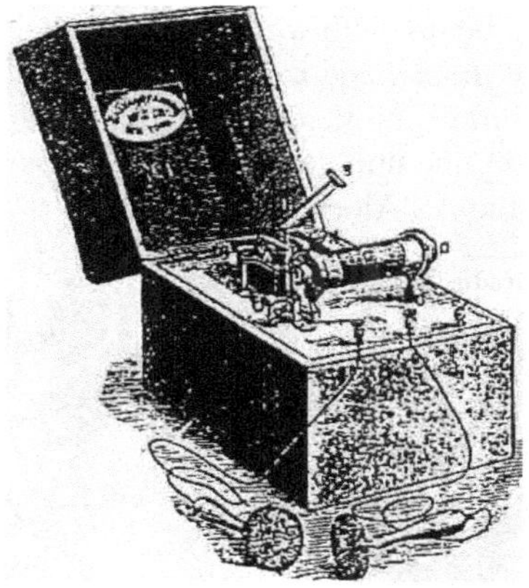

Fig G2. No. 1 Faradic Battery

No.1 Faradic Battery. The No.1 unit typifies (with some exceptions) the other faradic (electromagnetic) apparatuses made by this company. This particular faradic battery was offered by The Galvano-Faradic Mfg Co in 1871, and was still a popular electrical medical battery (without design changes) in 1905 (34 years later) when Van Houten & Ten Broeck Co was selling the product line of their newly acquired company. The unchanged design was then continued until around 1914. This unit was powered by one Grenet type wet cell that may have delivered about 1.1 volts. The Galvano-Faradic Mfg Co redesigned the cap or lid of the glass jar. The jar cap has a graduated hinged brass rod that attaches at its lower end to the zinc element. The hinge permits the rod to fold to prevent the immersion of the zinc element when the cell is not in use. The rod lowers and raises the zinc element, and the graduated marks on the rod measures depth, thus an arbitrary battery output. The cap has a metallic seal between the cap and glass lip that was patented in May 1871 and called the Powell hydrostat by The Galvano-Faradic Mfg Co.

The hydrastat prevented liquid from leaking or spilling when the apparatus was carried by hand or by buggy by city and country doctors. The No.1 unit was designed for home use and was among the best for that purpose. The wooden face plate contained the induction coil with its metal end caps that elevate the coil above the plate; a sliding metal current controller, and to its left an adjustable screw spring lever, hammer vibrator (rheotome). Two or three metal receptacles are located on the front portion of the face plate to serve as connecting posts for primary and secondary current, and with three posts the addition of combined currents is available. The company sold its units with either nickel plated metal or with raw metal.

In 1871, the faradic apparatuses were housed in either black walnut or mahogany boxes with a hinged lid that is secured by a front located lock and key, hooks and eyes, and with metal carrying handles. The No.1, a small family unit, nickel plated, sold for $11.00 in 1871 through 1874. In 1893, the unit came in a polished oak box, and sold for $10.00 according to the AS Aloe catalog.[4]

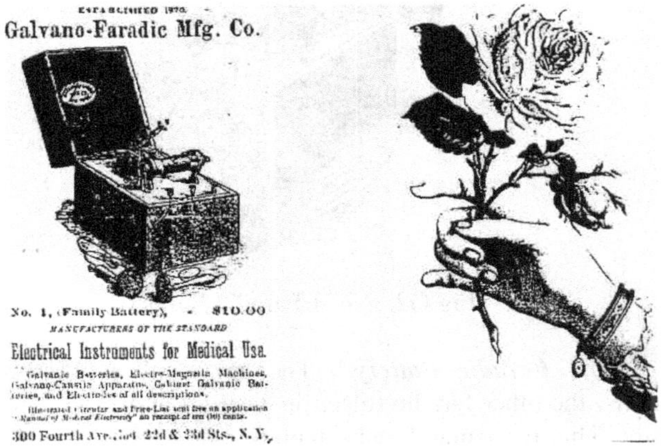

Fig G3. Trade Card (both sides)

Trade Card. The Galvano-Faradic Manufacturing Company also had a trade card representing this particular model of medical electrical battery. Such trade cards were passed out by sales people to attract customers. These cards were often 3 x 5 inches in size and were attractive (chromatic color). The No.1 Faradic Battery (Family Battery) was built in 1878, yet the address (300 Fourth Ave) shown on the card was that of Van Houten & Ten Broeck when they occupied that site in 1911 after moving from their original site from around the corner at 214-216 East 23rd Street, New York City. In 1911, Van Houten & Ten Broeck was selling the 1878 designed faradic electrical machine of The Galvano-Faradic Mfg Co pictured for $10.00.

Electro-Magnetic Machine No.2. A popular and well constructed faradic electrical battery in 1871 for family use (Fig G4) was the No.2 unit that used a single wet cell for power. The signature plate inside the lid of this particular unit reads "Galvano-Faradic Mfg Co, pats Feb 21, 1870; May 3, 1871, Mar 26, 1872, NY." The Company at this time was located at 300 Fourth Ave between 22nd and 23rd Streets. The unit was housed in either a black walnut or oak box (8.25 x 7.75 x 7.25 inches) that has a metal carrying handle on top of the lid. The corners of the box have diagonal wood wedge tongues, and all hardware are nickel plated. The face plate or panel is wood to match the wood of the box and has three sections (A = 2.5 x 3.37 inches to house accessories; B = 4.75 x 3.37 inches for a glass Grenet type wet cell with cover holding zinc and

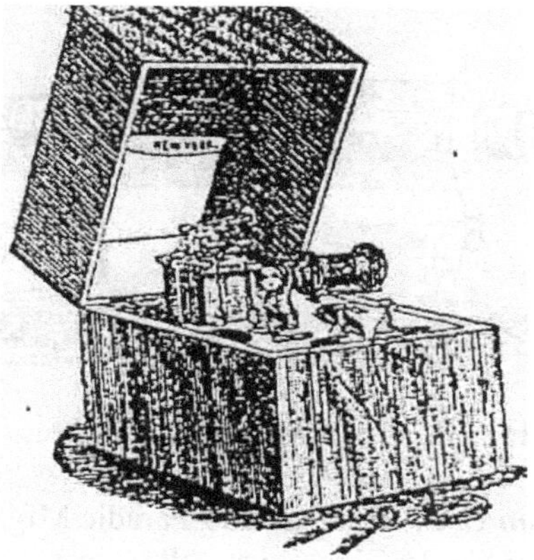

Fig G4. Electro-Magnetic Machine No. 2 (1871)

carbon elements and lever to raise and lower them; and C = 7.25 x 3.37 inches for the metal induction coil of 4.5 x 1 inches with nickel plated closed ends). On the left side of the induction coil is an adjustable screw spring lever, hammer interrupter; and on the right side is a sliding core tube rheotome (4 x 0.75 inches) that controls current amplitude. The face panel also has two connecting poles (posts) to the cell; three receptacle poles marked by plates "1, 2, 3" with primary between 1 and 2, secondary between 2 and 3, and combination between 1 and 3. The electrical components are mounted on top of a polished wooden base with the circuitry embedded underneath the wooden base.

The wet cell for this unit used a solution of bichromate potash (3 oz fine powder) in a mixture of sulfuric acid (3 oz) and water (1 pint boiling). When the solution was cool it was poured into the Grenet type jar. The Grenet cell consists of a glass jar that holds the electrolyte and fits into section B of the apparatus. There are two plates or elements, one zinc plate in the center with a connecting pole on the lid of the jar, and a carbon plate on each side and two connecting poles for them. The brass rod lever on the lid of the cell lifts and lowers the zinc plate from the electrolyte when the cell is not at work. Bichromate cells give an efficient current amplitude and an electromotive force of two volts. One No.6 dry cell or one Grenet wet cell was recommended for its power source, and the unit sold for $4.00. The cells sold separately for $0.40 and $2.50, respectively. The No.2 faradic battery was designed for family or home use, and was advertised as the medium size family unit. The machines were quality constructed compared with most units sold by major mail order companies. These two electro-magnetic or faradic apparatuses were patented in 1870. Like all of The Galvano-Faradic Mfg Co electrical batteries the metal was a dull polished steel finish. The company sold this unit for $16.00 in 1871, $19.00 in 1874, and $15.00 in 1893 (AS Aloe catalog).[4]

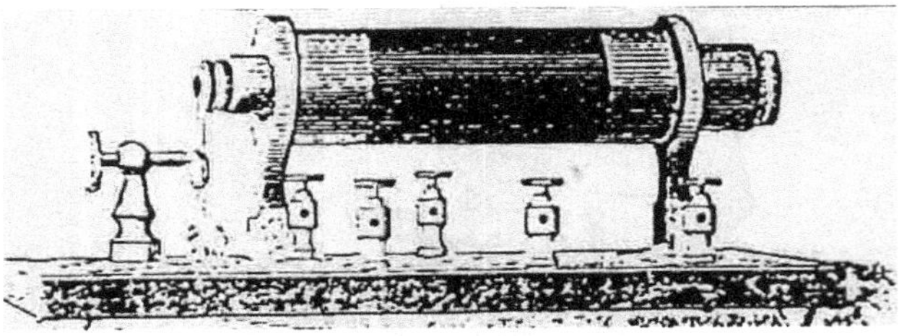

Fig G5. No. 2 Induction Coil

No.2 Induction Coil. The Galvano-Faradic Mfg Co also made a coil to be operated by a single Grenet wet cell or one dry cell. This unit probably became available in 1905, and sold for $4.00 without a cell. The price reflects a basic faradic unit without any frill (eg, a case to house the coil and cell). This coil is the epitome of the basic coil for The Galvano-Faradic Mfg Co's electrical batteries since 1871. The adjustable screw, spring lever, hammer, vibrating interrupter is vertical rather than horizontal to the face plate as seen on other brands of electrical batteries.

Faradic Battery No.3. This battery is similar to that of No.1 and 2 by The Galvano-Faradic Mfg Co except that its rheotome serves as two interrupters, and was designed for physician use. One interrupter is similar in design and operation as the conventional adjustable screw spring lever, hammer vibrator except in this No.3 model the hammer with its attachments are at right angle to the core of the coil. The vibrating interrupter controls fast faradic pulses. The other interrupter is a core mounted on a spring for vibration, a spring lever part is a "fork" that is adjustable for controlling the cone. An adjustable screw, connected to the circuit that contacts the cone to provide slow current pulses when the cone vibrates. The "fork" is an adjustable spring or elastic fork; its free

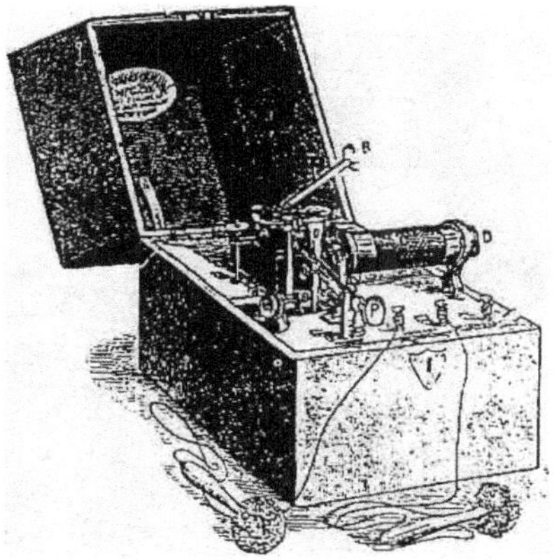

Fig G6. Faradic Battery No.3[4]

end embraces the hammer (vibrating armature) between the prongs to control vibrations. The upper end of the hammer vibrates freely when the fork is depressed. This fork design enables the operator to control the interval between each shock. The coil was designed with a coil output that was more powerful than those recommended for home use, and it offered three variations of current. The design makes for a versatile faradic battery. Like the No.1 battery, this unit is powered by one wet cell. The unit is housed in a black walnut or an oak box with a hinged lid, and metal carrying handle. It is secured by a lock and key in front, and on each side by a hook lever latch. Around 1893, it sold for $20.00 by AS Aloe, in 1905 Van Houten & Ten Broeck was selling the unit for $15.00. Its original cost in 1871 by The Galvano-Faradic Mfg Co was $22.00 without nickel plated metal, and $25.00 with nickel plated metal in 1872 through 1874. The face plate is matching wood like the case, and is divided into three compartments. The largest compartment houses the operational components; the smallest compartment with lid is for accessories; and the middle sized compartment is cutout to expose and contain the wet cell case. The cell case is exposed with its cap having attachments to connect with the circuit and an adjustable screw to raise and lower the carbon element. The customer had a choice of either a black walnut or polished oak case (8 x 7.5 x 7.25 inches), glued corners reinforced with corner pegs, otherwise the unit is the same as Nos.1 and 3. This model dates from 1871 (patented 1870), so in 1905 the unit had been marketed for about 34 years without design changes.

No.4 Double-Cell Battery. This faradic battery for physicians was offered by The Galvano-Faradic Mfg Co in 1871 for $33.00, and in 1874 for $37.00, but by 1895 the unit had been phased out. A reserve cell was carried in the unit to be used as a spare if the other cell became exhausted, and in combination with the other cell to increase the total voltage in cases of suspended animation (cardiac resusitation). The idea

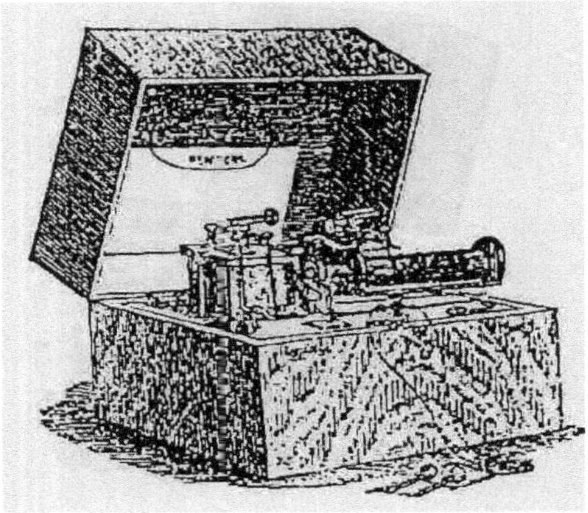

Fig G7. No. 4 Double-Cell Battery

for the extra cell may have been borrowed from Dr Jerome Kidder who manufactured some faradic electrical batteries with an extra cell. With this No.4 unit the company introduced its hard rubber cell casing that replaced glass jars for wet cells. The No.4 faradic apparatus also used the "fork" or lever device (like the No.3 Faradic Battery) for controlling slow and rapid pulse rates. Other than the Otto Flemming and Galvano-Faradic Mfg Co units, no other American company used the lever type of interrupter for slow pulse frequencies. A wooden box houses the apparatus; it has a hinged lid that locks with a key along with two hook lever latches in front. The induction coil has the metal end caps for elevating and supporting it, and is covered by fabric. Two metal receptacle connecting posts were also mounted on the front center part of the face plate.

Closed Cell Faradic Battery. This battery was designed for either physician or home use. This is a small compact unit enclosed in a polished black walnut or oak box that opens with a hinged lid that is cut into one fourth of the total box height to form an L- shaped box when open. The box is carried by a metal handle on top and has a self locking latch on front of the lid. The rear one fourth part of the box is used for accessories and the lower half of the box contains one wet cell as a source of power. The unit has a metal induction coil with a sliding metal tube (controller) on the right end for current amplitude control. Primary, secondary, and combined currents are provided by the induction coil. The left side of the coil is the conventional adjustable screw spring lever,

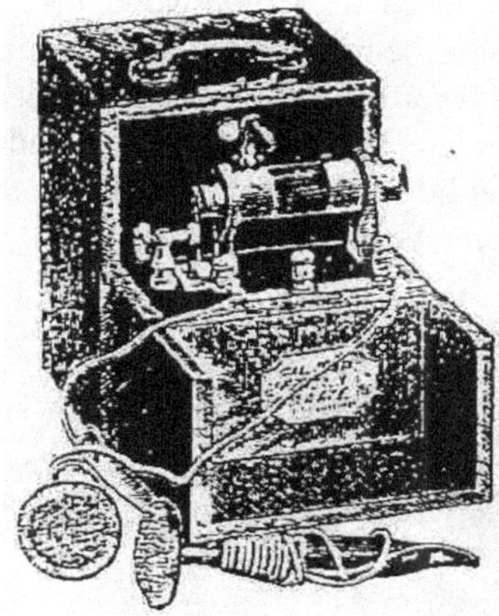

Fig G8. Closed Cell Faradic Battery[4]

hammer type of vibrating interrupter. Three adjustable screw connecting posts are also part of the face plate, like the other components. This unit was sold through the AS Aloe catalog in 1893 for $12.00.[4]

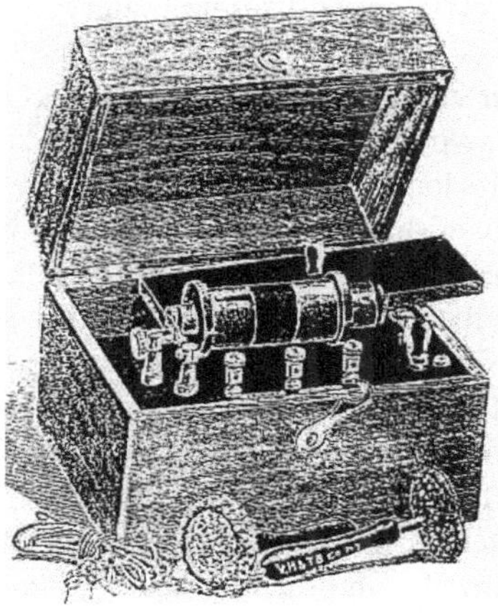

Fig G9. No. 5 Faradic Battery

No.5 Faradic Battery. The No.5 unit (Fig G9) was designed for home use and small enough to carry in the trunk of the traveler. The unit used a single standard dry cell that was located underneath the face plate. The face plate contains the metal induction coil with its sliding tube current controller; a lever On/Off control; three adjustable screw connection posts for providing primary, secondary, and combined currents; and an adjustable screw spring lever hammer, vibrator type of interrupter. The unit is housed in a birchwood box that has a wedge holding the glued corners of the box. The box has a heavy metal carrying handle and a heavy metal lever front latch to secure the hinged lid. A rear compartment of the face plate houses accessories, and has a metal knob post to remove its wooden lid. Around 1905, the unit sold for $7.00, and was relatively new that same year.

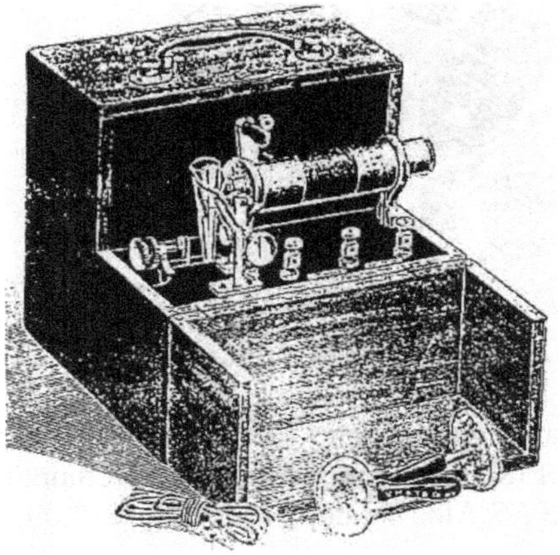

Fig G10. No. 6 Faradic Battery

No.6 Faradic Battery. The battery in Fig G10 was designed for physician use, and was powered by two No.6 dry cells (standard 2.25 x 6.25 inches) that were located underneath the face plate. The unit was encased in an oak box of different design. The box was built so that half of the upper portion of the box's width serves as a compartment for accessories, and the other half of the upper portion serves as the lid (the box is L-shaped on side view). The upper part of the box has a metal carrying handle and a lever latch on front to secure the lid. The face plate houses the metal coil with its sliding tube current controller; a cone shaped vibrator for slower and variable interruptions, and an adjustable screw spring lever interrupter for rapid current interruptions; a metal coil that supplies three currents; and three adjustable screw connection posts. All metal are heavy nickel plated. In 1905, the unit sold for $15.00 and dates from that time.

No.7 Faradic Battery. This unique faradic battery was designed for gynecologists for very rapid and very slow current pulses. The unit has three secondary coils that adjust to two primary coils with windings tapped by intervals to provide in effect seven coils. The secondary coils are wound with different sized wire and lengths to give effects of seven coils; the finest coils use No.36 wire and are wound with 1500, 1000, and 500 yards, respectively; No.32 wire wound by 800, 500, and 300 yards lengths provide medium coils; while No. 22 wire wound by 250 yards

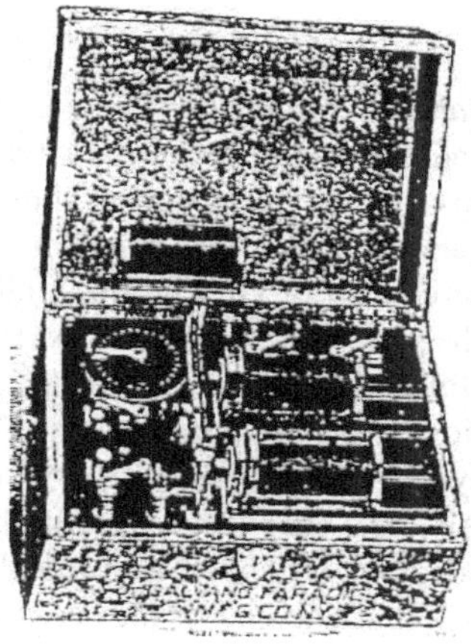

Fig G11. No. 7 Faradic Battery

provides a coarse coil. These coils adjust to two primary coils with one fitted to a cone shaped vibrator for slow muscle contractions, and two with a ribbon vibrator (singing rheotome). The ribbon vibrator was a new idea at the time to provide a wide range of interruptions per second. The design was to provide the most versatile of applications. The three coils are covered by black paper. The device is encased in an oak box with four No.6 dry cells (underneath the face plate) connected in series with a rheostat for fine control of current amplitude. The wooden box is hinged with a lid (1 coil mounted on inside lid); face plate has two coils; rheostat; lever On/Off control; two adjustable screw connecting posts; and two coil selector lever controls. The unit sold for $45.00 in 1905, and was the most popular electrical battery among physician customers of the company at the time.

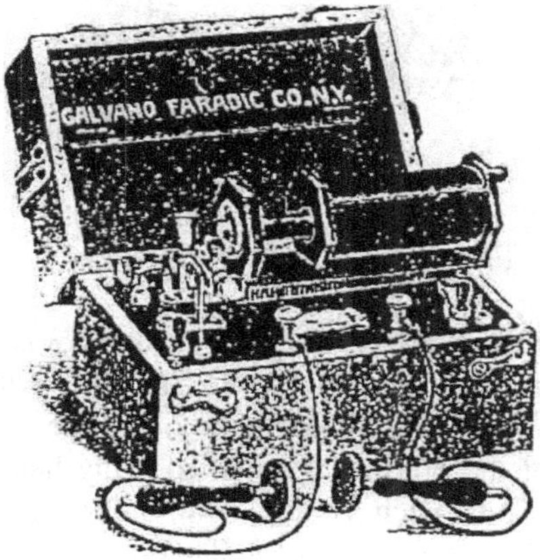

Fig G12. No. 8 Faradic Battery

No.8 Faradic Battery. Fig G12 shows a unit that was designed after the DuBois-Reymond prototype sledge inductorium. The design of the sledge inductorium has the secondary coil(s) sliding over the primary coil (in this unit over the soft iron core) which allows adjustments of minute increments or decrements of current amplitudes with the sliding toward or away from the zero position. This particular unit was the company's second most frequently sold electrical faradic battery because it was ideal for diagnostic and physiological study. The two interrupters (cone and spring lever type vibrators) permit very slow and very rapid current pulses, respectively. The secondary winding has No.36 insulated copper wiring, 1500 yards, and is tapped at intervals of 1000 and 500 yards. An adjustable switch at one end of the secondary coil allows the desired windings of the coil. The sledge inductorium type of electrical faradic battery allows secondary coils of different windings, other than those listed, to be used on the unit by changing the existing secondary coil and sliding the alternate one along the track. The unit is housed in an oak box; carried by a leather strap attached to the hinged lid; and the lid is secured by two lever type latches on the front of the box. The unit is powered by two No.6 dry cells, and sold for $25.00 in 1905.

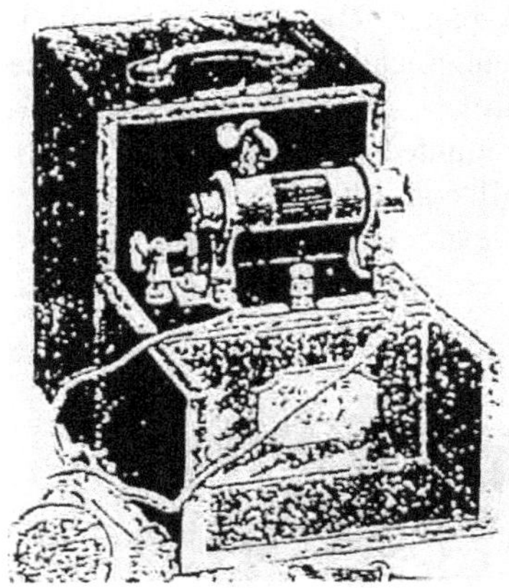

Fig G13. No.9 Faradic Battery[4]

No.9 Faradic Battery. The unit of Fig G13 is encased in an oak box designed like the No.6 unit (L-shaped) with an accessory compartment at the top rear half of the box, and the other top half is the lid. The rear top of the box has a metal carrying handle, and the lid is secured by a spring type latch. A single No. 6 dry cell was located in the rear compartment with the accessories. The face plate covers half of the opened box, and contains: the elevated metal coil with its sliding tube current controller; an adjustable screw spring lever vibrator type of interrupter; a lever On/Off control; and two adjustable screw connecting posts. The unit provides primary, secondary, and combined currents. Van Houten & Ten Broeck sold this Galvano-Faradic battery for $9.00 in 1905.

Goelet Faradic Battery. Dr Goelet was a local authority in New York on electrotherapeutics, and along with innovative ideas about rheostats designed medical electrical batteries. The faradic battery (Fig G14) was designed in 1894 or 1895 for the general practitioner. The unit has three secondary induction coils that provide different levels of current amplitudes for selective medical uses. Two coils are of the DuBois -Reymond or sledge inductorium design that slide over the

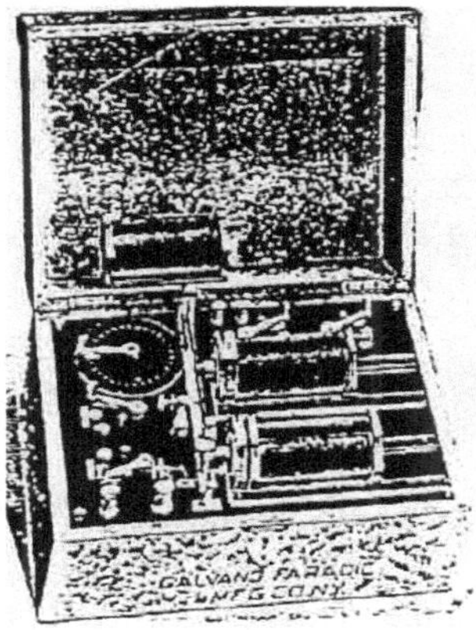

Fig G14. The Goelet Faradic Battery[4]

primary coil. Each of the three secondary coils is wound with different sized wires to provide the needed medical effect. The unit is powered by four dry cells located underneath the face plate. The face plate is flush with the top of the open part of the box. A wooden box houses the operating components, and it has a hinged lid that contains a metal carrying handle on its top and a lock and key for securing the lid. A dial rheostat is provided and is in series with the cells to offer smooth and small graduated increments of current. A coil selector switch is available, along with a lever On/Off control, two adjustable binding posts for cell connections, and two adjustable screw connecting posts complete the components on the face plate. The unit sold for $50.00 in the 1893 AS Aloe catalog.

Galvanic Batteries

Stohrer Galvanic Battery. At the time The Galvano-Faradic Mfg Co was founded (1870) the controversy whether to use faradic or galvanic electricity for treating various diseases still existed among those physicians using medical electrical batteries in their practices. Frederick Bartlett, then the vice president, first introduced an improved version of the famous Stohrer Galvanic Battery of Germany for sale. The Stohrer battery had a great reputation in the world, but it was inconvenient by design (shape and portability). Then 'Yankee' ingenuity prevailed.

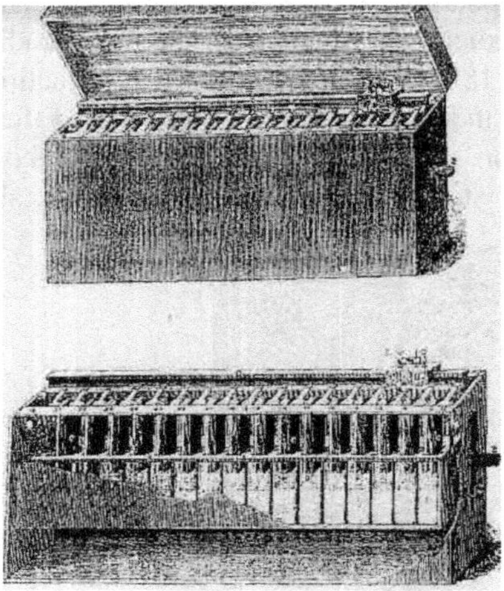

Fig G15. Improved Stohrer's Galvanic Battery

In 1870 and 1871, the general use 16-cell Stohrer (not available in 1877 by G/F) unit cost $30.00. For the addition of a leather strap for carrying the unit (portability) an extra $5.00 was added to the regular price ($35.00 total). Since physicians were using galvanic batteries for electrolysis, more tension or voltage was needed so a 32-cell unit was available for $50.00. Even in 1870, a commutator for current reversal ($3.00), a rheotome for current interruptions ($10.00), and a rheostat for current control ($10.00) were options for the extra cost (s).

Galvanic Unit. Bartlett then designed a galvanic battery (Fig G16) that eliminated the disadvantages of the Stohrer Galvanic Battery. He patented the ***Bartlett Galvanic Battery*** (later identified by its generic description as a 16-cell or a 32-cell or so forth cell galvanic battery) in 1871.

His newly designed galvanic battery was portable, but featured the idea of the "hydrastat" to prevent the spilling of cell fluid. The hydrastat is believed to have originated with F Bartlett and The Galvano-Faradic Mfg Co. Additionally, the Bartlett Galvanic Battery offered the convenience of portability, a commutator, and an electrical rheostat. The hard rubber (gutta percha) cell was also introduced in 1871 by The Galvano-Faradic Mfg Co for the price of $0.25.

The boxes came in polished oak or black walnut. The prototype for this particular galvanic battery was patented in 1870 or 1871, and originally was advertised in the 1874 catalog (ed 4) as "The Bartlett Galvanic Battery." The ***Bartlett Galvanic Battery*** in 1874 was offered with 12 wet cells for eye and ear treatments at $20.00; 24 cells for $ 40.00; and 36 cells for $60.00.

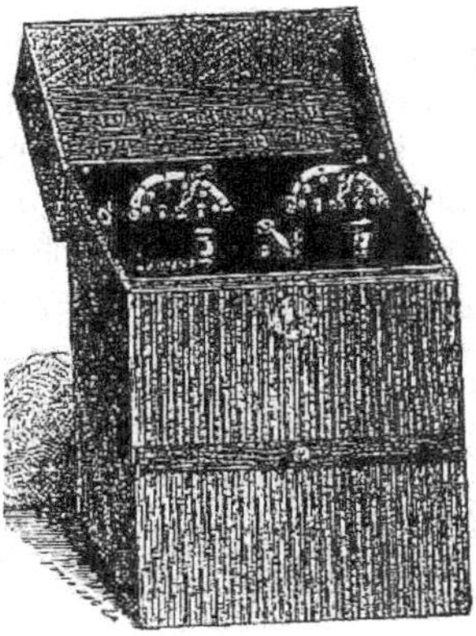

Fig G16. The Bartlett Galvanic Battery

Although patents are meant to limit and restrict copying, others (without patent) around the Fig G17, ***16-Cell Galvanic Unit***. A movable tray holding the cells (eg,12) is located in the bottom of the box (Fig 1). The adjustable rings (Fig 1) hold cells tightly against the hydrostat (Fig 2). Zinc and carbon plates form couples (Fig 3) and are fastened to the base over the cells. Similar features of the innovative item were being marketed in the 1870s.

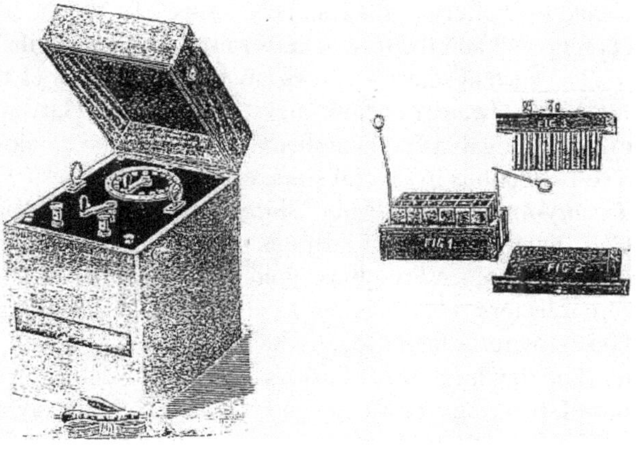

Fig G17. 16-Cell Galvanic Unit.

Between 1894 and 1897 The Galvano-Faradic Manufacturing Co produced the ***Portable Galvanic Battery*** that offered the physician consumer an option of the number of wet cells wanted to contribute to the unit's output. The option was 16, 20, 24, and 30 wet cells. The particular unit shown in Fig G17 has 16 glass jars for wet cells. The unit is encased in a wooden polished oak case (8 x 11 x 12.25 inches) weighing 20 pounds. In the front part of the case is a wooden tray (hydrastat) with an oak lip to match the case. The hydrastat was a paddle (10.75 x 5.75 inches), underside covered with rubber, that separates the glass wet cells from the zinc and carbon elements or couples to secure the battery when traveling in buggys or trolleys. The hydrastat was secured in the case by the nickel plated ring pins on either side of the hard rubber face plate. The top of the wooden case has a steel handle for carrying, and the lid of the case is secured with a pivot type latch that locks onto a disc on each side of the case. Inside of the lid is a small compartment with a hinged lid and pivot latch for storing accessories.

The face plate or panel (rubber) is framed with oak, corner joints are spline and brass reinforced. The face plate contains a 4.75 inches disc current controller with pivot (centered) mounted lever (handle); the disc has 16 buttons for each of 16 cells. Also included on the face plate are a polarity changer (commutator) with pivoting lever with poles acting as stops, and two connecting poles for electrode wires (cautery-electrolysis). The face plate is hard rubber table or panel housing the operating units; each side of framed panel has two lifting rings that screw tightly down to hold cells firmly against the hydrostat (bottom of panel has 16 zinc-carbon mounted couples). Each button corresponding to a cell (0 to 16) is connected to the elements within the disc on the rubber dial by buried wires. With the wire connections encased, the fumes from the fluid cannot reach the operator; no corrosion takes place and the battery is always ready for use. To use the battery, the hydrostat is removed and the tray of cells raised to immerse the elements in the fluid. The current selector allows any desired number (1 to16) cells to activate. All hardware is heavy nickel plated. The Galvano-Faradic Mfg Co offered the galvanic apparatus via the AS Aloe catalog of 1893 with plain cell selections in several sizes, options, and prices.[4]

Twenty-four Cell Galvanic Battery. The Galvano-Faradic Mfg Co's 24-Cell Battery (Fig G18) operates similarly as the 10, 16, and 20 cells units. The difference from these units is that the 24-cell unit has two circular cell selectors, each having 12 metal buttons. Having 24 cells makes all box structures larger (eg, hydrastat, oak box size, cell tray) than other units, but the face plate, besides two-cell selectors, has a lever On/Off control, two rings for raising and lowering the cell tray, and two

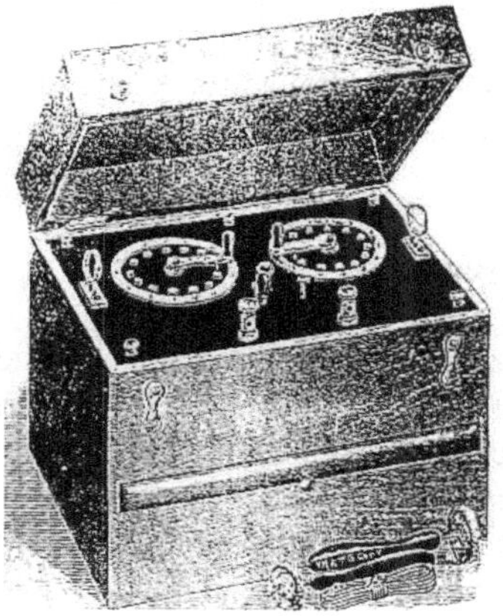

Fig G18. 24-Cell Galvanic Battery

adjustable screw connecting posts. Like the other units, all metal are nickel plated. Five adjustable screws secure the face plate to the box in addition to the rings on the rods. This 24-cell unit sold for $25.00, and a 30-cell unit for $30.00 in 1893.

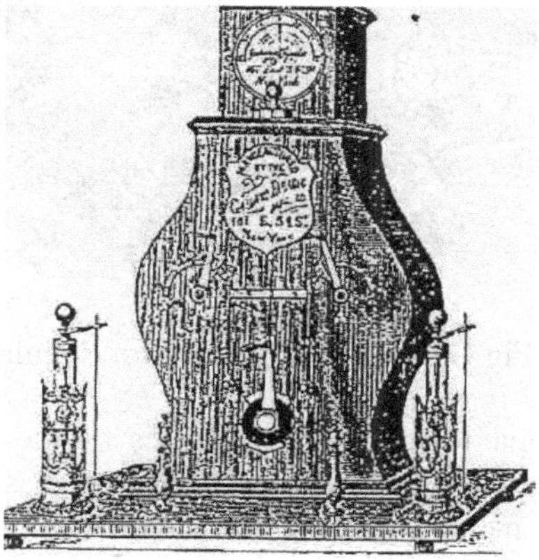

Fig G19. The Regulator

Regulator. The customer who did not want the operating accessories added to the medical electrical battery as one or more components could buy "The Regulator." The Regulator was a device that contained several electrical operating components for the galvanic battery but was not a feature designed in the galvanic batteries. In effect this unit was a rheostat for galvanic batteries. The Regulator contained a galvanoscope that indicated the presence and direction of current; a dial to vary the amplitude of the current; a commutator for reversing the polarity of the current; a water rheostat to smooth the patient's perception of the current; an electric rheotome for interrupting the current; and current selectors to operate selected cells. The Regulator was sold for $125.00 in 1874.

Combination Batteries

New Combination Regulator. This combined battery (Fig G20) contained The Regulator for use with galvanic current, and components to be used with faradic current. This combination regulator was designed for physicians having a large practice and desired convenience of application. The price for the deluxe unit with a Brenner type rheostat was $300.00 in 1874. Options were available to reduce the cost. The cost with a water rheostat was $225.00; 60 cells for $125.00; 100 cells for $225.00, and 125 cells for $275.00.

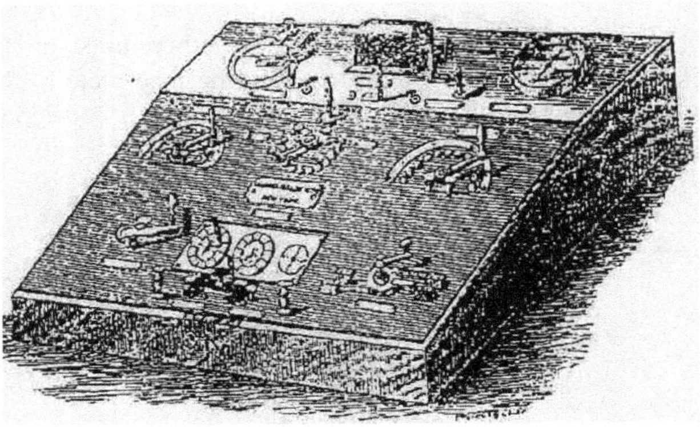

Fig G20. New Combination Regulator

The company provided the names of the 13 institutions and physicians having bought the combination battery and regulator at that time. A common method of providing creditability to a product in the 1870s was to list testimonials or the names of noted physicians (if possible) to the product's description. This approach to advertising was effective then.

Cabinet Regulator. Sometime as early as 1872 or 1873, Dr George M Beard (prominent electrotherapeutist of NewYork City) may have suggested to Frederick Bartlett of The Galvano-Faradic Mfg Co the idea of a desk or dresser for use with a combined electrical battery to provide both faradic and galvanic currents. The idea was to displace electrical cells from the basement or cellar to the physician's office by housing them in a cabinet (desk or dresser). The company responded with its Cabinet Battery or Cabinet Regulator and Batteries in 1874.

The connections of electrical wires to the cells are made at the rear of the drawer that houses the cells in the cabinet. The drawers can

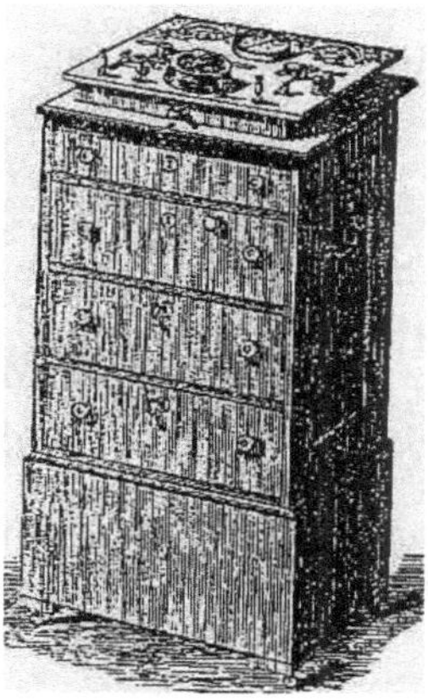

Fig G21. Cabinet Regulator and Batteries

easily be opened for periodic inspections of the cells and for replacement. The battery's face plate is placed on top of the mobile cabinet. The face plate of this particular early model contains a current selector for operating 1 to 60 wet cells; a current reverser, a commutator; a rheotome or interrupter with a push-pull metal rod; and On/Off switch; a short coil galvanoscope; a hydro- or water- rheostat; a faradic coil system; and connecting posts.

This cabinet unit was made with black walnut (38 x 17 x 13 inches) to house both the regulator and 60 cells. The cabinet has three full sized drawers for the batteries. The regulator contained: current selectors; a commutator; a rheotome, galvanoscope; a water rheostat; and a faradic coil system. The unit cost was $200.00 in 1874.

Sixteen-Cell Combination Battery. The company manufactured this 16 - cell unit that serves as both galvanic and faradic electrical

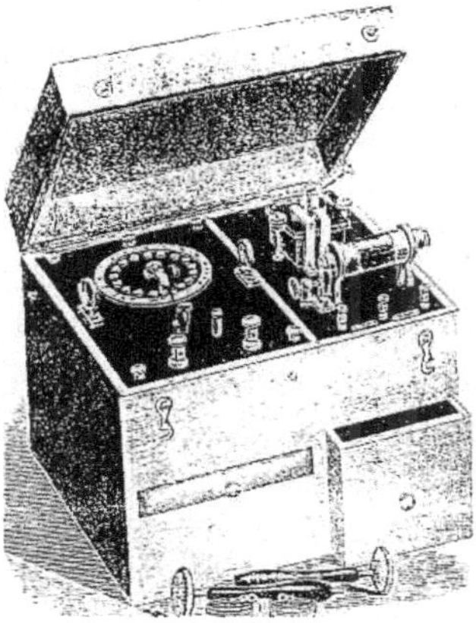

Fig G22. 16-Cell Combination Battery

batteries. The galvanic portion has 16-wet cells, while the faradic portion has a single wet cell; each current section operates independently. The oak box housing the two units looks similar to the units that have one or the other type of current except that two types of current batteries were combined into one box. That is, the right portion of the box is the same as the 16-cell galvanic battery presented, and the left portion of the box is similar to the No.1 Faradic Battery. A drawer from the front of the box is available for accessories. The 16-Cell Combination Battery sold for $28.00 in 1905.

The 24-Cell Combination Battery. This battery of Fig G23 is combined with the No. 1 Faradic Battery. Both the galvanic part and the

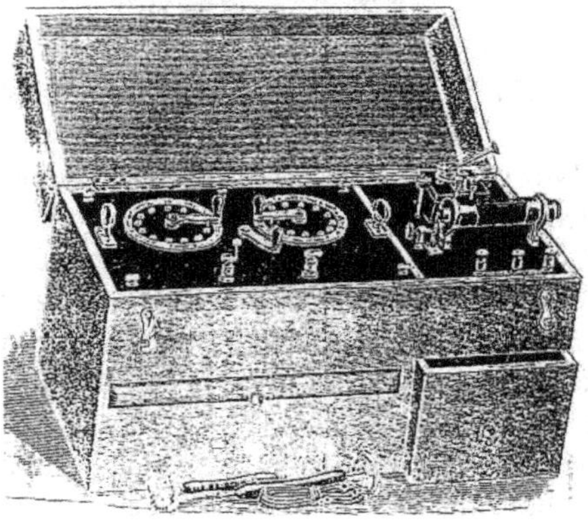

Fig G23. 24-Cell Combination Battery

faradic part in this combined battery are more powerful than the 16-cell combination unit. A drawer for accessories is underneath the faradic face plate, and the hydrastat is fitted from the front in the galvanic battery side of the oak case. This combination battery sold for $36.00 in 1905. The company also sold milliammeters for measuring and regulating current amplitudes during applications, cautery batteries, and office batteries, as well as influence machines.

Office Cabinet No.11. This polished oak cabinet measures 37 x 27 x 23 inches, has a large drawer for accessories, a glass cover, and two wood paneled doors on the cabinet. The cabinet contains two shelves that hold the "Fitch Perfect Battery" of 38 wet cells. The face plate contains two circular cell selectors with a lever control and metal buttons, a milliammeter, a DuBois-Reymond type faradic induction coil, a pole changer, lever On/Off control, a cone and spring lever interrupters, and two adjustable screw connecting poles. The cell selectors are designed so the levers slide from one button to another with one resting on one button to insure a gradual increase or decrease of current without a sudden

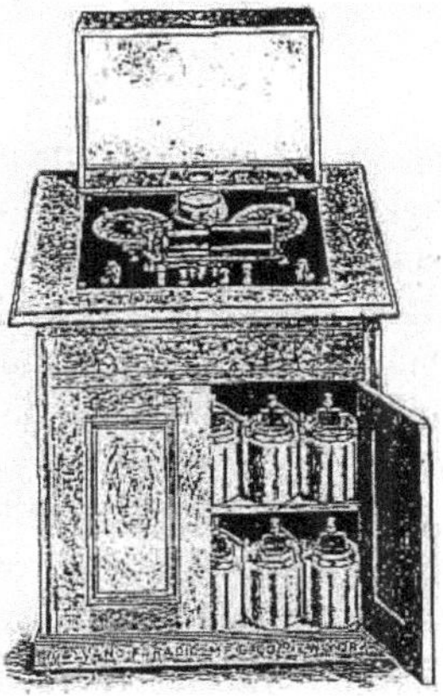

Fig G24. Office Cabinet No. 11

surprise shock. The maker used this method of controlling current amplitudes shock rather than a rheostat. The milliammeter ranges from 1 to 250 milliamperes. The faradic coil has a secondary coil that slides over a primary coil. The secondary coil is wound with 1000 yards of No.32 copper wire that is tapped at 500 yards that in effect serves as two coils, one at 1000 yards and one at 500 yards. The interrupters provide very slow to very rapid current pulses. The faradic battery operates independently from the galvanic battery, and is powered by two wet cells. The Office Cabinet No.11 is mounted on wheels for mobility, and in 1905 sold for $80.00.

The Galvano-Faradic Mfg Co also manufactured a wall battery, office table models, and a cabinet battery. These units offered the physician both faradic and galvanic currents so as to compete with other companies.

Galvano-Faradic Wall Cabinet. The battery of Fig G25 is an

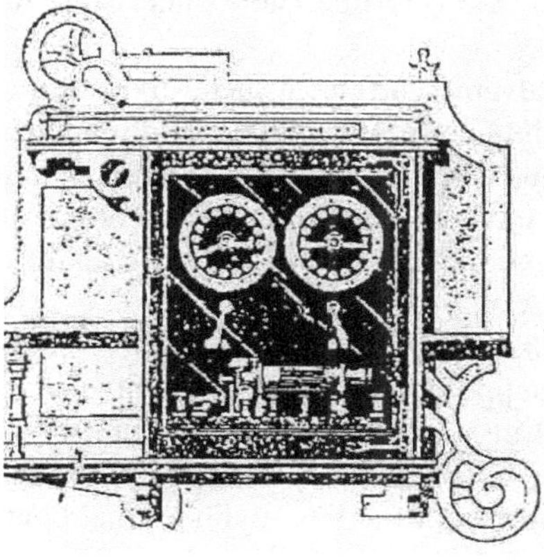

Fig G25. Wall Cabinet Battery[4]

an ornamental cherry or oak case (23 x 28 x 8 inches) with a hinged door of glass that opens on the right side. The face plate is enclosed within the glass door part, and is made of black polished hard rubber (12 x 14 inches). The face plate contains two cell selectors for galvanic cells, each having 12 metal selection buttons for 24 cells, and two lever controls for pole changing and faradic selection. On the horizontal shelf directly below the face plate is a panel that holds the metal induction coil with its metal sliding tube for current control; an adjustable screw spring lever, hammer vibrating type of interrupter; and two adjustable screws connecting posts. In 1893, the unit was displayed and listed in the AS Aloe catalog for $50.00.

Office Table Plate. This unit is encased in a polished oak case with a hinged lid that serves as a glass cover. The face plate is hard rubber (15 x 20 inches) that contains double galvanic current selectors; a

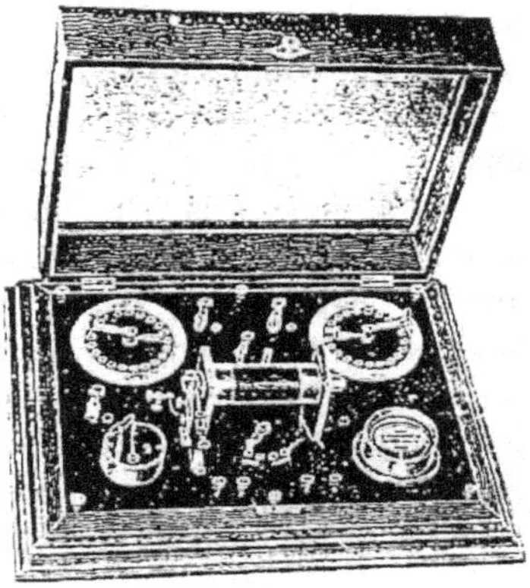

Fig G26. Office Table Plate, Style A[4]

pole changer for galvanic current; a metal induction coil with a Criado rheostat for controlling current amplitude; two interchangeable secondary coils; both rapid and slow vibrators; a faradic switch; a milliammeter (range of 0 to 250 mA); and an automatic rheotome for gradual current pulses. Complete, the unit cost $100.00, but without its wooden case it cost $75.00 by AS Aloe in 1893.

Criado Rheostat. The Criado Rheostat was a water type rheostat that was supposedly an improvement over the simple hollow metal tube that slid into and out of the coil, and the sledge inductorium (DuBois-Reymond) style of coil for control of current amplitude. The Criado Rheostat consisted of a glass cylinder that contained pure carbon filling for about 40 to 45 percent of the cylinder and water until touching a small sponge fitted to the end of a metal rod. The metal rod and sponge tip are lowered into the water to control current amplitude very effectively. This rheostat is used on a few of the Galvano-Faradic Mfg Co medical electrical batteries in 1895.

Perfection Office Cabinet Battery. This battery (Fig G27) manufactured by Galvano-Faradic Mfg Co provides both faradic and galvanic currents, and was designed for office use of physicians. The polished oak cabinet (37 x 27 x 23 inches) has a large drawer near the

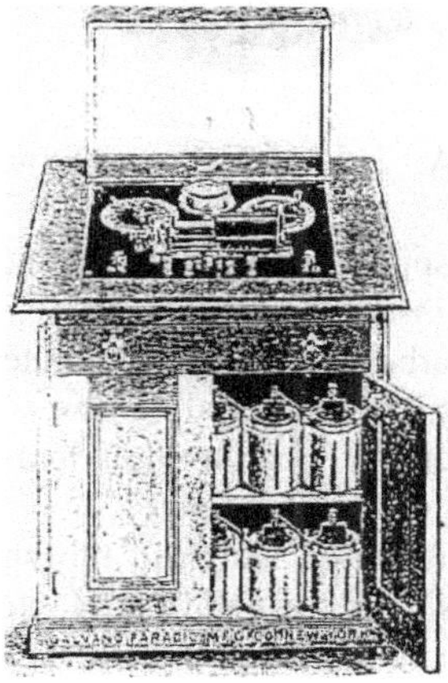

Fig G27. The Perfection Office Cabinet Battery[4]

top, a glass cover, two hinged doors that open in front below the drawer, and is mounted on wheels for mobility. The black polished hard rubber face plate contains the controls for its operation. These controls are: two double cell selectors, each having 20 metal buttons for the 40 Fitch Perfect Batteries; a DuBois-Reymond faradic sledge inductorium coil in which the secondary slides over the primary coil, a milliammeter (1 to 250 mA); pole changer; faradic switch; lever On/Off control; a water rheostat; an automatic rheotome; a wire coil rheostat; and four screw connecting posts. The metal parts are nickel plated. The 40 Fitch Perfect Batteries are located on two shelves hidden when the doors are closed. Circuitry is located underneath the face plate. The faradic secondary coil is wound with 1000 yards of No.32 copper wire, tapped at 500 yards to serve as two coils (one at 1000 yards and one at 500 yards). One rheotome is the conventional spring, hammer vibrator to provide rapid vibrations, and another interrupter for slow graduated vibrations. In 1893, this unit was sold by AS Aloe for $100.00.

Fitch Perfect Battery No.2 Chlorine. The Fitch Perfect Battery (3.9 sq base x 5.75 inches high including 0.34 inch neck that is 3.9 inches circular in diameter) may have bridged the gap between the wet cell that spilled when tipped, and the dry cell that omitted the spilling problem. The Fitch Perfect Battery was nearly the same as a wet cell except its lid was a screw-on glass jar lid that fitted the aqua glass neck jar snugly

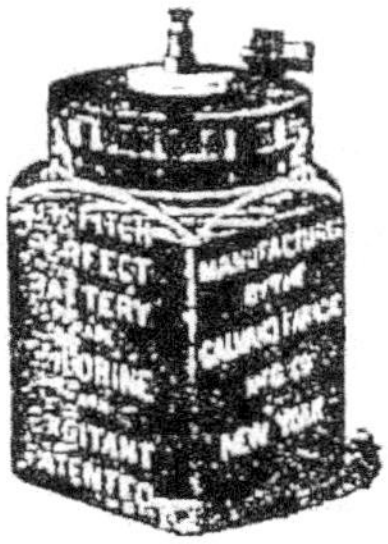

Fig G27A. The Fitch Perfect Battery

enough to prevent any spilling when tilted. The carbon element was 5.25 inches high, 3 inches in diameter with 2 inches center hole to fit the copper element. The carbon element is separated from the carbon by a 1.5 inches dia marble piece. The binding posts were mounted to the top of the carbon and copper. The operator only had to add solution ("Perfect Battery Excitant") and change the zinc element every two to four years. This battery was manufactured and sold through Galvano-Faradic Mfg Co (300 Fourth Ave, NY, address of Van Houten & Ten Broeck Co) in 1887, and was recommended for use with their cabinet and stationary office faradic and galvanic electrical apparatuses. The cost in the AS Aloe catalog for 1893 was a little higher priced than the conventional wet, dry cell, and chloride of silver dry cell. Each Fitch Perfect Battery cost $1.00.

Cylinder Top Cabinet Battery. This combination battery (Fig G27B) also used the "Fitch Perfect Battery" (40 cells). The electrical components include a DuBois-Reymond sledge inductorium that was interchangeable with three secondary coils of different capabilities (different wire length and sizes); a milliammeter ranging in scale from 1

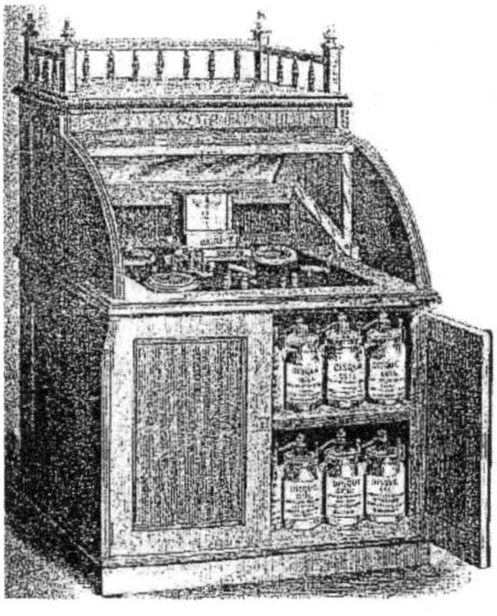

Fig G27B. Cylinder Top Cabinet Battery

to 500 millivolts; a German silver wire coil rheostat with coils of 5 to 5000 ohms of resistance (17,000 ohms total); an automatic rheotome; a pole changer; and double current selectors for whichever number of cells or series is to be chosen. Metal parts are nickel plated, and along with the electrical components are mounted on the black hard rubber face plate. The physician could select cherry or oak for the cabinet (39 x 25 x 54 inches). The cabinet is mobile with rubber encased wheels. The cylinder cover is of heavy glass front. In 1893, The Galvano-Faradic Mfg Co sold the deluxe unit for $230.00.

Static Machines

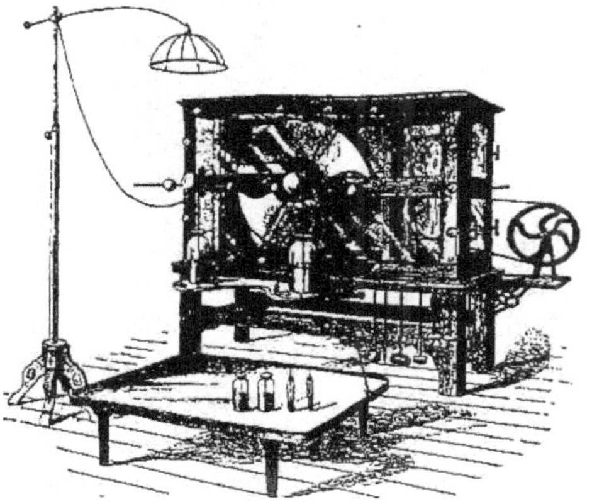

Fig G28. Electro-Therapeutical Apparatus (influence machine)[6]

Electro-Therapeutical Apparatus. This machine was the company's answer to the therapeutic use of the influence machine (Fig G28) with revolving plates of 30 inches in diameter, and the other unit with six revolving plates of 28 inches in diameter. In 1896, the 30 inches unit sold for $350.00, while the smaller 28 inches machine was bought for $300.00. The Wimshurst charger is located in the case with the plates. The earlier influence machines needed an electrical source to charge and get them started. Starting of this influence machine was by manual cranking, but a small Wimshurst was easy to crank and in turn got the larger unit operating easily before electrical motors were used for the same purpose. The operational components of the unit are mounted on dust proof ball bearings. The machine was used for therapeutic purposes and x-rays. Three pairs of Leyden jars were used in some operations of the machine. For additional information about medical electrical batteries of The Galvanic-Faradic Mfg Co after 1905 see Van Houten & Ten Broeck Co which may not have manufactured their medical electrical apparatuses prior to 1905. They apparently had a close business relation and under the direction of the Van Houten & Ten Broeck Co. When

Bartlett died in 1905 it was convenient and good business sense for Waite & Bartlett Co who had their own manufacturing facility to sell the Bartlett interest in the Galvano-Faradic Mfg Co.

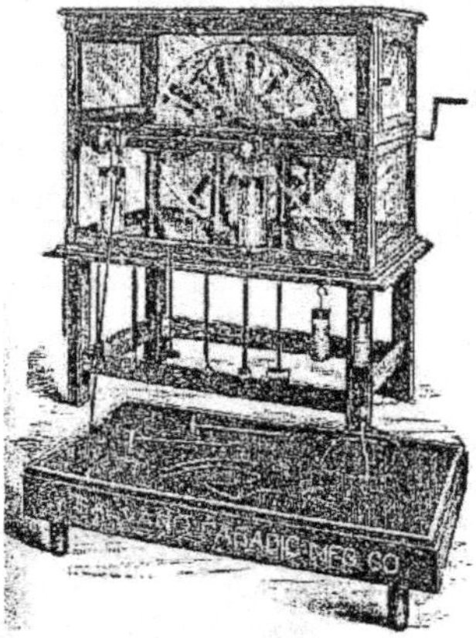

Fig G29. Improved Wimshurst Static Machine

Although the Wimshurst static machines were not commonly used by physicians in the United States, this improved and large model was marketed and sold in 1893 for $400.00. Improvements made by The Galvano-Faradic Mfg Co provided this static machine with the capability of operating in any weather (static machines collected moisture that caused them to malfunction). Therefore, this Wimshurst model was considered the most reliable at the time. This large machine was housed in an antique oak case (52 x 44 x 68 inches). A hand crank operated the six 27 inches revolving plates with three sets of Leyden jars. The accessories included an insulated platform, a crown for head breeze, and a set of hand held electrodes.

Miscellaneous

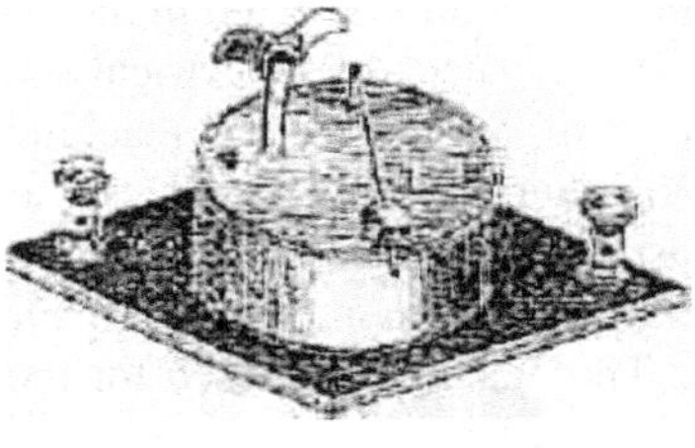

Fig G30. The Rheotome

Rheotome. The automatic rheotome was used with any of the galvanic units for producing rapid or slow monophasic pulses. This device eliminated the need of the operator or an assistant to manually interrupt the galvanic current to obtain monophasic pulses. This rheotome was introduced about 1905 at a cost of $10.00, and was contained on a wooden base. The wooden base has the company's signature and Powell's Rheotome embedded on the front.

Milliammeter. The Galvano-Faradic Manufacturing Co offered two milliammeters by 1905. The versions were vertical and horizontal.

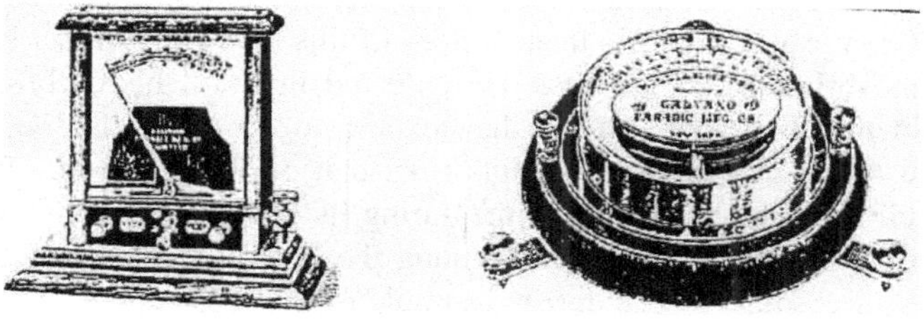

Fig G31. Milliammeters (vertical, horizotal)

A vertical milliammeter was introduced in 1905 at a cost of $12.00 if purchased through Van Houten & Ten Broeck Co, but if bought from Galvano-Faradic Mfg Co it cost $15.00. It was designed to measure galvanic current as it was delivered to the patient so that the practitioner could measure the amplitude accurately. Medical electrical batteries were not yet designed to contain devices to measure output so these were accessory items. Very few manufacturers of medical electrical batteries offered millimeters as standard equipment in 1900 to 1905. Milliammeters were often unreliable and added to the cost of equipment so were considered an accessory item. Chloride of Silver Dry Cell Battery Co of Baltimore, McIntosh Battery & Optical Co of Chicago, and the Frank S Betz Co of Chicago were pioneers for offering this device. Measurement of the quantity of galvanic current was an advancement in technology at the time. Known quantities of galvanic current are necessary to avoid burning the skin of patients from the excessive chemical effects of the current. Electrotherapeutists were skilled at judging current amplitudes through experience, the number of cells needed for a treatment, or the location of the rheostat during treatments. The particular unit had a scale ranging from 0 to 50 mA and another one ranging from 0 to 500 mA. A nickel plated lever control is moved to activate the desired scale. The scale could be calibrated, and two connecting posts are located on each side of the scale control lever. The scale is merely a cardboard hand drawn scale, but the unit was considered accurate. The moving parts are supported on jeweled bearings, and the pivots are ground, hardened, polished steel.

The horizontal milliammeter has leveling screws and a revolving case so the index needle adjusted to zero. The scales of the horizontal milliammeter ranged from 0 to 50, and 0 to 250, respectively. The device cost $20.00 through Van Houten & Ten Broeck Co, and $25.00 through Galvano-Faradic Mfg Co in 1905.

Summary

Frederick Bartlett was a pioneer in the mass production of medical electrical batteries in the United States. He founded his company in 1870 that was early for a manufactory of this type and product line. He was innovative and aggressive. He patented many of his early designs that did not then change over the next 35 to 40 years. The Galvano-Faradic Mfg Co held many patents (like that of The Chloride of Silver Dry Cell Battery Co of Baltimore) during its 35 years of business. The batteries were quality items and among the best in the business. These artifacts are some of the most desirable by today's collectors. These artifacts have withstood the rust of time that often is seen on some batteries.

The company offered a wide variety of batteries in its line ranging from the wooden case, to cabinet and wall models, to the large influence machines. Bartlett involved himself with Dr Henry Waite in 1879 or 1881 by forming a competitive company. Designs of medical electrical batteries manufactured by the two different companies varied to complement rather than out do each other. Both companies issued trade catalogs of their products that are revered and scarce. Bartlett was the businessman of each company with a flair for ideas in advancing electricity.

References

1. Davis AB, Dreyfus MS. The Finest Instruments Ever Made. Arlington, MA. 1986, p 141

2. Edmonson JM. American Surgical Instruments. San Francisco, CA, Norman Pub, 1997, p 218

3. Grigg ERN. The Trail of the Invisible Light. Springfield, IL, CC Thomas, 1965, pp 50-80

4. Catalog of AS Aloe Co, St Louis, MO, AS Aloe, 1893, pp 716-723

7. Catalog of Galvano-Faradic Mfg Co, New York, NY, Galvano-Faradic, 1871, pp 30-34, 74-75, 95

6. Catalog of Max Wocher & Son, Cincinnati, OH, 1896

CHAPTER 8. JEROME KIDDER MANUFACTURING COMPANY OF NEW YORK

Dr Kidder was a practicing physician who dabbled in the making of electrical batteries. This Chapter 8 outlines his success and the many quality products that his company made. The Kidder Co never reached the size of either the Frank S Betz or The Galvano-Faradic Mfg companies that were contemporaries. Jerome Kidder was a practicing physician (at some time in his career) whose interest in manufacturing was to produce quality medical electrical machines mainly for colleagues. Dr Kidder held patents for his electrical medical apparatuses in England and France in addition to the United States. (courtesy of Bakken Library and Museum, Minneapolis) The headquarters of his company was located at 820 Broadway, New York City, during the latter years of its existence (1879 through 1904 or later). While located on Broadway the sales office was in the Bible House, and his business was listed as manufacturing electricians.

In 1871, the Depot of Dr Jerome Kidder's Electrical Manufactory was "removed to NE cor of Fourth Ave. & 17th Street, New York, opp the Everett House" according to his trade catalog of 1871, Vitalizing.[1] This address of Fourth and 17th Street as cited in the company's catalog is in conflict with that of another source (544 Broadway, 1871 through 1872[2]). His catalog Vitalizing that illustrated and listed his product line of electromedical apparatuses was entered according to "Act of Congress in 1866 & 1867 in the Clerk's Office of the District Court of the United States for the Southern District of New York" and in 1871 "In the Office of the Librarian of Congress of Washington, D.C."

The company was the Jerome Kidder Manufacturing Co until sometime in 1881. In 1881, the company was assumed by Albert Kidder and was known for a brief period of time as the Albert Kidder & Company, but in 1882 it was again the Jerome Kidder Manufacturing Co. Jerome Kidder was well known and his name was better for business, after all, it had been known locally since 1859. The company remained at 820 Broadway during this name transition.

The company had changed addresses many times between 1862 and 1879. It was located at 429 Broadway in 1862 and 1863; 545 Broadway in 1864; 483 Broadway in 1865 and 1866; 480 Broadway in 1867; near Broadway in 1868 to 1871; 544 Broadway in 1871 and 1872; 50 Union Place (northeast corner of 17th and 4th Ave) from 1873 to 1878; 47 Lafayette Place in 1878; and then finally to its permanent location of 820 Broadway in 1879.[2] Kidder published a trade catalog of the company's products in 1862.

Dr Kidder established his company just prior to the Civil War in 1859 (1862 via Edmonson[2]). As mentioned, he registered his business with the United States government through the New York court in 1866 and 1867, and the Library of Congress in 1871 to copyright written materials (eg, trade catalogs). He immediately issued a catalog of his product line consisting of medical electrical batteries each consisting of six to 10 vitalizing currents and accessories. His apparatuses were known to be most complete in their construction, most perfect and simple in their operations, and most effective electrical machines for curing diseases. His first catalog was a 27-paged illustrated pamphlet of electrotherapeutic instruments and apparatuses, and appliances. His electrical equipment and accessories were higher in costs than many of those of his competitors.

In 1867 and 1871, his store on the corner of Fourth Avenue and 17th Street was known as Kidder's Electrical Depot. He was offering the highest premium, vitalizing, genuine six and nine currents medical electrical apparatus; or so his advertisements read. In 1874, the 22 paged catalog indicated that Dr Kidder was selling electro-allotrop (pertaining to one or two forms of carbon, sulfur, and phosphorus) physiological units that used different qualities of electricity to cure diseases.[1,3] Dr Kidder continued to sell and offer research data with his electro-allatropo-physiological batteries of different qualities to cure diseases between 1874 and about 1888.

In 1878, Dr Kidder issued an eight-paged folded brochure listing 64 items that included electrodes, an aesthesiometer, and a rheostat. Catalogs of the Kidder products were issued in 1887, 1888, and about 1895 illustrating and describing superior electrotherapeutic apparatus.[4] The company was still doing business and advertising medical electrical batteries in 1904.

Kidder manufactured an electromagnetic machine around 1871 to 1876 that contained a brass signature plate bearing the patent dates of 15 March 1860, 3 August 1865, and 10 October 1871. The machine was encased in an oak box (9.75 x 8.75 x 8 inches) that contained two compartments. The back compartment held a wet cell and a bottle of solution. The two glass jars were separated by a large and unusual brass cell holder that doubled as a positive connecting pole. Kidder's innovative wet cell was a tip type battery using quicksilver, amalgamated zinc, and sulfuric acid solution. Directions for operation are printed on a paper label glued to the inside of the lid. This particular unit was manufactured by Dr Jerome Kidder, North East corner of 4th Avenue and 17th Streets, New York, but sold through Max Wocher & Son Co, seller of surgical instruments, Cincinnati, OH. A 6.25 x 1.75 inches tin tube core was pushed and pulled over the induction coil (housed beneath the face plate) to control current amplitude. The face plate contained an On/Off switch, five brass connecting poles, and two brass poles that connect to the battery.

This unit of 1871 to 1876 was made from a patent of 1860 held by Jerome Kidder, MD. In 1861 and 1868 Dr Kidder obtained patents in which the patent officer, Dr Charles Page, insisted on Kidder meeting all patent requirements.[5] The process held up Dr Kidder's production in lost time that angered him. He later denounced Dr Page sometime after Page's death (see Davis/Kidder…in this chapter).

Meyer in his 1869 book accorded Dr Kidder a very favorable comment on his sledge type faradic medical battery. He stated that Dr Kidder's sledge machine was preferable because of "its compactness, its slight liability to derangement, the power of its several currents, and uniformity of its action." [6] It furnishes currents of 1st (current of primary coil) and 2nd (current of secondary coil) order. Galvanism is derived from either one or two Smee cells according to the size of the apparatus. The box contains the cells, also a bottle in which the spare dilute sulfuric acid used may be stored until needed.

Dr Kidder had dealings with Dr Charles Page of the United States Patent Office between 1861 and 1867. Page denied Kidder patents until his inventions met specific requirements of the Patent Office. History shows that Kidder was annoyed over these circumstances. In 1876, Kidder published a disclaimer about Page. Dr Kidder was a leading manufacturer of electrotherapeutics equipment between 1872 and 1898, and by then held several patents on components of his electrical machines. Kidder received negative publicity over his patent difficulties with Dr Page that probably cost him business losses. In 1876, Kidder attacked the dead Dr Page by denying that Page ever invented an electrical coil or any other device used in electrical instruments. Kidder posted such information in some of his equipment advertisements. Dr Charles Page is still credited for inventing an electrical coil despite Kidder's smear tactic.

Dr Kidder's catalog of 1871 was 14 pages in length and featured his electrical medical apparatus of six and nine currents. The catalog was prefaced by R Ogden Doremus, MD (professor of chemistry and physics in New York City College, and of chemistry and toxicology in Bellevue Hospital Medical College of New York), and the Reverend RW Oliver (professor of Divinity in the Protestant Episcopal Seminary, Nebraska City, NB). The catalog ended with numerous testimonials that endorsed the quality and efficiency of his electrical medical apparatuses. (Note: In the late 1800s testimonials of satisfied consumers were used rather than conducting research to substantiate claims and outcomes from treatments by medical electrical batteries.–ed)

The catalog contained the description and prices for his unique tip battery that he patented on 10 October 1871 and 7 November 1871. One battery and a four-coil helix unit sold for $25.00, while a 20-cell tip battery package sold for $40.00. Dr Kidder sold what today would constitute a power pack for supplying a medical electrical machine. He also produced a 12-, 18-, and 36-cell primary cell battery housed in wooden cases like those of the medical electrical machines of that period of time. Dr Kidder sold a galvanic-cautery unit using eight conventional wet cells with the metal elements (carbon, zinc) raised from the cells by cranking a compound bar attached to the metal elements for $75.00. In 1871, Dr Kidder also sold a current reverser to throw galvanic current rapidly from cells to alternate current in the opposite direction.

As mentioned most businessmen in electricity used testimonials in advertisement of their products. Dr Kidder used testimonials of individuals like: R Ogden Doremus, MD; and professor B Silliman, Jr, of Yale College whose name is often associated with the Davis & Kidder units endorsing the magnetoelectrical device. In Dr Silliman's letter to Dr Kidder on 23 December 1863 endorsing his products no mention is made of the Davis & Kidder magnetoelectrical device. (courtesy of Bakken Library and Museum, Minneapolis)

In 1878, Jerome Kidder, MD, offered an eight-paged booklet illustrating, describing, and pricing <u>Extra Appliances</u>. Items in this brochure were for electrotherapeutic use. His regular catalogs between 1872 and 1882 offered Galvanic electrical machines for various prices that were powered by 12 to 36 cells; Galvanic caustic apparatus; and Improved Pocket Induction apparatus. Dr Kidder recommended that his wet cells be filled with solutions of water (8 to 12 parts) and sulfuric acid (1 part). The average mixture was a 10:1 proportion, respectively. He further suggested that 1 teaspoonful of quicksilver (mercury) be added to the solution so that when the mercury touched the zinc elements the 2 metals would amalgamate to preserve the zinc element.[7]

Association of Kidder and Davis

By 1854, numerous patents and machines were using the principles of magnetoelectricity for patient treatments. One of the best quality and most known magnetoelectrical batteries of that time period was the so called Davis & Kidder design.

The Davis & Kidder names on a popular magnetoelectrical unit have been identified with Daniel Davis and Dr Jerome Kidder. Daniel Davis, the renown instrument maker of Boston, was retired by 1854 in which some Davis & Kidder units are labeled.

Ari Davis, the brother of Daniel, was a maker of philosophical instruments who worked in Washington, DC, in 1854 when he had two patents accepted. Patent No. 10,788 was issued for the joining of wooden boxes by brass angle corners, while patent No.11,415 was given for a compact magnetoelectrical machine. The latter device became very popular in the late nineteenth century (1870s-1890s), and was housed in the wooden box that was patented for its brass angle corners. Ari Davis' 1854 patent later became known as the Davis & Kidder Magneto-Electric

Machine which is still one of the most popular medical electrical batteries sold in antique shops and on computer auctions today. Soon after receiving his patents for the wooden box corners and his magneto

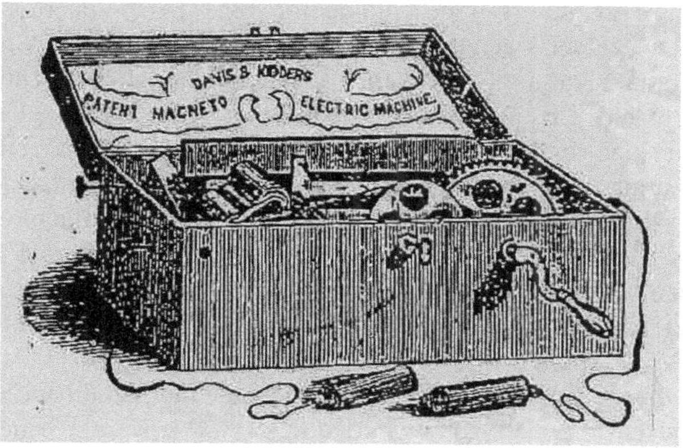

Fig K1. Davis/Kidder Magnetoelectrical Battery

-electric machine Ari sold his patent rights for $4,000.00 to Dr Walter Kidder. Dr Walter Kidder, a young medical paractitioner of Lowell, MA, saw the patent as a great investment opportunity. Without developing or producing the machine he then sold the patent rights after a year for a $6,000.00 profit. Walter H Burnap of New York City eventually got the patent rights, developed, and became the sole manufacturer of the Davis & Kidder magneto-electric machine.[8]

The Davis & Kidder machines sold today have the paper label "Davis & Kidder's Patent Magneto-Electric Machine" on the inside of the lid of the wooden box. Some of the earlier units have the date of the patent (1854) on the label, and apparently endorsed by the then leading scientists Dr Charles Page and Dr Benjamin Silliman. These earliest units may have been manufactured in the late 1850s or 1860s, but most likely were not manufactured until the 1870s. The units made in the 1870s and later do not have either the patent date nor the endorsements on their signature labels. All Davis & Kidder batteries are in wooden boxes with the brass angle corners.

As mentioned, the popular Davis & Kidder magnetoelectrical machine is often erroneously assigned credit to Daniel Davis a famous instrument maker of Boston (retired in 1854) and Dr Jerome Kidder, a physician of New York City. Dr Jerome Kidder went into the medical electrical business in 1859, and has emphatically denied any association in the manufacture of electrical machines with any Davis. The earliest of these units in question have the pictures and endorsements of Dr Charles Page and Benjamin Silliman on the paper labels. Dr Page did not invent or manufacture a magnetoelectrical machine of this type. Silliman often endorsed medical electrical machines in his publication The American Journal of Science and Arts but no record can be located of his endorsement for the Davis/Kidder unit.

Dr Kidder's trade catalog for 1871 (p 2) stated, "Those who desire Dr. Kidder's genuine improved machines, should buy none that do with a crank, and none unless they see the patent labels of 1860 and 1866 on the machine itself. Dr Kidder has never been associated in company with any one in business, therefore all machines that have the name of any other person associated with "Kidder" are not these machines."[1]

This magnetoelectrical machine was manufactured by WH Burnap Manufacturer of New York City at some time. JH Bunnell Co may also have made the unit at some time in the early 1900s. Units from 1854 to about 1870 had a bone handle on the crank for turning the brass gears with a pulley drive for the two small induction coils. The bone handle was replaced after 1870 with wooden and metal handles. The unit was housed in a mahogany wooden box (9.88 x 4.5 x 4.5 inches) with a hinged lid of about 1.5 inches high, and brass reeinforced corners of the box. The inside of the lid had a label with endorsements and information for treating diseases of the nervous system. The unit delivered crude faradic current and up to 400 volts from the rotating coils in conjunction with one or two horseshoe magnets. This unit was retailed by many vendors such as JH Bunnell; Manhattan Electrical Supply Company; Montgomery Ward & Co; and Sears, Roebuck and Co.

Awards

Dr Kidder was proud of his awards received from 1872 to 1882 at the Fairs of the American Institute held in New York, and the Franklin Institute of Philadelphia, PA. In 1870, he received the honorable mention award at the Fair of the American Institute for the value of his electrical machines as labor savers and for important additions to human comforts. Records do not reveal the specifics of these awards. In 1875, he received a gold metal for 'first order of performance.' He had five electrical medical batteries in the category. His apparatuses were ordered as: Improved No.1 for physicians' offices; Improved No.2 for physicians visiting patients and it had a turn down helix; Improved No.3 was another form of No.2; and Improved No.4 for office and a family's home use. His electrical medical batteries continued to win additional awards such as: 1876, the Highest Premium award at the Centennial Exhibition; and the silver medal at each of the Charleston, SC, Expositions of 1881 and 1882.

Commonalties of Kidder Medical Electrical Batteries

Dr Kidder's apparatuses were quality constructed whether for physician or home use. His apparatuses for home use were a little more costly than those sold by the other manufacturers of home or family medical electrical batteries that probably reduced his sales volume. Examination of the various home units will quickly verify this assessment as being of superior quality compared with those of competitors. Because of the Kidder prices and sales volume in the nineteenth century the artifacts are less commonly seen today in the antique market as are other cheaper brands.

Certain features of the Kidder batteries help to identify them. Most of the Kidder apparatuses used circular signature plates that usually are mounted on the face plate. Metal on the Kidder apparatus is heavy brass on earlier units and nickel plated on later units. The adjustable binding and connecting posts always had springs mounted to hold the adjusted positions (a unique quality feature). The coils of his faradic batteries are located underneath the face plate and have a large diameter metal sliding tube current regulator operating from the right side of the box. The sliding metal current regulators on Kidder faradic models appear to be tin or low quality metal compared with other components on his apparatuses. Because of the coils mounted underneath the face plate he used vibrating interrupters that were mounted parallel to and on top of the face plate that vibrated against a post on the face plate. Although Dr Kidder featured his faradic batteries as having variations of six to 10 currents accomplished by varying the windings on his induction coils, this feature did not alter physiological effects enough to gain continued use among colleagues. The varied windings may have been more of an electrical engineer's delight than that of physicians and physiologists. Historically, his use of tapped windings on the induction coils to affect physiological responses appears to have been a fad without clinical or scientific merit.

Faradic Batteries

Double Battery Physician's Office Electro-Medical Apparatus. Dr Kidder was a believer in current variations for the electrical treatment of diseases. He achieved current variations by wiring the secondary coil in sections so that one coil could serve as more than one. These current variations later prove not to have different physiological effects. This No.1 battery had nine different currents that varied by the combination wiring as four different coils, and using current changers to reverse the direction of all currents (primary plus 4 reversed currents). The current variations were achieved clinically by using five connection posts, and placing the secondary coil into the primary circuit. The unit comes in a polished walnut box (10.5 x 9 x 7.5 inches) with brass corners, and a hinged lid that secures by lock and key on the front. A sliding drawer is located on the left (rather than customary right) lower side of the box.

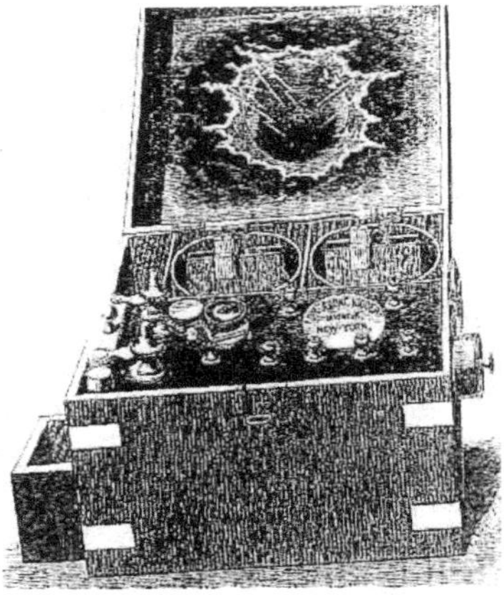

Fig K2. Double Battery Physician's
Office Electro-Medical Apparatus, No. 1

The face plate contains the five connecting posts, two binding posts to the wet cell, and an interrupter (rheotome). The coils are located underneath the face plate, and a large metal sliding tube current regulator (tin) was operated through the right side of the box.

Electro-Medical Apparatus No.2. In 1871, Kidder's No.2 (Fig K3) faradic electrical apparatus delivered six currents. The unit was

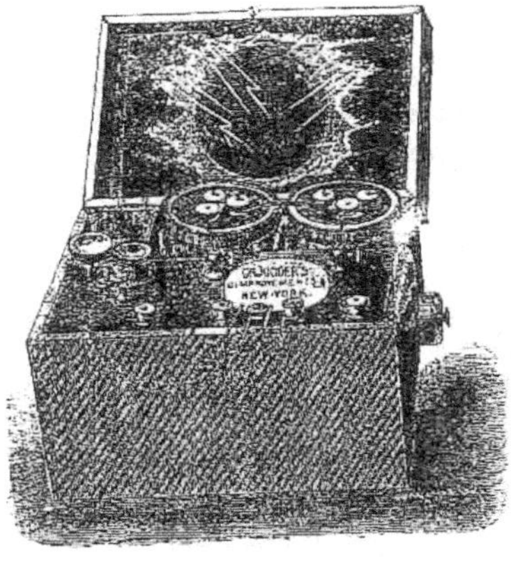

Fig K3. Physician's Visiting Electro-Medical Apparatus No. 2

encased in a mahogany or walnut box (8 x 6.25 x 6.75 inches) with a hinged lid, and a lock and key in front of the box. The face plate contained the Kidder signature plate, four metal receptacles for connecting to patients and providing the six currents, and the interrupter. The coils were mounted underneath the face plate so that the sliding metal tube current regulator was operated manually on the right side of the box. An open area behind the face plate is used for housing the two double stopper batteries that had rubber stoppers to prevent spilling of the fluid when being carried. The top of the box has a metal carrying handle. The metal was brass, and Kidder sold the unit for $25.00.

Kidder Faradic Apparatus No.2. This unit of Fig K4 differs from the conventional units by its construction and components. The unit is housed in a polished hard wood box (6 x 3.5 x 6 inches), hinged lid at the top that has a metal carrying handle, and a lever latch on the lower portion of the box. The right side of the box is hinged at the bottom, and when opened places the wooden face plate in the ready position for use. The face plate arrangement is the same as Kidder's Faradic Coil No.5A. Although smaller than other Kidder faradic apparatuses, the No.2 delivers 10 variations of current from tappings and varying the lengths and sizes of the wire windings on the induction coil. The unit has a single stopper type cell and sold for $27.00 in 1893 by AS Aloe. In 1895, the No.2 faradic battery of 1871 was no longer carried by Kidder.

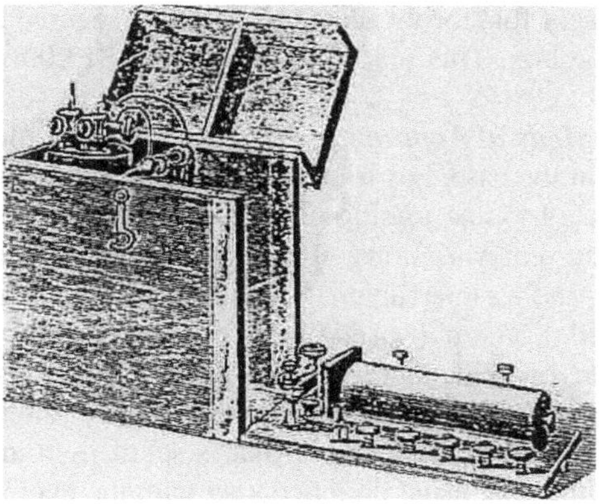

Fig K4. Faradic Apparatus No. 2

Physician's and Family Electro-Magnetic Machine No.3. Kidder encased this faradic battery (Fig K5) in a polished walnut box (12 x 4.25 x 7 inches). This unit carries a single rubber stopper cell that can be carried without spilling the fluid. The face plate occupies about 75 percent of the box area, and contains the Kidder signature plate, four metal receptacles for connecting with subjects, two binding posts for joining the wet cell, and the interrupter. Like his other faradic batteries the coils are arranged underneath the face plate. The sliding metal tube current regulator is operated manually from the right side of the box. The single rubber stopper cell is located on the left side of the box in an open

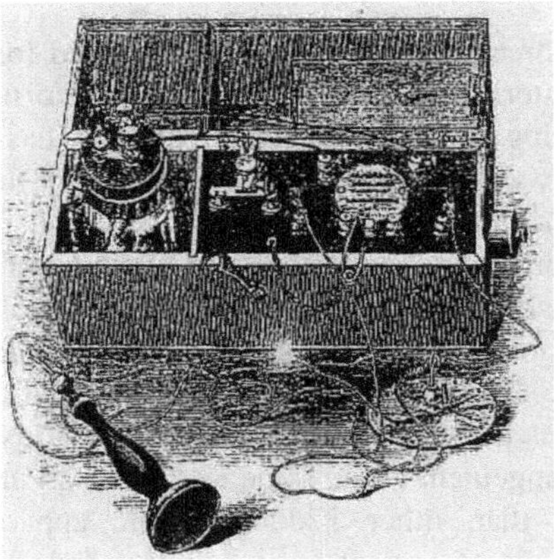

Fig K5. Physician's and Family Electro-Magnetic Machine, No. 3

area separated from the face plate. The lid of the box is hinged, contains a small compartment for storing accessories, and is secured by a lock and key in front of the box. This unit in 1871 sold for $23.00,[1] and was not available in 1895.

Electro-Medical Apparatus. In Fig K6 the face plate, is stained walnut darker than the case, has four metal receptacles (stamped A to D) to connect subjects by pins joining cloth covered wires to electrodes to provide the six current variations. It has two binding posts to connect with the wet cell, and an interrupter. A solution of sulfuric acid was used to activate the cell. The unit used one or two cells, but carried a glass beaker and bottle of acid solution. The glass vessels were manually blown with a pontil but were not embossed. The interrupter is an adjustable screw, spring lever hammer that is set at right angles indirect to the core rather than the usual direct contact with the magnetic core. All

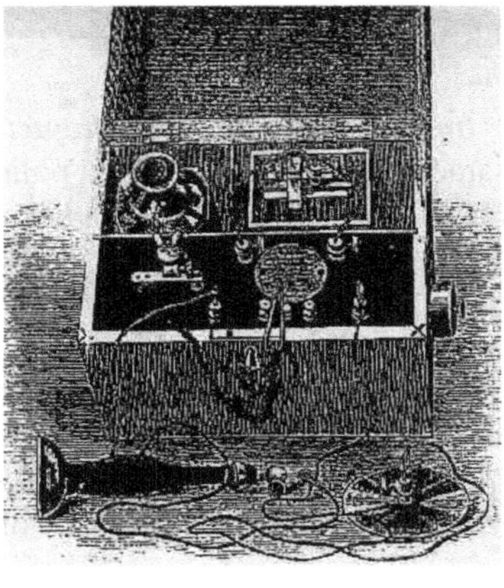

Fig K6. No. 4 Electro-Medical Apparatus for Physicians and Family Use

metal fixtures are brass, as well as the circular Kidder logo citing the address and the dates of various patents of improved features. The two American patents were issued in 1860 and 1864, while the English patent was issued in 1865, and those of France in 1865, 1866, and 1869. The patent dates suggest that this model dates to 1869. The coils are mounted underneath the face plate, are well varnished for insulation, and isolated in the case by its own enclosed wooden frame. The coils consist of a helix with combinations of windings with different diameters and lengths of copper wire, and a magnetic core. The coils provide six different currents that differ in magnetic, electrolytic, and sensational effects. Dr Kidder illustrates the relation of the six currents by a triangular diagram with the directions of the four poles and the various effects on the label. Also, the circuit is designed to use either one or two coils in the primary

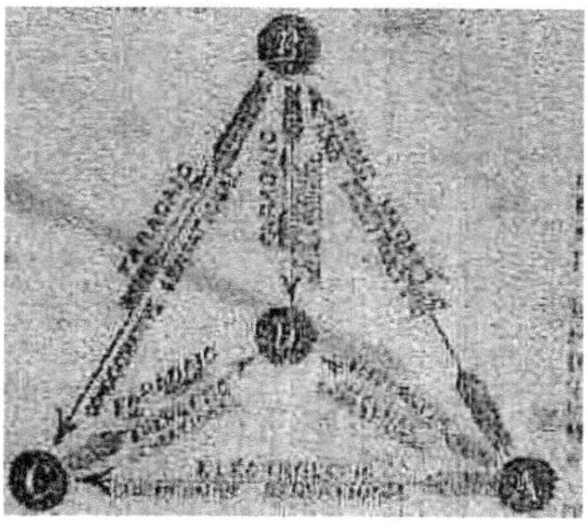

Relation of Kidder's Six Currents

circuit by closing the secondary coil in the primary circuit. The current regulator (sliding metal tube of copper and zinc) is operated manually from the right side of the box. The wet cell is a beaker with elements consisting of two zinc plates with a thin plate of platina between them. Platina is a silver plated alloy of platimum, palladium, iridium, and osmium that conduct electricity well but is of less value than pure silver. The chain holds the cramp that is inserted between binding posts and the negative brass marker to close the circuit. The walnut box (9 x 7.5 x 7 inches) has a hinged lid, no carrying handle, and is secured by a front located lock and key. Inside of the lid is a paper label of directions for operating and descriptions of the unit. The corners of the box are glued and have wedges (splines) inserted to strengthen them. The unit sold for $20.00 in 1871.

Faradic Apparatus No.4. This No.4 faradic apparatus of 1893 has some design changes from that of 1871. The face plate of this model has a lever On/Off control that was not present earlier. The wet cells of this model are made more secure in the box than that of the 1871 unit. This security is done by having a cut out panel over the wet cells.

Three variations of this faradic battery design were offered to consumers in the 1893 AS Aloe catalog.[9] Each of the three units delivered six variations of current from three coils operating from different lengths and diameters of wire windings. A single wet cell powered the unit but a second bottle of spare solution was packaged in the rear compartment of the case. The No. 4 unit is encased in a polished

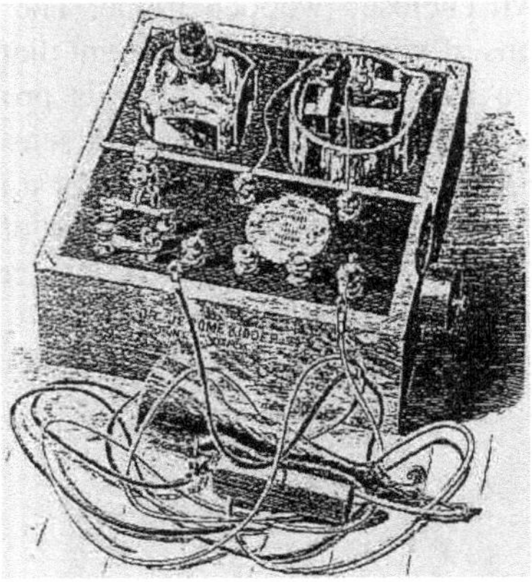

Fig K7. Faradic Apparatus No. 4[9]

hardwood box (8.75 x 8.25 x 7 inches). One variation in the Kidder Family Faradic Apparatus No.4 is that it does not have a switch for using the secondary coil in the primary circuit. It was the least costly unit in the series at $18.00. The second variation of this series is the Kidder Office Faradic Apparatus No.4 complete with the switch for using the secondary coil in the primary circuit. The addition of the switch and change in trade name cost $20.00. The third variation is the Kidder Tip Faradic Apparatus No.4 with a hydrostat for tipping the spare bottle of solution in use with the exhaustion of the first wet cell. The addition of this Kidder innovation, switch, and another trade name cost $24.00.

Six Current Electro-Medical Apparatus. This unit is a compact portable unit that is housed in a polished mahogany box (9.75 x 4.75 x 2.25 inches). This small unit has the effect of three coils (1 primary, 2 secondary) that deliver six current variations through four metal receptacles located on top of the box. No conventional face plate is used with this model. The sliding metal tube, current regulator is manually operated from the right side of the box. The operating components are approached by lifting a hinged lid that opens an area about one third of the total top of the box. Another small compartment on the right side of the box is for accessories. The single wet cell was carried externally to the apparatus. The unit sold for $18.00 in 1871.[1]

This model of Fig K8 is housed in a smaller box of polished walnut (7.5 x 6 x 6.25 inches) than most other Kidder batteries. The

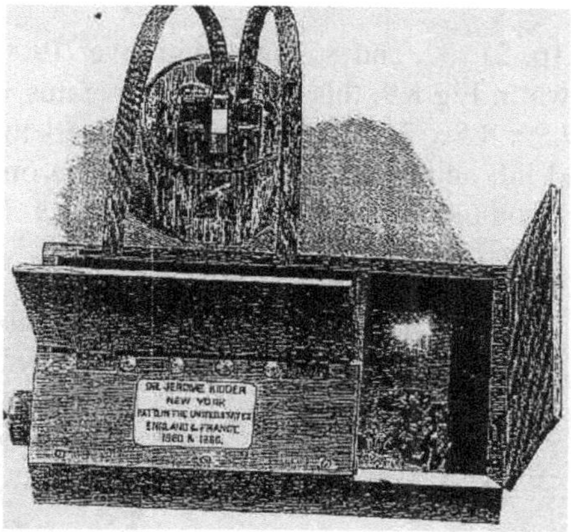

Fig K8. Family and Traveler's Six-Current Electro-Medical Apparatus

model was designed for family or home use and sold for $18.00 in 1871.[1] This unit is very similar to the No.2 unit of 1871. The unit has a single primary coil, but the secondary coil is wired with different diameters and

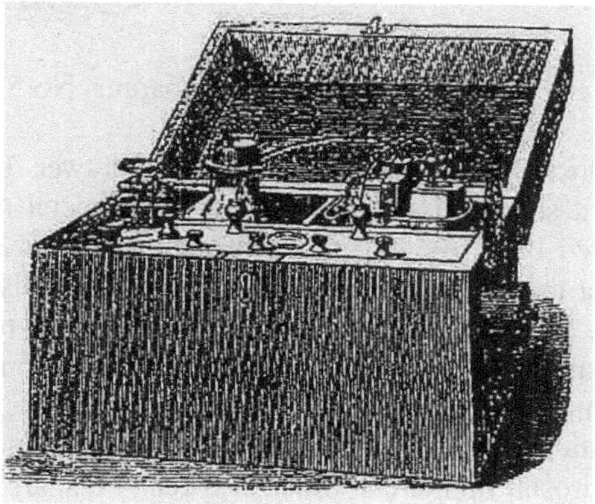

Fig K9. Six-Current Electro-Medical Apparatus

lengths of wire to serve as three coils. The four metal receptacles are used in combinations to provide the six current variations to the subject. The face plate covers the front half of the box, while the rear half houses two wet cells. The face plate has the signature plate, the interrrupter, and two binding posts in addition to the four connecting posts. The coils are located underneath the face plate, and the sliding metal tube, current regulator is manually operated from the right side.

Office Faradic Apparatus No.5. This Office Faradic electrical battery is the same unit as above, and listed in the 1893 catalog of AS Aloe for $24.00. It provided 10 different current combinations through four conditioned coils (coil wound and tapped to serve as 4) that consisted of Nos.16, 21, 32, and 86 wires with over 1900 feet in length. Like the unit shown in Fig K9, this particular apparatus was housed in a hard wood box (9.5 x 8.5 x 7.25 inches), glued corners that have wedges (splines), a hinged lid, and carried by a metal handle on top. No.5 also had an open cell compartment (wet cells, 1 spare, 1 to power using

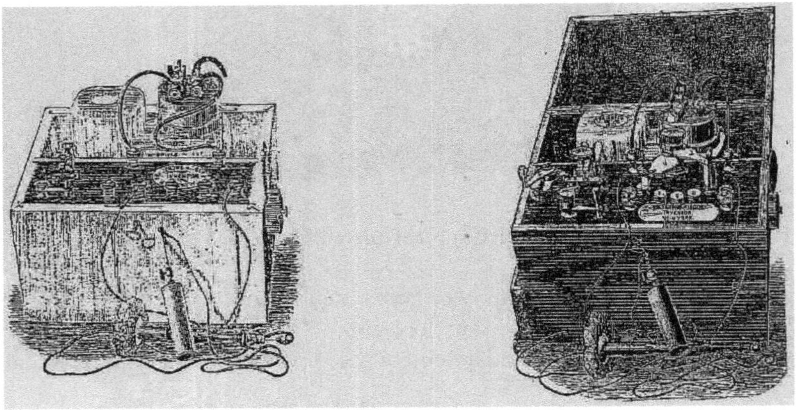

Fig K10. Kidder Office Faradic Apparatus No.5[9]

commercial sulfuric acid and 11 parts of water), a drawer for accessories on the lower right side, and above it is the sliding metal tube from the coil that is secured by a pivoting disc. The interrupter is an adjustable screw spring lever mounted parallel (rather than horizontally) on the hard rubber face plate. A lever On/Off control is located next to the interrupter on the face plate along with five adjustable spring screw connecting posts on the center-right side. All metal on the face plate are brass.

A variation of the No.5 Kidder Office Faradic Apparatus contained the hydrostat tip battery which was really a spare cell jar filled with fluid ready for use when the one in use is exhausted. According to the manufacturer the No.5 Tip Faradic Apparatus could be carried from place to place in a buggy without danger of spilling. The tip apparatus and battery unit complete sold for $27.00 in the 1893 AS Aloe catalog.[9]

An earlier model of No.5 (1871) used the tip cell arrangement that Kidder patented in that same year. This particular model was sometimes referred to as a continuous coil that used different sized wires in the windings to vary the currents (5 to 10 currents). A rotary lever switch was used in this model in combination with the five connector posts to vary the current to the patient. Although Kidder introduced this concept of continuous coil with current variations from the different windings on the secondary coil, the physiological effects never measured up with the engineering design. This early model was phased out by 1900 and its description was not included in the textbooks on electrotherapeutics thereafter. This 1871 model is displayed on the right in Fig K10.

Family Faradic Apparatus No.6. This faradic apparatus has two coils that provide three variations of current. A hollow metal tube (6 x 1.75 inches) was slid in and out of the coil from the outer right side of the box; a metal disc pivoted over the hole of the controller tube to secure when not in use. The unit was boxed in a polished wooden case (8 x 5 x

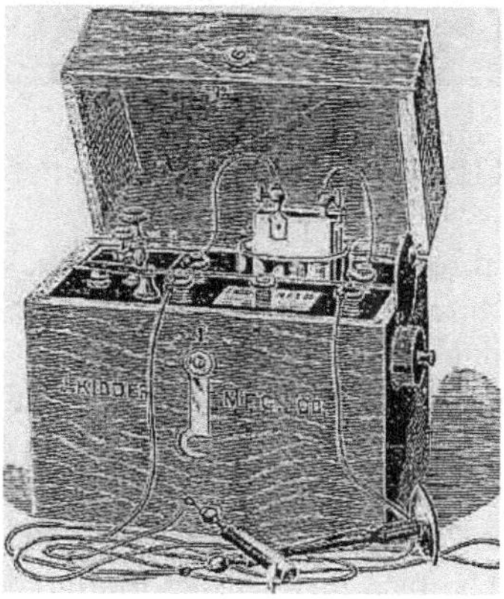

Fig K11. Kidder Family Faradic Apparatus No. 6

7.75 inches) in which corners were glued and wedged (splined) for sturdy construction. This wooden box is smaller than that of No. 4 but is a better unit. The box was hinged with a lid that has a metal carrying handle and a lever latch covering a lock and key arrangement. A single wet cell powered the unit and is kept in a rear open compartment with accessories. The cell jar space accommodates a jar of 2.5 x 5.25 inches. The black hard rubber face plate is flush to the lower open box portion, and contains the Kidder arrangement of a parallel adjustable screw spring lever vibrating interruper, two adjustable spring screw binding posts to the wet cell, and three adjustable spring screw connecting posts in the fore portion of the face plate. It sold for $15.00 in the 1893 AS Aloe catalog,[9] and $15.00 in the 1893 catalog of the Truax, Greene & Co of Chicago.

Faradic Coil No.5A. This faradic apparatus is really the face plate of other Kidder units in that it does not have any case. The coil is wound with four different lengths and diameters of wire to provide 10 variations of current. A switch is available for selecting the second coil in the primary circuit. The horizontal or conventionally mounted adjustable screw spring lever vibrating rheotome is on the left of the coil where the hammer strikes the core. A metal tube or sleeve slides over the coil to manually adjust current amplitude. Two adjustable spring binding posts for connection with an external power source are at the rear of the face plate, and five adjustable spring screw connecting posts are in front of the

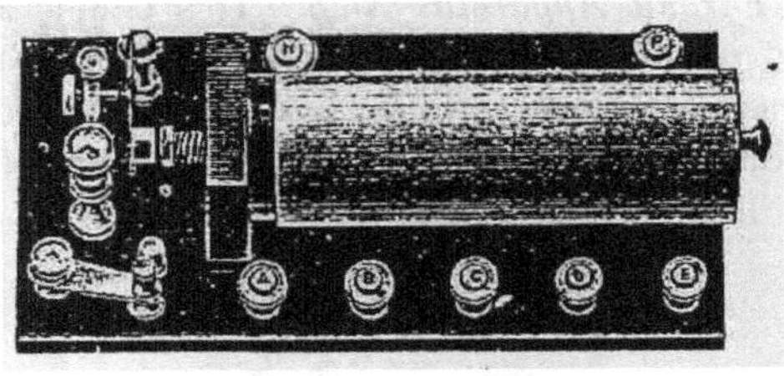

Fig K12. Kidder Faradic Coil No. 5A

coil on the black hard rubber base. A sheet of buckram covers the circuit on the bottom of the base and serves as a pad. The unit sold for $20.00 in the 1893 AS Aloe catalog.[9]

Small Office Cabinet. The cabinet of this faradic and galvanic office apparatus (Fig F13) is made of hard wood (37 x 25 x 14 inches), and sits directly on the floor. The top of the cabinet has a hinged lid, but no doors. Entry to the 22 wet cells (muriate of ammonia type) is from the rear of the cabinet. The face plate is like the faradic apparatus No.5, but in addition contains sliding devices for activating and deactivating cells on the galvanic side. The faradic coil is wound to provide 10 current

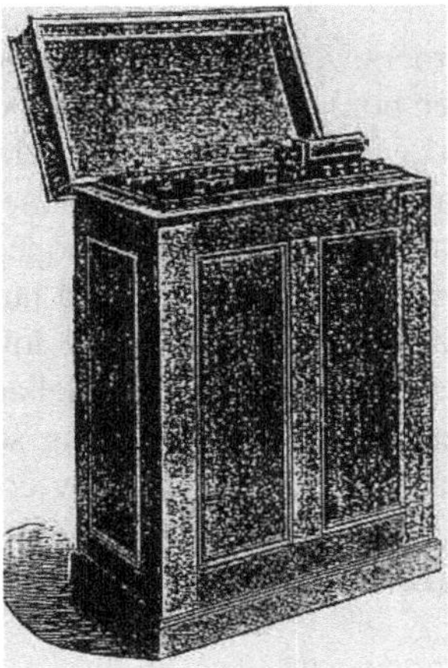

Fig K13. Kidder Small Office Cabinet[9]

variations. A pole changer is available on the galvanic portion along with an instant cutoff of the current when desired. This unit listed for $90.00 in the 1893 AS Aloe catalog.[9]

Sledge Inductorium Battery. Another medical electrical battery manufactured by Dr Kidder was his sledge inductorium or "sledge" style unit of 1876. (Fig K14) This particular sledge style (coil slides over soft core 4.75 x 0.75 inches to control current amplitude) unit was a faradic electrical machine that was powered by two cells. The unit is encased in a mahogany box (9 x 6.5 x 7.5 inches) with a heavy metal carrying handle on the lid, and a pivot latch type receptacle on front to secure the lid. A small lock and key locked the front latch. A signature plate is mounted inside the lid that reads "Dr Jerome Kidder,patented Mar 15, 1864; Jan 16, 1866; Sept 1866; Aug 10, 1869; re-issue Jan 4, 1876......., New York." Corners of the wooden box are reenforced with wooden wedges (splines).

The face plate is black painted wood that contains an induction

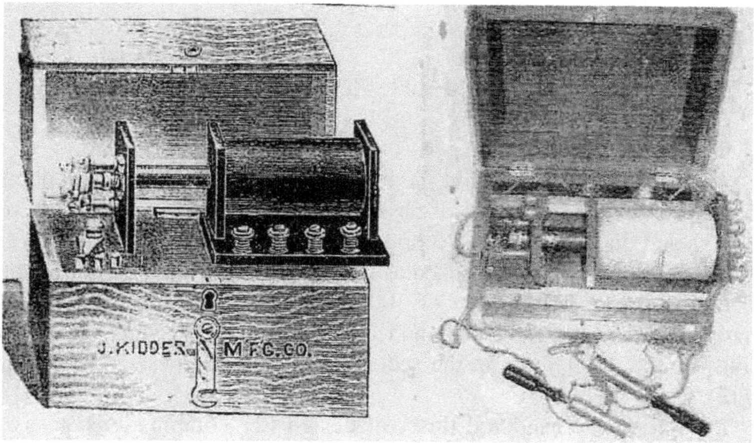

Fig K14. Kidder Sledge Inductorium Battery

coil (4.75 x 2.5 inches) with two hard rubber end blocks (3 inches sq); four connecting posts labeled from left "P, No.300, 32/500, Wire 700" on top, "Yards" on bottom. The bottom of each unit has runners to slide between two wooden runners; the right end contains an interrupter (rheostat) that adjusts hammer and spring; and an On/Off switch. The wooden runners are light colored wood, the front runner is scaled "0 to 5" inches and the rear is marked "P" & "N"; the rear of panel also contains two connecting posts "P" & "N". Accessories are stored with cells underneath the face plate. This unit was considered one of the finest American faradic electrical machines of its time.

Portable High Tension Apparatus. In 1896 through 1904, a sledge inductorium type faradic battery was featured by the Kidder Mfg Co in its catalog (1896), and in a general advertisement of electrical apparatus in 1904 (Fig K15). This unit is different than other sledge inductorium units, and was probably designed by Dr William J Herdman, a medical professor of neurological electrotherapeutics at the University

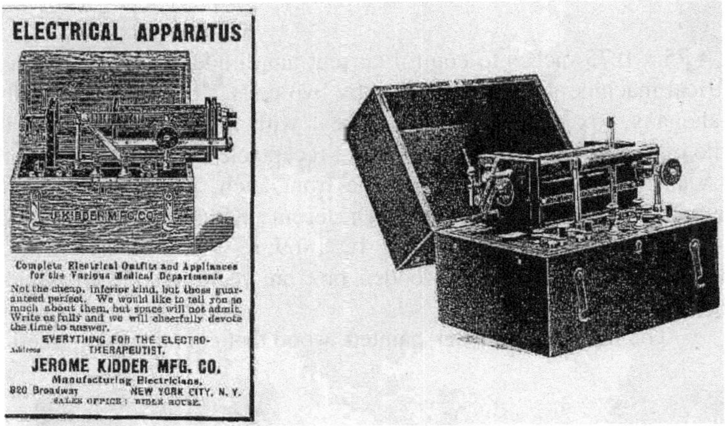

Fig K15. Kidder's Portable High Tension Apparatus

of Michigan.

Kidder liked to build the induction coils of his faradic apparatus to provide several variations of faradic currents by using wire of different lengths and diameters in the secondary coil or helix. In this particular unit No.21 wire of 84 yards was used as the first division and 154 yards in the second division; No.32 wire of 300 yards in the first division and 500 yards in the second divisiion; and No.36 wire of 500 yards in the first division and 1000 yards in the second division (total was 2538 yards of wire).

Kidder considered this coil design (21 combinations) to avoid the removal of secondary coils an advantage by replacing another coil for a specific treatment. A rheostat is a component of the unit to control electromotive force on the primary coil or field; a gear movement regulates the coil movement; an interrupter to control rapid frequencies and another one to regulate slow current frequencies; a switch to select the frequency of choice; and a pole changer to select the wire of choice and reversing direction of primary current. These components were mounted on a polished rubber face plate.

The unit uses four dry cells for power supply in portable operation, but for office work sol ammioniac batteries were recommended with the back contact posts. The wooden case (12 x 9 x 9.25 inches) has a self lock on front along with two hook lever latches, and a metal carrying handle on top. It sold for $40.00 in 1896. The Kidder Co advertised the unit with endorsements by leading electrotherapeutic physicians: Apostoli, Goelet, Rockwell, and Tripier.

High Tension Coils. The Kidder Co offered other portable high tension faradic batteries for family use. One such High Tension Coil was shown in the 1893 catalog of The Truax, Greene & Co of Chicago. This model is housed in a hardwood case (8.5 x 5 x 2.5 inches). The battery was then powered by either two closed bisulfate of mercury cells, or by

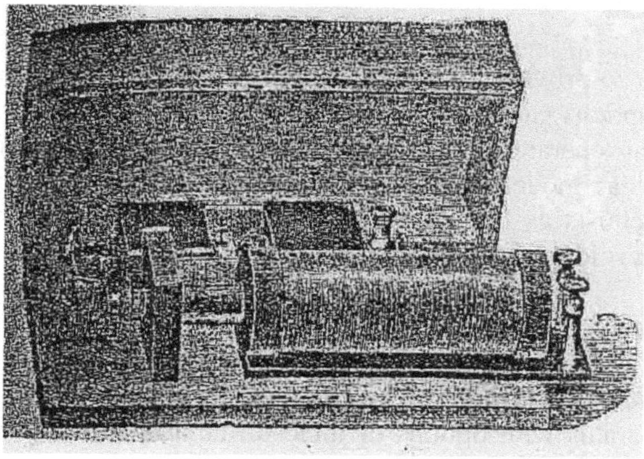

Fig K15A. High Tension Coil

another cell (dry or wet). Two binding posts are available to connect cells to two conductor posts on the base of the coil. The secondary coil is moved over the primary coil to provide gradated current amplitudes (principle of DuBois-Reymond). The coils combined were wound by about 4500 feet of wire. Although the secondary coil could be substituted with others, different coils were not included in the basic price of $30.00.

The **Portable High Tension Coils** model (Fig K15B) for family use was designed somewhat after the principle of DuBois-Reymond (ca 1845), and carried by The Truax, Greene & Co catalog of 1893. The unit has a wooden case (9.25 x 8.5 x 5 inches). This model has four different diameters and lengths of wire for use in combinations. The wire contained is about 8000 feet in length. The primary coil is moved in this model and during its moving (sliding) the current amplitude varies. In most models the secondary coils slide over the primary coils to gradate the current amplitude. The circular end plate or cap of the primary coil

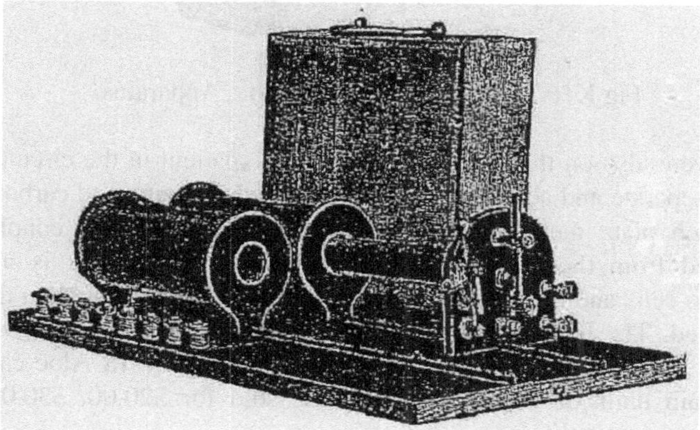

Fig K15B. Portable High Tension Coils Apparatus

has a vibrator to provide medium to rapid rates of current, interruptions. These interruptions can also be slowed by a second interrupter. One or more cells can operate the model. This electrical battery was designed similarly to a model used by such eighteenth century renown electrotherapeutists as Drs Apostoli, Goelet, Rockwell, and Tripier. In 1893, the unit sold for $65.00.

Galvanic Batteries

Portable Galvanic Apparatus. Kidder offered his portable galvanic apparatus with options of three different number of cells and two variations of quality. This galvanic unit of 1893 was redesigned from the basic models of 1871. The apparatus was enclosed in a hardwood box that has a hinged lid with a metal carrying handle. The case is hinged in the middle of the box and on top. Thus, the case has two hinged sections. The open top lid exposed the face plate with its slides for engaging the number of cells activated, and a pole changer for polarity selection of a specific connecting post. Two metal adjustable spring screw connecting

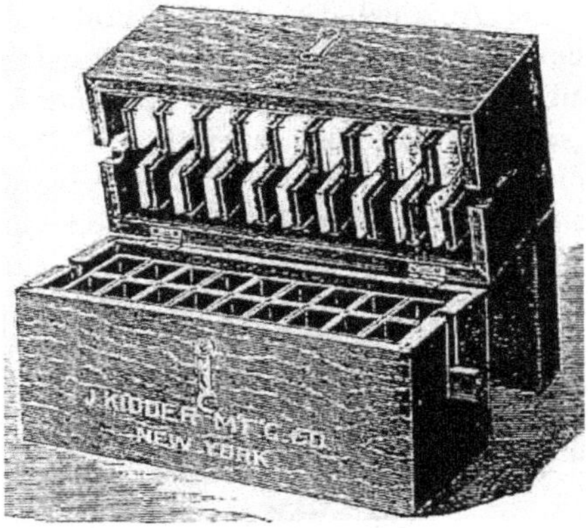

Fig K16. Kidder Portable Galvanic Apparatus[9]

posts were also on the face plate to place the patient in the circuit. Each cell is separate and accepts a couple composed of a zinc and carbon plate that each plate measures 5.25 x 1.5 inches. The sets of couples are removed from the cells when the lid opens. A hydrastat is inserted between cells and elements to keep cell fluid from spilling when the unit is carried. The better units came in 12, 18, and 24 cells, and sold for $26.00, $36.00, and $48.00, respectively in the 1893 AS Aloe catalog.[9] The plain units of 12, 18, and 24 cells sold for $20.00, $30.00, and $42.00, respectively.

Primary Cell Batteries. This battery of Kidder in Fig K17 is a galvanic unit offered as a 12- and 18-cell unit in 1871. The basic design is a number of individual cells (each 2.5 x 1.38 x 4.5 inches) inserted in a wooden box that is hinged with a hook lever latch on front to secure the lid. The connection to the subject is by two metal posts on the sliding current regulator. The current regulator was moved over the cells to increase or decrease the number of cells desired at a particular time. This 12-cell galvanic battery sold for $20.00 in 1871.[1]

In the unit of Fig K 18 the cell elements were couples of carbon

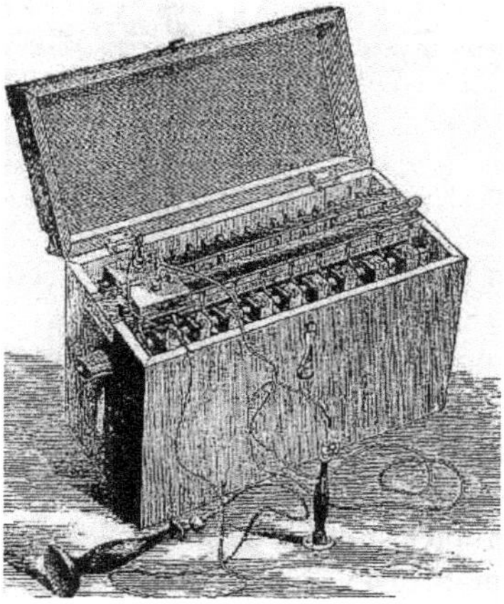

Fig K17. Primary Cell Battery, 12 Cells

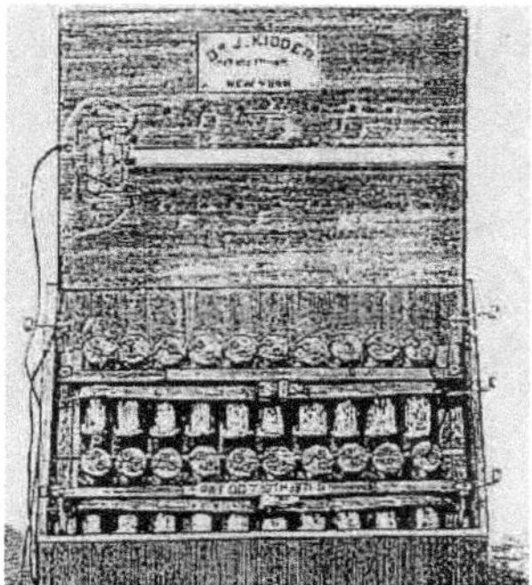

Fig K18. Primary Cell Battery, 18 Cells, 1871

and zinc contained in a polished mahogany box (15 x 7 x 11.5 inches).

Like the basic unit it also had a sliding device to engage the number of wet cells in series. Each unit has a cell saving device (a lever) that interrupts the flow of current when the slide is moved to engage the desired number of wet cells. The unit was designed so that two 18-cell

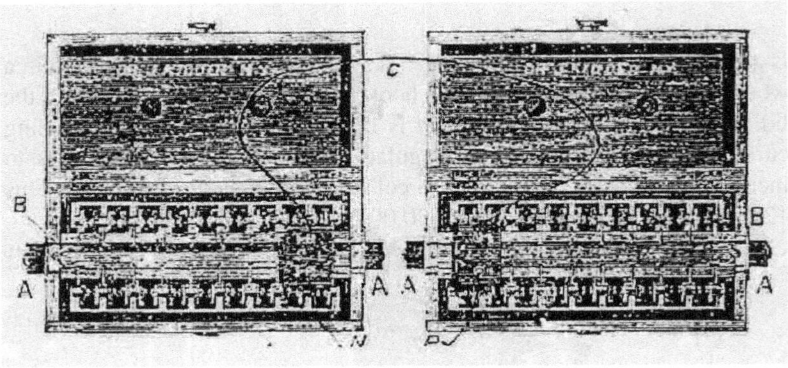

Fig K19. Kidder's Batteries joined

batteries can be joined to create a 36-cell battery. This 18-cell galvanic battery cost $30.00 in 1871.[1]

Although the operator could save money by investing in two 18-cell primary cell batteries to obtain the output of 36 cells, Kidder sold a separate 36-cell primary battery for $175.00. The battery offers several functions that the others cannot. This unit has a double switch current reverser; a wheel interrupter, and Kidder's great wheel-armed compound switch to select any number of wet cells at a time. This wheel is capable

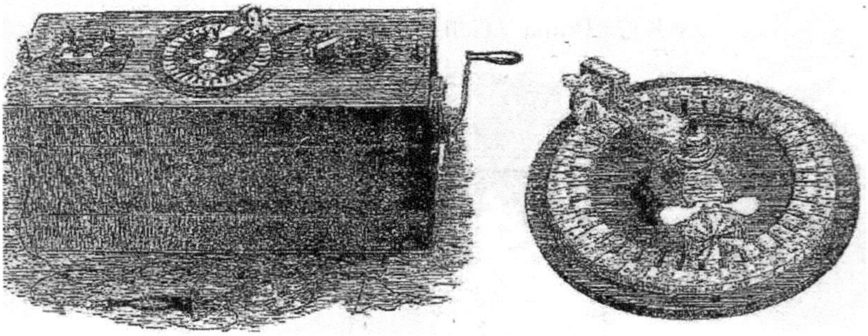

Fig K20. Primary Cell Battery, and Wheel-Armed Compound Switch

of decreasing or increasing the number of cells with or without breaking the circuit. Kidder added a newly patented device of his that changes the large current amplitude (cautery) to large current voltage. The crank and pulley system raises and lowers the elements from and into the cell fluid.

The unit is housed in a polished mahogany box.The idea of the **tip battery** (cell) is to have spare cells available when a set becomes exhausted in the middle of a treatment session. The tip battery has a series of metallic pins mounted in the lid. When the lid is closed and secured the pins engage with the elements to complete the electrical circuit. Two rows of cells are contained in separate trays so that either

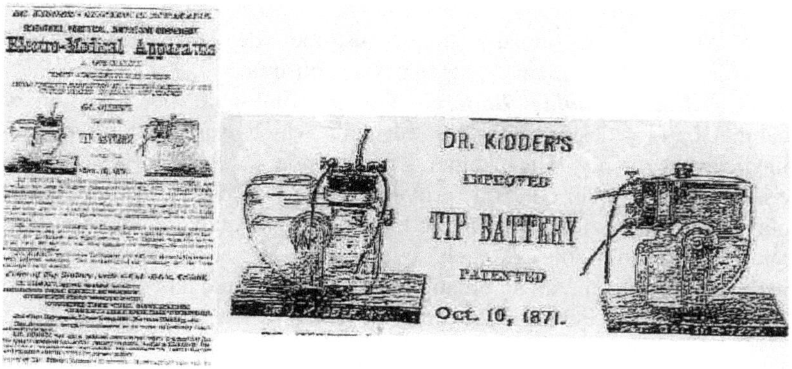

Fig K21. Tip Battery of Kidder

can be lifted from the box by leather straps. Kidder sold this unit in 1871 for $40.00.[1]

At the time (1871) the design of this cell was unique. The design allowed for charging or discharging on demand by tipping the cell, the sealed cap prevented the spilling of the acid when transporting the battery, and the tipping prolonged the life of the zinc and carbon elements. Kidder's cell was known as the hydrostatic tip battery.[8]

Miscellaneous

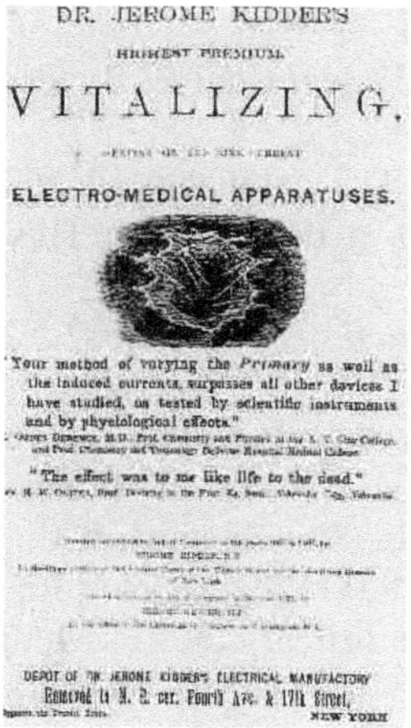

Fig K22. Booklet

By 1898, the Jerome Kidder Manufacturing Co was making x-rays that continued for awhile in the twentieth century. The company's success was its manufacture of quality medical electrical machines (particularly faradic coil machines) for physicians from 1865 to around

1898. Although the company's major customer was the physician, it also sold medical electrical machines to public consumers.

Kidder Cabinet Battery. The unit of Fig K23 is a stationary cabinet battery designed for 60 wet cells which was ideal for certain medical treatments. The cabinet has an open face plate (no lid) that contains: a faradic coil for providing 10 different combinations of currents; switches for selecting the faradic and galvanic current variations and reversing the poles of each; switches for operating the faradic coil and galvanic current; an automatic interrupter for rapid and slow galvanic currents and a switch for its operation; a water rheostat; a galvanscope

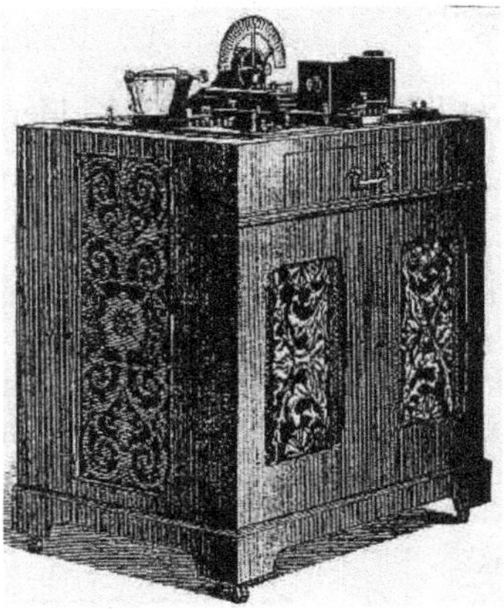

Fig K23. Kidder Cabinet Battery

and cord connecting posts. The cabinet is elaborately carved, and the furniture helped to serve as a deluxe unit. This unit was introduced around 1890.

High-Tension Induction Apparatus. The Kidder Mfg Co described this unit in 1894 (Times Register 25 Aug) and 1895 (Medical Record 21 Dec), respectively. The unit was designed by Dr SH Monell, a leading electrotherapeutist and x-ray physician of New York City. Monell called it an upright switchboard with a hidden compound induction coil having about 8,000 feet of Nos.36, 32, and 21 wire coils fixed permanently over the primary helix. Monell also designed the secondary current controllers, and primary rheostat. Six interior dry cells

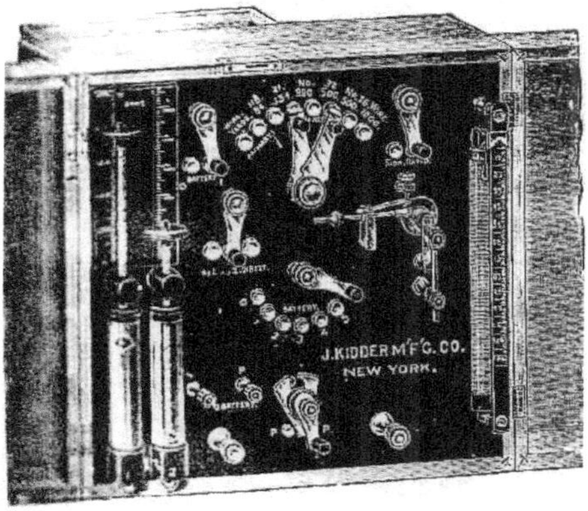

Fig. K23A. High-Tension Induction Apparatus

powered the unit, and the cells were controlled by a selector switch. The unit can deliver rapid and slow faradic pulses. The face plate also has a pole reverser, and adjustable magnetic field switches. The unit is housed in an oak box that has a split lid hinged on two sides of the box. When the lids are closed they are secured by a self locking device.

Wall Cabinet. The Kidder Mfg Co introduced this model (Fig K23B) around 1895 or 1896. The induction coil used the sledge induction principle and pulses could be controlled for rapid and slow

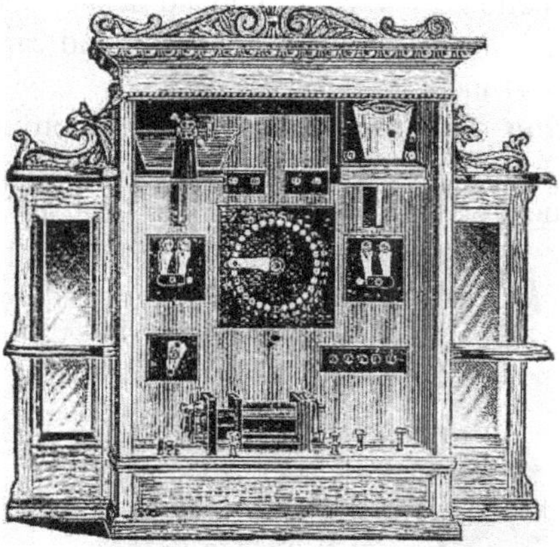

Fig K23B. Kidder Wall Cabinet

rates. The Kidder Mfg Co used its compound circular switch, a switch for galvanic current, a milliammeter, and various other switches.

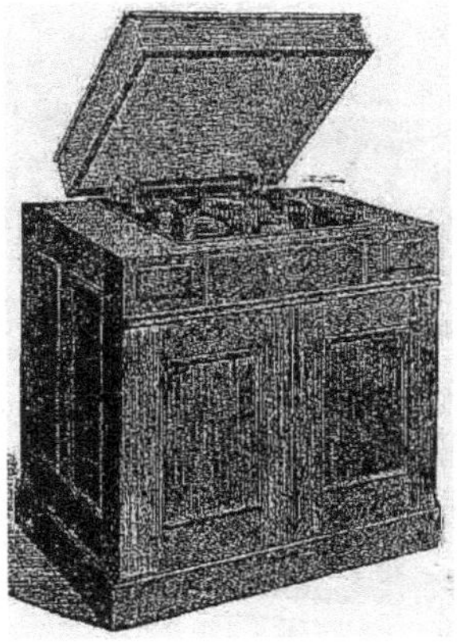

Fig K23C. Cabinet Apparatus

Cabinet Apparatus. This Kidder model (Fig K23C) contains a polarity changer, an automatic interrupter, a cut off switch, switches for faradic and galvanic currents, connecting posts, and a faradic coil providing 10 current variations. These electrical components are mounted on a black inlaid hard rubber face plate. Also, the unit has a compound circle of 40 cells that prevents defective cells from interfering with the galvanic current in the circuit or causing unwanted electrical shocks to the patient. Coil selectors are also included. Three cells are also included for the faradic functions. The cells supplied at the time delivered about 1.5 volts each. The unit cost $140.00 in 1893, and came in a hardwood cabinet (30 x 22 x 37 inches).

Continuous Coil Machine. The coil provides 10 different faradic currents from its coil functioning as that formed by different windings. The model was introduced between 1900 and 1907.

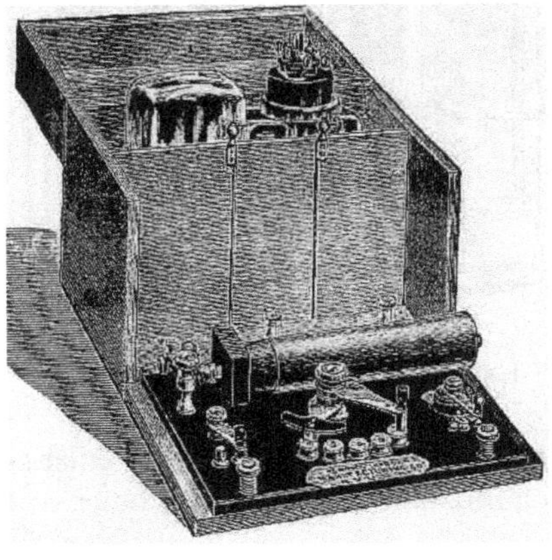

Fig K24. Continuous Coil Machine with Tip Battery

Physicians's Visiting Pocket Battery. The small battery (Fig K25) is compact and designed to fit into a coat pocket. Modeled after the

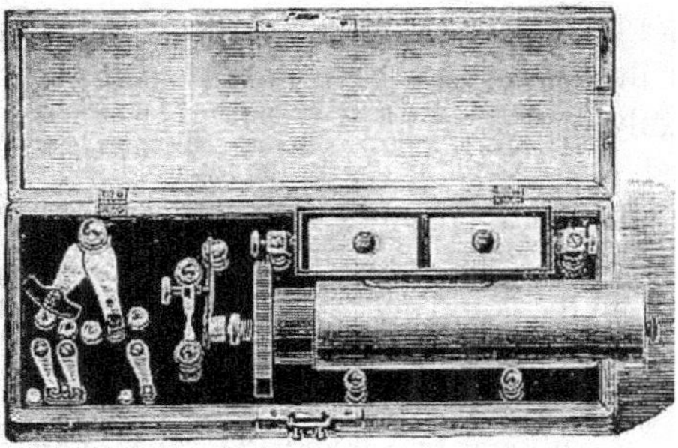

Fig K25. Physician's Visiting Pocket Battery

unit by Gaiffe of France, it is superior to Gaiffe's unit in workmanship and voltage output from its coil. The wet cell that powered the battery was a double, open, bisulfate of mercury cell. The coil is wound by four different lengths and diameters of wire that can deliver voltage equivalent to the batteries having larger coils. The wooden case (10 x 3 x 2 inches) has a self lock on the front. The style of the coil is of the sledge inductorium, has a spring lever adjustable contact screw type of interrupter, switches to select different windings or voltages of the coil, and an On/Off switch. The model was introduced around 1900. The coil is of common (Kidder) size, voltage, and is housed in compact form with a hydrostat tip cell.

Summary

Dr Kidder's apparatuses were quality constructed whether for physician or home use. His apparatuses for home use were a little more costly than those sold by manufacturers of home or family medical electrical batteries. Examination of the various home units will quickly verify this assessment. Certain features of the Kidder batteries help to identify them. Most of the Kidder apparatuses had a circular signature plate identifying the equipment with the Kidder name. Metal on the Kidder apparatus is heavy brass on earlier units and nickel plated on later units. The adjustable binding and connecting posts always had springs mounted to hold the adjusted positions. Most interrupters (rheotomes) were mounted parallel to and on the face plate of the apparatuses, since the coils were mostly located underneath the face plates. The sliding hollow tubes (tin) in the coils were usually larger (1.75 inches dia) than most by other companies (0.75 to 1.0 inch in dia). Accessories to the

Kidder apparatuses are of quality metals and woods, also. The wooden boxes are of hard wood, corners glued, and wedges (splines) inserted into corners make for sturdy and attractive cases.

The Jerome Kidder Manufacturing Company was founded as early as 1859 and Dr Kidder remained in charge until sometime in 1881. During most of these years Dr Kidder, MD, had an active role in the company (probably in designs of medical electrical batteries) since as a clinician he used various electrical batteries in his practice. Dr Kidder offered some innovative and unique features on his electrical batteries (eg: hydrostat tip cell, wheeled arm compound switchs, different coil windings). Although the company is among the earliest manufacturers of medical electrical batteries in the United States, artifacts of the Kidder manufactory do not generally appear before 1872 to 1875.

Dr Kidder authored two books. The first book Electro-allotrop-physiology. Uses of Different Qualities of Electricity to Cure Diseases was published in 1873. Editions two and three were published in 1877 and 1891, respectively. The second book was published in 1878 and reflected his views on health, The Vital Resources Contributing to Capacity, Health, and Longevity, including, also, The Great Law of Evolution and Progression of the Human Species, By the More Comprehensive Inheritance Resulting from Duality of Parentage.

In 1861 and 1868, Dr Kidder attempted to patent some of his electrical battery apparatuses that did not fully comply with patent regulations. Dr Charles Page, a noted physician-inventor of a type of induction coil and also in electrotherapeutics, was the patent officer and withheld approval until patent regulations were met. The process apparently delayed and cost Dr Kidder time and money. Some years after Dr Page had died Dr Kidder posted advertisements in an attempt to discredit the inventor of a type of induction coil. This situation is a very unusual event in the history of electrotherapeutics in the United States.

The Kidder Mfg Co changed ownership in 1881 and continued to at least 1904 or even to 1910. History of the company after 1904 has not been located. The owner (s) of the company after 1881 through 1904 did not adapt the product line to the then modern commercial electricity to power the apparatuses. Also, physician interest in electrotherapeutics began to wane. Thus, like some other manufacturers of medical electrical batteries the owner (s) were content to close out the business and fade into history.

References

1. Vitalizing, catalog of Jerome Kidder Mfg Co. New York, NY, Jerome Kidder, 1871

2. Edmonson JM. American Surgical Instruments. San Francisco, CA, Norman Pub, 1997, p 222

3. Davis AB, Dreyfus MS. The Finest Instruments Ever Made. Arlington, MA, Med Hist Pub Assocs, 1986, p 181

4. Romaine LB. A Guide to American Trade Catalogs 1744-1900, New York, NY, RR Bowker, 1960, pp 235-241

5. Warner DJ. Everything from Watch to Locomotive. Rittenhouse 5:81-93, 1991

6. Meyer M (trs Hammond WA). Electricity in Its Relations to Practical Medicine. New York, NY, D Appleton, 1869, p 127

7. Morrill SE. A Treatise of Practical Instructions in the Medical and Surgical Uses of Electricity. Kalamazoo, MI, Kalamazoo Pub, 1882, pp 78, 253

8. The Kidder hydrostatic tip battery. The Mfg Builder, 22 May 1890, p 116

9. Catalog of AS Aloe. St Louis, MO, AS Aloe, 1893

CHAPTER 9. McINTOSH BATTERY AND OPTICAL COMPANY OF CHICAGO

McIntosh medical electrical batteries were quality products in the industry. A brief sketch of Dr McIntosh, his success, and that of the company that he founded are reviewed in Chapter 9.

Lyman McIntosh (born 1840s, Sheboygan, WI?) finished his medical education in 1863 at the Caledonia, VT Medical College. He then served as a surgeon in the army for about one year, and then returning to Sheboygan to enter private practice. He practiced medicine for 15 years during which time he gained a deep interest in medical electricity, as well as many other science concerns. In the 1870s (ca 1878), he moved to Chicago to start his manufacturing business, the McIntosh N.U. Supporter Co.[1]

He incorporated his medical electrical business as The McIntosh Galvanic Belt and Battery Company in 1879. The company was first located at 192 Jackson and 194 Jackson,[2] but it took over additional space in 1880 by relocating to 300-302 Dearborn St,[3] Chicago, IL. The company was apparently managed by Harris L Emmert and Charles F Berg until about 1886. Dr McIntosh pledged his business to offer physicians the utmost in science and faradic battery development. The McIntosh Company soon became a leader in the manufacture of electrotherapeutics equipment. Dr McIntosh was also interested in other scientific and mechanical instruments so directed his company into manufacturing dental and optical instruments, stands for microscopes, and various types of microscopes.[1]

The company manufactured and sold medical electrical batteries (apparatuses) for use by physicians and for home use by public consumers. Over time the company became foremost in the medical electrical battery business. Additionally, the company sold respirators, bullet probes, electrical belts, electrical baths, larynoscopes, and microscopes. The illustrated catalog of 1881 emphasized various electrical bath apparatuses; electrodes; galvano-cautery batteries; galvanometers; medical electrical apparatuses; a stereopticon; "milliamperemeters;" and solar microscopes. The name of the company that was entered in the Office of the Librarian of Congress, Washington, DC, in 1881, and of its catalog for that year was the "McIntosh Galvanic and Faradic Battery Company Illustrated Catalogue."[3]

McIntosh issued trade catalogs that in addition to illustrating and listing its products contained valuable information such that they would be worthy of libraries of physicians as references. Competitors also published trade catalogs just as worthy, and today many of these catalogs are available in special medical oriented libraries as well as being sold as collector items. According to the McIntosh catalogs the company set policy to provide the lowest prices possible to physicians, but did not have discounts unless orders were cash and then a 20 percent discount was given.

The catalog of 1881 also served to educate physicians about electricity, its history, its uses, and a variety of treatments by electricity as advocated by leading physicians through their published articles in major medical journals. The educational section of the catalog also provided a glossary, while the business section contained descriptions and illustrations of each electrical battery listed in the catalog.

From its beginning the company was basically a manufacturer and retailer of equipment for physicians. A particular item of the company would be designed and manufactured that differed slightly from similar products of others and then patented in the same year. Once marketed, a product might be featured in McIntosh catalogs for many years without improvements or modifications. In some instances improvements and modifications were made, while in others a product might be dropped or its replacement added. The McIntosh Co, although the foremost leader, did not have the number of patents for its products as did some competitors (eg, The Chloride of Silver Dry Cell Battery Co, Galvano-Faradic Mfg Co, Waite & Bartlett). The McIntosh company survived for more than 73 years, and outlived all of its early competitors. The company survived as a formidable business because of its quality product lines, business and marketing practices, and of course its personnel.

LD McIntosh started making the Combined Galvanic and Faradic Batteries and galvanic belts when he incorporated the business in 1879 as the McIntosh Galvanic Belt & Battery Co. From this battery model he developed the Table and Wall Plates for use with wet and dry cells. The face plates and elements of these batteries changed from hard rubber and nickel plate to marble and slate plates and later chrome to accommodate the use of 110 volts direct "dynamo" or current developed by a motor. With the development of commercial source currents to control rheostats and allow for reliable meters it was not long until the sliding metal controllers of induction coils and arbitrary scales were replaced. McIntosh developed the MacLagan "shunt milliamperemeter" or wire rheostat around 1907, and the company offered 110 volts alternating "dynamo" current on many of its electrotherapeutic models. The alternating current (AC) units then required the use of transformers and rectifiers.

By 1885, the McIntosh Optical and Battery Co moved to 192 Jackson Street, and in its 13 paged catalog for that year were advertised solar microscopes, stereopticons, and combination of both; microscopes, achromatic objectives, optical lanterns, and ether oxygen lime lights.[3]

Late in 1885, McIntosh brought out another trade catalog advertising the combination of galvanic and faradic batteries, electrotherapeutic appliances, electrical bath equipment, and other electrical items. The catalog contained 64 pages this time with illustrations.[9] Additionally, at this time the company had been and was selling the electrical static (influence) machines to and for physician use along with faradic coil and galvanic electrical machines in wooden boxes. The faradic coil and galvanic electrical machines in wooden boxes were also being sold by the company to public consumers, but these units were of poorer quality than those for physician use.

In 1888, the McIntosh Galvanic and Faradic Battery Co moved to 141 and 143 Wabash. The company's name changed to McIntosh Battery & Optical Co in 1889, and had John S Emmert as president and Hugh McLachlan the secretary and treasurer. Alfred Smith became the secretary in 1890, and in 1891 Charles W Bassett was the president and C Alfred Smith was the secretary.[2]

The McIntosh catalogs of 1889 (No.16, revised, 200 pages), 1890, 1897 (illustrated with 288 pages), and 1899 (No.19 with 272 pages) seemed to emphasize the company's line of galvanic and faradic coil electrical machines or therapeutic uses more than previous catalogs.[3] The 1890s turned out to have been the peak years for wooden cased medical electrical batteries in the hands of physicians. With each new issue of catalogs the company appeared to be growing in sales for machines for electrotherapeutics. Dr LD McIntosh was still writing the preface of the company's catalog in 1890 as shown by the 10-paged illustrated catalog of that year.

The catalog of 1890 was the twelfth edition (114 pp) and offered a wide range of electrotherapeutic machines, accessories, equipment (batteries, instruments), electrical chair, electrical belts, microscopes, lamps, methods of treatment, and abstracts of published literature on electrotherapeutics directed to physicians and surgeons. Dr LH McIntosh prefaced that little advancement of technology had taken place in electrotherapeutics in recent years. (ed, That probably accounts for electrical apparatuses being sold for 20 years or more without design changes.)

While electrotherapeutics was at a standstill commercial electricity was advancing with its electrical lighting, power capacity, furnaces, telegraphs, and telephones. Mathematics had recently been applied in the manufacture of electrotherapeutic apparatuses and the results were milliammeter ("milliamperemeters") devices. The catalogs stressed the use of galvanic batteries for gynecology and surgery. For surgery at least 12 cells were needed to operate but if they were the chloride of silver type than 20 cells were required.

Most of the company's cells (batteries) delivered 1.6 volts each. The McIntosh Co's best acid cell was called the "plunge." This acid type cell consists of two large plates arranged on a base, and when activating the plates were immersed in acid. The storage cell, however, was considered ideal for electrotherapeutics since it could be recharged.

Dr LD McIntosh was involved in a series of lectures in Fumale, FL, on 1 March 1892 when he died.[1] During his professional career, he was involved not only in promoting medical electrical batteries but many scientific instruments. Dr McIntosh was a member of the American Medical Association, the American Microscopical Society, and the Illinois State Microscopical Society. He also had served on a committee for a World's Fair. He frequently lectured at educational conventions, while president at the American Dental College of Chicago.[1] Whether Bassett and Smith played a role in the McIntosh Co after Dr LD McIntosh's death is unknown. Under Dr LD McIntosh's control the company maintained a progressive atmosphere with up-to-date technology and science. The company provided updated instruments to physicians since its founding, and offered educational instruction to physicians about electrotherapeutics prior to any inclusion of the subject in the curricula of medical schools. The firm existed 60 more years.

The illustrated catalog of 1893 was No.16 (200 pp) and contained electrical batteries and electrotherapeutic apparatuses. This catalog shows that the company's name had changed (1889) to the McIntosh Battery & Optical Company from the McIntosh Galvanic and Faradic Battery Co, and at the time was located at 141 and 143 Wabash Avenue. Catalog number 18 (288 pp) was issued in 1897 and No.19 (272 pp) in 1899.[3] The McIntosh Battery & Optical Company of Chicago in 1897 wanted exposure in the east so had the Oelschlaeger Brothers of 42 E 23rd St, New York, represent them for electrotherapeutic equipment and supplies only. The Brothers had a set of elegant show rooms for physicians to visit. Their line of products included: office cabinet batteries, storage batteries for galvanic cautery, electrical and thermal baths, electrodes and electrotherapeutic specialties, controller for use with commercial currents, Jewel graphite rheostats, "milliamperemeters," and dental appliances. The Brothers also sold books on medical electricity. They made available reprints of leading published articles on medical electricity to physicians and other customers.

The 1893 catalog of the AS Aloe Co, St Louis, still offered a variety of McIntosh medical electrical batteries that were enclosed in wooden boxes, wooden cabinets, and plain units without cases but of mostly metal construction. The company was sold in 1897.[1] Dr McIntosh's son John remained associated with the company, and engaged in the x-ray business.

The McIntosh catalog for 1900 cited its location as 92-98 State Street, Chicago, IL. Its trade catalog (edition 21) was reduced to 96 pages that year, and listed mostly batteries and electrotherapeutic apparatuses.[3]

The year 1896, apparently transformed the electrotherapeutic industry from the more traditional faradic coil and galvanic electrical machines in wooden boxes to the manufacture of the newly invented x-ray machine. This transformation was a natural move for the manufacturers of the electrical static (influence machines), like McIntosh, and Waite & Bartlett, because these machines could power the x-ray that demanded high frequencies, high voltages, but small current amplitudes for operation. By 1905, the McIntosh company was advertising its new Hogan silent x-ray transformer in a 10-paged brochure. This catalog was showing the address of 322 West Washington St, Chicago. The McIntosh catalogs of 1907 (edition # 29, 158 pages), and 1909 (edition # 30, 158 pages) continued their emphasis on electrotherapeutic apparatuses and supplies. Items advertised were usually illustrated.

Like so many of its competitors, the McIntosh Co cautioned readers of its advertisements and literature not to buy cheapened versions of electrotherapeutic equipment. In the 1907 trade catalog Illustrated Catalog of Electro-Therapeutical Apparatus the company boosted using electricity in its factory for operating special machines in the manufacture of electrotherapeutic apparatuses. Also about this time, some of the faradic, galvanic, and combined batteries that used one or two dry cells were encased in a morocco covered box that was cheaper to

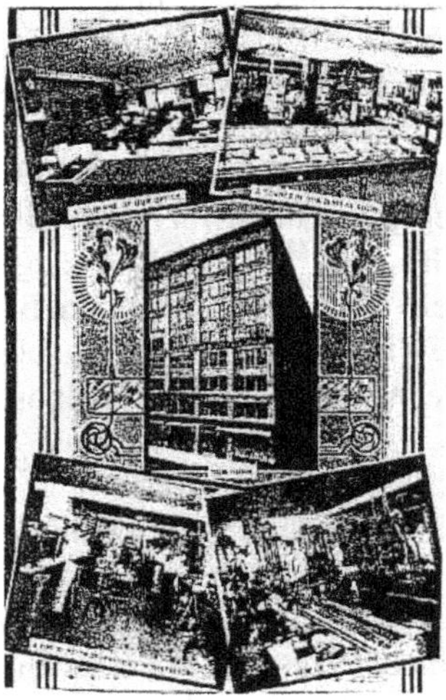

Fig M1. McIntosh Factory, 1907

produce than the customary hard wood boxes. In 1907, the McIntosh Battery & Optical Co was located at 227-229 Washington Street, Chicago.

In 1910, the McIntosh catalog, although still concentrating on selling electrotherapeutic apparatuses, indicated another change of address to 217-223 North Desplaines St, Chicago. The company seemed to emphasize its improved alternating current rectifier and potential equalizer. The 1911 catalog (edition #32, 192 pages) illustrated electrotherapeutic equipment. The 24 paged catalog of 1912 offered suggestions to spondylotherapists who were physicians specializing in back problems and using electrotherapy to treat their patients. The catalog of 1917 was dealing with the Simtech, simple Roentgen, Tesla and d'Arsonval technologies. Sometime between 1917 and 1922 the McIntosh Battery & Optical Co relocated to 223-233 North California Avenue, Chicago.[3]

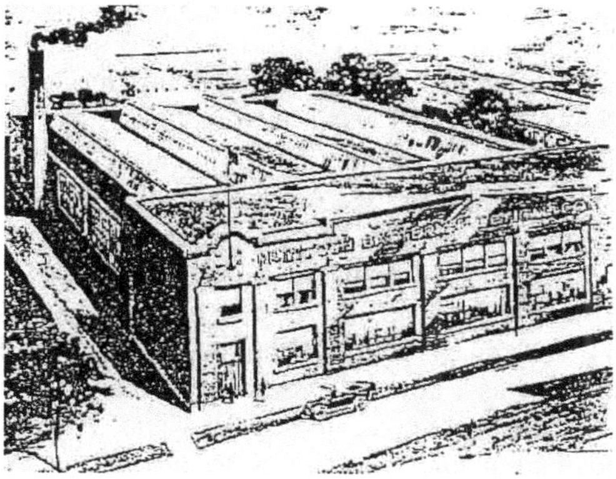

Fig M2. McIntosh Factory, ca 1920[4]

The McIntosh Battery and Optical Co was doing well in two areas of business so the company divided itself in 1922 to further promote specific science products that Dr LD McIntosh had promoted earlier during his career. The company was divided into the McIntosh Electrical Corporation and the McIntosh Battery and Optical Corp with the Stereopticon Division. Both companies seemed to do business from 223-233 North California Ave, Chicago.[3]

Around 1922 (no specific date), the McIntosh Co began publishing a monthly bulletin The Therapeutics of High Frequency in concert with the technologies of Nikola Tesla and Jacques d'Arsonval that were introduced in its catalog of 1917. The purpose of the bulletin was to educate potential consumers of its product. In 1923, the McIntosh bulletin of electronics offered electromedical and physical therapeutics equipment (note change in wording from electrotherapeutics). This equipment continued to be offered through its catalogs of 1926 and 1929.

In 1929, the McIntosh Electrical Corporation began publishing Polysine Philosophy as a manual to accompany each sale of the Polysine generator. The Polysine unit at this time had been marketed for 21 years. The manual was a catalog of 80 pages that served as an operating manual for the polysine generator (viz, generator #1158), but also as a text on the subject of electrotherapy. The manual covered galvanism, medical ionization, sinusoidal currents, electrodes, various uses in patient treatments, and it closed by serving as a price and illustrated catalog of the McIntosh line of electrotherapy products. The catalog also included the physical and physiological effects of various currents. In 1929, the corporation's main office address was still 223-233 North California Ave, Chicago, IL. Factory branches in 1929 included: 303 Fourth Avenue, New York, NY (note: 300 was address for Galvano-Faradic Mfg and Van Houten & Ten Broeck); 857 Boylston St, Boston, MA; 2116 Jenkins Arcade, Pittsburgh, PA; 318 Stewart Street, Seattle, WA; and 312 Medical Arts Bldg, Fort Worth, TX.[4]

The McIntosh Electrical Corp was thriving during the period of 1929 through 1933.[6] Catalog #59 was issued in 1948,[5] and the McIntosh Co was still manufacturing electrotherapy stimulators in 1952. Although the company divided itself into two companies in 1922, the McIntosh Electrical Corp appeared in the Illinois Secretary of State List of Domestic and Foreign Corporations as a foreign business because it incorporated in a state other than Illinois. The company was still located at 223-233 North California Avenue, Chicago. The McIntosh Battery and Optical Corp was listed as a domestic company at the same address, and George R Hogan was cited as its agent. The latter corporation manufactured and sold medical apparatus to physicians.[7] Early in its history McIntosh was often recognized at world fairs as the foremost manufacturer of electrotherapeutic appliances.

Electric Belt and Wet Cell

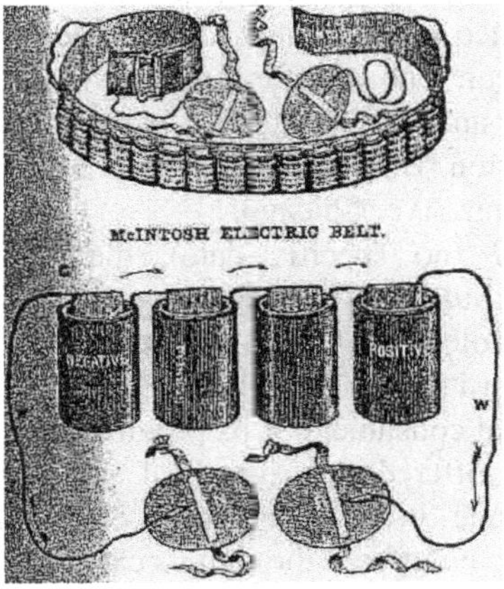

Fig M3 McIntosh Electric Belt

The McIntosh Co was still manufacturing electric belts in 1893, although the company did not emphasize them in its own catalogs. The retailer Truax, Greene & Co also of Chicago sold the McIntosh Electric Belt through its catalog of 1893. The belt was advertised as the perfect galvanic battery with quality workmanship. Under the direction of a physician the belt was suppose to provide relief for diseases that would indicate the use of a mild galvanic current. The basic belt sold for $10.00, but with the suspensory attachment it cost $12.50. These costs were high compared to competitors who sold similar belts for $2.00 to $5.00. The McIntosh Co of course cautioned buyers against purchasing cheap belts that would cause them disappointments.

In 1881, the company was promoting its combined faradic and galvanic wet cell that consisted of a container made of hard rubber, and divided into a larger section (fluid mixture) and a smaller section (drip

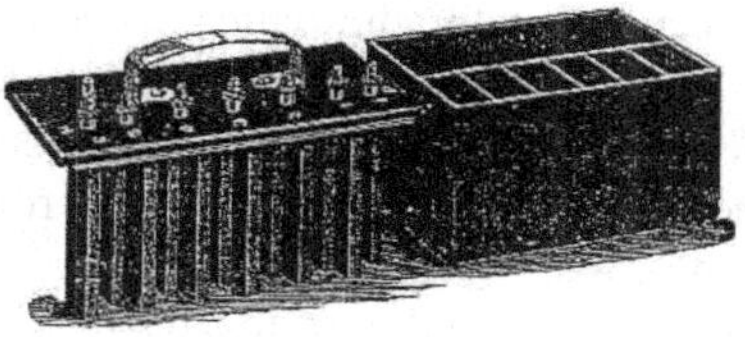

A. Galvanic Cell

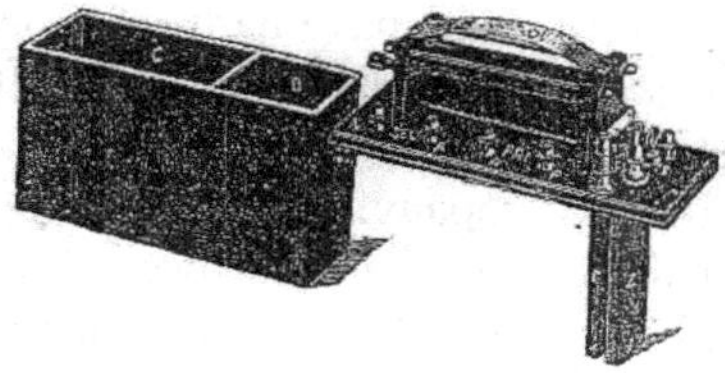

B. Faradic Cell

Fig M4. The McIntosh Wet or Fluid Cell Battery

cup). The face plate of the McIntosh faradic batteries was designed so that with its rotation the plate would align the carbon and zinc elements with either the fluid mixture section to activate the cell, or the drip cup that then would be aligned to store the elements when not in use. Customers who purchased medical electrical batteries were given directions for both mixing the cell solution and the operation of the unit. By 1905, the wet cell was being replaced on new models by the standard dry cell (2.5 x 6 inches) of the time. The McIntosh company was then promoting the Columbia No. 4 dry cell (Union Carbide Co, Chicago; smaller than standard, today's D) for use with its medical electrical batteries.

The McIntosh catalog of 1907, however, continued to devote two full pages to describing and illustrating the wet cell that was then called the "fluid" battery by the company. The exhausted zinc and carbon couples could easily be replaced by manipulating a screw arrangement. McIntosh recommended a solution of sulfuric acid, bichromate of potash, bisulfate of mercury, and water. Each cell of the battery delivered an electromotive force of two volts. After some usage the cell continued to deliver an electromotive force of 1.5 volts. These fluid cells in 1907 were being used mostly with models designed many years earlier.

Commonalties of McIntosh Electrical Apparatus

The most common characteristic on the McIntosh face plates of faradic and galvanic batteries was the nickel plated lifting handle on the face plate or on top of the faradic induction coil. The section of the apparatus having the attached handle could be raised, rotated, and lowered to activate or deactivate the carbon and zinc elements of the wet cell(s). The induction coils of the faradic batteries were capped at each end by a hard rubber square plate (similar to GP Pillings & Son of Philadelphia). The difference in induction coils between McIntosh and Pillings is that the former often used two nickel plated rods on top of the coil to join the squared end caps.

The wooden boxes had metal carrying handles mounted on top of the box, and self locking latches to secure the lid to the box. The induction coils on faradic apparatuses have hard rubber square blocks at each end that characterizes McIntosh models. There are exceptions to these marked characteristics in the McIntosh product line.

Usually the McIntosh company fixed its signature on the box lid or face plate when sold directly from its factory. However, when the McIntosh product was sold through medical suppliers, like other manufacturers, the name of the supplier was often substituted on a label for the McIntosh name. This practice of allowing the seller's name on the product often confuses collectors as to who was its manufacturer.

Until dry cells were introduced, the wet cells (ca 1879-1905) were composed of a specially designed (by McIntosh) hard rubber with compartments to function for the cell solution and drip cup. Quality wooden cases and quality nickel plated hardware are qualities associated with McIntosh. As advancements came to electrical apparatuses in the twentieth century the commonalties between units decreased or disappeared. McIntosh batteries can also be identified by their signature and by their designs.

Faradic Batteries

In 1881, McIntosh's only electrical battery for home treatments by public consumers was the Family Battery. McIntosh wholesaled products to distributors and medical equipment retailers so its name does not always appear on this battery.

Family Faradic Battery. The battery of Fig M5 has a polished black walnut boxed unit (6.25 x 5 x 6 inches), and a self lock with a key to secure the lid on the front of the box. The box (6.5 x 6 x 5 inches) has a metal carrying handle on top, hinged box-like lid, and a hook pivot latch on each side for securing the lid. The black hard rubber face plate has an induction coil with polished hard rubber square blocks at each

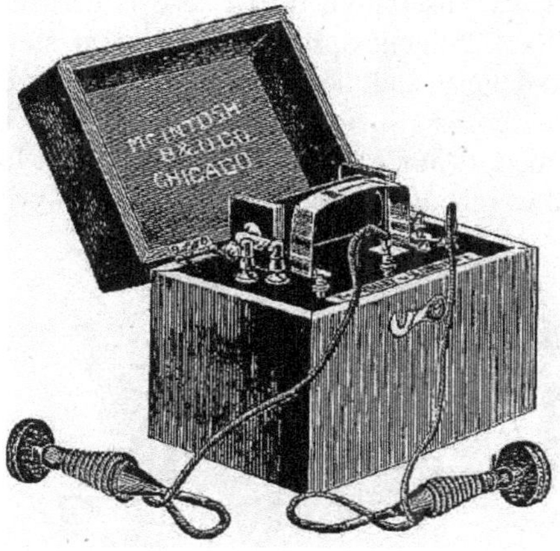

Fig M5. McIntosh Family Faradic Battery

end; a sliding hollow metal tube current controller; an adjustable screw spring lever, hammer vibrator type of interrupter (left side); three jack receptacles connecting posts to select current variations (fore part); and an On/Off lever control (right side). A nickel plate for "P, primary, N, secondary, P" is attached to the front top of the face plate. All metal is nickel plated. The face plate lifts by the nickel plated handle on the coil, and when lifted reveals carbon and zinc elements (1 pair forms a couple) that are permanently attached underneath the face plate. When the face plate is removed the elements can be removed from the fluid of the cells, rotated or reversed, and placed in a drip cup section of the cell to store. The bottom of the box underneath the face plate is a vulcanized rubber insert cell with two sections; one for cell fluid and one for a drip cup. Underneath the face plate is a soft rubber cover that prevents cell fluid from spilling when the face plate is secured in the box.

This unit in 1890 was marketed by the McIntosh Co as a quality family battery in answer to the "cheap" models being sold by competitors for public use. The latching of the lid of the box changed between 1890 and 1895. In 1893, the box had no lock on the front, but rather a single hook pivoting lever latch. Models from 1881 to 1890, had the lock on the front of the box and a hook pivoting lever latch on each side otherwise the model was the same in 1893. The unit sold for $18.00 in the catalogs of McIntosh in 1881 and 1890, and that of AS Aloe in 1893.[8] Amazingly, the cost was held to $10.00 during this span of time. It dates to around 1881 or before, and without any changes it was still available in 1886 for $9.00, and in 1907 for $6.00. Complete, this model weighs 10 pounds.

The McIntosh family battery of 1881 was redesigned slightly and sold as the ***Domicile Battery*** in 1907 for home use. The metal lifting handle on the coil was discontinued, the case is dark Old English oak finish (8.75 x 7.13 x 3.25 inches), is powered by one standard sized (2.5 x 6 inches) dry cell battery, and the lid is secured by a lever latch in front. Inside of the lid is a compartment for accessories. The On/Off switch is designed to be in the Off mode before the lid is closed. In 1907, the unit sold for $5.00 and weighed nine pounds complete. Its price in 1918 was

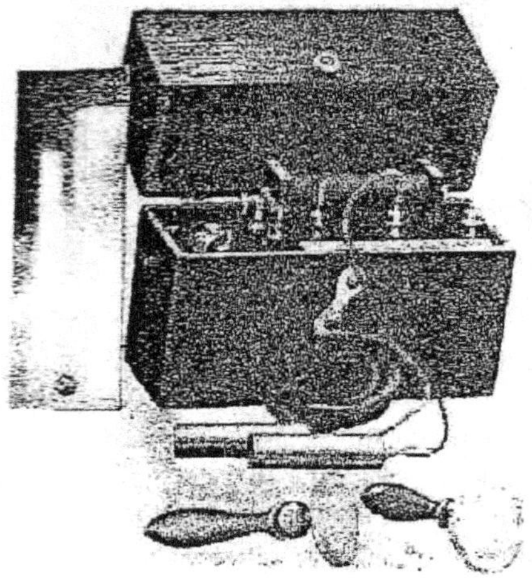

Fig M6. The McIntosh Domicile and Masseuse Battery (1881 & 1907)

$7.50 complete with a booklet of instructions.[9]

This same model was also marketed as the McIntosh ***Masseuse Battery*** to hair dressers and dermatologists who wanted appliances for facial and scalp applications. Thus, the difference between the Domicile and Masseuse Batteries was the number and types of accessories. The Masseuse Battery had eight appliances rather than six for the Domicile, but cost $6.75 and weighed 10 pounds in 1907.

No.44 Faradic Battery. This unit is identical to that of the Domicile Battery of Fig M6. Like the Domicile Battery the lifting handle on the induction coil has been discontinued so the No.44 unit dates to about the same time (1907) as the Domicile. The No.44 is contained in an oak case (7.25 x 6.5 x 5.25 inches) that has a metal carrying handle on top of the lid, and the lid is secured in front by a heavy brass pivoting latch. Directions for operation are cited (black print on yellow) on a paper label glued inside of the lid. Like similar McIntosh faradic batteries the induction coil is capped at each end by a square black hard rubber plate. Also, like other McIntosh models of the same period of time the sliding metal current regulator is on the right of the coil while the spring hammer type of vibrating interrupter is on its left. Three output posts are on the front part of the hard rubber face plate to provide primary, secondary, and combination currents. These posts are labeled by a nickel

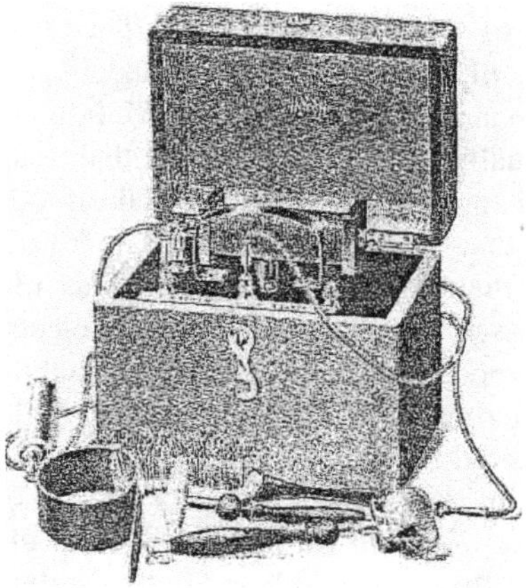

Fig M7. The McIntosh No. 44 Faradic Battery (1907)

plate, characteristic of McIntosh faradic batteries. The lever On/Off switch is on the front left side of the face plate. This unit was designed for family use.

The McIntosh Co manufactured the No.44 Faradic Battery (Fig M7) as early as 1900 to 1902 for family use. This unit's design departs from the series produced from 1881 to 1893 in that the metal lifting

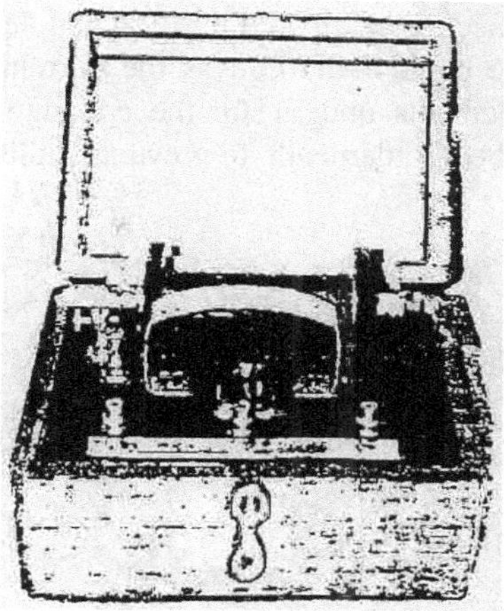

Fig M8. The McIntosh No. 44 Faradic Battery (1900-1902)

handle for the face plate is located on the face plate in front of the coil rather than on the square end caps of the coil. Also, the two nickel plated rods connecting the end caps above the coil are eliminated. Unlike the latter version (1918) of the No.44 Faradic Battery of Fig M7 the sliding metal current regulator is on the right side of the coil while the spring lever hammer type of vibrator is on the left. The On/Off lever is centrally located on the face plate, and the three connecting posts with the nickel plate label are similar in all No.44 units by McIntosh. The oak case (7.5 x 5.25 inches) is actually smaller in total size than that of the latter (1918) version. The metal carrying handle is located on top of the lid, and is of better quality than that of the 1918 model. The lever latch on front of the case is similar to that of the 1918 model. This unit was designed for family use and masseurs who wanted to apply electricity to the face and head after a shampoo. In addition to the usual accessories this unit included an electrical hairbrush, massage roller, and wrist electrode. The unit was then powered by two standard dry cells, weighed nine pounds, and sold for $7.50 in 1907.

Physicians' Faradic Batteries. Several electrical batteries for physician use were illustrated and listed in the McIntosh trade catalogs of 1881 and 1890, and the AS Aloe catalog of 1893.[8] These electrical units included: Physician's Faradic Battery (Fig M9), and Physician's Faradic Battery No.3 (Fig M11). Some differences are noted between these two batteries.

In the first unit (left), Physician's Faradic Battery, the polished black walnut box (9 x 6 x 7 inches) with a hinged lid has a self locking latch on front and on each side a hook pivoting lever latch. A metal carrying handle is located on top of the lid. The face plate is hard rubber; it contains a faradic coil with square hard rubber end caps stabilized by two metal rods connecting them, and a lifting handle on its top; a sliding metal tube over the core of the coil as the current regulator, attached carbon and zinc elements underneath the coil and face plate that are covered by soft rubber underneath to prevent spilling of battery fluid;

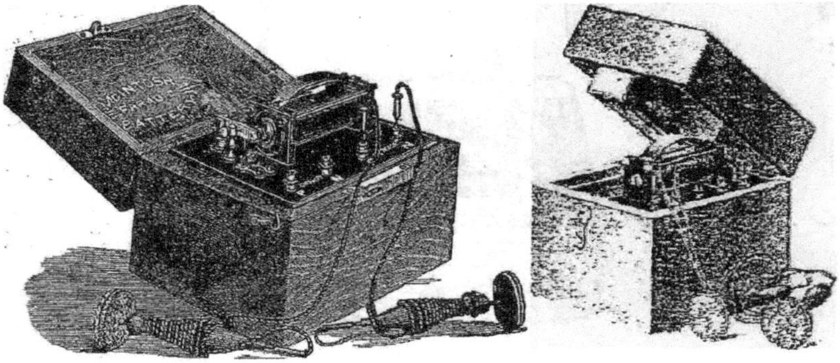

Fig M 9. McIntosh Physicians' Faradic Battery

four connecting posts with the wording for two "primary (P, N)" and for two "secondary (P, N)"; and a spring lever, hammer type of vibrating interrupter. Two fixed metal fixtures are near the interrupter and connect with the circuit. This unit was powered by a single hard rubber cell with a drip cup (sectioned cell) that is activated and deactivated with the carbon and zinc elements inserted and lifted by the handle on top of the coil, and rotating the face plate, respectively. The cost was maintained from 1881 to 1895 as $18.00 complete with accessories (weighs less than 6 pounds complete). In 1896, the cost was dropped to $16.00, and weighed less that six pounds. This battery, like most of the McIntosh Co batteries, has a signature plate on top of the box, and a metal plate giving the patent date and serial number on the face plate. Also, a box number is indented on the box edge near the face plate. This battery was patented on 29 November 1881.

The faradic unit for 1907 (Fig M9, right) changed in its orientation. That is, the coil was rotated to coincide with the depth of the wooden case rather than the traditional position with the box's length. The case was enlarged (7 x 8.25 x 7.25 inches) to accommodate a glass cell casing and drip cup of its fluid cell. The cost was only $10.00 and it weighed about nine pounds. This model is pictured in Fig M9.

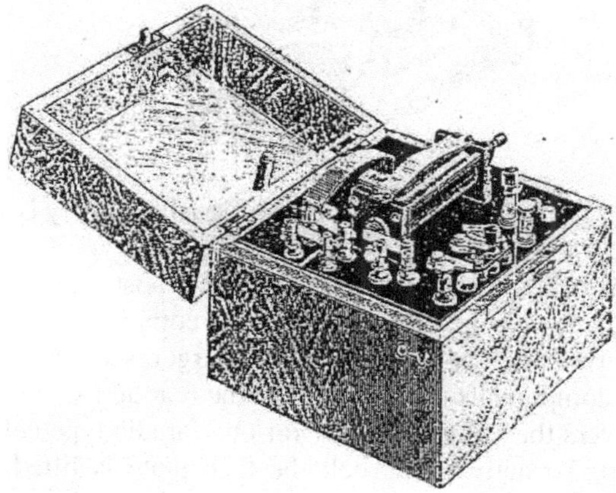

Fig M10. McIntosh No. 66 Practitioner's Faradic Battery[9]

No.66 Physician's Faradic Battery. By 1918, the No.66 Practitioner's Faradic Battery was changed to accommodate two standard dry cell batteries located underneath the face plate, and was then the McIntosh No.66 Practitioner's Faradic Battery. The unit is encased in a finished quartered oak box (9 x 6 x 7.5 inches), has a metal carrying handle on top, and a lever latch on the front. The coil is finished in polished hard rubber with two metal rods, connecting each end cap, and hard rubber squared end caps. The face plate is enameled slate.

Accessories are housed in the lid compartment. The complete unit cost $12.00 in 1918.

Physicians' Faradic Battery No.3. This battery or second physician's battery is a step up from the Physicians' Faradic Battery (Fig M9). It is housed in a polished black walnut box (8 x 8 x 6.5 inches) with hinged lid and metal carrying handle. Each side of the box also has a lever pivoting latch, and a self locking device on the front secures the lid when in the proper position. The black hard rubber face plate contains the coil with its lifting metal handle, two metal rods, and a sliding hollow tube current controller. Each end of the coil has a square black hard rubber block. The coil has a polished hard rubber spool and cover. The

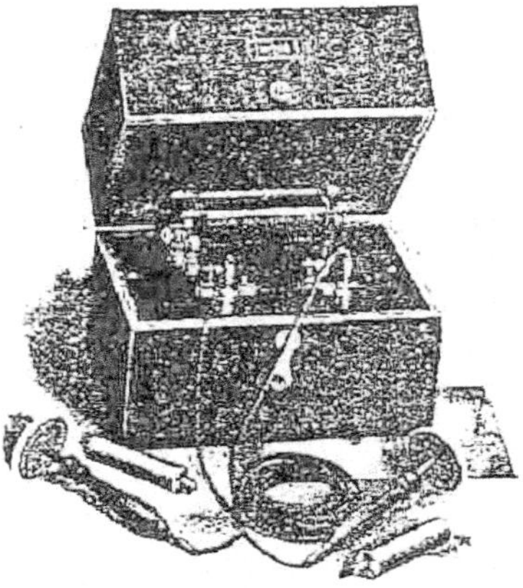

Fig M11. McIntosh Physicians' Faradic Battery No. 3

face plate has two adjustable screw connecting posts, a pole changer, and switches to connect primary, secondary, and combined currents. The face plate forms two sections; the front and larger section (7 x 5 inches) contains the components mentioned, and the rear and smaller section (7 x 2 inches) covers the vulcanized tray for one faradic type cell with a fluid and drip cup. To activate the cell the face plate is lifted, rotated, and lowered; the reverse procedure deactivates the cell. The soft rubber undercoating of the face plate prevents fluid from spilling when the box is carried. The carbon and zinc elements are permanently attached to the face plate. Accessories are stored underneath the larger section of the face plate. The unit cost of the No.3 Physician's Faradic Battery was $30.00 from 1881 to 1893 (AS Aloe[8] and McIntosh[10] catalogs, respectively).

Although this model was patented in 1881, it was still marketed without design changes between 1917 and 1920. This fact is based on the observation of individual units having a signature plate on the top of the lid of the box citing the location of "223-233 N California Ave..." from which the company operated after 1917 (or between 1917 and 1920).

Faradic Coil. An induction coil similar in design and power to that of the Domicile and Masseuse Batteries is mounted on a wooden base that serves as a face plate. The buyer only needed one dry or fluid

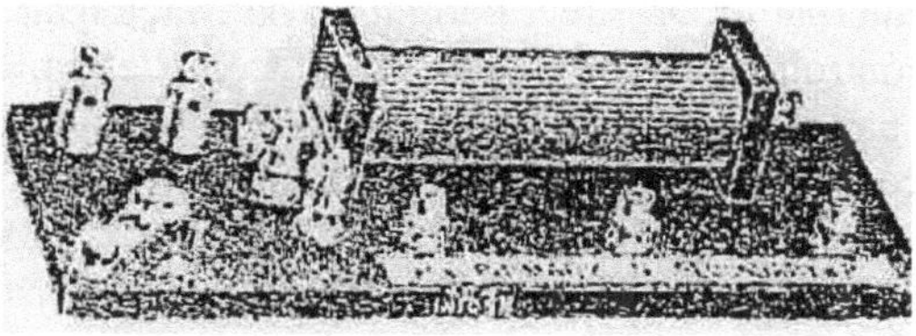

Fig M12 McIntosh Faradic Coil

cell to power it, and the unit functioned as any faradic battery. A vibrating type of spring hammer interrupter was present along with an On/Off lever, and connecting posts to the cell and to the patient. A nickel plate labeling "P, N, P" was located on the front part of the face plate. This unit cost $3.50 in 1907 and included accessories.

High Tension Faradic Battery. The 1907 trade catalog of the McIntosh Co listed its new high tension unit designed for physician use. This unit is portable and contains all new features for that year. The induction coil's windings were featured in the new design as having 230 feet of No.20 wire in the primary winding, and 4500 feet of No.36 wire in its secondary portion. The secondary coil was tapped at 1500 feet, and at 3000 feet to provide its operators a selection in voltage output. This coil continued to be made with the two nickel plated rods connecting the two square end plates. This battery has two rheotomes; one is a singing

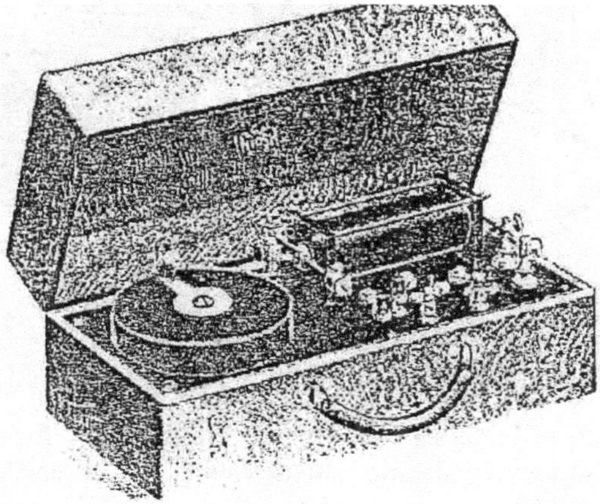

Fig M13. McIntosh High Tension Faradic Battery

ribbon vibrator type and the other is a slow vibrator. These rheotomes provide a variety or full range of vibrations possible in 1907. The unit is powered by three standard sized (2.5 x 6 inches) dry cells, but when used in the physician's office the unit was capable of being powered by either 110 volts of alternating or direct currents. The MacLagan wire rheostat was used to control current amplitude. The face plate is black enameled slate, and the unit is housed in a quarter sawed golden oak box. The box has a leather carrying handle on front with a latch lever at each end of the box front. The unit weighed about 28 pounds and cost $25.00 in 1907.

Gem Dental Battery. The McIntosh company made an electrical battery especially for dentists. This particular unit was made available around 1893 for use by dentists and physicians to test for sensitive teeth. The unit came in a black buckram (Morocco style) covered wooden box (5 x 7 x 2.75 inches) with a self locking device in front and a metal carrying handle on top. The induction coil with rods connecting the square end caps matched that used in the No.3 Physician Battery (Fig M9). The face plate is hard rubber; the metal is nickel plated; a spring lever adjustable screw contact vibrating type interrupter is used to control pulse frequencies, and a sliding metal tube controller is used for controlling current amplitude. A control switch and binding posts are also on the face plate. A Grenet cell came with the unit, along with accessories for $18.00 in 1893.

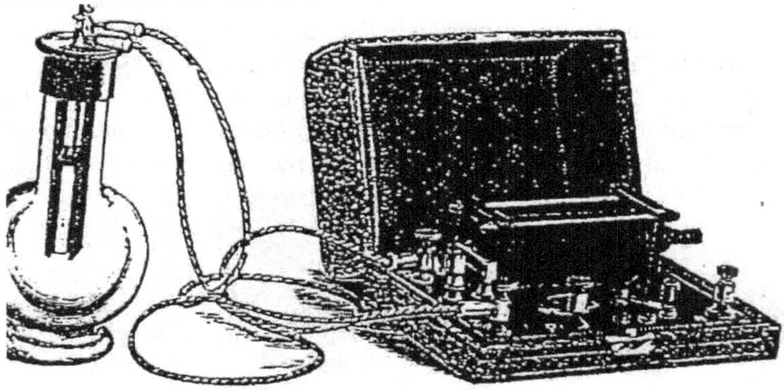

Fig M14. The Gem Dental Battery[8]

Galvanic Batteries

Electrical batteries made by the McIntosh Co for physician use included the series of galvanic batteries with 12, 18, and 24 cells from 1881 (probably 1879) to 1895 or later. These wet cells were modular in style, McIntosh used mostly dry cells after 1905. The basic design of the wet cells was similar for each unit with the size of the box varying with the number of cell packs. Each wet cell pack contained six cells (basic vulcanized rubber with two sections), a metal lifting handle, a lever hook latch on each side, and self lock; 12 wet to 24 metal jack receptacles, and a cell pack switch. One connecting post is contained on two of the wet cell packs. Each galvanic unit has a hard rubber electrode box mounted on the lid. The 12-Cell Galvanic Battery (upper left) formed the basic unit with two wet cell packs, is contained in a polished black walnut box (10.5 x 8.25 x 7.25 inches); sold for $30.00 in 1881 through 1895; and weighs 11 pounds. The price dropped to $28.00 in 1896. The black plates

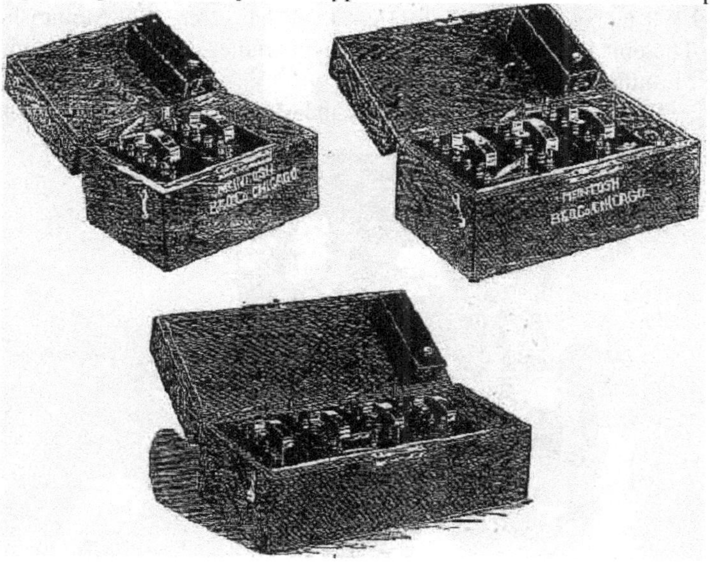

Fig M15. Galvanic Batteries of 12 (A), 18 (B), and 24 (C) Cells

covering the wet cell packs are hard rubber. This unit cost $15.00 in 1907.

The 18-cell unit (upper right) has three wet cell packs, two cell pack switches, a polished black walnut wooden box (14.25 x 8.25 x 7.25 inches); two connecting posts (1 post on each of 2 cell packs); and two cell pack switches. The unit sold for $40.00 (1881 to 1895; $36.00 in 1896) and weighed 15 pounds. By 1907, the price was cut in half ($20.00). George Tiemann & Co of New York listed the McIntosh 18-cell battery in its catalog of 1889 at the same price (with McIntosh signature), but was encased in a slightly larger polished walnut case (12 x 8.5 x 7.5 inches), yet weighed slightly less (~14 pounds).

McIntosh's 24-cell galvanic battery (lower center) contains four wet cell packs, each serving as a hard rubber face plate with six metal receptacles and a metal lifting handle. The wet cell-packs along with their corresponding vulcanized cell (fluid and drip cup sections) are joined by a cell connecting switch. The galvanic components are housed in a polished black walnut box (18 x 8.25 x 7.25 inches) with a metal carrying handle on top, a lever hook latch on each side, and a self locking device in front. The complete unit weighs about 20 pounds and listed for $55.00 in the 1881 and 1890 McIntosh catalogs[10] and in the 1893 AS Aloe catalog.[8] It cost $48.00 in 1896 (20 pounds), and in 1907, the unit cost $25.00 and weighed about 28 pounds. The George Tiemann & Co listed and illustrated the McIntosh 24-cell battery as having the same style wooden case as others in this series of wet cell batteries. The case is 15 x 9 x 8 inches or slightly different than that offered by McIntosh in 1881. The unit listed as weighing 20 pounds rather than 28 pounds cited in the McIntosh catalog of 1881.

Electrolysis Battery. In 1907, the McIntosh Co offered this unit

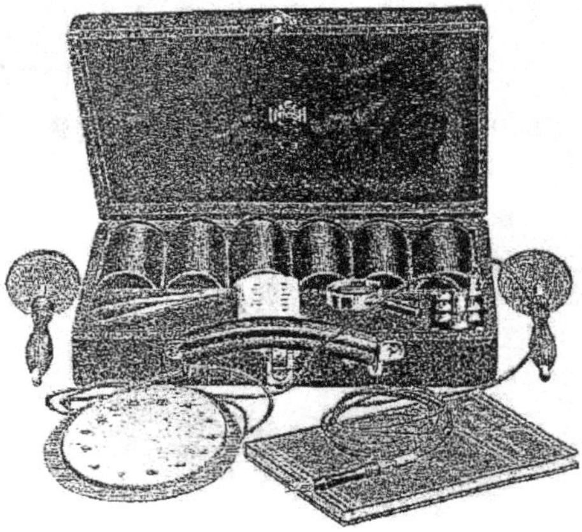

Fig M16. McIntosh Electrolysis Battery

(Fig M16) for $12.00. This galvanic battery was used by dermatologists for treatment of skin problems and removal of superfluous hair. It was powered by six No.4 dry cells (1.5 x 4 inches vs standard size 2.5 x 6 inches) that are easily removed. The flat type of case is covered in morocco, has a leather handle in front, and a snap latch to secure the lid. A compartment for accessories is provided. Operation receptacles for the six batteries are located on the right front of the face plate. The unit weighs about 10 pounds.

Also in 1907, the McIntosh Co manufactured a six-cell (fluid) galvanic battery. This galvanic battery sold for $10.00, and weighed about 10 pounds.

Combination Batteries of Box Style

Twelve, Eighteen, and Twenty-Four-Cell Combined Galvanic and Faradic Battery. McIntosh combined faradic units with galvanic units to form the combined units (Fig M15). Like the company did for its galvanic units, it built units from the basic 12-cell combined battery, but added its six-wet cell battery pack to the appropriate apparatus. In reality, a faradic electrical circuit was added to the basic galvanic units to form a modular type of an arrangement that at the time was an innovative manufacturing idea.

The 12-cell combined galvanic and faradic unit (upper left) was enclosed in a polished black walnut box (13.5 x 8.25 x 7.25 inches),

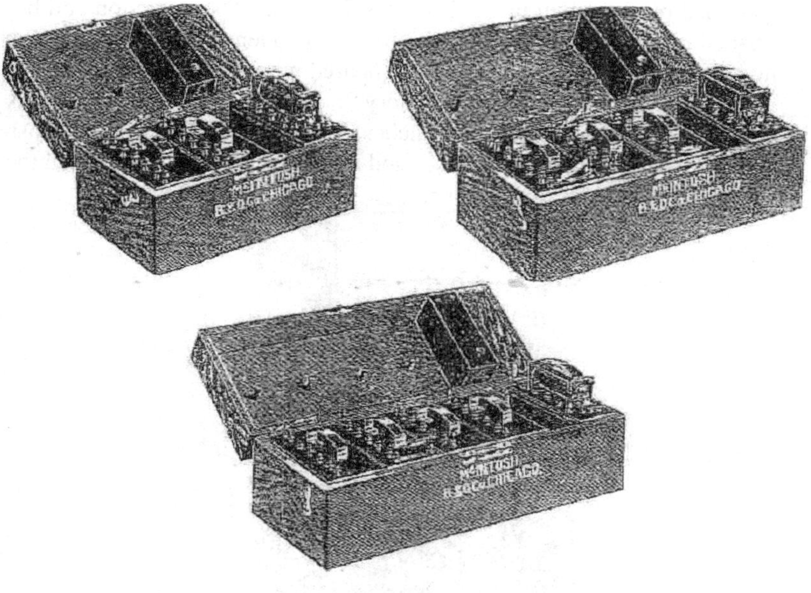

Fig M17. McIntosh Combined Galvanic and Faradic Batteries

hinged lid containing a box for sectioned accessories, a metal carrying handle, and a self locking latch. Additionally, a lever hook latch that pivots is located on each side of the box. An operating components part of the face plate (2 cell packs, accessory box) along with the cell packs forms the faradic battery. The typical McIntosh induction coil (but orientation changed) with two metal rods joining the hard rubber, square end blocks of the coil along with an adjustable screw spring lever, hammer vibrating interrupter are included on the operating components section. A sliding hollow metal tube current controller is attached to the coil along with three metal connecting posts to comprise the faradic section. The faradic battery has its own power supply (2 wet cells) independent of the galvanic section. The complete unit sold for $40.00 between 1881 and 1895. This unit sold for $20.00 and weighed 22 pounds in 1907.

The 18-cell combined battery (upper right) has three wet cell packs with a faradic section the same as with the 12-cell combined battery. The case is the same style but larger than the 12-cell unit, being 17 x 8.25 x 7.25 inches. Two cell pack connecting switches connect the three cell packs in series. The unit sold for $52.50 from 1881 to 1895, but dropped to $25.00 in 1907. It weighs about 28 pounds. The George Tiemann & Co listed this same combined battery with wet cells in its 1889 catalog. Like the other sized batteries in this series it was encased in a polished black walnut box (17 x 8.5 x 7 inches). The induction coil has polished hard rubber end caps that are square. Tiemann unlike McIntosh cited the weight as only 18 pounds compared with 28 pounds.

The 24-cell combined battery (bottom center), polished black walnut case (20.75 x 8.25 x 7.25 inches), has the characteristic McIntosh coil (lift, rods, squared end caps), and an extra large wet cell to run the

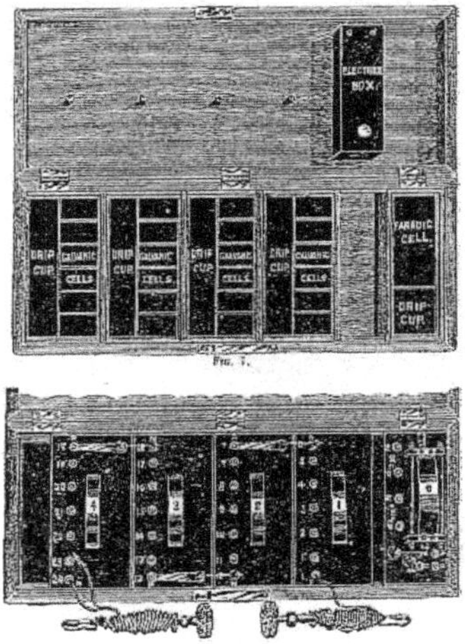

Fig M18. Location of Cells in Combined Batteries
(top, Galvanic; bottom, Faradic)

coil. It weights 24 pounds, is portable with its metal carrying handle on top, lever hook latches on each side, and a self locking device on front. In 1881[10] to 1893[8] the unit sold for $67.50 and in 1907 it cost $30.00. It weighs 33 pounds. The 1889 catalog of George Tiemann & Co cited the dimensions of the McIntosh 24-cell combined galvanic and faradic battery as 17 x 9 x 8 inches or different sized than that listed by McIntosh in its 1881 catalog. The unit's weight was given as 22 pounds with the same price ($67.50).

McIntosh Combined Galvanic and Faradic Batteries. These units were redesigned by 1907 with the replacement of wet cells by dry cells. They were offered in either 14 or 27 dry cells units in 1918.

The McIntosh 14-Dry Cell Combined Galvanic and Faradic Battery (left) used 12 small No.4 Columbia dry cells for the galvanic operation, and two cells for the faradic portion. The number of galvanic cells operating are controlled by a selector dial switch while specific

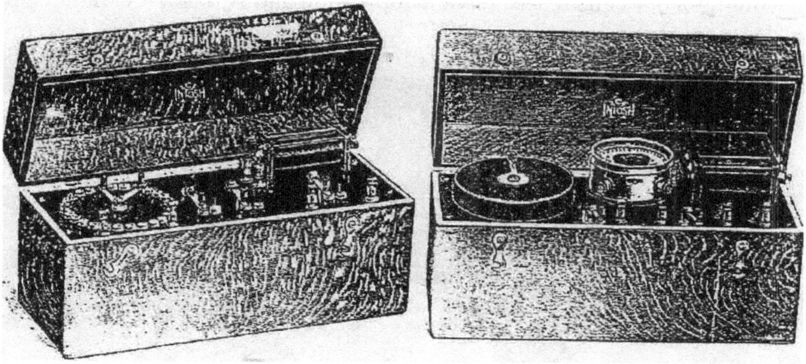

Fig M19. McIntosh Combined Batteries

power was recommended for treatments for removing of superfluous hair and facial blemishes (moles, naevi, warts), and for lighting diagnostic lamps. The case is black buckram (leatherette like and typical style for early twentieth century), a leather carrying handle on top, and two lever hook latches on the front. The metal rods on the squared end caps of the coil were used for this model. In 1918, the consumer had the option of buying it for $20.00 with standard accessories, or for $25.00 with electrodes for electrolysis and massage.

The 27-dry cell unit (right) was named ***"Simplified"*** 27 Dry Cell Combined Galvanic and Faradic Battery, and sold for $27.50. Twenty-five No.4 Columbia dry cells were used for the galvanic operation, and two were used for faradic currents. The galvanic operation has a selector dial switch, and an interruption switch for diagnostic work. The faradic operation has the characteristic induction coil of McIntosh mounted on the enameled slate base or face plate with its two metal rods, square hard rubber end caps, and sliding metal current controller. The unit is encased in a quarter-sawed golden oak case (17 x 9 x 7 inches). The top has a carrying handle and two lever hook latches on the front. In 1907, this same unit sold for $25.00 and weighed about 33 pounds for the 27 cells units.

The ***"Elaborate"*** or variation of the 27 Dry Cell Galvanic and Faradic Battery is essentially the same as the "Simplified" 27-cell unit except that it is more elaborate (like its name) with the improved McIntosh "milliamperemeter" (range of 0 to 150 mA), and the MacLagan wire rheostat. A switch removes the meter from the circuit when the battery is used to light diagnostic lamps. The wooden case is the same as above, as are other components. It sold for $35.00 in 1907, but $37.50 in 1918[9]. It weighs about 36 pounds.

"Universal" portable combined battery. The "Universal" (Fig M20) was designed for physician use, and was powered by 43 No.4 Columbia dry cells in the galvanic operation and two No. 4 Columbia dry

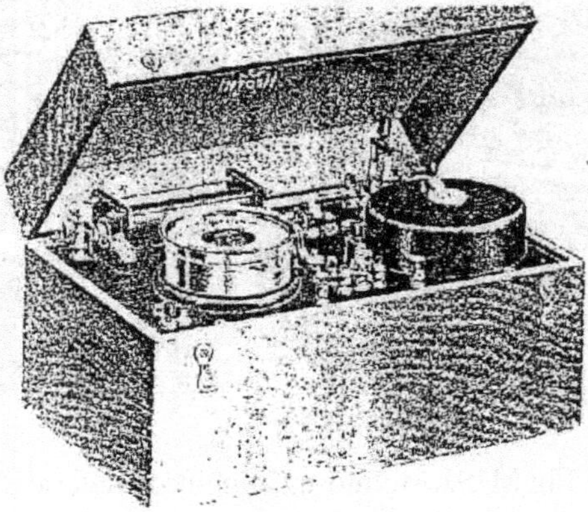

Fig M20. McIntosh "Universal" 45 Dry Cell Combined Galvanic and Faradic Battery

cells for the faradic operation. These cells are easy to remove. The McIntosh Co considered it as a powerful model. Its face plate is polished black enameled slate, and contains a MacLagan wire rheostat, a McIntosh "milliamperemeter" that ranges from 0 to 100 mA on its scale, a faradic coil with a singing rheotome and a slow vibrator, a pole changer, and several switches to operate its functions. Also, on the face plate are binding posts to connect with the patient. In addition to being powered by dry cells the unit can be powered by a 110 volts direct current source (that was commercial current in 1907). The unit delivers galvanic, primary faradic, and secondary faradic currents, and current to light a diagnostic lamp. This combined battery is contained in a quarter sawed golden oak case (18 x 11 x 9.5 inches) that has a leather carrying strap on top of the lid. Operating instructions were enclosed with the unit that weighs about 60 pounds and cost $50.00 in 1907.

Dry Cell Combined Galvanic and Faradic Battery (Fig M21). In 1907, McIntosh redesigned this 14 cells combined unit. This physician use battery used 12 Columbia No.4 dry cells in the galvanic section and two cells in the faradic section. A cell selector served the galvanic section for control of current amplitude and the number of cells activated. The galvanic current was supposed to be sufficient in this model for treatment of all skin problems, and for use with a diagnostic lamp. The galvanic and faradic sections can be combined. The nickel plated rods connecting two square caps at the ends of the induction coil that were characteristic with McIntosh batteries from 1881 to 1905 were eliminated in this model. An On/Off switch controls the operation of the faradic coil, and

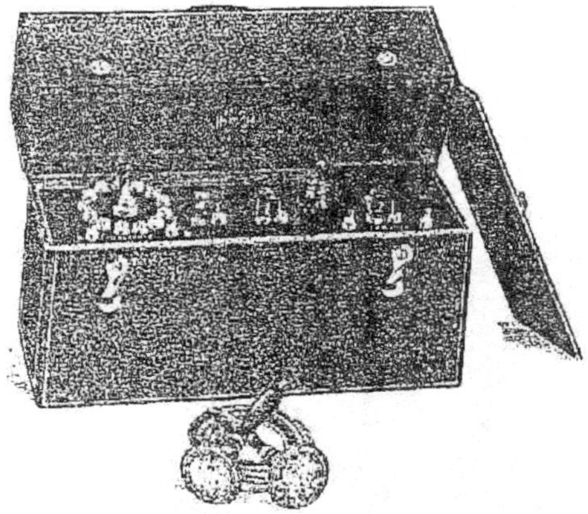

Fig M21. 14 Dry Cell Combined Galvanic and Faradic Battery

another switch enabled the selection of either the primary or secondary currents from the coils. The cells are located underneath the face plate. The case is lined and covered in morocco. A leather carrying handle is on top of the hinged lid that is secured in front by two lever latches. Accessories are located in the lid compartment. This 18 pounds model cost $17.50 in 1907.

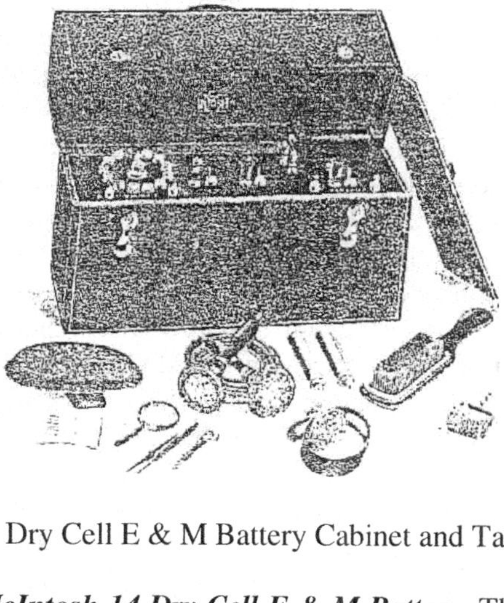

Fig M22. 14 Dry Cell E & M Battery Cabinet and Table Models

The McIntosh 14 Dry Cell E & M Battery. The E & M battery of Fig M22 was designed for electrolysis (galvanic) and massage (faradic) treatments. The model was used by various operators who treated skin blemishes and removal of superfluous hair, and provided electrical massages. The number of accessories increased for this battery otherwise it is the same as the 14 Dry Cell Combined Battery of Fig M19, left. This model weighs about 22 pounds and sold for $22.50 in 1907.

Cabinet, Plate and Table Models

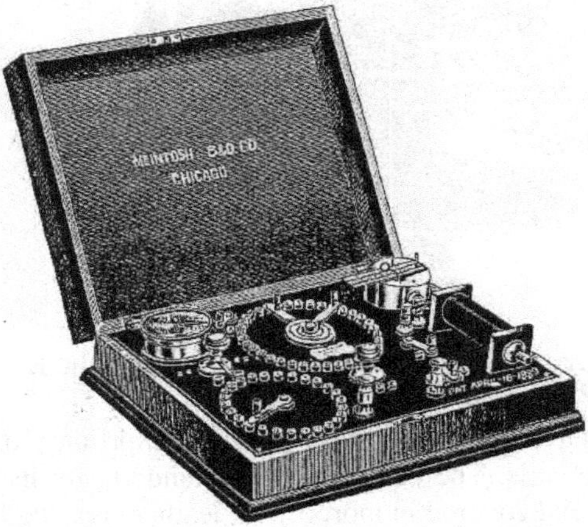

Fig M23. McIntosh Table Battery and Plate

Table Battery and Plate. Dr McIntosh designed the compact unit of Fig M23 as a complete office apparatus for physicians. The office unit is housed in a wooden box having a face plate of polished rubber, 12 x 16 inches. The face plate contains a galvanic switch for 32 to 60 cells; an automatic rheotome for rapid and slow galvanic pulsed current, a galvanometer; a pole changer; a current indicator; two binding posts; a McIntosh type coil (hard rubber cover, hard rubber square end blocks, no rods); and a circular coil rheostat of 25 coils (each 100 ohms) to range from 100 to 2500 ohms resistance for either faradic or galvanic circuits. This unit operated with a 32-cell gravity battery, and cost $150.00 in 1881. This model of 1890 was an upgraded unit from that of 1881, and was patented in 1889. Beginning in 1890 this model contained the milliammeter and the automatic rheotome for galvanic pulses that the earlier unit did not have. In 1890, the physician customer had a choice of polished walnut or oak for the case. It cost $110.00 with a wooden case in 1890, or $106.00 without the wooden case.[10] In 1896, it cost $108.00 with and $100.00 without a case. Although this table and plate model was marketed in 1881,[10] it was not until 1889 that it was patented as the No.1 Office Table Plate (Fig M25).

Table Battery and Plate. McIntosh introduced a similar model to that of Fig M23 in 1886 (Fig M24) with a table and plate battery. The difference between the two models is that the earlier unit (Fig M23) was patented on 17 May 1886, and has an earlier type of automatic rheotome for controlling galvanic current pulses. The 1886 model's rheotome (upper right) was designed to reduce the previous need of changing wires

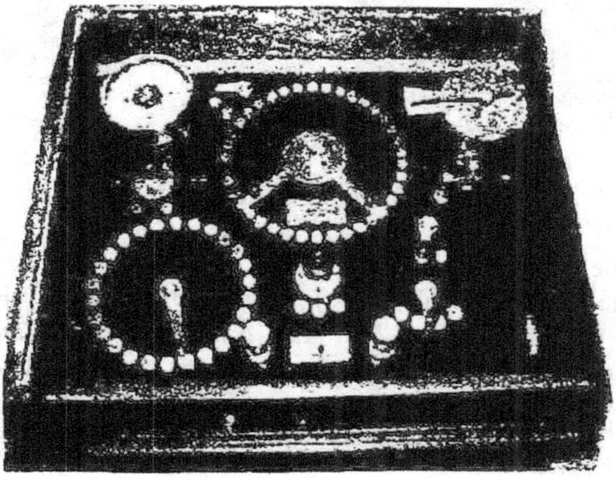

Fig M24. McIntosh Table Battery and Plate of 1886

or connections between the battery and selective elements to deliver slow and fast interruptions. The rheotome contained on the unit shown in Fig M20 is more sophisticated than that of the 1886 unit. The 1886 model is housed in an oak case (17 x 14 x 6 inches) that has a hinged and glass lid. This unit of 1886 provides faradic and galvanic (continuous and pulsed) currents.

No.1 Office Table Plate. The McIntosh Table Battery and Plate of 1881 to 1890 became the No.1 Office Table Plate by 1895 (Fig M23), and was designed and patented by Dr McIntosh on 16 April 1889 (date embossed on the face plate) to give the physician a complete electrical apparatus. A wooden carrying case (same as Table Battery and Plate of Fig M23) enclosed the electrical components for faradic and galvanic currents, and was offered in either polished oak (new for 1890 and 1895) or black walnut as a cabinet or table model. The black polished hard rubber face plate measured 12 x 16 inches and contained: a galvanic double switch for 32 or more cells; an automatic rheotome for fast and slow pulsed galvanic (monophasic) current frequencies; a milliammeter (replaced the galvanometer of 1881 to 1890); a pole changer; current indicator; two binding posts; a faradic coil with hard rubber square end blocks; and a circular rheostat that uses 25 resistors of 100-ohms each for a range of 100 to 2500 ohms for either faradic or galvanic circuits controlled by a circular switch. Cells to power the combined battery are

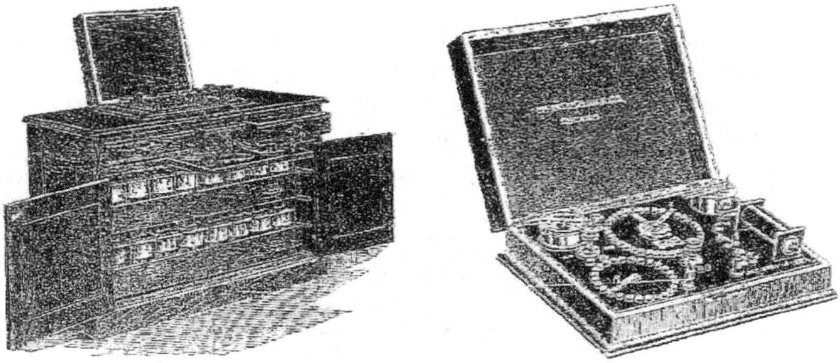

Fig M25. No. 1 Office Table Plate

kept in the cabinet portion of the unit that could hold up to 36 gravity cells. The complete unit sold for $185.00 in 1881.[10] By 1890, the identical unit became the McIntosh ***No.1 Cabinet Battery***. This unit could also hold 48 Diamond carbon cells, or 48 Gonda Leclanche cells, or 42 Law batteries, or 42 Disque Leclanche cells. The battery sold for $105.00 with a case or $100.00 without a wooden case in the AS Aloe catalog of 1893.[8]

This No.1 combined apparatus was also offered in a wooden cabinet (8 feet x 22 x 40 inches for the top), antique oak or black walnut, cell drawers that hold 42 Fitch's Perfect Batteries or 42 Law batteries or 48 Gonda Leclanche batteries (all wet cells). The No.1 cabinet style combined battery unit sold for $150.00 in the 1893 AS Aloe catalog.[8]

No.2 Table Battery. In 1890, McIntosh offered a modified version of his Table Battery (Fig M26, left) that was a less expensive

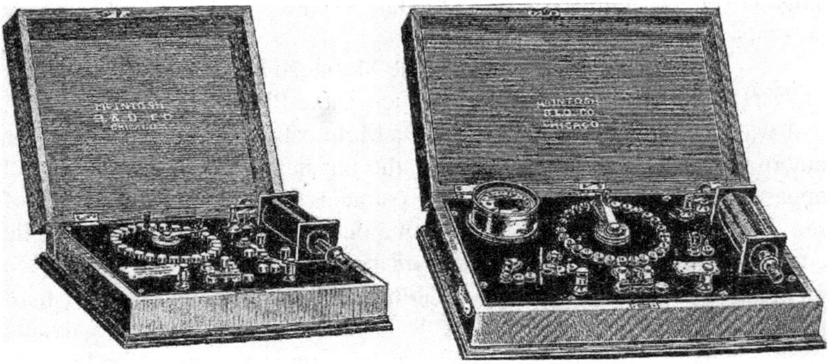

Fig M26. McIntosh No. 2 Table Battery

unit. The hard rubber face plate is 10 x 12 inches and is enclosed in a polished walnut box with a front self locking device.

The unit has a double galvanic circular switch that permitted the operator to use any number of desired cells. This switch is arranged with

25 metal buttons or more for the each number of cells needed by the operator. The face plate also has the McIntosh faradic coil with hard rubber cover and square end blocks; a pole changer; two binding posts; a switch to select faradic primary and secondary currents, and galvanic currents; and a switch to connect the coil with the cells. This unit sold for $35.00 with the wooden case or $30.00 without a case in 1890,[10] but it cost $38.00 and $30.00, respectively in 1896.

Also in 1896, McIntosh offered the No.2 model as the ***No.4 Office Table Plate*** (Fig M26, right). The No.4 model is the same as the No.1, but the face plate was enlarged (15.5 x 9 inches) to accommodate the addition of a milliamperemeter. The selector switched was increased to 40 buttons for 40 or more cells. With case the model cost $68.00 and without the case it cost $60.00. This particular unit is difficult to obtain by collectors.

No.2 Cabinet Battery. The cabinet battery of Fig M27 incorporated the Table Battery and Plate of Fig M23 into a cabinet in 1890 for the physician who liked furniture in the office. The McIntosh No.2 Table Battery was encased in a table-cabinet unit. The battery section was the same as that of the Table Battery of 1890[10] and has a wooden cover. The cabinet portion has two drawers for accessories; two

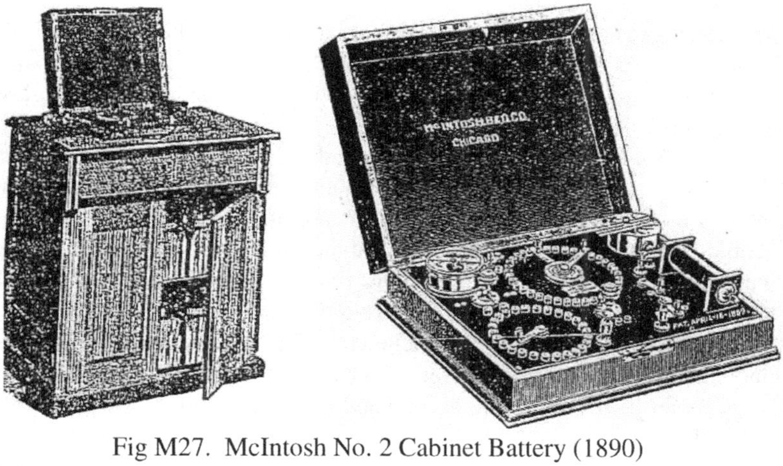

Fig M27. McIntosh No. 2 Cabinet Battery (1890)

doors when closed hide the two shelves holding batteries. The unit sold for $100.00 complete with 36 Diamond carbon cells (each cell has 1.75 volts). The unit was not available in 1895.

Office Battery. This combination faradic and galvanic cabinet battery was the deluxe unit of the McIntosh Co's electrical battery product line. It cost $225.00 complete with 36 gravity cells in 1881 and ranged between $223.00 to $235.00 depending on one of four types of batteries desired in 1890. The exact unit was not available in 1895. The type of electrical circuitry and components was similar to that of the McIntosh Table Battery. The base of this finished black walnut cylinder cabinet is 34 x 19 inches; it has a cylinder cover that rolls down to cover

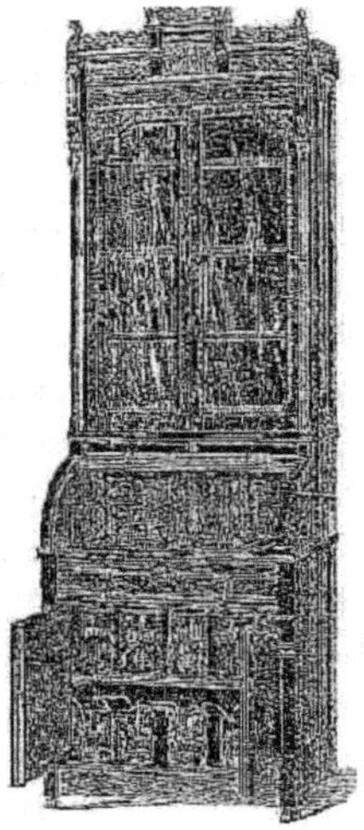

Fig M28. Office Battery in Cabinet Case (1881-1890)[10]

the electrical components. The cabinet has a full sized drawer, and solid wooden doors hiding the two shelves of cells (36 to 48). A four-shelf bookcase is mounted on top of the wooden base, and it has two glass-wooden doors.

No.4 Cabinet Battery. McIntosh's No.2 (left) and No.4 (right) Cabinet Battery (Fig M29) are combined faradic and galvanic apparatuses, and are the exact operational components of No.2 and No.4 Table Batteries of Fig M26. No.2 cabinet sold for $90.00 without any cells or for $80.00 without cells and rheostat by AS Aloe in 1893.[8] In 1896, it sold for $64.00 without cells; $100.00 with 36 Diamond Carbon cells; and $84.00 with 30 Leclanche cells. The polished oak cabinet was table height with two top drawers and two solid doors. The shelves inside the cabinet held 40 or more cells. The black hard rubber face plate (12 x 10 inches) with wood and glass cover contains: a faradic coil with hard rubber end blocks and cover; pole changer; two binding posts to deliver primary, secondary and combined currents; a switch to select the currents; a milliammeter; and a controlling switch. The No.4 unit (right) is the same as No.4 of Fig M26 with a face plate of 15.5 x 9 inches to accommodate the milliamperemeter. The No.4 has the McIntosh carbon rheostat that was new at the time. The cabinet was highly polished oak with a plate glass cover. The No. 4 Cabinet Battery cost $100.00 without

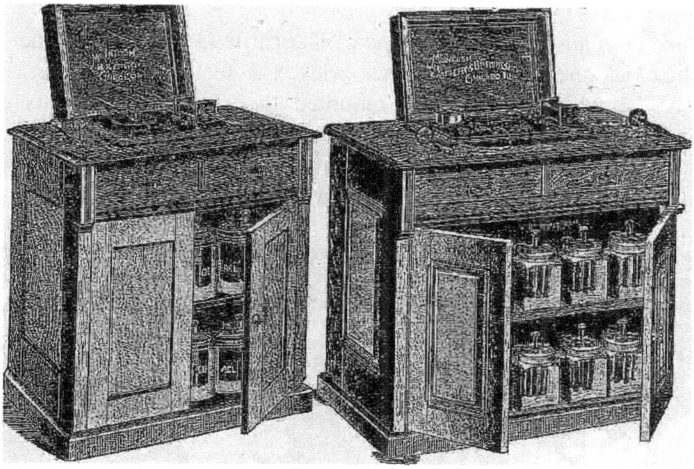

Fig M29. McIntosh No. 4 Cabinet Battery

cells for $90.00 or without rheostat for $90.00.

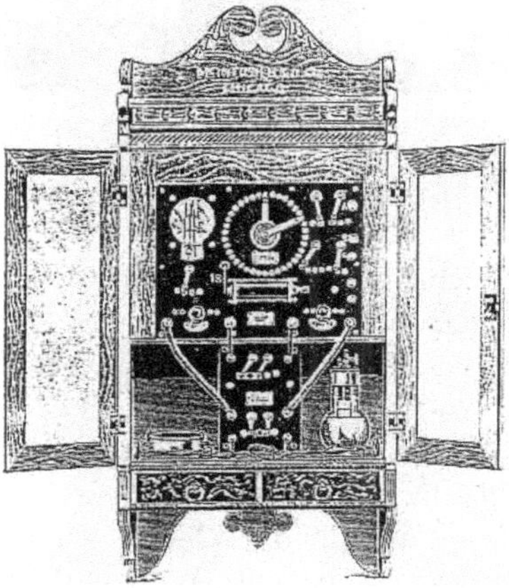

Fig M30. McIntosh Complete Wall Plate with DeWatteville Current Combiner in Wall Case

Complete Wall Plate. The McIntosh Complete Wall Plate of 1893[8] (Fig M30) is a combined faradic and galvanic apparatus with a large polished oak or walnut cabinet having beveled plate glass doors. Three variations were offered: unit in case with hydro platinum rheostat and milliammeter sold for $140.00; the unit in a case without rheostat or milliammeter sold for $95.00; and the unit in a case with a carbon rheostat cost $130.00. The cells were sold separately for this model.

Little Gem Cabinet. The combined faradic and galvanic current apparatus of Fig M31 (left) is a cabinet model and because of its completeness and utility was named "The Little Gem." The cabinet is of polished oak measuring 20 inches wide x 5 feet high. The back hard rubber face plate is vertically mounted to display components of: a double galvanic circle switch board for two independent 20 cells; a cell selector switch; an automatic rheotome for either faradic or galvanic currents ranging from a single pulse every 10 seconds to 66 pulses per

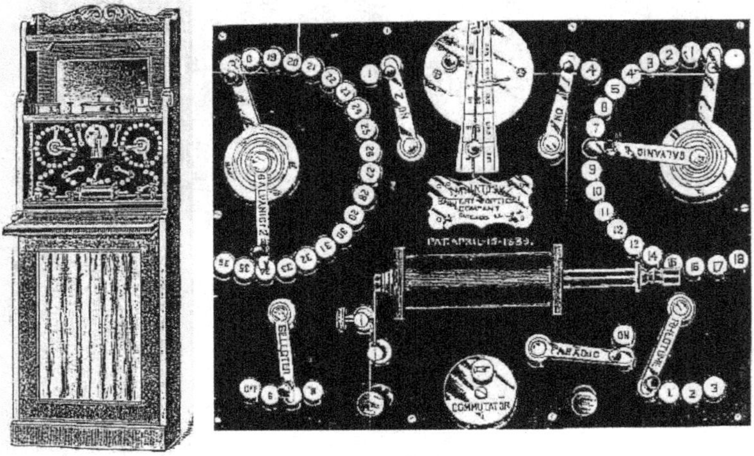

Fig M31. The Little Gem Cabinet[8] and Its Components[11]

second; a faradic pole changer; a galvanic pole changer; a milliammeter switch; a rheostat switch; and two binding posts. A shelf above the face plate is a galvano-cautery rheostat and binding posts for cautery. The unit can accommodate 43 No.1 Samson cells that can be placed in the cabinet underneath the face plate. The cautery unit uses two 35 ampere storage cells located behind the face plate. This unit was McIntosh's show piece for 1893 and was sold by AS Aloe for $240.00 with reflecting mirror and glass plate doors to protect components. Without the glass plate doors the unit sold for $210.00.

In 1899, the Voltamp Electric Manufacturing Company of Baltimore introduced its "Little Gem." The Voltamp version was a small, one dry cell powered, boxed faradic unit for home use. The Little Gem sold for $5.00. (see Voltamp in Chapter 19).

The close-up view in Fig 31 (right) of a face plate contains operating components similar to those of The Little Gem Cabinet model. Circular discs with buttons allowing activation of any number of cells to deliver galvanic current are available, and controlled by rotating levers. An automatic regulator for monophasic pulses (galvanic current) is present to operate the disc controls. An induction coil is available to produce faradic pulses at rates controlled by a vibrating interrupter. Faradic current amplitude is controlled by a sliding metal controller. A controller switch permits the operator to select sections of the coil for producing a variety of faradic characteristics. A selector switch varies the number of cells operating in the faradic electrical circuit. This face plate dates between 1890 and 1894.

No.3 Wall Plate. The Wall Plate model of Fig M32 was available in 1896, and was designed for treatments requiring high intensity (voltage) with the power from 50 or more cells. The current is

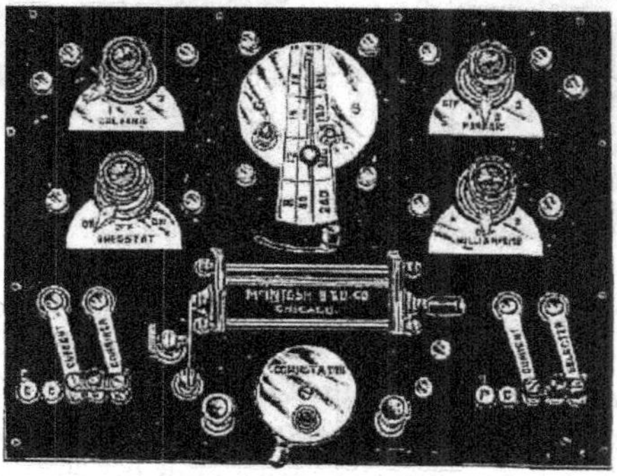

Fig M32. No. 3 Table or Wall Plate

controlled by a hydroplatinum rheostat (mid left) or a McIntosh current controller (coil end), and a registered milliamperemeter. The faradic coil operates from three cells independent of the galvanic circuit. The galvanic current can be pulsed (6 to 600 per minute) by a graduate automatic rheotome (upper center) through a switch. A current selector is used to arrange galvanic, faradic (primary, secondary), or combined faradic and galvanic currents. The basic unit without the meter and hydroplatinum rheostat cost $44.00, and when both meter and rheostat were included the unit cost $88.00.

Wall Plates. The unit of Fig M33 was developed by the McIntosh Co between 1895 and 1900. The MacLagan rheostat was not yet developed, although lamps were used in series with the carbon-button type rheostat. The face plate is mounted on a golden oak base (15 x 11 inches). The face plate contains lamps; coil with sliding metal current controller and a spring lever, hammer vibrating interrupter; pole changer; button rheostat; switches to control the number of cells or 110 volts direct current; single throw switch; and binding posts to connect to the patient.

The advertisement in Polk's medical directory of 1904 shows another wall model (No.6 Plate, Wall Cabinet) of a combined faradic and galvanic battery.[12] Although this unit was not listed in the catalogs cited, it is one of the combined current batteries that improved yearly. As technological developments took place the McIntosh Co incorporated them.

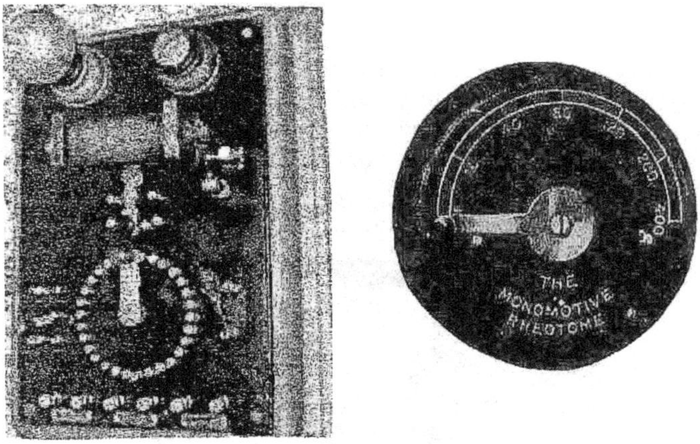

Fig M33. McIntosh Wall Plate and Monomotive Rheotome

Wall Plate. This McIntosh Wall Plate (Fig M34) represents the company's model of about 1905 to 1907. This model may have followed the No.6 series. The lamps were in series with the rheostat to help with the resistance alterations and patient safety, and could use either direct current or dry or wet cells as its power source. This combined battery offered features of the earlier models (eg, The Gem) but has the "milliamperemeter" (a McIntosh improvement) and the MacLagan rheostat.

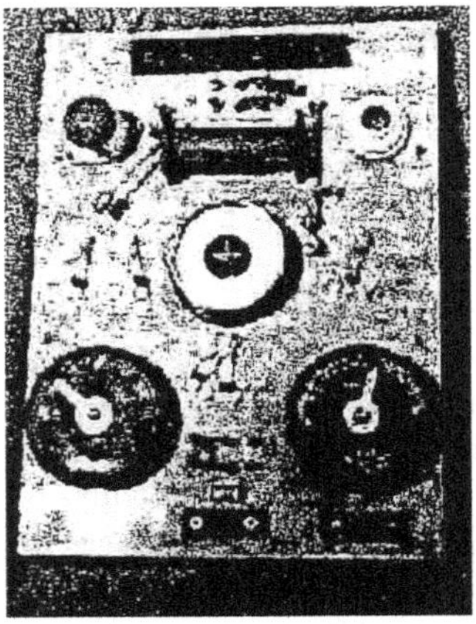

Fig M34. McIntosh Wall Plate

Around 1900 to 1904 concern centered on ways to power medical electrical batteries in a physician's office. The medical electrical apparatus was capable of delivering faradic, galvanic, and in some models sinusoidal currents. Extra electrical power was needed for units delivering current for applications of electrolysis. Some buildings were equipped with constant current (direct) at 55 or 110 volts. The sources of current power for street cars, arc lighting, and high frequency applications were too dangerous for use in the physician's office. Therefore, the McIntosh company, like other manufacturers of the period of time, designed medical electrical batteries to accommodate a variety of electrical power sources. Medical electrical batteries between 1900 and 1910 were designed to adapt to the power sources of 55, 110, 200, and 500 volts direct current, and to that of batteries comprising 10 to 100 dry or wet cells in series.

No. 6 Plate. With the advertisement of 1904[12] a series of wall plates was introduced. The No.6 Plate came in several models. The unit in Fig M35 (left & right) is a combination apparatus that is powered by direct current from a wall supply. The vertical face plate contains the electrical components of a graphite disc rheostat, a milliammeter, an automatic galvanic rheotome, a faradic coil, a variety of control switches, pole changer, and binding posts. The cabinet is made of golden oak with a beveled glass plate in the door. A drawer below the door houses accessories. The light bulbs are resistance lamps. This 1904 unit (left) has the graphite rheostat that was the precursor of the MacLagan rheostat.

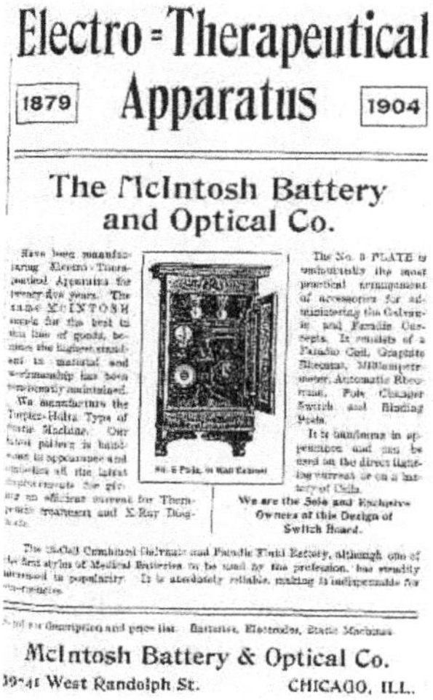

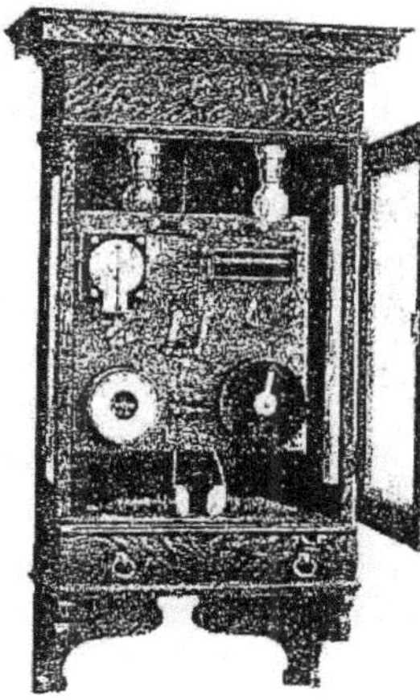

Fig M35. McIntosh No. 6 Plate

In 1907, the model to the left came with one of four power options: 1) 110 volts direct current or cells for $50.00; 2) 220 volts direct current for $52.50; 3) 500 volts direct current for $55.00; and 4) 110 volts alternating current with a switch for sinusoidal current for $52.50. The MacLagan rheostat dates the units from 1905 to 1907.

MacLagan Rheostat. This rheostat was developed after 1900, perhaps around 1904 to 1907 (shown in Figs M19 & 20, also). Unlike the carbon resistance rheostats marketed at the time, the MacLagan rheostat used a variety of wire resistances that were durable and reliable. It was developed to control sinusoidal current when the unit was powered by a 110 volts alternating current source. The rotating lever permits gradual increases and decreases of current amplitudes while protecting the patient from any sudden shock. Some faces of dials are marked with a range of 0 to 70 volts.

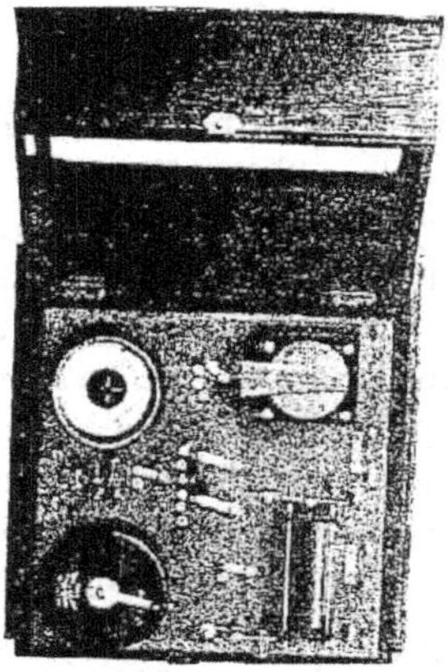

Fig M36. McIntosh No.6 Plate, Style "B" Case

No.6 Plate, Style "B". This No.6 unit (Fig M36) is housed by a quarter sawed golden oak case (19 inches square x 11 inches) that was designed for placement on a table top or wall. The lid or door has beveled plate glass. The unit is powered by 18 dry or wet cells placed externally to the unit, or by 110 volts direct current, or 110 volts alternating current. It weighs about 88 pounds and cost $45.00 in 1907.

Basic Table Plate. In 1900 to about 1907, the McIntosh company made the Basic Table Plate model of Fig M37 (left) available to provide faradic and galvanic currents. The above figure shows such a basic Table Plate without cabinet or table encasements. The slate face plate contains all of the electrical components for the unit's operation. These components were: the automatic rheotome for pulsed galvanic (monophasic) current; the induction coil with its attached interrupters to regulate fast (vibrator style) and slow (lever style) faradic pulses; the graphite, octagonal style rheostat to control faradic current amplitudes; the milliammeter displayed the amount of galvanic current flowing during an application; binding posts to connect the unit with cells connected in series; and switches for On/Off and current functions.

The company further reduced costs to the consumer for a basic wall plate. Fig M37 (right) offers the consumer a wall model for faradic and galvanic currents that could be operated using 120 volts Edison (direct) incandescent mains (source current). The model (right) came

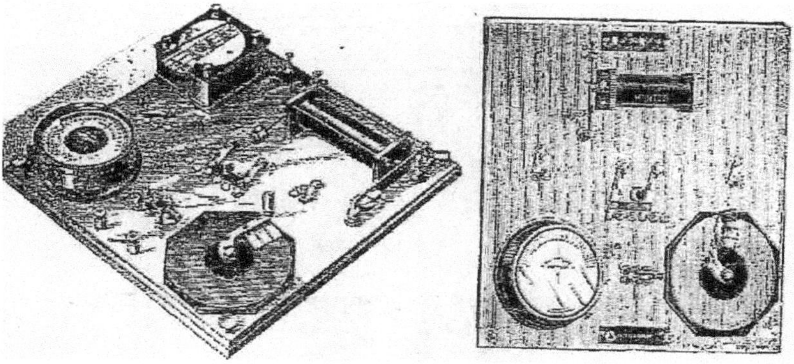

Fig M37. Basic Table Plate

without the automatic rheotome for galvanic monophasic pulses, but for unidirectional galvanic current. The model offers a shunt circuit (divided reduced current) to protect the patient as well as the option of powering the model by Edison or a battery of cells for direct current source. The models shown in Fig M37 are the 1902 models.

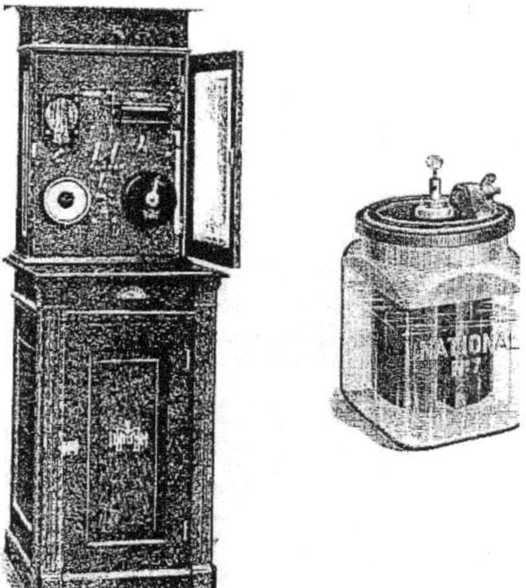

Fig M38. No. 6 Plate in Style "C" Upright Floor Cabinet & Cell

No.6 Plate, "C" Style. The unit of Fig M38 has the same electrical components as models (left and right) of Fig M35 but differs by being a full sized cabinet (25 x 24 x 70 inches) weighing about 290 pounds without cells; 330 pounds with National cells; and 400 pounds with dry cells. The basic unit with accessories but without cells cost $70.00; $82.50 with 43 National No.7 cells; and $80.00 with 43 Columbia No.6 dry cells in 1907.

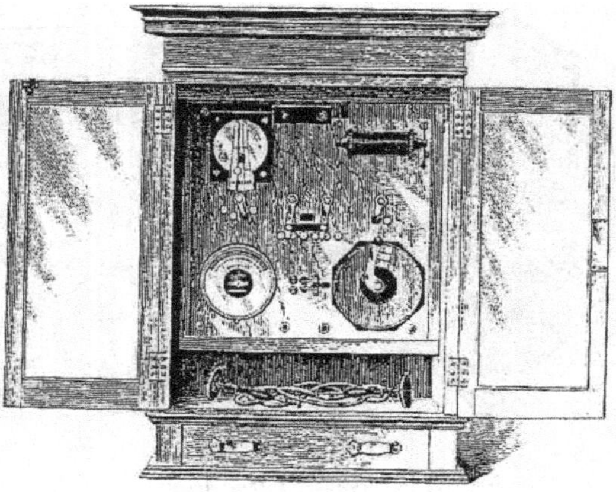

Fig M39. Wall Plate Cabinet

Wall Plate Cabinet. This unit of 1900 to 1907 (1902 unit in Fig M39) is very similar to the Table Plates of Fig M37, but is encased in an oak cabinet with double glass plate doors. A sliding drawer is for accessories. This unit was powered by direct current sources (cells or electrical grid).

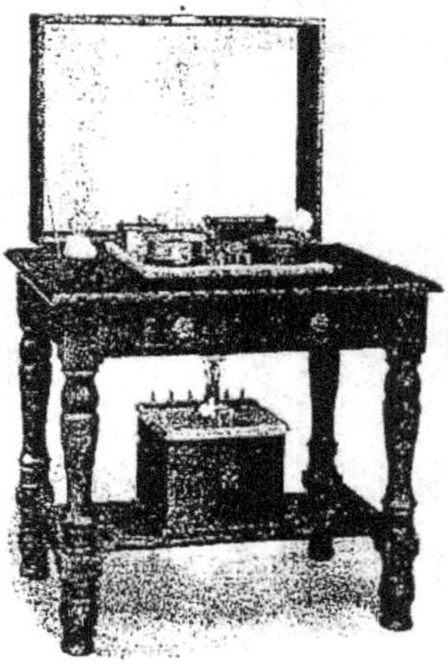

Fig M40. McIntosh No. 6 Plate in Style "E" Table Cabinet

No.6 Plate, "E" Style. This unit of Fig M40 is especially wired for operating with alternating current source by using a current rectifier that sold for $70.00. When wired for 110 volts direct current the unit cost $60.00. The electrical components of this unit are similar to all other No.6 Plates in the series. It offers faradic, galvanic, and sinusoidal currents. The table is made of quarter sawed dark golden oak (32 x 26 x

36 inches) and weighs 240 pounds with the rectifier and 200 pounds without the rectifier. The table has casters to provide mobility.

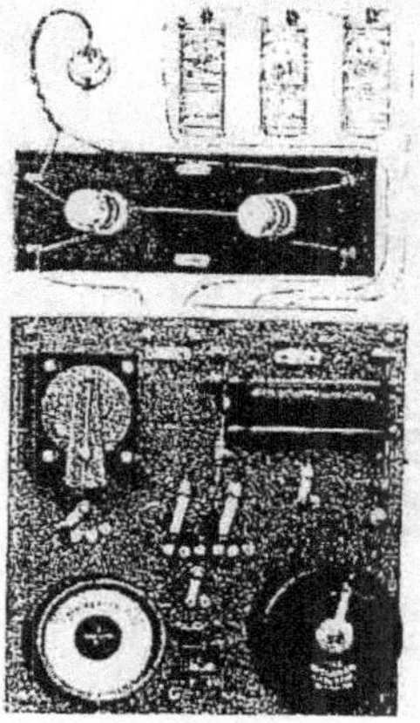

Fig M41. McIntosh No. 6 Plate for 220 Volts Current

No.6 Plate, 220 Volts. The No.6 Plate model of Fig M41 was sold in 1907 with only the basic electrical components for use with 220 or 500 volts direct current. The 220 volts version sold for $39.75 and included a reduction board, and three No.6 Columbia dry cells. The complete No.6 Plate for 500 volts cost $40.75. The reduction board contains and operates with two and five power lamps, respectively.

The No.6 Plate model also came in a version that used either 110 volts direct current, or 110 volts alternating current with a rectifier, or 43 dry or fluid cells. The plate has a polished marble face plate (16 inches square) that contains the MacLagan rheostat, McIntosh "milliamperemeter" with shunt, graduated automatic rheotome, a large induction coil with rapid and slow frequencies by the spring lever hammer vibrating interrupter, a pole changer, current selector, a single throw switch, and binding posts. Its shipping weight was 45 pounds and its cost was $35.00 in 1907.

This updated wall plate in Fig M42 was available around 1906 and was still being sold in 1918. The cabinet is quarter-sawed golden oak with a glass door and accessory drawer below the door. The face plate is a 16 inches square aseptic porcelained steel (also, this steel unit was known as type 12 asceptic porcelain plate). The vertical face plate comprises a MacLagan wire rheostat that consists of a solid block of porcelain wound with high grade resistance wire; it has a moving tip contact that increases and decreases the amplitude of faradic, galvanic, and sinusoidal currents. The ranges of the two scales of the milliamperemeter are 0 to 20 and 0 to 400 mA, respectively.

The rheotome is monomotive. About 1915 or 1916 McIntosh

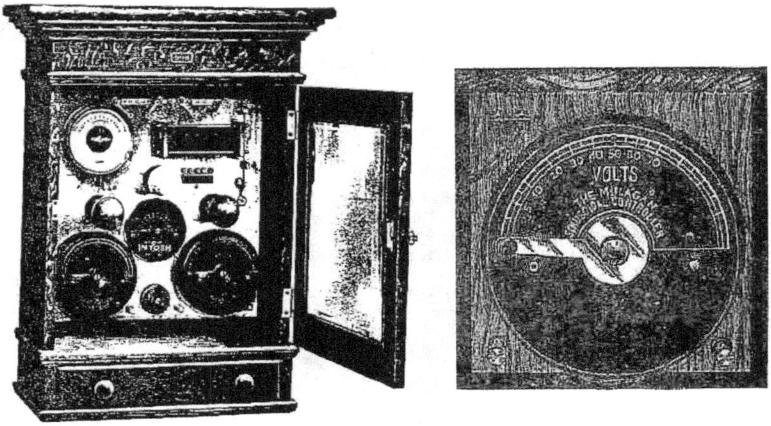

Fig M42. McIntosh No. 6 Plate for 220 Volts

manufactured a so called ***"monomotive rheotome"*** to interrupt or set pulse rates for faradic, galvanic, and sinusoidal currents. This unit was a disc that rotated like the rheostats to function over a range from 20 to 400 pulses per second. The rheotome functions with a clock works mechanism; wound by a key; and runs for 45 minutes. It has platinum tip contacts (all with equal resistance) inside of the dial; the operator selects the frequency desired which in turn sets the rate and closes the circuit. Returning the lever arm to zero opens the circuit. The rheotome is in series with the battery and the patient when operating.

The faradic coil of the Wall Plate has a primary winding of 230 feet of No.20 coarse wire, and the secondary coil is wound with 1300 feet of No.30 fine wire. The unit has a transformer for cautery and sinusoidal currents; a pole changer; three resistance lamps, and a dial selector that with a turn of its knob immediately makes all connections for any available modality. These electrical components provide: galvanic current, diagnostic lamp current; fast primary faradic current; fast secondary faradic current; slow primary faradic current; slow secondary faradic current; combined faradic and galvanic currents; rapid sinusoidal current; and current for cautery. In 1918, this basic unit sold for $100.00. The basic unit with a rectifier and potential equalizer for 100 to 120 volts alternating current or direct current sold for $125.00. Other options with fewer components were also available (eg, AC, DC, or 50 wet cells).

In 1915 through 1918, the source current in physicians' offices was alternating. In the case of a wall plate, the alternating current often had to be changed into direct current, and this was by means of a rectifier or a rotary converter. The use of a rectifier was more common than use of a rotary converter because of the reduced cost. When the wall plate is used with direct current sources the faradic and galvanic circuits are supplied by the direct current. The motor generator is used to transform the direct current to an alternating current to supply the power for the transformer used in cautery and sinusoidal currents. The rectifier with a pressure equalizer was necessary to transform alternating current source to direct current for use with the faradic and galvanic currents.

No.9 Cabinets. The McIntosh company introduced a series of wall cabinet apparatuses that it labeled as No.9. This series of Wall Cabinet models was similar in appearances to those of Fig M35, but this new series contained improved electrical components and operational features. The improvements in the No.9 series include: a high tension faradic coil, "milliamperemeter" with shunt, a "monomotive rheoton" dry cell cautery switch, an energy changing switch, a pole changer, and a current condenser (capacitor). The unit provides the following currents: interrupted (monophasic) galvanic, combined faradic and galvanic, high tension faradic, primary faradic, combined primary and secondary , and cautery currents. Current was available for diagnostic lamps. The unit could be powered by direct currents of 110, 220, and 500 volts; by dry or

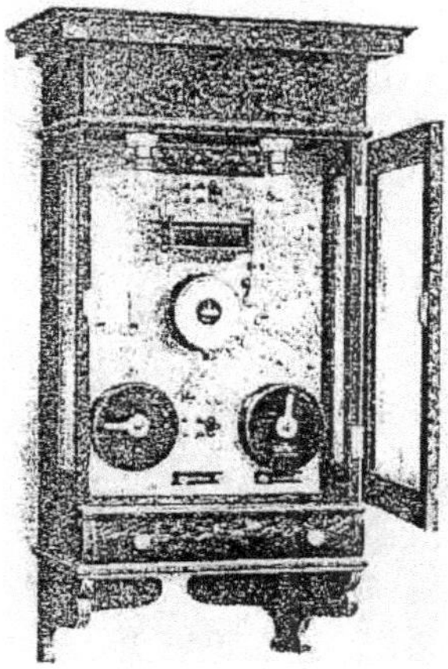

Fig M43. Therapeutic Wall Cabinet No. 9

fluid cells of chloride of ammonium; and by alternating current using a rectifier. The unit's shipping weight was 165 pounds. It cost $75.00 with 110 volts direct current or cells, $77.00 for 220 volts direct current, and $80.00 for 500 volts direct current in 1907.

The No.9 unit of Fig M44 has the same electrical components mounted in an upright floor cabinet (25 x 24 x 76 inches) as other No.9 models in this series. The basic unit with accessories and with 43 National No.7 cells, shipping weight of 315 pounds, cost $95.00. Weighing 575 pounds shipping weight it sold for $107.50; and with 43 Columbia No.6 dry cells at 425 pounds it sold for $105.00 in 1907.

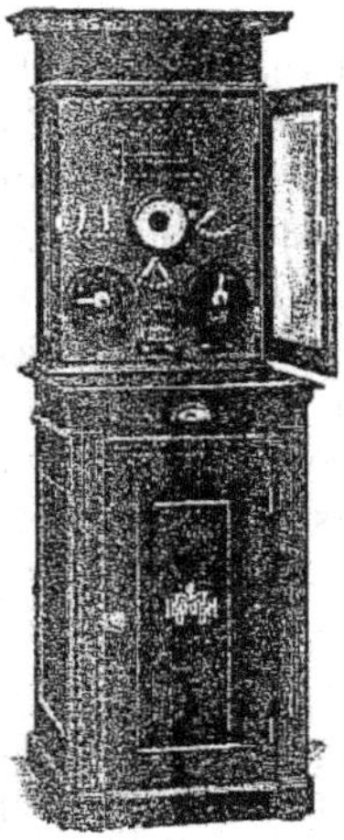

Fig M44. No. 9 Therapeutic Plate, Style "C" Upright Floor Cabinet

This No.9 unit (Fig M45) was wired especially for alternating current while using a rectifier. The model sold for $100.00 and was shipped weighing 265 pounds in 1907. When wired for 110 volts direct

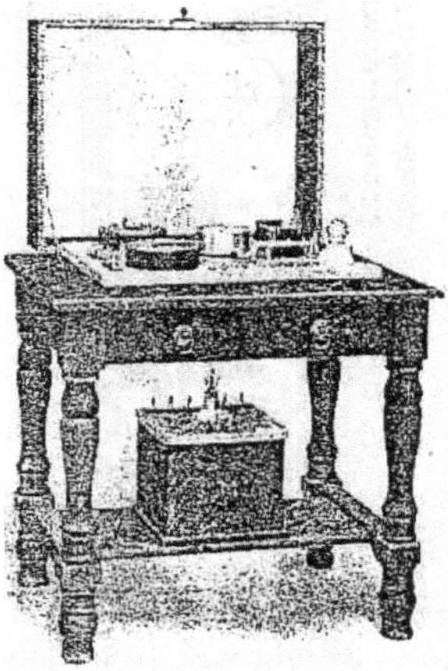

Fig M45. No.9 Therapeutic Plate in Style "E" Table Cabinet

current and shipped at 225 pounds the cost was $85.00. It has the same features as other No.9 Plate units, but is mobile on a table having casters. A variety of faradic and galvanic currents are produced by this model. The quarter sawed oak table has a beveled plate glass cover and is 32 x 26 x 36 inches in size.

This full sized cabinet model in Fig M46 resembles Style "C" of series No.9 (Fig M44) in the construction of the cabinet. The difference in the two units is that No.8 provides galvanic, high tension faradic, sinusoidal, cautery, and diagnostic lamp currents. The dimensions of the

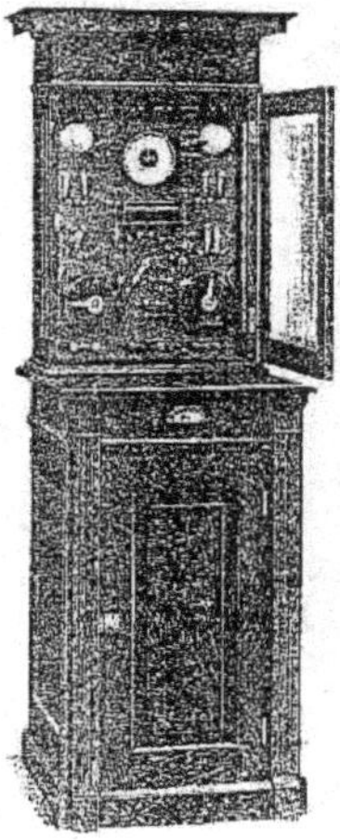

Fig M46. Universal Wall Cabinet No. 8

two cabinets are similar. The No.8 model operates with 110 volts alternating of direct currents. The unit's shipping weight was 325 pounds, and it sold for $120.00 in 1907.

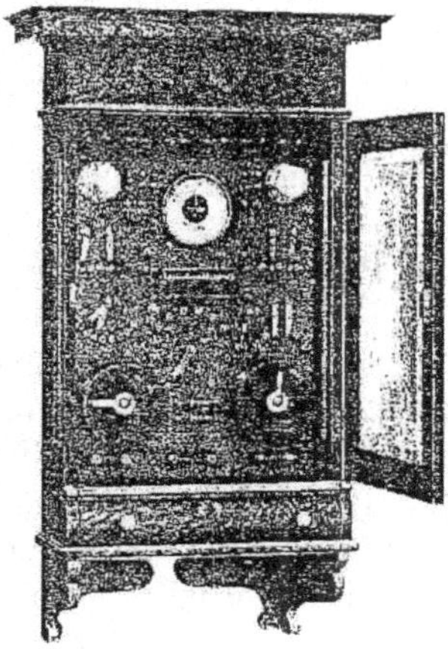

Fig M47. Combination Wall Cabinet No. 10

Combination Wall Cabinet No.10. The model No.10 (Fig M47) contains similarities of both that of No.6 and No.9 Wall Cabinets in case design, and that of No.8 in electrical components and functions. The basic wall mounted unit with accessories for 110 volts alternating current was $115.00 (with rectifier, weight of 245 pounds), and for 110 volts direct current was $130.00 (with motor generator, weight of 209 pounds) in 1907.

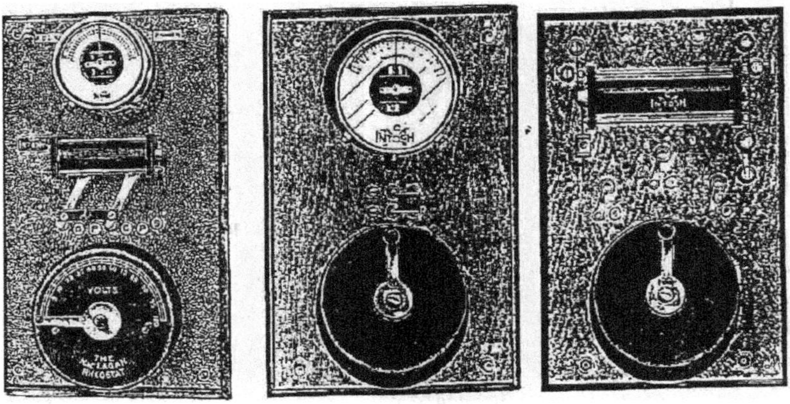

Fig M48. McIntosh Simplified Wall Plates[9]

Simplied Wall Plates. To the left is a basic type plate offering faradic and galvanic currents. It has a MacLagan wire rheostat, a "milliamperemeter," a faradic coil, and a current selector. The plate is a marble base (9.5 x 16 inches). Without a wooden case the unit cost $35.00, and with a case it was $40.00 in 1918. The polished marble base (10 x 15 inches) of 1907 differed slightly from that of 1918. The unit of 1907 has a double pole, a double throw switch, and a lamp wired in series with the rheostat. The unit could be connected to 110 volts direct dynamo (motor derived) direct current or 20 to 40 cells for power. The unit could also be adapted for sinusoidal current if 110 volts alternating current was available. Complete with accessories, weighing about 20 pounds, it cost $15.00 in 1907. No "milliamperemeter" is available on this model.

In the center is a plate for only galvanic current. The marble plate has the improved McIntosh "milliamperemeter" with shunt, a MacLagan wire rheostat, and a pole changer. The unit was used with cells located externally, 110 volts alternating current, or with an alternating current rectifier. In 1918, it sold for $24.00. In 1907, the marble base was 9.5 x 16 inches. The unit was then powered by 110 volts direct current, as well as with a rectifier for alternating current, and a battery of cells. It weighed about 20 pounds and cost $18.00 in 1907. A series tap with cord was available for an additional $1.25.

To the right is a faradic switchboard. The 9.5 x 16 inches marble face plate has a faradic coil with two vibrators. One vibrator gives coarse current (massage), and the other is for high rate pulses (anesthesia via a ribbon or singing rheotome). The plate also has a wire rheostat, and switches for selecting primary and secondary faradic currents, and binding posts. Binding posts connect to the patient and to the power source. The model cost $21.00 in 1918.

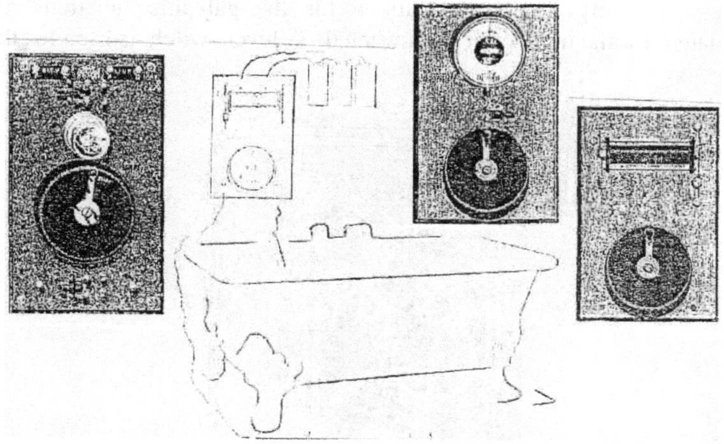

Fig M49. McIntosh Switchboards of 1907

In addition to serving as a vibrator and massage unit, this model in 1907 was also designed to be used in electrical baths with three cells for power. It weighed about 24 pounds and sold for $16.00. Additional attachments were available for this unit (eg: current tap, bathtub electrodes, and waterproof cords).

McIntosh Batteries for Truax, Greene & Co

In 1892 or 1893, The McIntosh Co manufactured electrical batteries for the Charles Truax, Greene & Co using designs proposed by the Chicago seller. Truax, Greene & Co called its models the Columbian, the Exposition (not shown), and the Chicago. The names of these models are named for the Columbian Exposition of 1893 held in Chicago and were no doubt made just prior to the Exposition. (On the occasion of the Exposition's convened group of experts many of the electrical terms used today were defined and adopted.)

Columbian Electrical Wall Cabinet. The model in Fig M50 has features common to McIntosh's The Little Gem that was made and marketed in 1881 to 1890 (Fig M31). The Columbian manufactured and marketed in 1893 was an improvement of The Little Gem model yet not offering power circuits for direct or alternating currents. The Columbian used two faradic coils, each having its own sliding metal current controller but sharing a screw adjustable interrupter. A second vibrating interrupter was also shared. The two interrupters offered pulsed frequencies of slow and rapid rates. This wall cabinet used 38 cells for the galvanic functions and three cells for the faradic functions. The cells were located in an adjoining area (eg: a basement, closet, or room). Each function had button switches that controlled the number of cells operating at any time. The buttons for the galvanic functions are graduated for the number of cells wanted. A lever switch is used for the

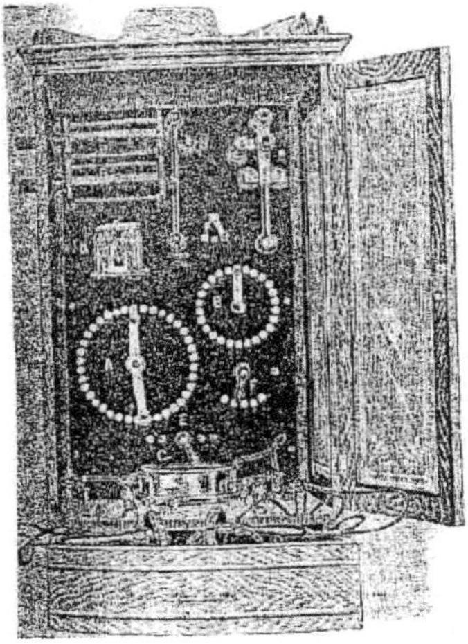

Fig M50. The Columbian Electrical Wall Cabinet

three buttons for faradic functions. A double switch is used to allow all or any number of cells to be switched into the circuit. Switches allow the patient to be placed in and out of the circuit without being shocked. A McIntosh "milliamperemeter" is located on the face plate. This wall cabinet was made of antique oak (15.5 x 11.5 x 34 inches) that has a beveled glass door and a drawer for accessories. All metal are nickel plated and the face plate is hard rubber.

"Chicago" Electrical Office Cabinet. This particular unit (Fig M51) for Truax, Greene & Co in 1893 was styled somewhat after McIntosh's No.4 Cabinet Battery of 1881 to 1890 (Fig M29). Each unit has similar electrical components to the McIntosh No.1 cabinet unit. The cabinet of the "Chicago" is made of antique quarter-sawed oak (47 x 22 x 33 inches). The face plate of the unit is hard rubber inlaid on the top. The electrical components are contained on the hard rubber face plate, drawers were rearranged from two in the No.1 Office Table Plate to four in the "Chicago." A wooden partition divides the drawers in the "Chicago." The "Chicago" contained 40 cells in its cabinet and cost $195.00 in 1893. Additional cells could be used if housed externally to the cabinet. Casters mounted on the corners of its base allows for mobility of the cabinet.

The "Chicago" also came in a horizontal table plate housed in a wooden book type case (22 x 12 x 5 inches) for $130.00. The customer could buy the same unit housed in a glass top case for only $76.00, also

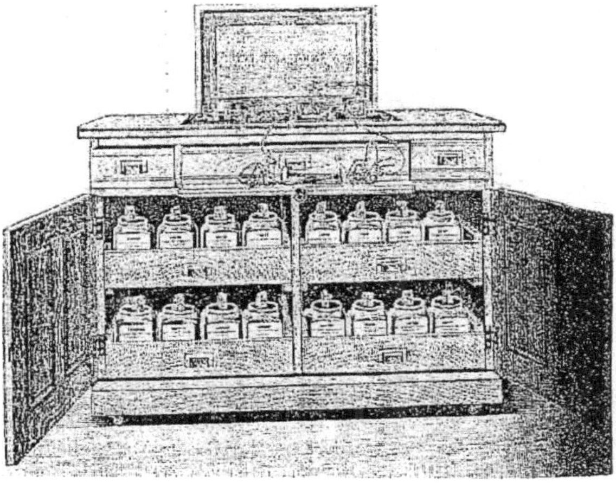

Fig M51. "Chicago" Electrical Office Cabinet

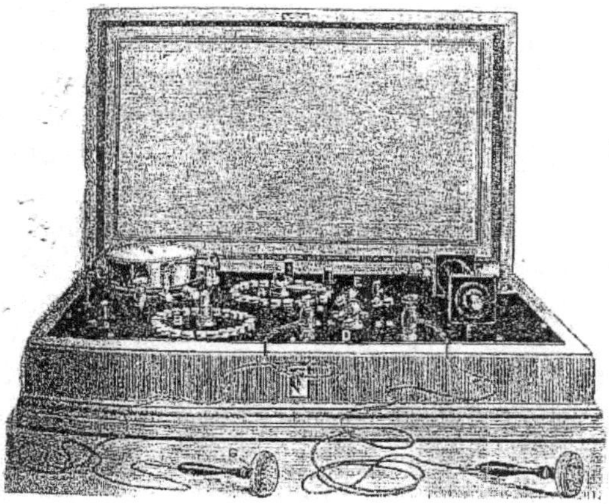

Fig M52. "Chicago" Table Plate

in 1893. Forty cells external to either unit were used to power it. A double galvanic switch of 25 buttons, a 25 button German wire rheostat, a pole changer, switches for current selection, a McIntosh "milliamperemeter," and a coil offering two faradic currents of variable quantity and voltage (tension) are contained on the hard rubber face plate. All metal are nickel plated. The hinged lid is secured by a self locking latch in front. This particular unit is similar to the McIntosh

Table Battery and Plate of 1881 to 1890 except that it does not have an automatic galvanic interrupter that is shown in Figs M23-M25.

Combination Batteries, Bath Models

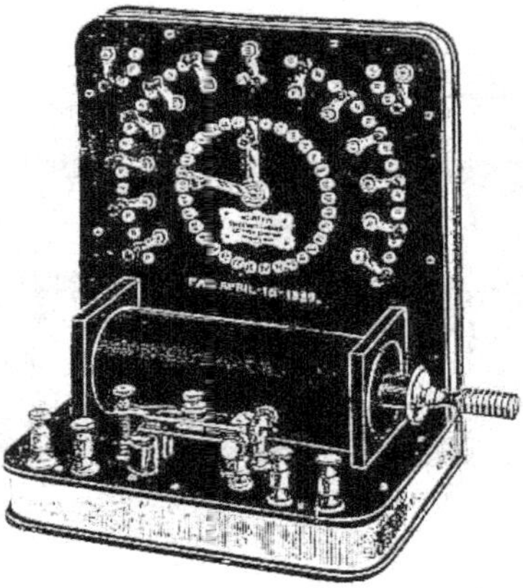

Fig M53. Combined Galvanic and Faradic Bath Apparatus No.1

In addition to the three switchboards of Fig M49 the McIntosh Galvanic and Faradic Battery Co manufactured a special faradic and galvanic electrical battery for use in treatments involving a bathtub (limbs immersed in water). The No.1 model is ornamental and is a L-shaped device made of hard rubber components, and vertical (or shield) and horizontal face plates. The vertical face plate has 12 lever switches that change poles of 12 cells, and a 12-switch galvanic double control with buttons connecting each cell. In each upper corner of the vertical plate is a lever switch that connects one of the two currents to either binding post. The shelf or shield of the L-shaped apparatus contains the induction coil with polished square hard rubber ends and cover. The coil has a sliding tube current regulator. The interrupter is horizontal to the shelf and operates with two small coils and an adjustable screw spring lever that has a bar that vibrates with the two coils. The shelf also has four binding posts.

One wood bathtub or tub of soapstone could be purchased with the battery unit for an additional $25.00, or an indurated (hardened) fiber tub for an additional $15.00. The cost of the wood tub separately was $160.00. With 36 gravity cells it sold for $250.00 (without the cells for $200.00) in 1881. The unit in 1890 sold for $214.00 with cells and $200.00 without cells. If all cells were desired by the customer the case was $200.00 ($160.00 without cells) through the AS Aloe catalog of 1893.[8] The vertical or shelf part of the unit was patented in 16 April

1889. One might speculate that this particular unit's manufactured date ranges from 1889 through 1893 and later.

The 24-cell unit weighs about 24 pounds and sold for $67.50 from 1881 to 1893. The same design of circuitry, the same style of wooden case (except size of 20.75 x 8.25 x 7.25 inches) and the same style cell pack (4 cell packs) are used in the Twenty-Four Cell Combined Galvanic and Faradic Battery of the McIntosh Battery and Optical Co in 1893.

Bath Apparatus No.2. The design of the unit in Fig M54 is very different than that of No. 1. No changes of design occurred between

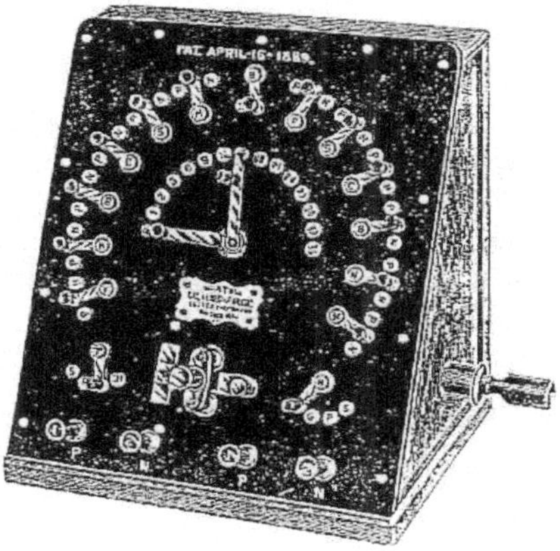

Fig M54. Combined Galvanic and Faradic Bath Apparatus No.2

models of 1881 and 1893. The face plate of this apparatus is a triangular, polished black walnut case. The induction coil is located in the triangular case and has a sliding current regulator tube that protrudes outside of the case for ease of operation. The face plate is of hard rubber and contains 12 switches for controlling the cells, four binding posts for choosing polarity, a rheotome, an On/Off lever control, and a current selector. It cost $85.00 for only the face plate version, but the regular unit without cells cost $125.00 in 1893.[8] Two options were available in 1881 ($175.00 for face plate and cells and without cells for $140.00), and in 1890 ($140.00 and $126.00, respectively).[10]

"Extra". In 1897 (via catalog edition 18 of McIntosh), a new battery for baths was introduced for sale to physicians (Fig M55). The unit was designed for two of the largest sanitariums in the United States. The vertical portion of the L-shaped unit contains the same electrical components as the bath apparatus No.1. The horizontal portion face plate also contains the same electrical components as No.1, but additionally it has a small faradic coil, an automatic rheotome for use with galvanic current, a "milliamperemeter," and a circular coil rheostat with resistances ranging from 100 to 15,000 ohms. A complete unit that

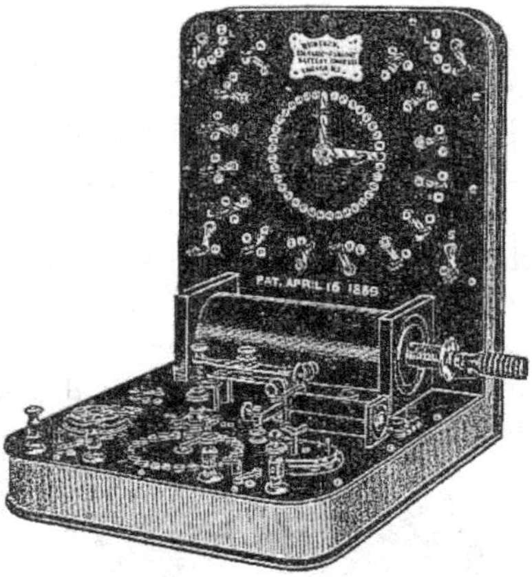

Fig M55. Combined Galvanic and Faradic Bath Apparatus, "Extra"

included the combination battery, an indurated fiber bathtub with a special large cell for powering the bath coils, and 60 galvanic cells cost $300.00. For the plate only the price was $200.00.

Influence Machines

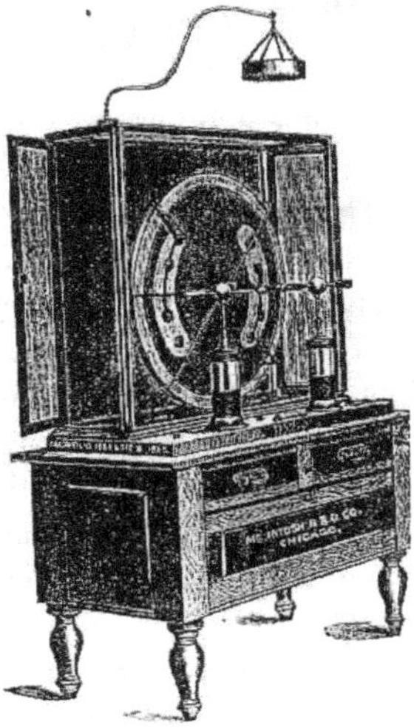

Fig M56. Atkinson's Toepler Electric Machine

Atkinson-Toepler. The Atkinson model of influence machines was made only by the McIntosh Battery & Optical Co, and the model had a glass protecting case. The Atkinson patents for the machine were granted on 10 April 1883 and 8 December 1885. Static electrical machines like the Atkinson model were popularized in the United States in the 1880s by Dr William Morton of New York City. The popularity of the influence machines, as they were called, ran from the 1880s through the 1890s, and waned gradually to about 1930 when they ceased to be marketed. The Atkinson machine has two or four circular plates, while many have only two plates. The glass plates of this machine came in different sizes and numbers. A machine with two plates of 16 and 18 inches in diameter cost $60.00, and with plates of 25 and 28 inches cost $125.00. The four plate model cost $100.00 for 16 and 18 inches, while one with 25 and 28 inches cost $200.00 (AS Aloe, 1893).[8]

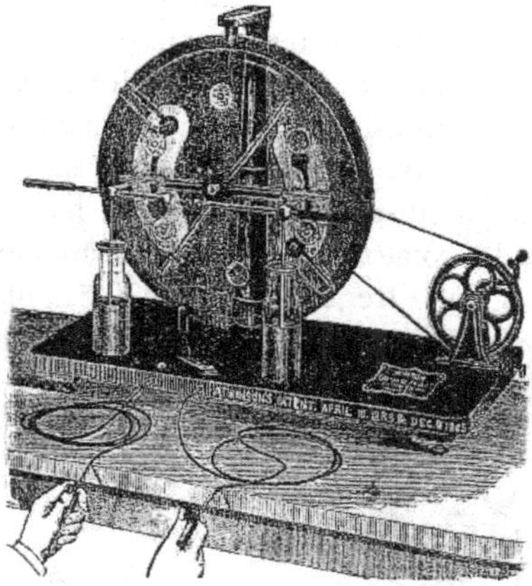

Fig M57. Atkinson's Toepler Table Model

Miscellaneous

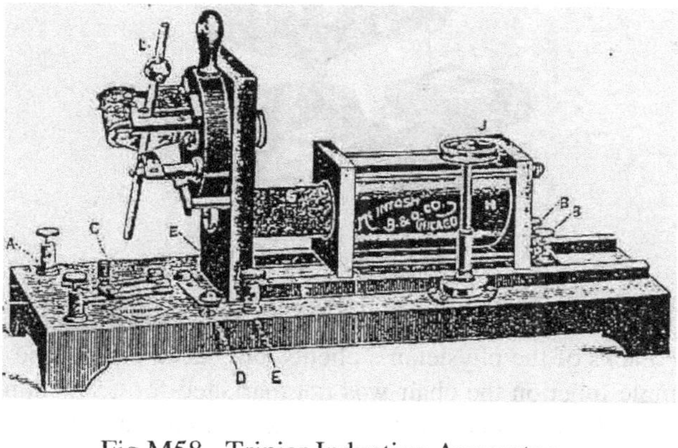

Fig M58. Tripier Induction Apparatus

Tripier Induction Apparatus. This unit is somewhat like that designed by DuBois-Reymond of Germany and France in the 1840s. This faradic electrical apparatus was used successfully and endorsed by well known gynecologists Drs Apostoli and Ranvier of France. By special windings of different lengths and sizes of wires the induction coil delivers currents from three different coils (similar method used in batteries by the J Kidder Mfg Co). This unit does not have a wooden box for a case, but the coil and electrical components are mounted on a base that in part serves as a sledge inductorium for the secondary coil to slide over the primary coil. A rack and pinion helps the secondary coil to slide forward and backward over the primary coil, and is uncommon in medical electrical batteries. The base has a pole changer or commutator on the left side along with two binding posts for connecting the apparatus to power cells, two connecting posts, and a contact button that opens and closes the circuit manually. The interrupter or rheotome is also rare for faradic electrical apparatuses. The rheotome has two small coils, an adjustable lever, and a rotator with a handle. Movement with the handle increases or decreases the frequency 50 to 3000 pulses per minute. The Tripier apparatus was used to control pain by stimulating sensory nerves. Along with three cells the unit sold for $80.00 in the 1893 catalog of AS Aloe.[8]

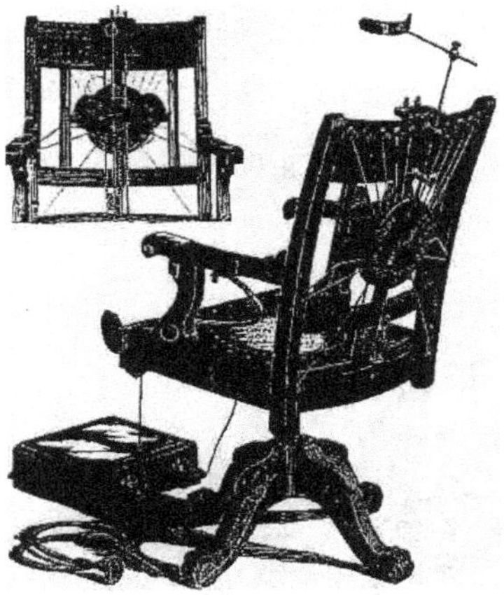

Fig M59. Electrical Chair[10]

Electrical Chair. The Electrical Chair was designed to treat the aching backs of the physician's clients, but because it was so focused for that single function the chair was not marketed for a very long period of time. Sore backs could easily be treated without an electrical chair by available medical electrical batteries purchased for a large variety of ailments, and physicians most often were conservative when buying batteries. The Electrical Chair was available through the McIntosh company's catalogue of 1890.

The chair came in walnut with embedded heavy nickel plated electrodes. Current is regulated by a switchboard mounted on the back of the chair, and through a selector the current can be directed to most areas of the body as desired (neck, back, seat, arm(s), and feet). The chair is adjustable to accommodate the various sizes of clients. A wheel-pulley system can lower or raise the electrodes to the spine of the client, and spacing between electrodes can be altered. Also, the neck electrode is adjustable. The foot stool serves as an electrode for one or two feet and when inverted the stool serves as a tray for water electrical treatments of the entire foot or feet. This ingenious electrical chair sold for $90.00 in 1890.

Sinusoidal Current Apparatuses

Officials of the McIntosh company kept abreast with technological changes that aided its progression over 50 years to make it a leader in the manufacture of physical therapy apparatuses. From time to time the McIntosh Co would issue publications for physicians on various specialized electrical treatments. In 1902 (perhaps as early as 1900), the company was manufacturing apparatus to produce sinusoidal currents that were in demand then by physicians. In 1909, McIntosh's engineers designed what they called an ingenious apparatus for producing various forms of sine waves with controlled frequencies by mechanical speed reduction devices (the Polysine series). Up to this time the apparatus producing sinusoidal currents appear to be converted into combined electrical units to accommodate the components needed to provide the smoother form of alternating current (sine vs faradic). The McIntosh Co considered this newly designed product to be the result of its continued principles of high standard design, workmanship, materials, and latest scientific development that was initially pledged in 1879 when Dr LH McIntosh opened his business for the medical community.[5]

In 1911, the company published Sinusoidal Technique: A Working Manual of the Sinusoidal Current, about 1912 Suggestions for Spondylotherapists, about 1917 Sinusoidal Therapy, in 1922 The Therapeutics of High Frequency, The Electron in 1923, and around 1929 Alternating Current Therapeutics,[3] and along with the directions for operating the Polysine units the Polysine Philosophy.

Dr John Harvey Kellogg of Battle Creek, MI, around 1891 produced a magnetoelectrical machine that delivered satisfactory pulses similar to that published by Jacques D'Arsonval of France in 1892. Graphically, pulses produced by machines of Kellogg and d'Arsonval were perfectly smooth and uniform curves. The pulses were alternating currents of sinusoidal form which D'Arsonval named correctly, and has subsequently been the accepted term. Kellogg called the sinusoidal shaped pulse his "characteristic of excitation," but his term never became acceptable. Kellogg performed clinical trials using the new waveform, and found that the sinusoidal pulses produced less sensory discomfort than that produced by apparatuses using induction coils and similar current amplitudes.[13]

Kellogg first experimented with this form of pulse in 1882 by using a telephone generator of Western Electric Mfg Co of Chicago (magnetoelectrical) that could produce strong muscular contractions with apparent little pain. He used the generator in his clinical practice and presented findings at professional meetings between 1882 and 1889. Kellogg also modified and improved his magnetoelectrical apparatuses during this period of time so that by 1902 or earlier McIntosh Battery and Optical Co was manufacturing sinusoidal machines similar to prototypes of Dr JH Kellogg.[13]

Independent Sinusoidal Model. The sinusoidal unit of Fig M60 was designed in 1902 for wall mounting that requires a pulley to be connected to the sinusoidal apparatus and to a motor (diagram). This is the only known unit designed in the United States to use a pulley in the operation of the unit. The Independent Sinusoidal Apparatus was built to

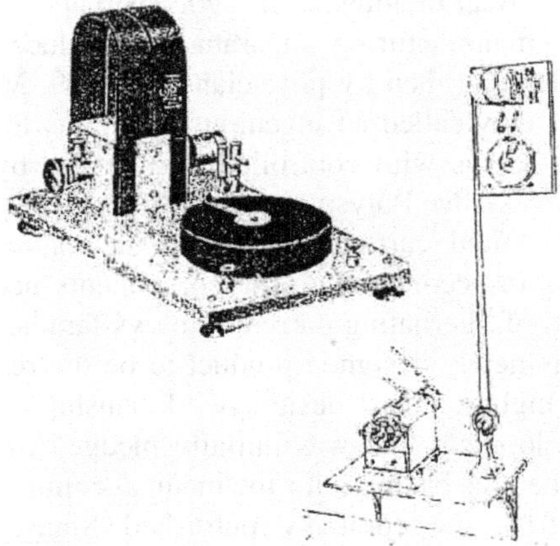

Fig M60. McIntosh Independent Sinusoidal Apparatus

accommodate 110 volts direct current by a water motor, a direct current motor, or motor to operate static machines. The complete unit had a shipping weight of 42 pounds in 1907. The basic unit with accessories but without a motor could be bought for $30.00, but if a motor was wanted with the basic unit the cost was $34.50.

Early Sinusoidal Apparatus. McIntosh Co designed its improved sinusoidal apparatus of Fig M61 rather early in time (perhaps 1905) to be used with a 110 volts direct current source. The direct current source was connected to the small motor (dynamo, left) wound to receive the source current in the motor circuit that is controlled by a rheostat.

The MacLagan rheostat used with this model was an improvement over the unit in Figs M62 & 65 that still used the graphite, octagonally shaped rheostats. The sinusoidal unit (right rear) consists of an armature carrying the coils of wire revolving between two permanent magnets in the patient circuit. The sine waves are uniform and the current is controlled by a rheostat. The motor circuit rheostat controls the rapidity of the alterations. With the black enameled slate base the unit weighs nearly 72 pounds, and with all accessories it cost $50.00 in 1907.

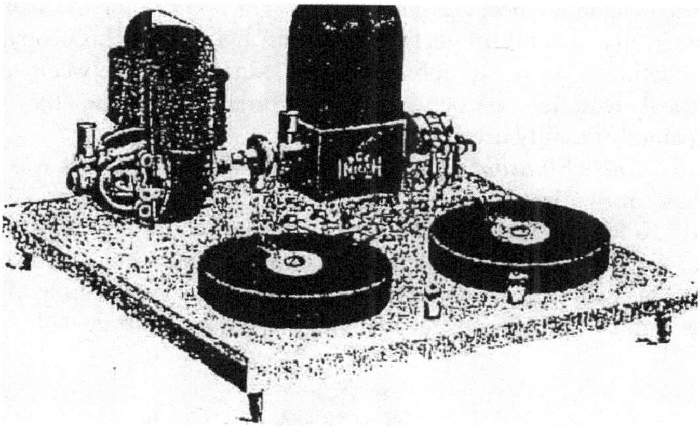

Fig M61. McIntosh Improved Sinusoidal Apparatus

The McIntosh company also offered the consumer an option with the model in Fig M62. Rather than using the upgraded rheostat (MacLagan) the consumer could benefit from the design of the sinusoidal apparatus by using the Jewel type graphite rheostats at a lower cost.

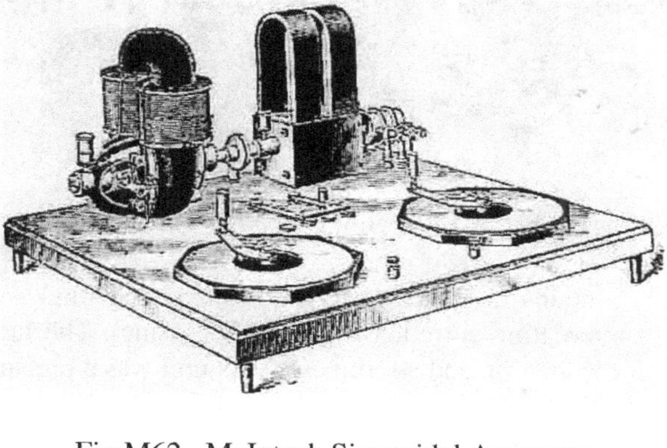

Fig M62. McIntosh Sinusoidal Apparatus

Sinusoidal Apparatus. The model of Fig M62 is nearly the same as that of Fig M61 except that it is an earlier version. This model dates from 1900 and 1902 (above unit is 1902 model), and probably was still being manufactured until the improved units having the MacLagan rheostat were available around 1905 to 1907. This model has the graphite, octagonal style rheostat that preceded the MacLagan rheostat, and an earlier style direct current motor.

The McIntosh company kept the construction of the MacLagan rheostat a secret as long as it could (wire resistances rather than graphite). Copying was rather rampant then among manufacturers of medical electrical batteries because patents were not applied for the many new features that would protect against infringement. This copying by manufacturers accounts for the many similarities between medical electrical batteries, particularly those produced among the smaller companies of family use apparatuses.

Early Sinusoidal Unit. By 1909, sinusoidal current was the "in current" of the time. Although first invented between 1882 and 1889 by Dr JH Kellogg of the Battle Creek, MI, Sanitarium and of Cornflakes fame, it took some time to make apparatuses that were practical while using alternating and direct current motors. This model is a McIntosh early sinusoidal apparatus for mounting on top of an office table or desk.

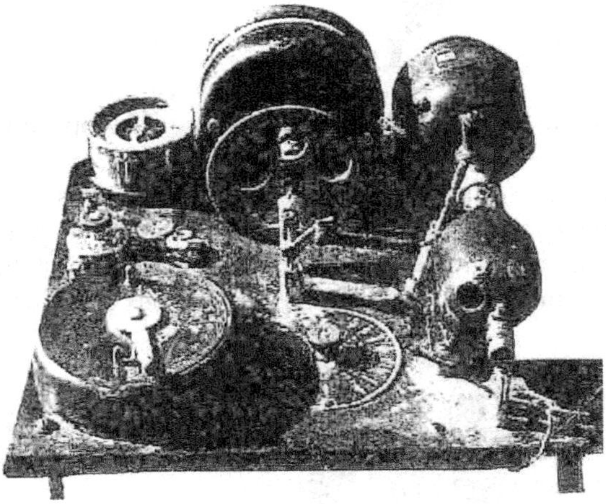

Fig M63. Early Sinusoidal Current Unit

The model contains a MacLagan rheostat, meter, and switch for variations of alternating current waveforms (polysine). The face plate is heavy slate for insulation and adornment. This unit was a precursor to the Polysine.

Polysine No.4. Although sales of the Polysine began with the catalog issue of 1909, it was in 1910 that the polysine was really officially introduced by the McIntosh Co personnel to the medical profession at the American Medical Association meeting in St Louis. Leading electrotherapeutists of the day such as: Neiswanger, Rice, Snow, and Tousey quickly adopted the Polysine unit in their medical practices, and the McIntosh Co was quick to announce this in its catalogs.

During World War 1, the Polysine apparatus was used by the United States Army's Medical Corps in its hospitals, and it proved to be of considerable value to patient treatment. In the World War I period of

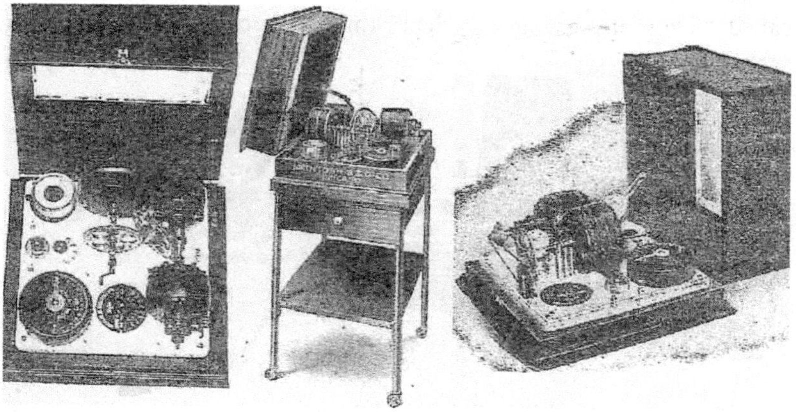

Fig M64. McIntosh Polysine No. 4, 1918[9]

time mostly non-physicians (eg, physical therapists) were used to administer the electrical treatments to patients when physicians worked more in diagnostics and triage.

About 1920 to 1922, the McIntosh company upgraded its Polysine unit of 1918 by replacing the "monomotive" rheostat used with faradic current (left, Fig M64) with the MacLagan rheostat used to control sinusoidal current. The Polysine units in Fig M64 (center and right) are the same except the consumer then had the option to buy the model with or without a mobile stand. The upgraded model offers sinusoidal pulses ranging from 2 to 30 per second; a pulse that has the two rates superimposed; a slow surging galvanic current on a 30 per second surging sinusoidal current; conventional galvanic current; combined galvanic-sinusoidal current; and a current for diagnostic lamps.

The McIntosh company manufactured other medical electrical apparatuses that produced sinusoidal currents. As noted, sinusoidal currents were introduced by Dr JH Kellogg in the 1880s, and in 1906 or

1907, McIntosh made a unit patterned after the 1889 design of Kellogg (Fig M65).

1907 Apparatus. This model of 1907 (left) consists of a face plate comprising a direct current motor to produce the sinusoidal currents by means of the circuit connection with a rotating coil between a set of three permanent magnets. A disc rheostat controls the current amplitude while connecting the circuit with the patient. This model is similar to that of Fig M61, but has three permanent magnets rather than two. Three magnets made this model slightly more powerful than those in Fig M61 and M62. The model in Fig M65 (left) was so designed that the axis of the armature is wound and directly attached to the axis of the motor. This arrangement eliminates use of a belt that is part of others (eg, AE Kennelly & M60). Two additional brushes from the motor generate a so called "interrupted galvanic current" (monophasic pulses) that is then

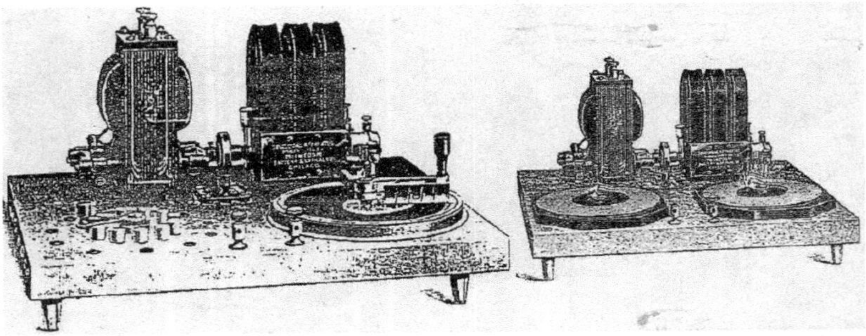

Fig M65. Sinusoidal Apparatus[14]

converted to the sinusoidal current by a switch. Thus, the operator has either pulsed galvanic or pulsed sinusoidal currents as treatment choices.

The rheostat of this model (left) is a graphite controller that puts the patient into a shunt circuit (divides current to reduce amplitudes). The rheostat could be used with 120 volts Edison (direct) current or that of a battery of cells. The switch on the left of the face plate operates the number of cells for selecting voltage with galvanic current.

The McIntosh company offered this same unit with a choice of a rheostat, rather than a switch, to control galvanic current. The rheostats in this model (right) are of the Jewel graphite controller type that also puts the patient into a shunt circuit.

The introduction of the sinusoidal apparatuses in the early twentieth century brought design changes to the medical electrical battery models. The hard rubber and wooden face plates were replaced by metal, porcelain, marble, and slate. Traditional electrical components seen on the face plates also changed. The induction coil was replaced by alternating and direct current motors and permanent magnets. Additional switches and dials were used in circuits as well as meters. The wooden cases were replaced by metal and porcelain mobile stands or table top models. Rectifiers were being used to convert direct current to alternating current.

Universal Mode. This unit was an apparatus that offered a variety of electrical currents and multiple functions. The original concept and design was that of Dr JH Kellogg of the Battle Creek Sanitarium. Although Dr Kellogg's first apparatus for multiple currents was the development of sinusoidal current around 1893 or 1895, this unit was manufactured and sold by McIntosh in 1916 or before as its Universal Mode. This model used a mobile stand to hold the apparatus and allow for mobility. It performs several functions that include 16 effects (physiological) according to the manufacturer. Nine effects are provided through its sinusoidal currents. The unit produces slow and rapid sinusoidal currents that are controlled by a knob on a friction device.

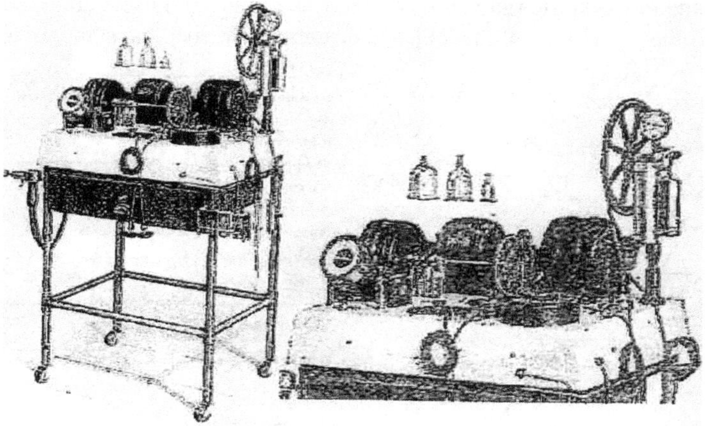

Fig M66. McIntosh Universal Mode[9]

The face plate is enameled porcelain steel that holds a: rheostat, faradic coil, motor, direct current generator, cautery unit, transformer, dial selector, and pole changer. The MacLagan wire rheostat controls the galvanic current functions for electrolysis, and gynecology. The galvanic current is measured by the "milliamperemeter."

The Universal Mode delivers combined faradic (primary or secondary with various frequencies) and galvanic currents; combined galvanic and sinusoidal currents of 1800 periods per minute; rapid sinusoidal currents at 1800 per minute; galvanic monophasic pulses at 3 to 88 per minute; diagnostic lamp; cautery; combined faradic and galvanic currents at 3 to 88 per minute; superimposed waves at 3 to 88 per minute; surging sinusoidal current at 6 to 176 periods per minute; primary faradic current at 3 to 88 per minute; secondary faradic 3 to 88 pulses per minute; and slow sinusoidal pulses at 3 to 88 per minute.

Electrocautery points, loops, and snares may be heated with the unit. Vibratory massage is available for spinal stimulation; and inhibition or local effects are possible when fitting the massage cable to the shaft of the motor. The unit also performs nasal drilling; electrical heated air; pneumomassage of the ear, eye, or skin; vaporizing or nebulizing of oils; and deep suction. The spraying of oils or liquids is done with the pump that provides up to 50 pounds of pressure by turning a thumb screw. The unit also provides endoscopic lamps for diagnostic uses.

The basic unit without the stand was $250.00 in 1918. A stand was $25.00, and other options were additionally priced. A complete unit with all options was $386.00.

The McIntosh Universal Mode unit delivered 16 different waveforms. Fourteen of these waveforms are shown in Fig M66A, while the diagnostic lamp and cautery modes of the unit also used the monophasic galvanic waveform above. Basically, the faradic, sinusoidal, and the monophasic (galvanic) waveforms produced muscle contractions. The other variations of the pulsed currents performed the same function

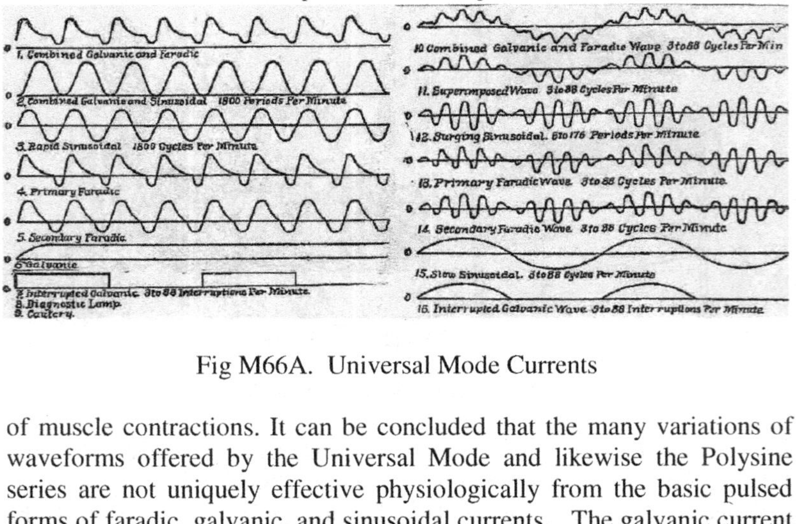

Fig M66A. Universal Mode Currents

of muscle contractions. It can be concluded that the many variations of waveforms offered by the Universal Mode and likewise the Polysine series are not uniquely effective physiologically from the basic pulsed forms of faradic, galvanic, and sinusoidal currents. The galvanic current (unidirectional, positive in Fig M66A, 2nd from bottom, left) produced chemical effects physiologically, and is uniquely different from the pulsed currents.

Since the Polysine series was designed and manufactured later than the Universal Mode, many of the currents have been eliminated that were once available on the Universal Mode (Fig M66A vs Fig M68). Waveforms seen in these two figures may seem to be different than those presented earlier in Part 1, Chapter 1 (Fig 6 through Fig 12). Faradic pulses or waveforms are similar; the difference is in the methods of recording them. Earlier waveforms were recorded by slow oscillating

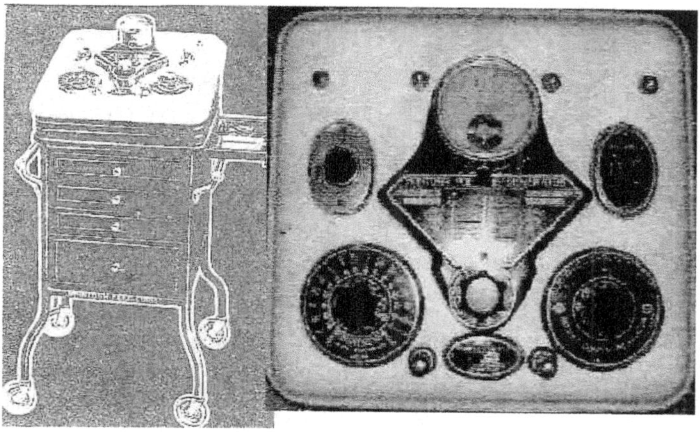

Fig M67. Polysine, 1929[5]

graphic recorders, while those shown in Chapter 1 were recorded by an oscilloscope that displays the true form instantly.

Polysine model of 1929. The Polysine unit in 1929 was an improved electrical generator, and perhaps the successor to the Universal Mode. The face plate is metal that was introduced in medical electrical batteries around 1910 to 1912, and contains: a current selector dial for any of the 16 current forms; a frequency regulator; a "milliamperemeter" with a range of 0 to 150 mA; a voltage regulator; and an electrode heater. The metal stand (18 x 19 x 42 inches) has large rubber tired casters for easy mobility; four drawers; and a face plate of enameled porcelain (17.5 x 18.5 inches). This model is the 1929 design of an apparatus that had been marketed by then for 21 years.

The Polysine is a generator that delivered five forms of galvanic current, five forms of sinusoidal current, and six forms of the currents combined. The unit provided a slow sinusoidal pulse ranging from 12 to 120 hertz; a rapid sinusoidal pulse of 1800 per minute; a superimposed or combined pulse of the 1800 per minute rapid sinusoidal form imposed upon the slower sinusoidal form; a surging (ramping) sinusoidal form similar to the former; a slow ramping galvanic current; a rapid ramping galvanic current; a conventional galvanic current; a combined galvanic and sinusoidal current; and a current for use with the diagnostic lamps. Sinusoidal pulses are superior to faradic pulses because of the reduced sensory irritation. This Polysine offers 18 various forms of sinusoidal pulses. Fig M68 shows five of the sinusoidal waveforms of the Polysine. These waveforms depict modifications of the sinusoidal current through variations in pulse durations, frequencies or rates, and amplitudes. These modifications alter the sinusoidal current shape, and subsequently change their affect on muscle tissue. The most notable change on muscle behavior is those variations occurring from singular to tetanic (fused) contractions.

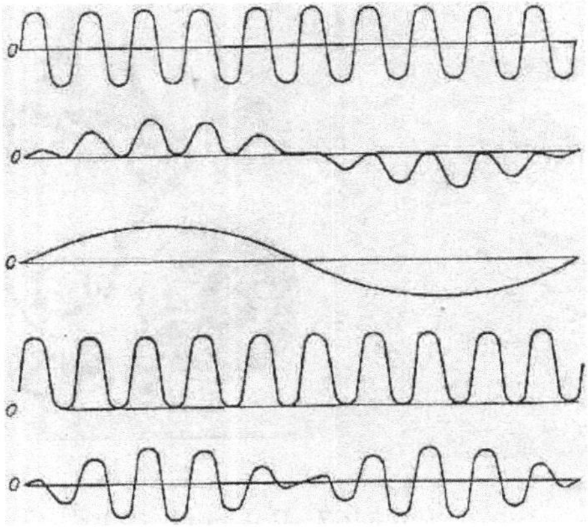

Fig M68. Example of Polysine Waveforms

Polysine No.5005. This Polysine model (Fig M69) was still in production in 1932 by the McIntosh Co. The manual Gleanings of Low Voltage Therapy by Dr GA Remmington accompanied each Polysine model sold in 1932.

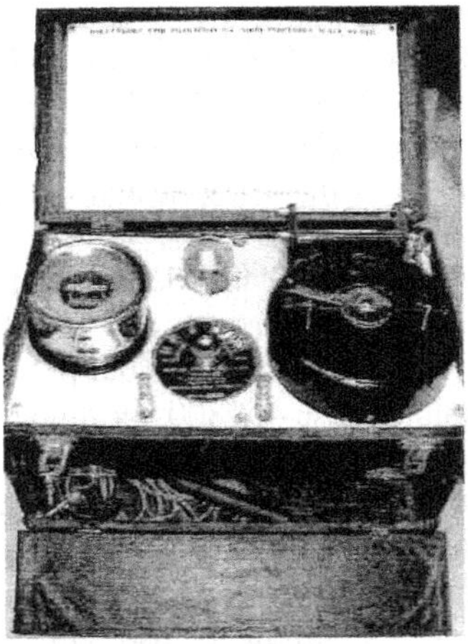

Fig M69. McIntosh No. 5005 Portable Wall Plate

The wall plate models were very popular among physicians between 1905 and into the 1920s. This particular unit is believed to be the last model by McIntosh that still used the traditional induction coil to provide faradic currents along with galvanic and sinusoidal currents. The faradic current was being replaced by the sinusoidal current from about 1902 to the 1920s because of the reduced sensory stimuli by sinusoidal pulses. Still some physicians were demanding the capability of both faradic and sinusoidal currents. This portable wall plate was advanced enough to eliminate the motors and magnets of the earlier sinusoidal units to produce sinusoidal pulses. This No.5005 Portable Wall Plate used a four pronged B-H Raytheon vacuum tube to serve as a rectifier to convert current types. Since this unit was manufactured by the McIntosh Electrical Corp of 223-233 N California Ave, Chicago, it dates from 1929 just prior to the introduction of the Polysine No.1156 unit of 1929. Use of permanent magnets, and alternating with direct current motors was being replaced in the 1920s by vacuum tubes.

This unit is powered by 100 volts AC. The case is wooden (15 x 9.38 x 10.25 inches) but covered with black buckram. The hinged lid is secured by two snap latches on the front and when opened displays the directions and the McIntosh locations. The top of the lid has a leather carrying handle that is anchored at each end by a chain link. The lower front half of the case opens the accessories compartment that is secured by two snap latches. The face plate is painted slate and holds the electrical components: an induction coil with 1.75 inches hard rubber square end caps that are connected by two metal rods, an adjustable spring lever vibrating interrupter, two adjustable connecting posts marked N and P, a lever selector control for AC (galvanic from rectifier, earth free sinusoidal, and secondary faradic currents) and DC (galvanic from line, primary faradic, and secondary faradic currents), a six inches MacLagan rheostat measuring 0 to 100 volts, and a milliammeter graduated 0 to 150 mA each for negative and positive polarities. The unit weighs about 40 pounds.

Summary

The McIntosh Co was founded in Chicago, IL, in 1879 as the McIntosh NU Supporter Co by physician LH McIntosh. During its more than 73 years (1879-1952) of operation, it became the most dominant manufacturer of electrotherapeutic apparatus in the United States. The company also outlived most of its competitors while being recognized as one of the best in its field. Many trade catalogs, educational publications, apparatus operating manuals, and a newsletter were published by company personnel to inform consumers about products but also about specific technologies as educational tools. During its many years of operation the company changed its name and address on several occasions. It expanded into other major cities so as to form a national network of offices that could easily be within the grasps of practicing physicians. Electrotherapeutic products made by this company were of superior quality, reliability, and durability. The latest technologies were incorporated in its products as well as its personnel developing new technologies. The McIntosh company offered the widest variety of apparatuses among its competitors. The company manufactured and sold the batteries, cells, accessories, and electrical belts. Electrical belts were part of the company's name between 1879 and 1881. Dr LH McIntosh was an innovative physician who kept abreast of the technological developments, and incorporated the latest improvements in the company's products.

McIntosh batteries have endured well, and sold well when measured by the availability of artifacts in antique shops and eBay auctions today. The products of The McIntosh Co were quality items and sold well that accounts in part for their survival as artifacts.

The trade catalogs of The McIntosh Co educated the physician who was not schooled in electricity, at least up to the early twentieth century. A physician could deliver effective medical treatments with electricity by reading the catalogs, perhaps an acquired textbook on the subject, or by attending an annual meeting of the electrotherapeutics organization.

References

1. Obituary, Dr.LD McIntosh Am Monthly Microscopical J, 1892(http:www.americanartifacts.com/smma/micro/mcinobit.htm), 2001

2. Edmonson JM. American Surgical Instruments. San Francisco, CA, Norman Pub, 1997, p 180

3. Davis AB, Dreyfus MS. The Finest Instruments Ever Made. Arlington, MA, Med Hist Pub Assocs, 1986, pp 221-223

4. Romaine LB. A Guide to American Trade Catalogs 1744-1900. New York, NY, RR Bowker, 1960, p 253

5. Polysine History. Polysine Philosophy, Chicago, IL, McIntosh Electrical Corp, 1929, p 7; (courtesy of David Rickert)

6. Grigg ERN. The Trail of the Invisible Light. Springfield, IL, CC Thomas, 1965, pp 50-80

7. (www.Google.com;www.zianet.com/sparks/sparkmakers2.html), p 13

8. Catalog of AS Aloe. St Louis, MO, AS Aloe, 1893, pp 734-742, 772

9. Brooks Denhard Illustrated Catalogue of Surgical Instruments and Allied Lines. Louisville, KY, 1918, pp 518-524

10. Catalog of McIntosh Battery and Optical Co. Chicago, IL, McIntosh, 1881, pp 26-35; 1890, pp 32- 40

11. McIntosh H. Practical Handbook of Medical Electricity. Boston, MA, Therapeutic Pub, p 79

12. Polk. Medical Registry and Directory of North America. Chicago, IL, RL Polk, 1904

13. Kellogg JH. The Physiological Effects of a Magneto-Electrical Current of Regular Variations. JAMA 20:420-424, 1893

14. Rockwell AD. Medical and Surgical Uses of Electricity. NewYork , NY, EBTreat, 1907, pp 50, 288

CHAPTER 10. FG OTTO & SONS OF NEW YORK CITY

A maker of other such items as clocks, and musical and surgical instruments, FG Otto played a role in the golden era of medical electrical batteries. Chapter 10 reviews his career and role as a maker of electrical batteries, and features many of those products.

Ferdinand G Otto was a maker of quality medical and surgical instruments before and during the Civil War, and was one of the fine German craftsmen in New York City in the mid to late nineteenth century. FG Otto was in business as an instrument maker with Augustus Koehler, another fine craftsman from Germany, from 1853 to 1860.[1]

Perhaps as the largest and best known surgical instrument company in the United States in 1850, George Tiemann of New York City trained men through apprenticeships and then hired them as employees to make instruments. Several men left the employ of Tiemann at different times to begin their own instrument making business. Both Ferdinand G Otto and August Koehler are examples of men leaving Tiemann to form a competitor company. In 1853 or 1854, the two German born former employees of Tiemann formed their own shop at 58 Chatham Street on the same street as the George Tiemann Co. (Chatham St was in the vicinity of the medical community of New York City at the time) Their shop offered a variety of surgical and orthopedic apparatuses for sale. The company of Otto & Koehler was dissolved on 15 February 1860 when Koehler left the partnership. FG Otto then went into partnership with John Reynders in 1860. John Reynders, like his new partner, was another former employee of the George Tiemann Co.[2]

The Otto & Reynders company was formed at the same 58 Chatham Street location where Otto worked since 1853. In 1864, Otto & Reynders moved a few doors away to 64 Chatham Street. Otto & Reynders then successfully promoted the idea that by keeping abreast of the latest surgical literature and technology they could serve the surgeons of New York City better than others. Their products soon vaulted them as leaders of surgical instruments in the New York area. In 1867, the company began making custom orthopedic shoes for Dr Lewis A Sayre, father of American orthopedics. By 1870, the business had grown to where Otto & Reynders employed seven men and one apprentice. At that time the business was selling $20,000.00 of surgical instruments yearly. They expanded the business by becoming importers of surgical items (eg: laryngoscopes, syringes, transfusion apparatus) for Josef Leiter of Vienna, Austria, in that same year. They also specifically imported German devices for the local surgeons who immigrated from Germany. Otto & Reynders, however, continued to manufacturer most of the products sold by the company, and started to make instruments locally for dentists, orthopedists, and local laryngologists. In spite of their great success the partners split after 15 years of partnership on 15 February

1875.[1] Perhaps Otto's desire to include his sons in the partnership had something to do with the dissolution of Otto & Reynders, and form the FG Otto & Sons firm.

After the dissolution of Otto & Reynders in 1875, Reynders formed the John Reynders Co, a company located at 303-309 Fourth Avenue, NY. The Reynders Co became a supplier of medical and surgical equipment and instruments. Later he compressed his business to 303 Fourth Avenue where he sold anatomical preparations, orthopedic apparatuses, skeletons, surgical instruments, and veterinary items. The company issued an illustrated and price list of its orthopedic apparatuses and trusses, and surgical instruments in 1880. This particular catalog was the third edition (262 pp) of the company since its founding in 1875. Sometime in the early 1880s (ca 1882) John Reynders sold his business to his son Charles.[1] The John Reynders Co closed its operation in Chicago (1 May 1884), then the New York firm became the only John Reynders & Co through 1898. Reynders may have manufactured a limited number of medical electrical batteries, but son Charles probably dropped the electrical battery line by the mid 1880s. This company issued catalogs of its products line until 1896 after which time no further trade catalogs are found that carry medical electrical batteries with that name. In the 1890s, Reynders was selling camera cams, microscopes and accessories, microtomes, and optical equipment.[3]

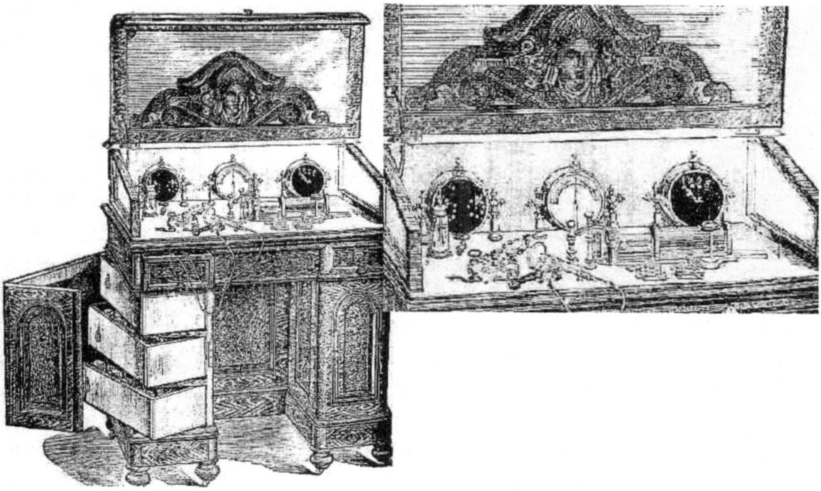

Fig JR. Combination Faradic-Galvanic Desk Cabinet Battery

This large wooden combination faradic and galvanic battery was made by John Reynders & Co about 1876. The unit was shown by Beard and Rockwell in the fifth edition of their book in 1881.[4] The wooden cabinet was hinged from the top and closed over the face plate. It has drawers for batteries (12, 24, or 60 zinc-copper type wet cells), and accessories. The face plate contains a sledge inductorium coil for faradic current, but it could be placed in the circuitry of the galvanic current to serve as a rheostat. The unit has a current reverser, a current interrupter, and a galvanoscope. The sledge inductorium has many windings so as to deliver a pleasant current. The unit can be secured by a lock and key on the front of the desk when not in use, and it is mobile with leg casters.

This 1876 desk cabinet battery of Reynders became the prototype for Otto Flemming's Cabinet Battery of 1886 or earlier. The electrical components of the two cabinet batteries are identical. The face plate as well as everything about the two cabinet models below the face plate are identical. A difference occurs in the lid or desk top covers. Both top covers are elaborate with carvings but the carvings are different. Flemming either copied the cabinet style or acquired the pattern from Reynders when he dropped the electrical battery line in the mid 1880s.

FG Otto, in the meanwhile (1875), went into business with his two sons, Albert and Gustav. The sons of FG Otto did learn to make surgical instruments, but when and where is unknown. Otto probably took his two sons on as apprentices and when they had completed their training they showed enough competency to be partners with dad.

Between 1875 and 1883, FG Otto & Sons were located in the same building at 64 Chatham, New York City, while in 1880, they also located at 39 Centre.[1] FG Otto & Sons expanded their business in 1880 and founded a factory in Jersey City Heights, New Jersey. The factory was equipped with state-of-the-art machinery and tools, and employed 50 skilled workers.

The 1871 patented glass wet cell casings bearing the name "FG Otto & Sons" were made in New York, and then again between 1886 and 1888, and in 1895 at 44 Sherman Street.[1] During the period of time between 1889 and 1900, FG Otto & Sons manufactured a variety of fine clocks, mandolins, and music boxes in their Jersey City plant. The FG Otto & Sons manufactured mandolins in Hoboken, NJ, around 1900 to 1904. The company is most famous for its surgical instruments (early), and its clocks and music boxes (after 1880s). The company was expert in making music boxes, and at one time even made coin operated music boxes for arcades. In 1890, the company made obstetrical instruments. The sons were challenged twice over patent infringements in the 1890s. The competitor, Regina Company, claimed infringements on two music boxes that FG Otto & Sons changed.[5] No trace of the company after 1905 has been found.

Commonalties of Otto Batteries

FG Otto & Sons manufactured faradic batteries for the physician and the public consumer. The faradic batteries were contained in wooden boxes made of cherry with glued corners. The top of the lids have metal carrying handles and mostly hook lever locks on the front of the box. The face plates are made of matching cherry and contain the electrical components. The components consist of an induction coil that is characterized by having a square wooden end cap on each end and preceded by a metal sleeve or band; coils have a sliding metal controller; a spring lever vibrating interrupter is adjacent to the coil; and the boxed faradic batteries contain a single Otto & Sons wet cell. The top of the wet cell is connected to the circuitry by two nickel plated rotating levers. The top of the wet cell is exposed by means of a cut out space on the face plate while the base of the cell rests underneath the face plate. The quality of workmanship is generally good. Inside of the lid of each unit is a cloth banner diagonally to the lid that gives the name of the battery. One of the major accessories to the faradic batteries is the Otto & Sons wet cell, and all styles are embossed with the company's name and location.

Glass Wet Cell Casings

FG Otto & Sons produced wet cells in 1871 that were made at least in two different sizes. The glass cases, although patented in 1871 by FG Otto, were probably manufactured in 1875 when Otto & Reynders became the FG Otto & Sons Co. The casings were made in both New York City and Jersey City with the New York City units preceding the other in time.

The larger glass wet cell (5.75 inches overall height with 3.75 inches square base; sides 2 inches tall, offset neck 3 inches high and 2 inches square) is embossed (raised) on the neck with "LD Patented July 4 1871" and with the company embossed on one side (same as neck) as "F.G. Otto & Sons New York." Otto cell cases between 1871 and 1879 were made in New York and are so marked. The glass is aqua (light greenish blue). The smaller glass cell, also believed to be of the 1871 patent, but made in 1880 in New Jersey (not dated) has a 3-inch square base, 2.5-inch high sides with offset circular neck (1.75 inches high and 1.75 inches diameter) is embossed on one side as "F.G. Otto & Sons Jersey City." The smaller glass wet cell case is also aqua. Both cell cases are designed after a Grenet style.

Both glass wet cell cases are bimal type of bottles. These bimal type bottles were blown from a two-piece cast iron mold. The mold probably had a snap bottom that was used in blowing the bottle in the mold, but removed to leave a smooth bottom on the glass bottle. The cast iron mold is made so that the embossed lettering is raised on both bottles. The cast iron bimal mold was used in the United States between 1830 and 1920 in an effort to make the bottles uniform in shape and size. (This method was mostly replaced after 1902 when the automated glass making machines were introduced.) A glass blower could produce many

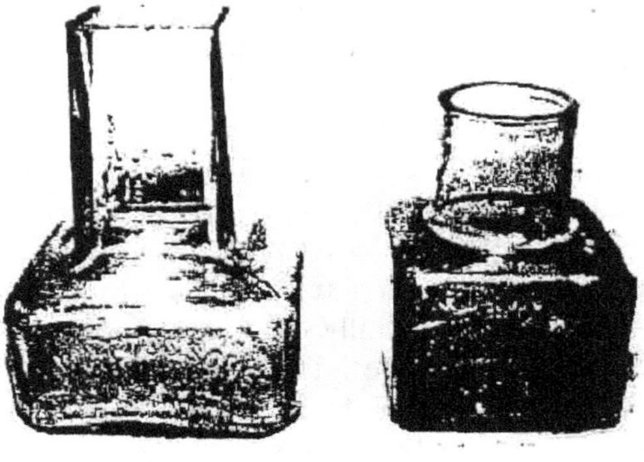

Fig O1. Otto Wet Cell Case: A. Large, B. Small

of these cases in one day. Seams are formed in the two-piece mold along two sides of the bottle up to the neck. The upper body and neck of the bottle were added when the mold was removed. As the seams moved higher along the neck of the bottle the date of manufacture also became later (eg, 1870 vs 1830). Once the upper body and neck are placed on the bottle a metal insert is placed in the neck and rotated. This operation makes the neck and its lip smooth. Often bubbles are seen in the glass that are caused when the melded glass meets the sides of the cast iron mold. The color, aqua, results from the iron content of the crude silicate of lime and soda from the sandbanks of New Jersey. The aqua glass was the cheapest form of bottle to make. The New Jersey area at one time had many glass factories that used the cheap and available sand.

In 1875, the company issued a 24-paged illustrated catalog and price list of its line of batteries, surgical and orthopedic instruments.[6] FG Otto & Sons issued their trade catalogs to about 1886.[3] In the 1880s the company was selling bandages, druggists' sundries, orthopedic appliances, trusses, and surgical instruments in addition to their wet cells and a small line of medical electrical batteries.

Electrical batteries, orthopedic appliances, and surgical instruments[3] were listed in its catalog of 1884 that was similar to the 1875 catalog except more text and more instruments were included in the 1884 issue. The company remained at 64 Chatham Street, New York City, in 1884.[5] In the later years of the company (very early 20th century) medical electrical batteries may have been manufactured by Otto & Sons mostly for medical suppliers or sellers.

FG Otto is believed to have designed and manufactured wet cells prior to dissolving with Reynders in 1875, however, the four faradic boxed units described here have definitely been traced to 1894 through 1905. The Otto faradic batteries were designed for a cut out space on the wooden face plates for the Otto & Sons wet cell. Electrical batteries were being redesigned by most manufacturers at the turn of the nineteenth and twentieth centuries to accommodate the dry cell. Otto batteries remained designed mostly for the wet cell and only the Drescher units used the dry cell. Also, the name of Otto & Sons was continued on its designed batteries sold by The Smith & Shaw Electric Co and AS Aloe in 1893. The Smith & Shaw Electric Company was an outlet retailer of many FG Otto & Son products.[7]

Alpha Faradic Battery. This unit (Fig O2) has been traced to 1894 when it was listed in the catalog of Montgomery Ward & Co.[8] The unit was then sold for $5.00. The Alpha Faradic Battery was also

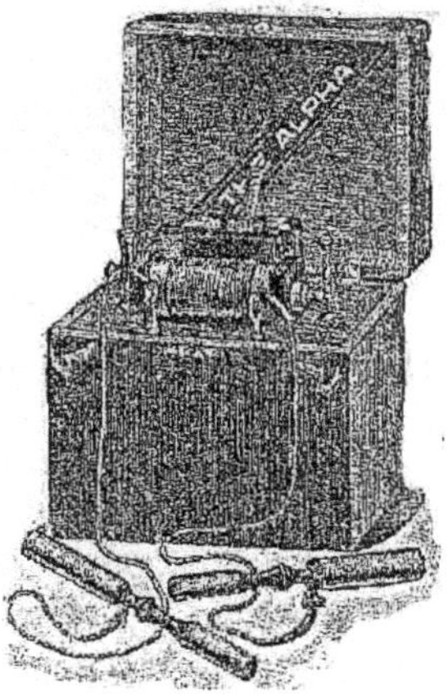

Fig O2. The Alpha Faradic Battery[7]

illustrated and listed in the catalogs of Max Wocher of Cincinnati (1896)[9] and of AS Aloe and The Smith & Shaw Electric Co in 1893 for $ 5.50.[7] The cherry box has a hinged lid that bears a ribbon or banner "The Alpha" across the inside of the lid. The lid has a latch that snaps into place on the front along with two hook lever latches, and a metal carrying handle on top. The wooden face plate (cherry) contains the induction coil (square blocks at each end) with its sliding metal controller, an adjustable screw spring vibrating interrupter, and a slot cut for the top of the Otto & Son wet cell. Two swivel arms, each on metal posts, connect with the battery top to activate the circuit. Two connecting buttons are also contained on the front of the face plate. The unit is powered by a single

Otto & Son wet cell. The complete unit weighs 8.5 pounds. This same unit is believed to be ***The Nonpareil Faradic Battery*** when sold through Max Wocher & Son in 1896.

Phoenix Faradic Battery. The Phoenix (Fig O3) is similar to other Otto & Son batteries, but was designed for physician use. The unit is contained in a cherry box, glued corners, with a metal carrying handle on top, and a lock and key on the front along with two hook lever latches.

The right bottom side has a sliding wooden drawer to house

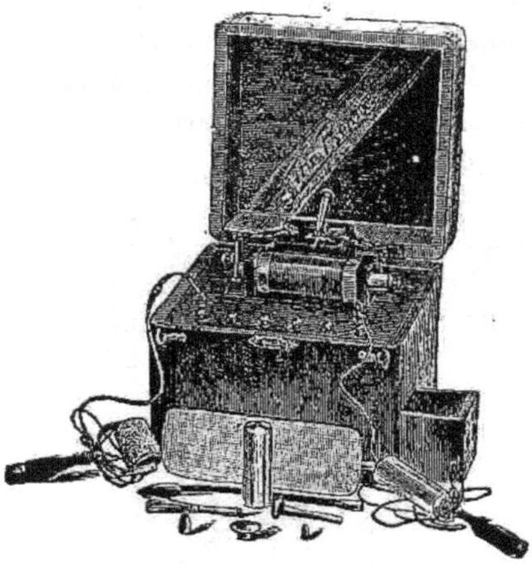

Fig O3. The Phoenix Faradic Battery

accessories. The induction coil has square end caps, a sliding metal controller, and the coil possibly delivers a higher voltage than that of The Alpha and The Nonpareil Faradic Batteries. The electrical batteries designed and sold to physicians customarily contained more powerful electrical outputs than those units sold to the public. An adjustable screw spring vibrating interrupter is to the left of the coil. This unit was sold through AS Aloe (1893),[7] and Max Wocher & Son (1896).[9] The unit sold for $10.00, and came with a set of 10 electrodes which is a larger selection than offered with most batteries in 1896. In 1893, The Phoenix Faradic Battery was selling for $16.00 (AS Aloe).

In 1885, the "Phoenix" faradic battery was also made by Otto & Sons and sold by the national seller Whitail Tataum Co (Chicago, New York, Philadelphia, San Francisco). The name was altered for sale by other sellers. The Phoenix has six button type connectors for current variations. The metal current controller is on the right side of the coil.

Climax Faradic Battery. The unit of Fig O4 was manufactured by Reynders (after Otto & Sons original design), but was sold through Sears, Roebuck and Co. The Climax was designed for home use. The 1897 catalog of Sears, Roebuck and Co listed the unit for $4.00.[10] In

1893, The Smith & Shaw Electric Co sold the same model for $4.50. The unit was powered by a single Otto wet cell with carbon and zinc elements, and was encased in a cherry box (ca 7.25 x 6.5 x 5.75 inches). The lid has a metal carrying handle on top with a cloth ribbon ("The

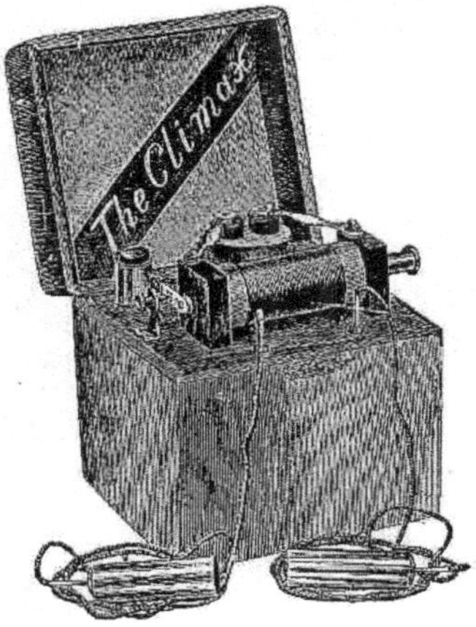

Fig O4. The Climax Faradic Battery

Climax") across the inside of the lid. A lever latch secures the lid. Like Otto faradic batteries, the face plate contains an induction coil with the square wooden end caps and metal bands or sleeves, a sliding metal current controller; an adjustable screw spring vibrating interrupter; and connecting buttons. The wet cell is exposed at the top and connected to the circuit by two nickel plated rotating levers.

Drescher Pocket Battery. FG Otto & Sons designed a pocket battery (Fig O5) after that of Drescher of Germany and Gaiffe of France. The pocket battery was a series of three models, and was in demand for physicians who traveled to their patients (The Chloride of Silver Dry Cell Co of Baltimore also made similar models). No.1 (left) was designed for the public consumer, while Nos.2 (right) and 3 (center) were designed for physician use. No.1 was powered by a single small dry cell and Nos.2 and 3 used two small dry cells each. The induction coil of No.1 did not produce as high a voltage as the other two. No.1 and 2 had a single hinged lid and snap latch on front of the cherry box. No.3 has two hinged lids that fold toward each other and locked by a snap latch on top. Each unit controlled current by a sliding metal controller that slid in and out of the coil through the box in front. The common adjustable screw spring vibrating interrupter was available on each unit to control current frequencies. In 1893, the AS Aloe sold the three pocket batteries for $5.00, $7.50, and $9.00, respectively.

The Smith & Shaw Electric Company of 168 West 34 Street, New York City, was selling the Otto electro-medical apparatus in 1893,

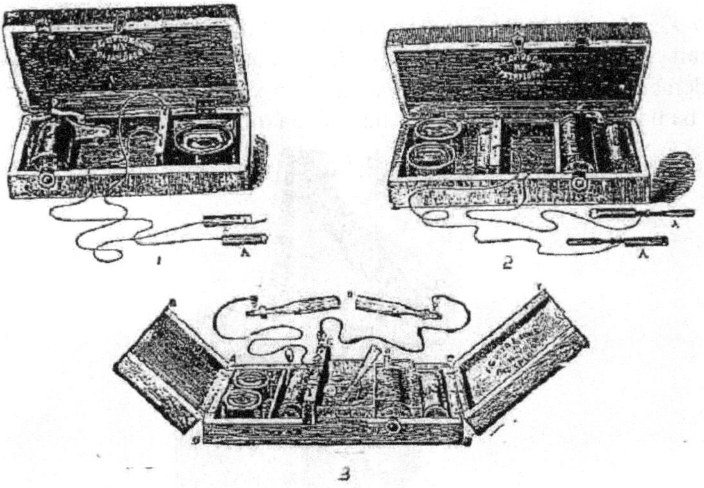

Fig O5. The Drescher Pocket Battery, No.1, 2, 3

and perhaps after 1895. These units have induction coils that deviate from the customary Otto characteristics of wooden square block end caps and a metal sleeve or band around the coil and adjacent to the square block cap at each end. Supposedly in keeping with the Drescher influence, Otto & Sons designed the induction coils of these three faradic batteries using circular wooden end caps that were slightly larger than the coil (offsetting style). This style of faradic battery did not have the common style face plates, but rather appear as electrical components spread around in a wooden case. The basic style of this battery series permitted it to be carried in a pocket of a coat. Smith & Shaw were a major retailer of products of Otto & Sons.

"The Florence" Faradic Battery. This battery used the same wet cell of Otto & Sons of 1871, but this particular electrical battery was patented August 18, 1885. The unit was encased in a cherry box (6.5 x 5.5 x 6.5 inches) with a hinged lid. The corners of the box were grooved and glued. The inside of the lid has a diagonally placed red ribbon with "The Florence" lettered in yellow. The face panel is matching wood of the box with 2.5 inches square cut in front to fit the top of the wet cell and connect with two rotating levers of nickel plate from near the induction coil. The face panel has two circular holes of 0.875 inch to hold the nickel plated hand held tube electrodes. The induction coil on the panel is 3 x 1 inches in size with black wooden blocks at each end. The right end of the coil has an adjustable screw spring type interrupter, while the left end has a nickel plated tube (3.25 x 0.75 inches) to slide over the core of the coil so as to control the current amplitude. "The Florence" was perhaps the best selling medical electrical battery of Otto & Sons,

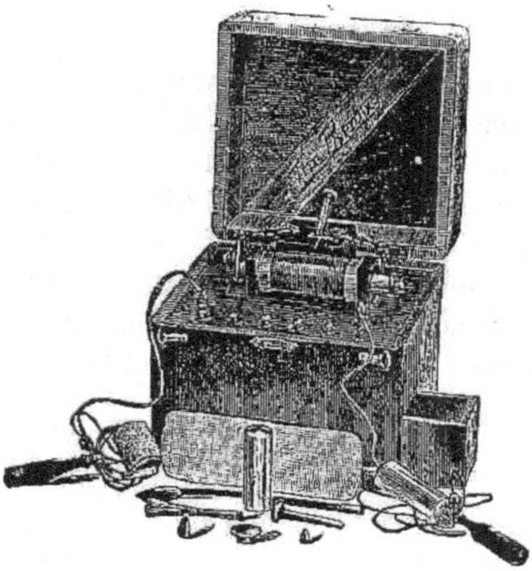

Fig O6. The Florence Faradic Battery

and is seen more frequently in antique shops and eBay auctions than any of the other models by Otto & Sons.

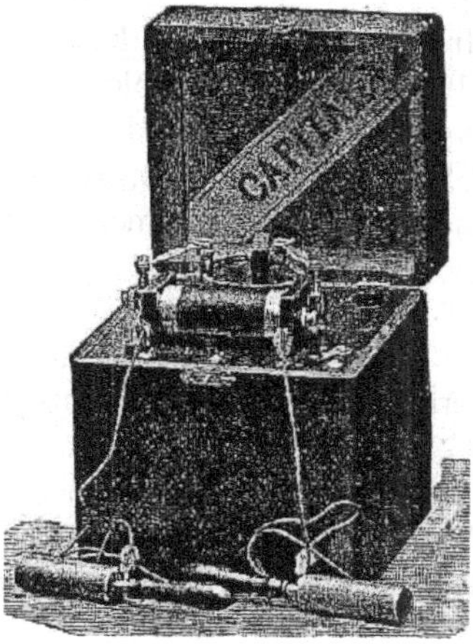

Fig O7. The Capital

Capital. Another faradic battery for home use by Otto & Sons was The Capital. This battery was encased in an imitation mahogany box (6.5 x 5.75 x 7.25 inches) with a metal carrying handle on top and a locking device on the front. This faradic battery is powered by a single wet cell (Grenet style) that rests on the bottom of the box underneath the face plate. The top or neck of the cell is exposed through a cut space in the face plate, and is connected in the circuit by two metal rotating levers. In front of the wet cell, and mounted on the face plate is the induction coil with its sliding metal controller on the right. On the left of the coil is the adjustable screw spring lever vibrating interrupter. The metal buttons connect the patient to the battery for providing primary, secondary, and combined currents. This battery was sold and listed by the Sears, Roebuck and Co catalog of 1897 for $4.50. Max Wocher & Son Co of Cincinnati sold The Capital faradic battery for $7.00 in 1906. The complete unit weighed almost five pounds. All metal parts are nickel plated. A banner is diagonally placed on the inside of the lid and reads "The Capital." The Capital is a similar unit to that of the "Climax."

Summary

Ferdinand Otto was one of the outstanding German instruments makers who settled in New York City during the 1850s and 1860s. He preceded the mass production process and therefore his custom made instruments are highly prized today among collectors. The medical electrical battery aspect of his business may have been a sideline for adding to the company's revenue. His medical electrical batteries appear to have been popular among public consumers, since some models are frequently found in antique shops and on eBay auctions. Otto made glass wet cells that are also frequently found on the antiques market. These medical batteries and cells both appear durable and of moderate quality. Otto's best quality items were the clocks and music boxes that bear his trademark. Early in his business FG Otto made thermometers, and in 1877 the company was manufacturing pulse measuring devices.[11]

References

1. Edmonson JM. American Surgical Instruments. San Francisco, CA, Norman Pub, 1997, pp 93-94, 208, 227

2. George Tiemann & Co. American Armamentarius Chirurgicum, 1889, reprinted. San Francisco, CA, Norman Pub & Printers Devil, 1989, pp 26, 49

3. Davis AB, Dreyfus MS. The Finest Instruments Ever Made. Arlington, MA, Med Hist Pub Assocs, 1986, pp 249, 271-272

4. Beard GM, Rockwell AD. A Practical Treatise on the Medical and Surgical Uses of Electricity, ed 5. New York, NY, William Wood Pub, 1881, pp 314-316

5. (Mechanical Music Digest Archives http:foxtail.com/ Archives/Digests/2000.02.08.01.html)

6. Romaine LB. A Guide to American Trade Catalogs 1744-1900. New York, NY, RR Bowker, 1960, pp 235-241

7. Catalog of AS Aloe. St Louis, MO, AS Aloe, 1893, p 758

8. Catalog of Montgomery Ward & Co, Chicago, IL, Montgomery Ward, 1894-1895

9. Catalog of Max Wocher & Son. Cincinnati, OH, Max Wocher, 1896, p 143

10. Catalog of Sears, Roebuck and Co. Chicago, IL, Sears, Roebuck, 1897

11. Davis AB. Medicine and Its Technology. Westport, CT, Greenwood Press, 1981, pp 69, 128

CHAPTER 11. GEORGE P PILLING & SON COMPANY OF PHILADELPHIA

The medical electrical batteries and the history of the company's founder are presented in Chapter 11. George P Pilling, Philadelphia, PA, was a manufacturer and retailer of medical equipment and instruments. Pilling formed his business in 1854 at 3451 Walnut St[1] or NE 4th and Chestnut[2] as a silversmith until 1860 when he began making excellent silver surgical instruments. He moved his shop in 1855 to 7 Gold Street, and then again in 1858 to 214 Gold Street. He relocated his business to 21 S 7th Street in 1864, to 701 Chestnut Street in 1867, and to 111 S 10th Street in 1877 to 1887. After a time Pilling was regarded as an outstanding instrument maker. He made and sold surgical instruments with masonic marks, sold jewelry, and fine cutlery.[2]

The manufacture of cutlery and jewelry was started in Philadelphia on Dock Street in 1814 by Jacob Stockman who made and retailed emblems and jewelry. Stockman got into making surgical instruments through specific requests from local surgeons. George P Pilling first served as an apprentice under Stockman then gained a partnership until he assumed full ownership in 1854. Kelly assigned the founding date of 1814 (as does Pilling catalogs) for the George P Pilling & Son Co (in spite of his ownership from Stockman in 1854), and cited 3451 Walnut Street as its location.[1] Pilling remained at the original location when he assumed the ownership in 1854.

George P Pilling gained a creditable reputation for his fine craftsmanship of medical instruments, and became well known. Pilling received an award from the Franklin Institute in 1858 for his work with mechanical devices, and another award in 1874.[3]

Pilling's son was apprenticed to JH Gemrig who was also a well known local maker of fine surgical instruments, and who was making surgical instruments during the time of the Civil War. There was a family relation between the Gemrigs and the Pillings so the two instrument makers often shared trade technology.[4]

Jacob H Gemrig after emigrating from Germany established business at 109 South Eight St, Philadelphia, PA, in 1839.[4] From 1840 to 1844 he worked at his shop at 143 N 6th Street, and also at 48 N 6th between 1841 and 1844. Initially, he was in cutlery but then began medical instrument making.[2] In 1840, Gemrig issued a catalog featuring surgical instruments; orthopedic appliances; apparatus for deformities, dislocations, and fractures. His shop was located on S 48th Street between 1845 and 1880.[2] He also published catalogs in 1865, 1867, 1870, 1876, and 1879.[4] In 1867, Gemrig's son Charles joined his father and that firm was then known as JH Gemrig & Son.[2] In the same year the company expanded its products to include veterinary instruments. Gemrig and Gemrig & Son remained makers and sellers of surgical instruments, and apparently never sold medical electrical batteries.[4] Jacob Gemrig retired in 1881, and the sons continued the business until 1900 when they sold the business to William H Richter who after 25 years closed the business in 1925.[2]

The Pilling business meanwhile became George P Pilling & Son when his son finished his apprenticeship with Gemrig, and moved to the North East Corner of 23rd and Arch Streets.[4] George P Pilling & Son were located at 117 S 11th from 1888 to 1896 and at 1229 Callowhill Street from 1897 to 1900.[2]

German instrument makers immigrated to New York and Philadelphia to establish and control the surgical instrument business in the United States between 1840 and 1890. Prior to 1840 and after the 1890s European instrument manufacturers (viz, German) dominated the surgical instrument business in the United States by making and importing them in great quantities.[2] Many instrument makers in Philadelphia went out of business during this time, but Pilling kept abreast with the latest technology and survived the German imports by adopting new manufacturing and marketing approaches. In 1891, he and HK Mulford designed the first antitoxin syringe.[3] In 1907, GP Pilling & Son Co also got involved in making apparatus for cardiovascular specialties. The company introduced the Bowles stethoscope in 1907, and in 1919 in association with Dr Chevalier Jackson it began its line of bronchoscopy, larngoscopy and esophagoscopy instruments.[3] Pillings learned to mass produce its product lines that then contributed to his success.[2] The Pillings Co continued business throughout the twentieth century with a wide variety of items in their shop that included cases made of wood and leather to box their surgical instruments.[3] George P Pilling & Son also made and sold veterinary instruments and supplies.

The Pilling trade catalog of 1909 indicated that the company exported dental, surgical, and veterinary instruments. Surgical instruments and hospital supplies were listed in the catalogs of 1921, and of 1932-1933. Also in 1932, the company listed bronchoscopic, eye, ear, nose, and throat instruments. In 1950, a catalog listed surgical instruments and hospital supplies. The GP Pilling & Son Co continues to make surgical instruments today.

Pilling & Son began selling blood pressure items in 1901 according to its 24 paged catalog for that year. The company issued a catalog in 1904, and in 1905 offered the Complete Guide for Domestic Home Treatment of Electricity that accompanied the sale of certain electrical batteries. The company continued issuing catalogs but in 1914 it added a special catalog for surgical instruments. In 1920, the company added dental products to its inventory. A catalog with surgical instruments was published in 1921 to 1922. In 1925, the company published three catalogs, and one catalog was published in 1926. The catalog of 1927, listed apparatuses for eyes, ears, and throat. The company again published three catalogs in 1928, and single issues in

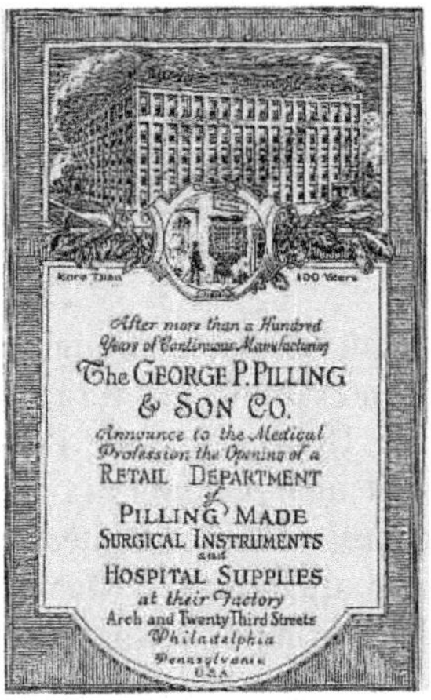

Fig P1. The George P Pilling & Son Company, ca 1920s

1929,1932, 1937, and 1939.[4] The company maintained a huge inventory of medical items that included a wide variety of general hospital, medical, and surgical equipment and accessories.

The George P Pilling & Son Co sold medical electrical batteries to both physicians and public consumers, although their dominant business was with physicians emphasizing surgical instruments. Pilling was one of the few companies still selling battery powered medical electrical apparatus as late as 1932 that were aimed toward public consumers for home use. Most units at that time were powered by alternating current (AC), and the Pilling & Son Co offered limited galvanic models that used the commercial current power source (Figs P8 & P9).

Pilling obliged the public consumer who seemed to prefer the violet ray units between 1915 and 1950s. These high frequency electrical stimulators used glass electrodes that glow as a violet light when activated. The demand for the box style medical electrical batteries, however, decreased after the 1920s.

The George P Pilling & Son illustrated and listed a Congress medical electrical battery in its catalog of 1932 that is often seen today for collectors in antique shops. The company was still located at Arch & 23rd Streets.

Commonalties of Pilling Apparatus

The Pilling faradic electrical batteries do have specific features that decidedly differ from other manufacturers. The induction coils of

Pillings have ends capped with black square wooden blocks. The coils are covered by fabric but near the wooden square block ends are metal sleeves at each end. Three medical electrical batteries for home or family use have diagonally cut wooden cases (horizontal or vertical) that no other manufacturers have produced.

Faradic Batteries

The 1932 catalog illustrated and listed (p 317, P22824) a Faradic Battery under the categorical heading "Faradic Batteries Operational From Dry Cells." This 'Congress' style unit was claimed to be a high grade coil, adjustable current amplitude, and operated by one large (standard) dry cell.

'Congress' No.1. The faradic battery of Fig P2 is an exact replica of the unit shown by the 1905 and 1932 Pilling & Son Co catalogs. This is the only medical electrical battery in which the encased cherry (case of 1905 was mahogany) box opens on the diagonal and vertically to form two triangles when opened. The case is secured by a lever type latch on a fancy engraved mounting. The base of the box is slightly larger than the box when closed (6.25 x 5.75 x 0.38 inches). This particular unit has "Pat Apd For #1928" stamped into the bottom of the left base. The wooden box (5.5 x 5 x 9.75 inches) opens to show the operational devices on the left side along with the standard size dry cell. The face panel is partly hidden by the dry cell, but its upper part has the induction coil (2.25 x 1 inches) that has square wooden blocks at each end. The right side of the coil has a nickel plated hollow tube that slides

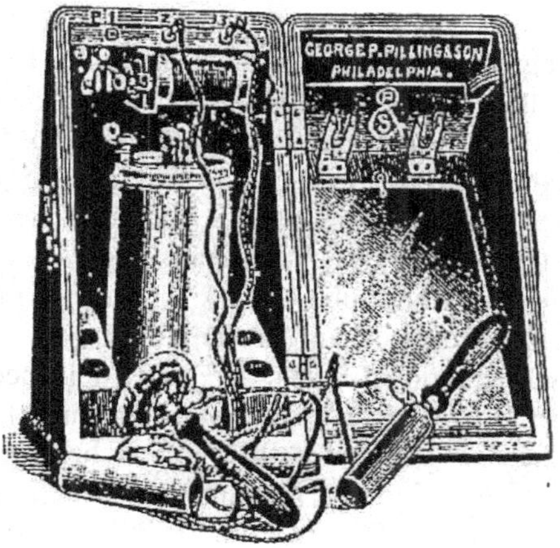

Fig P2. 'Congress' No. 1

over the core of the coil to control current amplitude. On the left side of the coil is an adjustable screw spring type interrupter to control frequency. The left half of the opened lid is lined with purple paper. The usual accessories are supplied with the unit.

The author labels this particular unit as The Congress No.1 for identification, although this was not cited by the Pilling & Son Co. In the 1905 Píllings & Son catalog this unit is called the "***Domestic Single Battery, No.1***,"[5] but in the 1932 catalog the unit does not carry any trade name.[6] The 'Congress' No.1 name cited by the author is based on the exactness of models and the use of the name "Congress" by items (viz, medical electrical batteries) retailed by George Frye of Portland, ME. George P Pilling & Son or their logo was stamped or embossed on the wood cases when retailed directly by them. However, since this company wholesaled medical electrical batteries to retailers over the United States, the retailers frequently had their signature plates or labels attached to units that they sold. Collectors should be aware of this practice when identifying manufacturers of medical electrical batteries, large manufacturers sold their products to many different retailers or agents at wholesale prices and the retailers placed their signatures on the products. (noted eg, Sears and Roebuck Co) Therefore, medical electrical batteries having a name and address on a label may or may not be the real manufacturer unlike statements by sellers on eBay. Commonalities in a product line associated with a particular manufacture are usually the most reliable means of identifying and dating electrical apparatuses.

'Congress' No.2. This unit (Fig P3) is the same as that described in Fig P2 ("P22826–Faradic Battery"). This unit is the same as that described in Fig P2 with the same accessories except that it has a more powerful coil, and is operated by two dry cells (not illustrated in the catalog). The Congress No.2 is printed on the label glued at the bottom of the unit. The 'Congress' No.2 faradic battery has a 3 x 1 inches induction coil mounted like the No.1 on the upper right side of the open triangular and vertically cut cherry (or mahogany) box (10 x 8.5 x 5.5 inches). The coil is larger in No.2 than in No.1 so as to increase the output. The coil has square wooden blocks (1.5 inches) on each end, while on its left is the adjustable screw spring type interrupter, and to its right side is a sliding chrome plated hollow tube (3.25 x 0.38 inches) that slides over the core of the coil to control current amplitude. Note that after about 1920 nickel plated operational items were often replaced with chrome. Also, on the upper left side is a lever switch for On/Off. The displayed unit in the figure has two standard (6.25 x 2.25 inches) dry cells to power it. Accessories were included and mounted and stored on both sides of the box. The 1905 trade catalog of George P Pilling & Son Co used the trade name of "***Domestic Double Battery, No.2***" for this particular unit.[5] Thus, the collector may find a Pilling No.1 or No.2 Electrical Battery labeled as either "Congress" or "Domestic……"

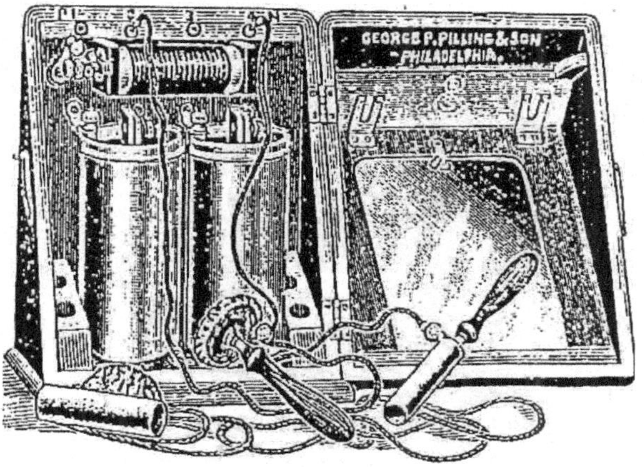

Fig P3. Congress No. 2

The directions accompanying the 'Congress' No.2 state that "Sockets Nos.1 and 2 give the primary or mild current; Nos.2 and 3 give the secondary or strong current; and sockets Nos.1 and 3 give the two currents combined very strong." Although these directions seem to be written for Congress No.1 unit with three sockets or outlet posts, the Congress No.2 has four outlets. By using the No.4 outlet post in combination with any of the others it "will give a greater variety of current." Actually, the same directions serve both Congress Nos.1 and 2 units.

Note that the use of "Congress" in the name of the unit suggests a link with George Frye of Portland, ME, and other retailers. Frye was a retailer of medical equipment and supplies and who sold Pilling & Son Co items as well as items from the Voltamp Electric Co of Baltimore, MD. Frye liked to have his name on the label of medical electrical batteries that he sold. He is known to have used "Congress" in association with some of the batteries that he sold. Pilling & Son Co did place "Congress" on some batteries retailed directly from their factory, but also placed other labels on units that were sold wholesale to suppliers around the United States. The Congress No.2 Double Cell faradic battery as presented here was also retailed and labeled with a plate signature of Max Wocher & Son, Cincinnati, OH.

George P Pilling & Son also illustrated and listed a Congress medical electrical battery in its catalog of 1932.[6] The Congress unit in question was the unusual triangular box lid faradic electrical battery.

Philadelphia Single Cell Battery. George P Pilling & Son Co manufactured a medical electrical apparatus for home use (Fig P4) that was similar in appearance to The New No.4 Home Medical Apparatus series that JH Bunnell & Co of New York City made and sold between

1880 and 1919. Thus, the first Bunnell battery of this series preceded the manufacture of that by Pilling that was not marketed until 1900.

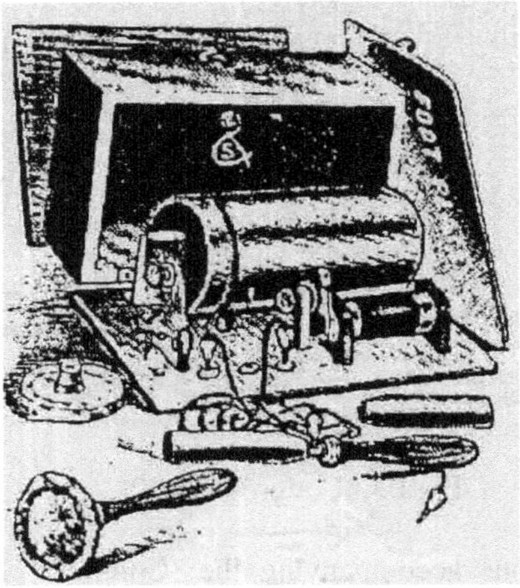

Fig P4. The Philadelphia Single Cell Battery

The Pilling unit, however, was made and sold from 1900 to 1932 (perhaps later), and had its name on a label inside the lid of each of its units between 1900 and 1905. The units from the two companies differed with Pilling having square wooden end caps on the induction coils (they have a red colored or nickel cylinder battery holder), while the end caps of the coils on Bunnell batteries were circular. The battery cylinder of the Pilling single cell unit is slightly shorter (exposing more battery) than that of the Bunnell unit. Both units are designed to use the standard dry cell (6.25 x 2.25 inches) of that time. Many of these single dry cell medical electrical apparatuses of exact design and dimensions were manufactured by two companies (Bunnell and Pilling). Each company accommodated the retailer by placing their names on the labels inside of one lid. JH Bunnell & Co of New York City was the major manufacturer of this particular series of Home Medical Apparatus.

This home faradic electrical battery of Pilling in 1900, The Philadelphia Single Cell Battery, was slightly smaller than that made in 1905. In 1900, the mahogany box was 8.75 x 4.5 x 4.75 inches, while in 1905 it measured 9 x 5.25 x 4.5 inches. The boxes are dovetailed and glued at the corners. The Philadelphia Single Cell Battery is encased in a polished mahogany box that has two hinged lids. The bottom lid (when case is open) also serves as a face plate to contain the electrical components. The top lid serves to secure the accessories in a separate section. The box has a metal carrying handle on top and a lever latch in front securing each of the two lids. Most metal are heavy style, and the unit of 1905 cost $5.00.[5]

Literature. The 1900 units, had the directions for operating the battery on the label inside one lid, while in 1905 and thereafter the directions were provided within the 34-paged booklet Complete Guide for Domestic Treatment by Electricity.[5] The booklet accompanied the sale of each family or home use medical electrical battery. In the Preface of the booklet the GP Pilling & Son Co claimed that most prior treatise, like theirs, offered the public consumer unwarranted treatments and cures by electricity. While chastising others over exaggerated claims they were doing the same in their booklet. They covered a wide variety of ills and conditions (abscesses to wounds), but some conditions covered by Pillings were of doubtful merit. The conditions discussed in the booklet that are questioned by the author are: ague (malarial fever), carbuncles (infected boils), chilblain (frostbite), croup (hoarse cough), felon (infected toe), general debility, measles, quinsy (infected tonsils), and scrofula (like tuberculosis). Treatment by electricity was offered in the GP Pilling & Son Co booklet as being different from competitors because their electrical apparatuses benefited patients in such ills; after all their vast experience enabled them to design and make only products that worked. Their improved facilities prepared them to produce quality medical electrical batteries. The George P Pilling & Son Co did offer an atlas of the body showing muscles and their names, some names were abbreviated. They correctly stated that only the faradic electrical batteries

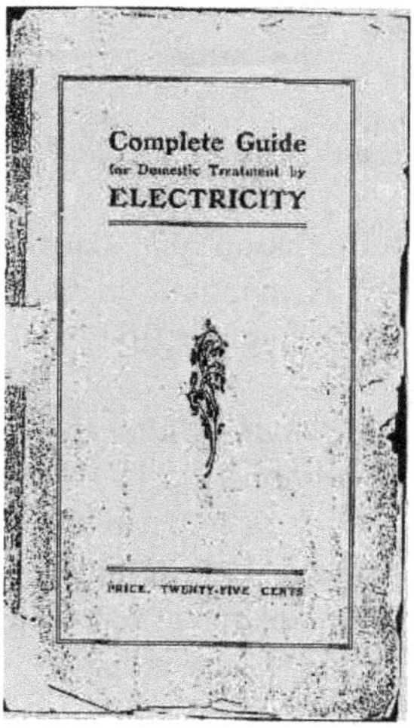

Fig P5. Treatment Booklet

should be used by families for home use. (while ignoring that galvanic currents may work better for alleviating some stated medical conditions, ed)

Landowne Single Cell Battery. This faradic electrical battery is the same in all aspects of design and structure as units No.1 and No.2 except the diagonally cut mahogany cases of Nos.1 and 2 open horizontally. The ***'Congress' or Domestic Battery*** units open vertically, and their circuitry are contained in only one section (the other section serves as a lid only). The horizontal arrangement in Fig P6 places the induction coil in the top section, the battery is located in the other or lower section. No face plate is needed with this arrangement, but a circuit connection between sections is required. The coil to subject connection is made from the top or coil section of the opened case by two buttons. The induction coil is enclosed on both ends with a square wooden block with adjacent metal bands. A sliding metal current controller moves from the

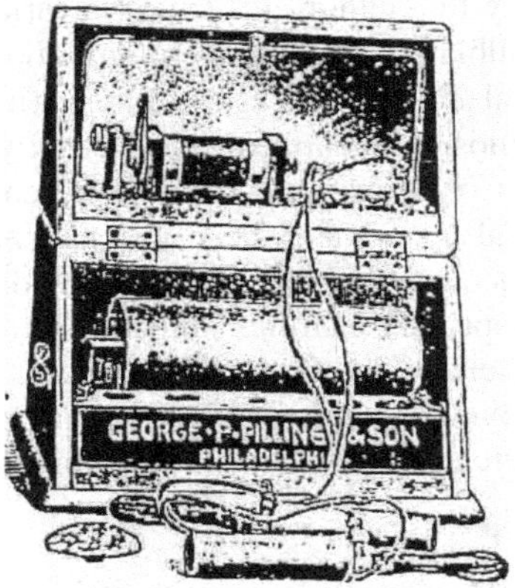

Fig P6. The Landowne Single Cell Battery

right side of the coil, while the adjustable screw contact and the spring hammer vibrating interrupter is mounted on the left side of the coil. It sold for $8.00 in 1905.[5] The triangular (diagonally) cut wooden box is cherry.

Faradic Home Medical Battery. Pilling & Son Co manufactured the faradic home unit (Fig P7) from 1900 to at least 1932 for retail by agents or distributors of medical equipment and supplies (eg, Detroit Battery Co, George Frye Co, Manhattan Electrical Supply Co (MESCO). This particular unit was made for a single or double cell. The above unit is a single cell battery in a polished oak box (8 x 4.5 x 4.5 inches) having an overhang lip (8.75 x 5.25 x 0.38 inches) for the top and the bottom of the box. The lid is hinged with a metal carrying handle on the top and a hook lever latch on the front of the box. A Pilling feature is a well made case that in this box has the corners dovetailed and glued. The face plate is black painted wood and is divided by a nickel plate for accessories in the rear section and the electrical components in the front section. The electrical components include: a 3 x 1 inches induction coil, covered by a black fabric, with a nickel plated sliding tube current regulator; the coil is mounted by its black square (1.25 inches) wooden end or cap blocks (a Pilling design or trademark); an On/Off lever control; three outlet connection eyes; and an adjustable screw spring lever, hammer vibrator type interrupter that is a single piece of metal. In

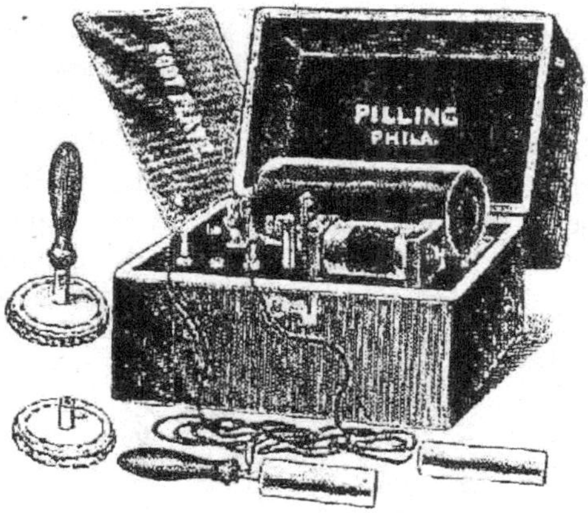

Fig P7. Faradic Home Medical Battery

1900, MESCO sold a similar unit for $6.50. The design of this unit resembles the single lid unit of JH Bunnell's 1880 or 1881 New No.4 Home Medical Battery, but remember the circular end caps of the induction coil was the design of JH Bunnell & Co.

Galvanic Batteries

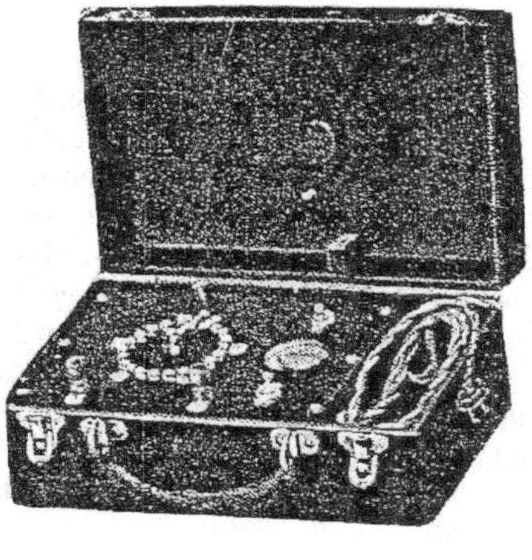

Fig P8. Galvanic Battery

Galvanic Batteries. GP Pilling & Son Co also illustrated and listed a galvanic current (Fig P8) apparatus on page 317 of their 1932 catalog. Some galvanic current apparatuses using alternating current for power used a new type of rectifier, no moving parts, no cell solutions, and no cell renewals. This unit generates current equal to 10 dry cells. It is complete in a leather cover case, 14 x 8 x 6 inches with leather handle, accessories needed for treatments, and it weighs seven pounds. One could buy the P22812 that was the same unit except that it could generate current equal to 20 dry cells. Another option was P22814 that was the same except capable of producing current equivalent to 30 dry cells, and had a milliammeter and pole changer for reversing polarity without changing connections. Buyers had to contact the company for price quotations on all of their medical electrical batteries and accessories.

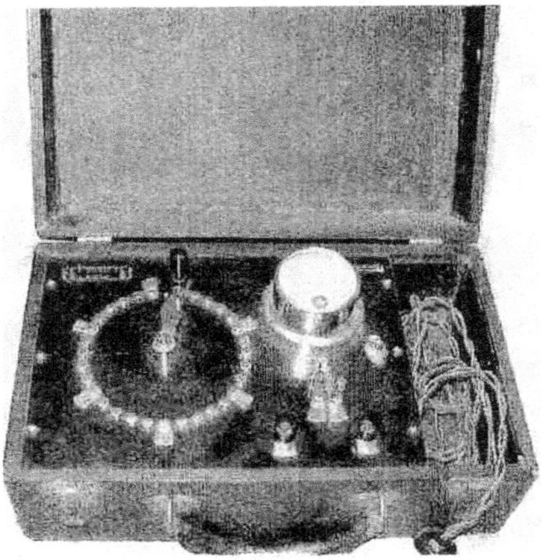

Fig P9. Galvanic Battery

The unit in Fig P9 is the same as that listed in the catalog as P22814 (Fig P8 with milliammeter and pole changer), although it may carry the signature plate of The EF Mahady Company of Boston. The case is wooden covered with buckram (leatherette like) and measures 14.5 x 8.25 x 6 inches. The weight is seven pounds. This unit is equipped for 110 volts AC, has an On/Off switch, and a large elaborate rotating controller for current marked 0, 5, 10, 15, 20, 25, and 30 DC milliamperes with four chrome posts in between each labeled marking. The face panel appears as a thin layer of bakelite. A small open compartment on the left side of the face panel houses the accessories and the connecting power cord. This unit dates to 1932 or earlier.

The EF Mahady Co of Boston, MA, was located on 671 Boylston Street. The company published its trade catalog between 1915 and 1920 (index, 416 pages) to illustrate its variety of surgical instruments, and physician supplies. In 1929, the company served as a distributor for standard surgical instruments, and published a separate section on Stille Hand-Forged surgical operated from street current in its 458 paged catalog. Its address was given as 851-857 Boylston St for that year. The catalog also illustrated and listed a variety of surgical instruments and physician supplies.[4] The EF Mahady Co did not manufacture any medical electrical battery.

The City Directory of Philadelphia for 1939[7] listed "Charles J Pilling, Jr, on 23rd and Arch Streets as a retailer of dental instruments. The same Directory listed George P Pilling of 232 W Willow Grove Ave and Franklin Terrace building as an engineer. Also, listed was George P Pilling, Jr, with locations in Physician office, Medical Arts Building and with residence on Hamilton Court. The George P Pilling & Son Co is still conducting a surgical instrument business as Pilling Surgical, and is located in Horsham, PA. The company claims to be the oldest surgical instrument maker in the world.[3] In the twentieth century the company in addition to manufacturing and selling medical and surgical apparatuses and supplies was also involved in selling instruments for treatment of cattle, horses, and poultry.

Summary

The company headed by George P Pilling was an early firm in the United States that was involved with the making of medical instruments. Although the company has been said to have started in 1814 when Pilling was associated with Stockman, Pilling's name appeared on the shop in 1854. George P Pilling first made cutlery and jewelry, but became involved in making surgical instruments with local demands. He won awards for his craftsmanship of medical instruments, and is best known for his work in that field.

The George P Pilling & Son company manufactured many of the medical equipment and instruments that the firm sold. The company also retailed dental, medical, and veterinary equipment and supplies made in the United States by others as well as retailing imported items.

The company's involvement with the manufacture of medical electrical batteries seemed to have started in 1900 and continued for more than 30 years. The company got involved in this field of manufacture at the end of the golden age in medicine. The company still sold a small selection of medical electrical batteries in 1932. The company continues in business today.

References

1. Kelly EM. The Business Founding Date Directory. Scarsdale, NY, Morgan & Morgan, 1954, p 100

2. Edmonson JM. American Surgical Instruments. San Francisco, CA, Norman Pub, 1997, pp 46-47, 64, 261

3. History of the Pilling Company. Pilling Surgical (http://www.pillingssurgical.com/history.html), 2002, pp 1-2

4. Davis AB, Dreyfus MS. The Finest Instruments Ever Made. Arlington, MA, Med Hist Pub Assocs, 1986, pp 142, 212, 258-259

5. Complete Guide for Domestic Treatment by Electricity. Philadelphia, GP Pilling & Son, 1905

6. Catalog of George P Pilling & Son, Philadelphia, PA, 1932, p 317

7. City Directory. Philadelphia, PA, 1939, p 475

CHAPTER 12. VAN HOUTEN & TEN BROECK COMPANY OF NEW YORK CITY

A modest attempt to piece together information about an early company in New York is made in Chapter 11. The Van Houten & Ten Broeck Company of 214-216 East 23rd Street,[1] New York City, was founded in 1870.[2] This company may at first have been a retailer of medical supplies. About 1893, the company was retailing the medical electrical batteries of the Galvano-Faradic Mfg Co, and displayed such in the AS Aloe catalog of that year. In 1896 or 1897, the company was manufacturing and selling the Morton-Wimshurst-Holtz machine as well as other influence static electrical machines. They, like so many other manufacturers of the influence static electrical machines got into the making of x-ray machines in and after 1896.

Static Machine

Dr William J Morton on 5 February 1896 published an article in Electrical Engineer claiming that he was able to produce roentgen rays with his high voltage influence machine. Dr Morton first stated that the x-rays were produced between the discharge rods of the static machine, but later he corrected himself by stating that he had placed a gas tube between the discharge rods to obtain roentgen plates. Manufacturers of

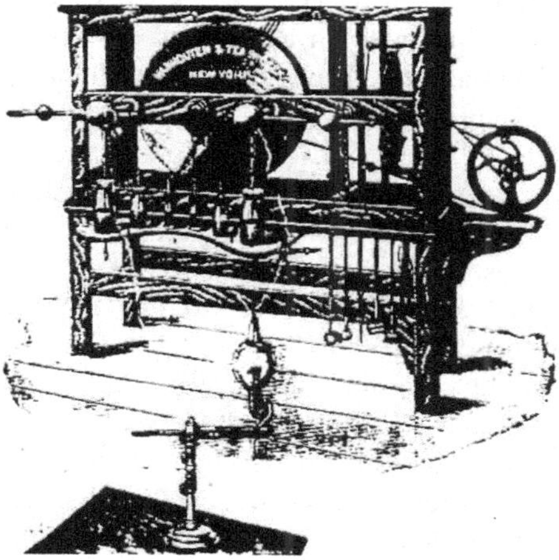

Fig V1. The Morton-Wimshurst-Holtz Influence Machine and Monell static tube

medical electrical apparatuses, in particular static machines, were in the business of making roentgen machines from their static units as soon as they read his paper.[2] The Morton-Wimshurst-Holtz Influence Machine was used for static electrotherapeutic treatments and for diagnostic x-rays along with the addition of a Monell static tube.

The AS Aloe Co of St Louis was still serving as an agent for The Van Houten & Ten Broeck Co in 1899 for selling the Morton-Wimshurst-Holtz Influence Machine. In 1899, the Van Houten & Ten Broeck Co was located at 300 Fourth Ave, New York[1] (same address as the Galvano-Faradic Mfg Co). Each manufacturer of the influence machines tried to maintain the latest technology so the machines were often very similar in construction. The company entered the x-ray business early, perhaps in 1896 or 1897, like others that were manufacturing influence machines that could power the x-ray tube. The x-ray machine imposed new requirements on manufactures. Manufacturers were faced with updating their machines every one or two years that added costs to their operations. Also, manufacturers were required to promote their machines so advertising became very competitive. Each company cautioned readers and potential customers in its advertisements against buying units other than their own. In 1903, Van Houten & Ten Broeck Co maintained through advertisements that its unit was best and that only cheaper quality units would end up in one's attic or barn.[3] These conditions of progress or time probably impacted on small companies, like Van Houten & Ten Broeck, that after several years exited the x-ray and electrotherapeutic fields. Van Houten & Ten Broeck was out of business in 1914.

The Van Houten & Ten Broeck Co trade catalog for the 28th edition listed and illustrated an assortment of Galvano-Faradic Mfg Co medical electrical batteries. The Galvano-Faradic Mfg Co was bought by Van Houten & Ten Broeck Co from Dr Waite of the Waite & Bartlett Co in 1905 after the death of Bartlett. Up to this time The Van Houten & Ten Broeck Co was manufacturing influence machines and x-ray units, and retailing cell powered electrical apparatus. A close relation between the two companies, apparently existed over a long period of time prior to the sale. The Galvano-Faradic Mfg Co may even have manufactured electrical apparatuses for Van Houten & Ten Broeck prior to 1905, and they shared the same address after 1899. The 28th edition of the trade catalog of Van Houten & Ten Broeck Co was expanded to two sections and 31 pages from the 15-paged catalog of around 1898. This particular catalog of Van Houten & Ten Broeck Co also used the 300 Fourth Avenue, New York, address that previously was that of the Galvano-Faradic Mfg Co. Purchase of the Galvano-Faradic Mfg Co in 1905 gave them the manufacturing capabilities for what was a continuing product line for them, the conventional faradic and galvanic medical electrical batteries.

The Van Houten & Ten Broeck Co became a manufacturer of conventional medical electrical batteries for the first time with the purchase of the Galvano-Faradic Mfg Co. The product line of medical electrical batteries powered by wet or dry cells was contained in Section I of the expanded 1905 catalog (40th or 41st edition), while their product line of influence machines and x-rays was contained in its catalog of about 1898. By 1905, however, the peak markets for these battery powered electrical apparatuses used by physicians had passed, although considerable volumes of these apparatuses continued to be sold to public consumers for home use. Section 1 of this catalog listed: faradic batteries, galvanic batteries, combined batteries, cautery batteries, "milliampere meters," and electrodes. By 1905, many of the medical electrical apparatuses were powered by alternating or direct current from commercial sources. The sinusoidal current was beginning to replace faradic current in 1905. The sinusoidal current was an improvement over the faradic current to the comfort of the patient because of its equal electrical force and smooth waveform in each direction of a pulse. The faradic pulsed current was rather crude with unequal force between negative and positive directions of the pulse which made for uncomfortable sensory effects. However, apparatuses powered by commercial electricity to produce sinusoidal current did not peak until about 1910 or 1912.

Commonalties of Van Houten & Ten Broeck Co

The faradic and galvanic battery line of this company is also that of The Galvano-Faradic Mfg Co. Major identifying features of the faradic apparatuses are: 1) the induction coils have adjacent metal sleeves to metal end caps that raise the coil above the face plate; 2) use metal signature plates or recessed lettering on the inside lid of its apparatuses that bear the name of Galvano-Faradic Co; 3) have vertical rather than horizontal (to face plate) spring lever, hammer vibrating interrupters, and 4) use heavy quality metal (nickel plated) fixtures. The galvanic models are identified by: 1) use of metal signature plates or recessed lettering on the inside of the lid of their units; 2) have a circular metal ring with metal buttons for each cell; 3) use heavy quality metal (nickel plated) fixtures; 4) use two hinged ring rods that lift the cell tray; 5) use a lever device on the wet cell when pushed down to elicit slow pulses and when the lever is pulled up to attain rapid pulse rates; and 6) the hydrastat is located on the front side of the wooden box.

Faradic Batteries

No.1 Faradic Battery. This unit was offered by the Galvano-Faradic Mfg Co about 1872 (perhaps 1871) as a family battery, and was still a popular electrical medical battery in 1905 when Van Houten & Ten Broeck Co was selling the product line of its newly acquired company. This unit was powered by one wet cell that may have delivered about 1.1

volts. The unit was designed for home use and is among the best for that purpose. The unit was enclosed in an oak box with a hinged lid, and is secured by a front located latch. It sold for $8.00 in 1905, and for $10.00 by AS Aloe in 1893.[4]

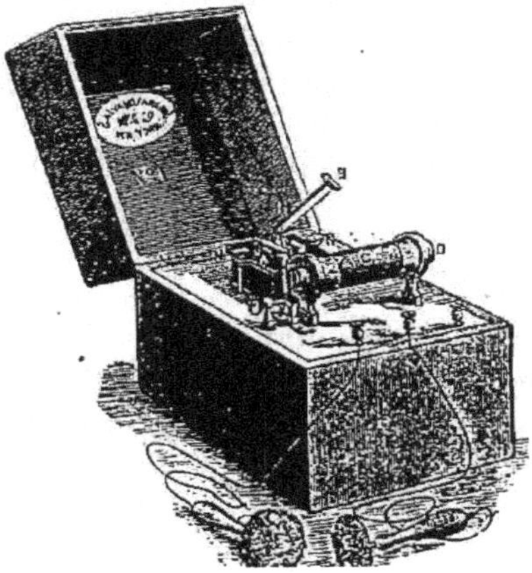

Fig V2. No. 1 Faradic Battery

No.2 Induction Coil. The faradic coil of Fig V3 is essentially composed of the components contained on the face plate of some of the other Galvano-Faradic Mfg Co electrical medical batteries (eg, No.1). It consists of the usual components of a faradic battery; ie, an elevated

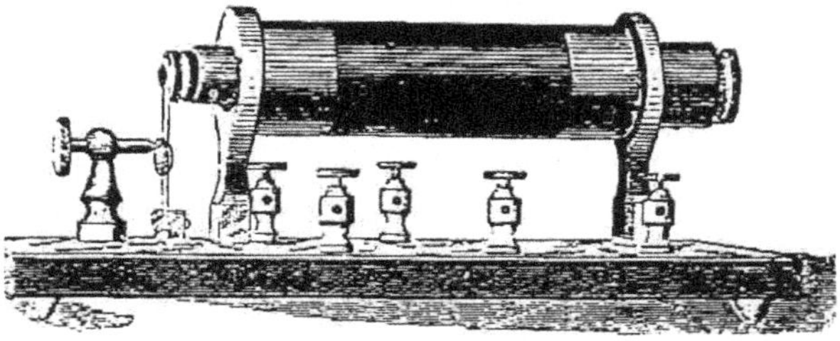

Fig V3. No. 2 Induction Coil

induction coil covered in fabric, capped at each end by a circular metal band or sleeve that elevates and supports the coil from the face plate. The coil is with a sliding tube current controller, an adjustable interrupter, two screw adjustable binding posts, and three screw adjustable connecting posts. Like all of the Galvano-Faradic Mfg Co electrical batteries the metal was a dull nickel plated (or stainless steel like) finish. The electrical components were mounted on top of a polished black walnut or oak base with the circuitry embedded underneath the wooden base. One No.6 dry cell or one Grenet wet cell was recommended for its power source, and the unit sold for $4.00. The cells sold separately for $0.40 and $2.50, respectively. This particular unit was sold by AS Aloe in 1893 as an electro-magnetic machine for $15.00.[4]

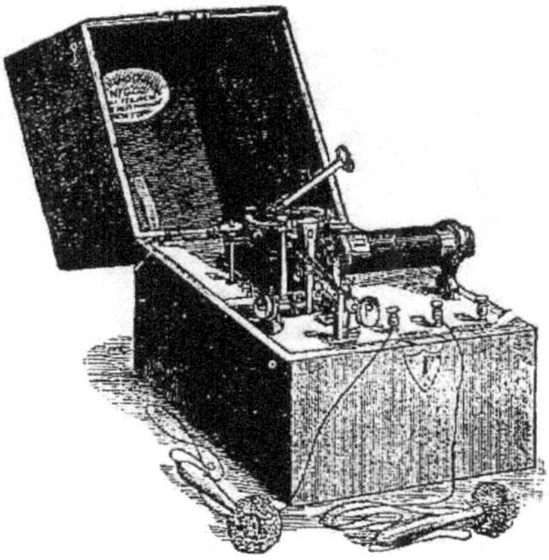

Fig V4. No. 3 Faradic Battery

No.3 Faradic Battery. This battery of Fig V4 is nearly like that of No.1, but designed for physician use. It was designed with a coil output that was more powerful than those recommended for home use, and it had two interrupters. This unit has the cone and the adjustable screw spring lever type interrupters for delivering very slow to very rapid current pulses, respectively. Thus, it is more versatile than those for home use. Like the No.1 battery, this unit is powered by one wet cell. The unit is housed in an oak box with a hinged lid, metal carrying handle, and secured by a lock and key. In 1893, it sold for $15.00 by both the Galvano-Faradic Mfg Co and Van Houten & Ten Broeck Co,[4] but in 1893 AS Aloe sold the same unit for $20.00.

No.5 Faradic Battery. The faradic unit of Fig V5 was designed for home use and for the traveler. It was small enough to carry in the trunk of the traveler. The unit used a single standard dry cell that was located underneath the face plate. The face plate contained the metal induction coil with its sliding tube current controller; a lever On/Off control; three adjustable screw connection posts for providing primary, secondary, and combined currents; and an adjustable screw spring lever hammer, vibrator type of interrupter. The unit is housed in a birch box that has a wedge or spline holding the glued corners of the box. The box has a heavy metal carrying handle and a heavy metal lever front latch to secure the hinged lid. A rear compartment of the face plate houses accessories, and has a metal knob post to remove its wooden lid. In 1893, the unit sold for $7.00. This faradic battery was not listed by the AS Aloe

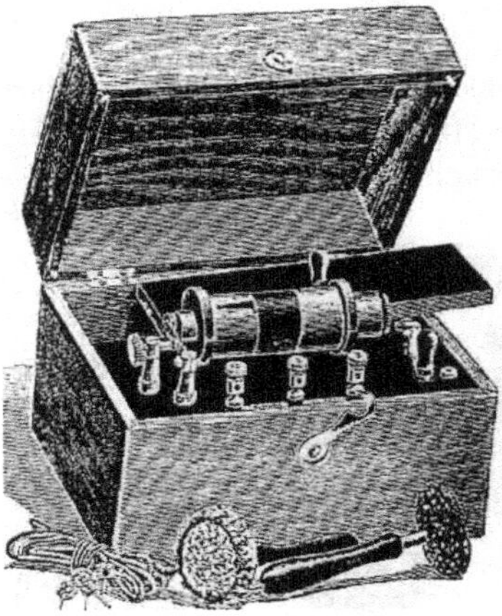

Fig V5. No. 5 Faradic Battery

trade catalog in 1893.

No.6 Faradic Battery. The unit of Fig V6 was designed for physician use, and was powered by two No.6 dry cells that were located underneath the face plate. The unit is encased in an oak box of different design. The box was built so that half of the upper portion of the box's width serves as a compartment for accessories, and the other half of the upper portion serves as the lid (the box is L-shaped on side view). The upper part of the box has a metal carrying handle and a lever latch on front to secure the lid. The face plate houses the metal coil with its

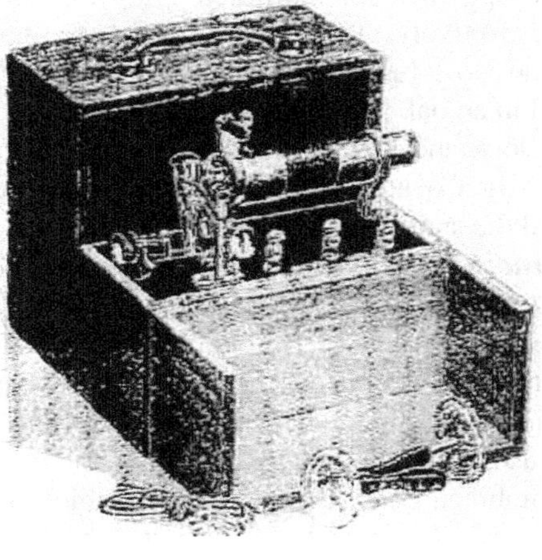

Fig V6. No. 6 Faradic Battery

sliding tube current controller; a cone shaped vibrator for slower and variable interruptions, and an adjustable screw spring lever interrupter for rapid current interruptions; a metal coil that supplies three currents; and three adjustable screw connection posts. All metal are heavy nickel plate.

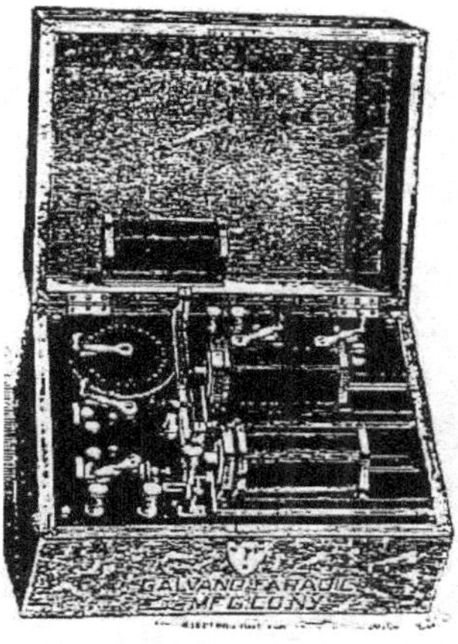

Fig V7. No. 7 Faradic Battery

In 1893, the unit sold for $15.00.[4]

No.7 Faradic Battery. The unit of Fig V7 is a unique faradic battery that was designed for gynecologists for very rapid and very slow current pulses. The unit has three secondary coils that adjust to two primary coils tapped by intervals to provide in effect seven coils. The three coils are covered with black paper. The secondary coils are wound with different sized wires and lengths to give effects of seven coils; the finest coils use No.36 wire and are wound with 1500, 1000, and 500 yards, respectively; No.32 wire wound by 800-, 500-, and 300-yard lengths provide medium coils; while No.22 wire wound by 250 yards provides a coarse coil. These coils adjust to two primary coils with one fitted to a cone shaped vibrator for slow muscle contractions, and two with a ribbon vibrator (singing rheotome). The ribbon vibrator was a new idea around 1890s to provide a wide range of interruptions per second.

The design was to provide the most versatile of applications. Encased in an oak box with four No.6 dry cells (underneath the face plate) connected in series with a rheostat for fine control of current amplitude. The wooden box was hinged with a lid (1 coil mounted on inside of the lid); the face plate has two coils; a rheostat; a lever On/Off control; two adjustable screw connecting posts; and two coil selector lever controls. The unit sold for $45.00 in 1893,[4] and was the company's most popular electrical battery among physician customers.

No.8 Faradic Battery. The unit in Fig V8 is designed after the DuBois-Reymond prototype sledge inductorium. The sledge design has the secondary coils sliding over the primary coil (in this unit over the soft iron core) that allows adjustments of minute increments or decrements of current amplitudes with the sliding toward or away from the zero position. In addition to the sledge style of induction coil arrangement the secondary coil was of different designs than is customary for the company. The end caps were shaped hexagonally of hard rubber rather than the customary circular metal end caps with adjacent metal sleeves. This particular unit was the company's second most popular electrical faradic battery because it was ideal for diagnostic and physiological

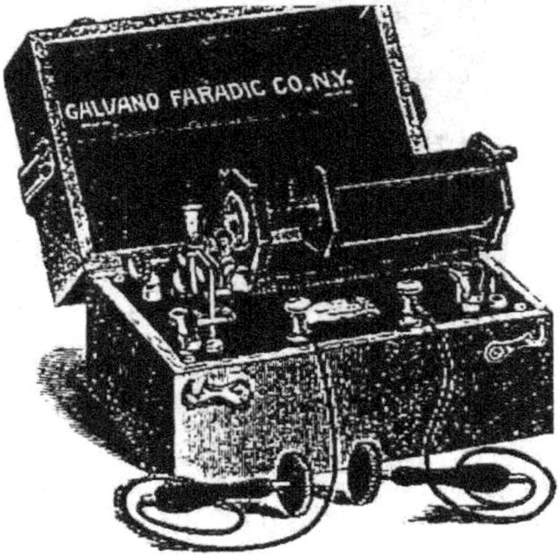

Fig V8. No. 8 Faradic Battery

work. The two interrupters (cone and spring lever type vibrators) permit very slow and very rapid current pulses. The secondary winding has No.36 insulated copper wiring, 1500 yards, and is tapped at intervals of 1000 and 500 yards. An adjustable switch at one end of the of the secondary coil allows the desired windings of the coil. The sledge type of electrical faradic battery allows secondary coils of different windings, other than those listed, to be used on the unit by changing the existing secondary coil and sliding the alternate one along the track. The unit is housed in an oak box; carried by a leather strap attached to the hinged lid; and the lid is secured by two lever type latches on the front of the box. The unit is powered by two No.6 dry cells, and sold for $25.00 in 1893.[4]

No.9 Faradic Battery. No. 9 is encased in an oak box designed like No.6 (L shaped) with an accessory compartment at the rear top half of the box, and the other top half is the lid. The rear top of the box has a metal carrying handle, and the lid is secured by a spring type latch. A single No.6 dry cell is located in the rear compartment with the accessories. The face plate covers half of the opened box, and contains: the elevated metal coil with its sliding tube current controller, an adjustable screw spring lever vibrator type of interrupter, a lever On/Off control, and two adjustable screw connecting posts. The unit provides primary, secondary, and combined currents. Van Houten & Ten Broeck sold this Galvano-Faradic battery for $9.00 in 1893.[4]

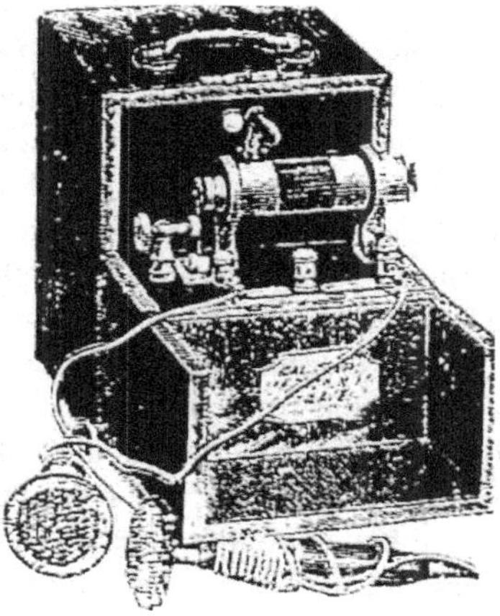

Fig V9. No. 9 Faradic Battery

Galvanic Batteries

The ***16-Cell Galvanic Battery***, like the other galvanic batteries, is housed in a rather large oak box (8 x 11 x 12.25 inches). A removable tray was located in the bottom where 16 glass jar cell cases are placed.

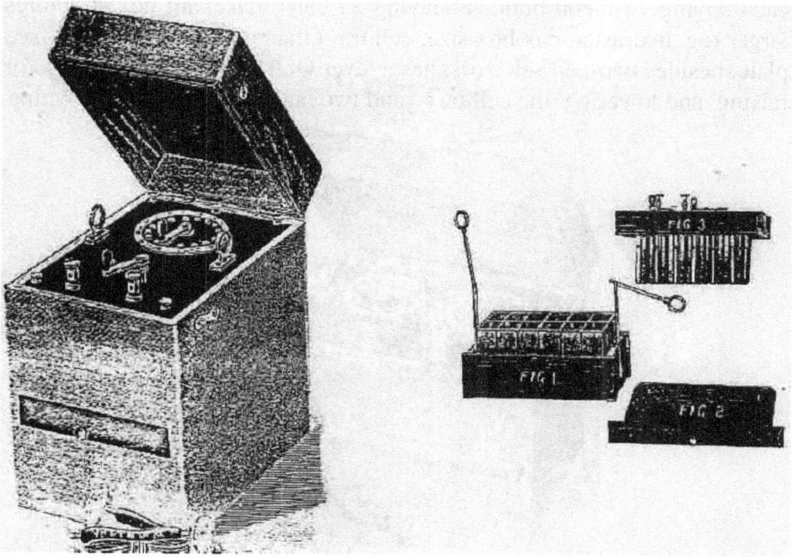

Fig V10. 16-Cell Galvanic Battery; cell tray, hydrastat, a plates

The tray was lifted and lowered by two-hinged metal rods attached to the tray, and with a ring at the top of each rod. Attached underneath the face plate (gutta percha or hard rubber) were 16 carbon and zinc plates that served as 16 electrical couples. (These features are pictured in figures to right.) Each couple was connected at its attached end to wires joining the 16 metal buttons (corresponding to a cell) on a circular controller. The buttons were controlled by a lever centered in the circular controller of the face plate. The carbon-zinc couples could be raised or lowered by the ringed-rod. When raised the elements or couples were removed from the acid battery solution. To insure that the couples were free or separated from the solution a hydrastat or rubberized tray was inserted through a slot in the front of the box. Once the hydrastat was inserted the unit could be transported without spillage of the battery solution. The tight fitting tray, hydrastat, and face plate also prevented the undesirable fumes of the battery solution from escaping to annoy the operator and others. Components on the face plates were fewer and operating the unit was easier than that of the faradic batteries. The face plate of this galvanic battery consisted of the circular current selector of 16 buttons, lever On/Off control, and two adjustable screw connecting posts. A 10-cell unit of this design sold for $15.00, the 16-cell unit sold for $20.00, and a 20-cell unit was $22.00 in 1893.[4]

24-Cell Battery. The Galvano-Faradic Mfg Co's unit of Fig V11 operates similarly as the 10, 16, and 20 cells units. The difference between these units is that the 24-cell unit has two circular cell selectors, each having 12 metal buttons. Having 24 cells makes all box structures larger (eg, hydrastat, oak box size, cell tray) than other units, but the face plate, besides two-cell selectors, has a lever On/Off control, two rings for raising and lowering the cell tray, and two adjustable screw connecting

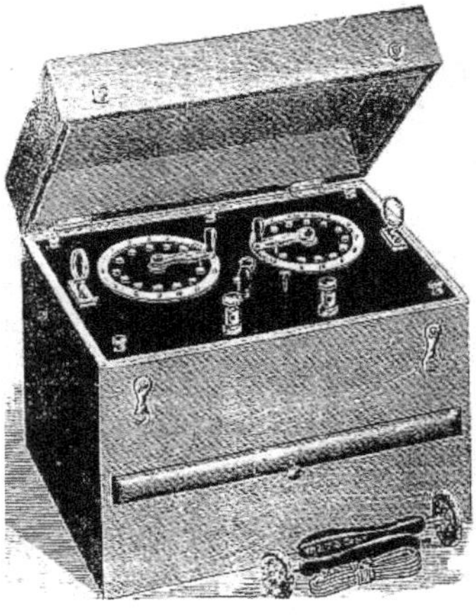

Fig V11. 24-Cell Galvanic Battery

posts. Like the other units, all metal are heavy nickel plated. Five adjustable screws secure the face plate to the box in addition to the rings on the rods. This 24-cell unit sold for $25.00, and a 30-cell unit for $30.00 in 1893.[4]

Combination Faradic and Galvanic Batteries

16-Cell Combination Battery. The company manufactured combination units that served as both galvanic and faradic electrical batteries. The galvanic portion has 16-wet cells, while the faradic portion has a single wet cell; each current section operates independently. The oak box housing the two units looks similarly to the units that have one or the other type of current except that two types of current batteries were

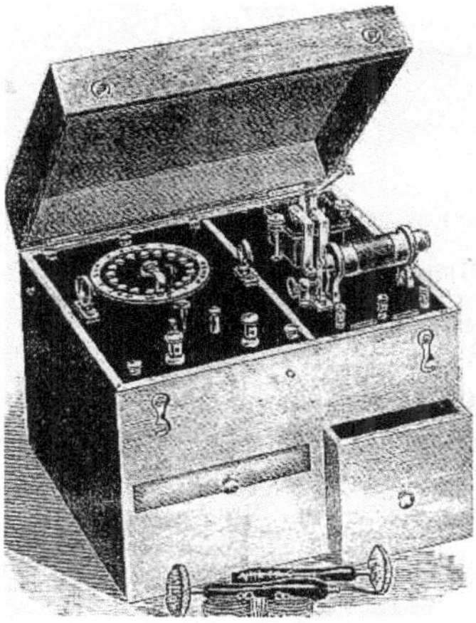

Fig V12. 16-Cell Combination Battery

combined into one box. That is, the right portion of the box is the same as the 16-cell galvanic battery presented and the left portion of the box is similar to the No.1 Faradic Battery. A drawer from the front of the box is available for accessories. The 16-Cell Combination Battery sold for $28.00 in 1893.[4]

24-Cell Combination Battery. The unit presented is combined with the No.1 Faradic Battery. Both the galvanic section and the faradic section in this combined unit are more powerful than the 16-cell combination unit. A drawer for accessories is underneath the faradic face plate on the right front, as well as the hydrastat fitted from the left side of the front underneath the galvanic battery of the oak case. This combination battery sold for $36.00 in 1893.[4]

The galvanic and combined galvanic and faradic batteries of the Galvano-Faradic Mfg Co sold for higher prices in 1895 than in 1893 through AS Aloe of St Louis. The regular galvanic 12, 16, 24, 32, and 36 cells unit ranged from $30.00 to $70.00, but with the rheotome the prices ranged from $60.00 to $80.00 for the 24, 32, and 36 units, respectively.

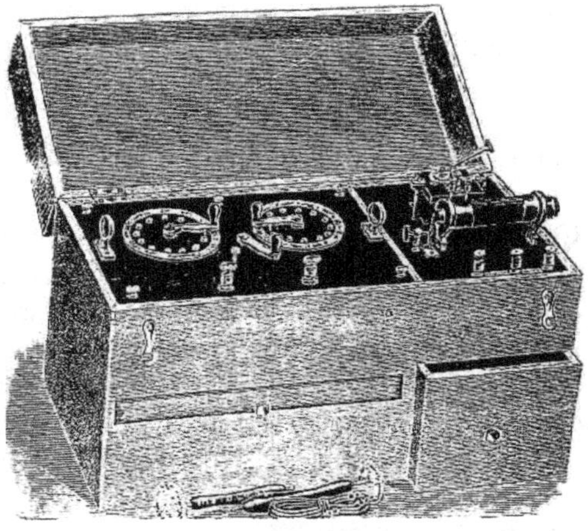

Fig V13. 24-Cell Combination Battery

AS Aloe in 1893 only handled the combined galvanic and faradic batteries for 16 and 24 cells for $45.00 and $60.00, respectively.

Office Cabinet No.11. This cabinet (Fig V14) is polished oak cabinet that measures 37 x 27 x 23 inches, has a large drawer for accessories, a glass cover, and two doors on the cabinet. The cabinet contains two shelves that hold the "Fitch Perfect (cells) Battery" of 38

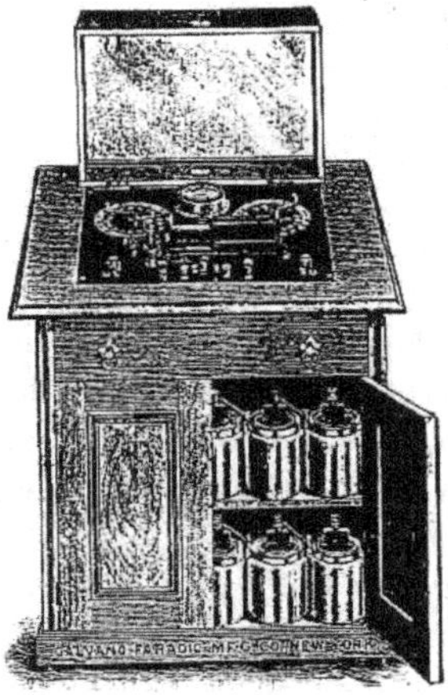

Fig V14. Office Cabinet No.11

wet cells. The face plate contains two circular cell selectors with a lever control and metal buttons, a milliammeter, a DuBois-Reymond type faradic induction coil, a pole changer, a lever On/Off control, a cone and spring lever interrupters, and two adjustable screw connecting poles. The cell selectors are designed so that the levers slide from one button to another with one resting on one button to insure a gradual increase or decrease of current without a sudden surprise shock. The company used this method of controlling current amplitudes rather than a conventional disc rheostat. The milliammeter ranges from 1 to 250 milliamperes. The faradic coil has a secondary coil that slides over a primary coil. The secondary coil is wound with 1000 yards of No.32 copper wire that is tapped at 500 yards, and another one tapped at 1000 yards which in effect serves as two coils. The interrupters or rheotomes provide very slow to very rapid current pulses. The faradic battery operates independently from the galvanic battery, and is powered by two wet cells. The Office Cabinet No.11 is mounted on wheels for mobility, and in 1893 it sold for $80.00.[4]

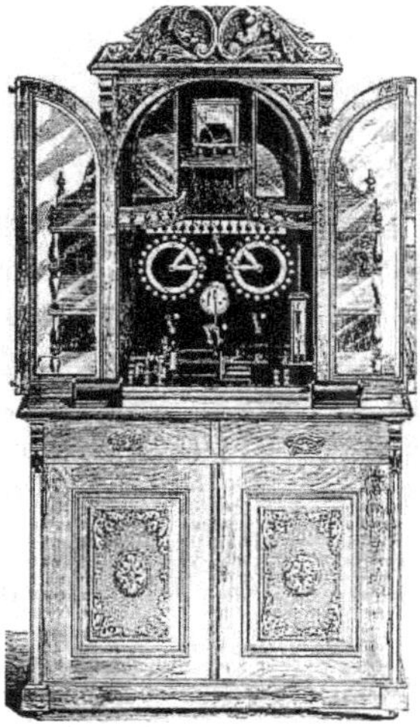

Fig V15. Cabinet Combination Battery

Cabinet Combination Battery. Sometime between 1905 and 1907 this unit was introduced by Van Houten & Ten Broeck. The large wooden cabinet was designed for the office of physicians with the upper portion containing the electrical components and the bottom part housing 40 or more wet cells of the Fitch Perfect Battery type for power. The face plates (vertical and horizontal) were made of black hard rubber. The vertical face plate contains: a pole changer; an automatic rheostat for galvanic current; various switches to bring the milliammeter, the automatic rheostat, and the water rheostat into the circuit; these three components can be operated with the meter to measure resistance of the patient; and two circular dials for selecting the cells. The dials are connected by heavy insulated copper wiring to connect with each button on each circular dial. The wiring passes behind the cabinet but is easily accessible. The vertical form of milliammeter is located upper most on the face plate. The meter is unaffected by magnetism, has a double scale of values, and measures 1 to 500 milliamperes. The horizontal face plate houses the faradic coil that can be interchanged with others to modify tensions (voltages). The faradic coils contain German silver wiring of 5 to 5,000 ohms resistance or a total resistance of 17,000 ohms; a water rheostat to modify (smooth) the current from any number of cells; binding posts; and an automatic rheotome. The rheotome provides graduated interruptions for galvanic pulses, and is built on the principle of a clock with a strong spring.

Milliammeters

The Van Houten & Ten Broeck Co also sold milliammeters for measuring and regulating current amplitudes during applications, cautery batteries, and office batteries, as well as influence machines. The milliammeter was a valuable component in the circuit between the medical electrical apparatus and the patient to determine the current amplitude. Knowing the current amplitude enabled the physician to set the dosage in treatment of patients and for recordation. Various forms of the milliammeter were manufactured as a separate component while some electrical batteries were beginning to be equipped with a milliammeter as an integral part of the circuitry by a few manufacturers in the early 1900s. Two such quality milliammeters are pictured.

The vertical milliammeter (left) manufactured by Van Houten & Ten Broeck, displayed in the 1908 catalog is an attractive vertical model framed in hardwood. The unit can be adjusted for two scales: 0 to 50, and 0 to 500 milliamperes by a switch. The face has two adjustable screw connecting posts. AS Aloe sold the unit for $15.00 in 1893.[4]

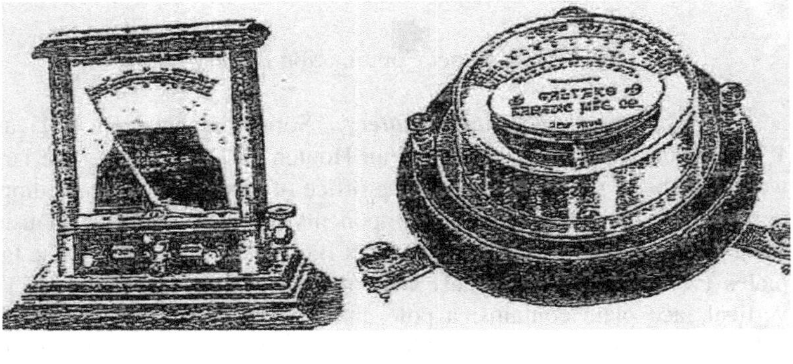

Fig V16. Milliammeter

The Galvano-Faradic Mfg Co made a metal circular milliammeter (right) that was horizontal to the surface, and that sat on three adjustable leveling screws. It had two scales ranging from 0 to 50 and 0 to 250 milliamperes, respectively. The needle indicator pivoted on a jeweled bearing. AS Aloe in 1893 sold the unit for $12.00.[4]

Summary

Much history about the company that was formed in 1870 and folded in 1914 remains a mystery. The early products of Van Houten & Ten Broeck do not surface in antique shops. Not until after 1905 and before 1914 do any medical electrical batteries appear as today's collectables, and these are models designed by the Galvano-Faradic Mfg Co. The Morton-Wimshurst-Holtz influence machine may be available to collectors but this unit is scarce. By 28 March 1916 the company's stock had no value,[3] and the company was closed for business and inheritance tax.[5]

References

1 Davis AB, Dreyfus MS. The Finest Instruments Ever Made. Arlington, MA, Med Hist Pub Assocs, 1986, p 326

2 Selling the tradition of innovation.(http:/www.xray. hmc.psu.edu/rci/ss3/ss3_7.thml, 6 March 2002, p 2

3 Grigg ERN. The Trail of the Invisible Light. Springfield, IL, CC Thomas, 1965, pp 50-80

4. Catalog of AS Aloe, St Louis, MO, AS Aloe, 1893, pp 1-15

5. Keane CP, Emmerich HJ (eds). Marvyn Scudder Manual of Extinct or Obsolete Companies, vol 1. Marvyn Scudder, New York, NY, 1926, p 1275

CHAPTER 13. VICTOR COMPANY OF CHICAGO

Chapter 12 covers the Victor Company's involvement with medical electrical batteries, some of its marketed batteries, and scant individual involvement. The Victor Co was founded in 1893 by Charles Francis Samms (1868-1934) and Julius Benjamin Wantz (1873-1952) at 87 Washington Street, Chicago, IL. This address may have been the home of Wantz where the two started their firm (in the basement[1]). Their first development in manufacture was to build an electrical dental engine along with their product line of high quality dental equipment and supplies, medical electrical machines, and surgical instruments. The company incorporated in 1895 to become the Victor Electric Corporation. The company's shop in 1896 was located at 218 Washington Street. In 1898, the company moved again, and this time to 418 Dearborn St. Each move was believed to constitute an expansion of manufacturing and retailing space because of their growing business, but frequent moves were common among the medical electrical battery industry in the 1870s through the 1890s because of costs, competition, and small profits. CF Samms was the president of the corporation and apparently was behind the company's early shrewd business ventures.

The Victor catalog (edition # 3, 48 pages) of 1898 shows a selection of high grade electrical, dental, surgical equipment, and specialties. Office equipment with dental engines was also offered in the well illustrated catalog.[2] In 1896, the company started producing static electrical machines of the Holtz variety for use in electrotherapeutics and for powering x-rays. The company experienced tragedy with an early x-ray model when wiring designs exposed the operators to 50,000 volts of electricity. This was enough electricity to electrocute the unknowing. Needless to say, the negative publicity was used against the Victor Electric Corp by competitors.

In 1903, the Victor Electric Corp was occupying two floors at 55-61 Market St, Chicago. In October 1910, the company advertised a high frequency coil for sale that was used in connection with x-ray apparatuses. Between 1910 and 1915, the company used both a Victor and a Wantz seal on some of its products.

The Victor Electric Corp in 1907 apparently bought the Macalaster-Wiggen Company, located in Boston, MA, to give the firm an electrical manufacturing presence in the Boston area. Along with the purchase of the Boston firm was the Macalaster-Wiggen Co's Chicago location at 737-739 W Van Buren St.[3] By late 1917, the company's office in Chicago was at 236 S Robey Street.[4] The Macalaster-Wiggen Co was established in 1897 and issued catalogs of its x-ray equipment and supplies from 1907 to 1916. Only the 1907 catalog listed electrotherapeutic items. The Victor Electric Corp also purchased the electrical manufacturer Snook Roentgen Company of Philadelphia.[1]

The company changed locations between 1907 and 1916 four times. Three of these changes of location were in the Sudbury Building of Boston, MA; 1907 at 210; at 605 prior to 1914; and in 1914 it moved to 79 Sudbury Building. Then about 1915 the company located at 66 Broadway, Cambridge, MA.[4]

The Victor Co overcame the earlier negative publicity in the x-ray business by producing the Coolidge high-vacuum tube known as the "hot-cathode" that became the standard of the industry for some time. The Coolidge high-vacuum tube (along with the autotransformer) enabled the operator of an x-ray to have better control of the voltage energy (gap) and of millamperage to establish a quality radiographic technique. So well received was the "hot-cathode" that the Victor Electric Corp became its lone manufacturer by 1913, and the company's contributions in the x-ray industry were sufficient enough to become the basis of today's general electric medical systems.[1]

No Victor made static influence machine has been found that was used in its x-ray business. The Victor Electric Corp seemed to concentrate its manufacture of medical electrical apparatuses on units that produced combined galvanic and faradic and later sinusoidal currents. By 1910, most medical electricians were abandoning apparatus producing faradic currents in their practices in favor of those delivering the sinusoidal currents. Also, the Victor Electric Corp's electrical apparatuses most often adopted the commercial power source (direct or Edison current) to operate its equipment.

Sometime in 1917, EC Jerman (1865-1936), later renown for techniques in x-ray applications and as the founder of the American Society of X-Ray Technicians, became associated with what was to become the Victor X-ray Corp. Through the urging of CF Samms. Jerman started the Victor Education Department in 1917 to help promote professional and technical activities among those engaged with the operation of x-rays. The Victor Electric Corp was recruiting talented personnel at this time to fend off the competition of the 1916 consolidation of x-ray manufactures.[1] In the same year, 1917, General Electric, a British firm, bought part interest in the Victor Electric Corp.

The Victor Electric Corp in the early twentieth century relied on dealers and agents for sales of its products. In 1920, the Victor Electric Corp became the Victor X-Ray Corp and with this change the company dropped its dealers so that the factory or main office coordinated all sales and service. As the General Electric Co of England acquired more and more of the Victor Electric Corp so did more changes occur. The General Electric X-ray Corp completed its acquisition of the Victor Electric Corp in 1926 because it wanted a company that made many electrical items. As in most company buyouts or mergers changes occur that alter the commercial structure of the smaller company. The Victor Electric Corp changed[1] with the merger by moving the x-ray business from Chicago to

Milwaukee, WI. In 1930, the name Victor was discontinued from the name, and thereafter it was the General Electric X-ray Corp (GEXCO). General Electric X-Ray Corp was selling physical medicine equipment in 1932 in which one of its advertisements cited "(formerly Victor X-ray Corp), 2012 Jackson Blvd, Chicago," in association with the equipment. In 1946, the General Electric Co closed its x-ray plant at 2012 W Jackson Blvd, Chicago (old plant of Victor), that ended the Victor Electric Corp.[3]

James Picker was with the company when the Victor Electric Corp was named, and contributed much to the x-ray part of the business. Just before General Electric began its association with the Victor Electric Corp, Picker left (1915) to form the James Picker Company in New York City. The James Picker Co bought the Waite & Bartlett Co of New York City from Harry Fuller Waite, MD, in 1929. Between 1937 and 1967, the Waite Manufacturing Division of the than Picker X-Ray Corp was located in Cleveland, OH, where it occupied three floors of a building.

Although the corporation's main product by 1920 was the x-ray, it continued to manufacture and sell many of its previous electrotherapeutic products. Victor was still selling its Multiplex-Sinusoidal Apparatus under the name Victor in 1929.

The company marketed its Victor No.10 fulguration and high frequency diathermy unit in 1916. In 1918, the corporation's electrotherapeutic products for physicians included: the Victor No.2 Wall Plate that offered galvanism, primary faradism, secondary faradism, combined secondary faradism and galvanism, and endoscopic light current; the Victor Combistat that provided cautery current, nasal drilling, compressed air, suction, pneumatic massage, and vibratory massage in addition to the traditional electrical currents of No.2; the Victor Multiplex-Sinusoidal Apparatus; and the Victor No.1 electrolytic rectifier for converting alternating into direct current.[5] The Victor Electric Corp manufactured and sold forms of its electrotherapeutic wall plate style apparatus from 1893 into the 1920s. The evolution of these wall plate apparatuses grew with updated faradic-galvanic units to the more modern Polysine apparatus that could produce a variety of sinusoidal and galvanic currents. During the early twentieth century (1915 to 1920s), apparatuses for delivering sinusoidal currents replaced the faradic units because the newer alternating (AC) current waveforms were more acceptable or comfortable than faradic currents to patients when their sensory nerves were electrically stimulated.

Commonalties of Victor Apparatuses

The Victor Co (Victor Electric Corp) started rather late during the golden period for the medical electrical battery business. Since most manufacturers in the United States were already established (1870s through the 1880s), the Victor Co, at first, seemed to concentrate on quality medical electrical batteries (combined faradic and galvanic) for the physician and powered by dry cells. Sometime around 1910, perhaps earlier, the company was producing medical electrical batteries that were powered by the commercial current (Edison DC, AC) of the time period. By 1918, all Victor batteries were electrically powered (power grids) using state-of-the-art electronic tubes and switches. Most of its units were encased in wooden boxes covered by black buckram. The company continued, however, using induction coils with some units producing alternating currents into the 1920s.

The Victor signature is always located on its equipment, however, the company did wholesale to medical suppliers who then had signatures, other than Victor, located on the unit they retailed (eg, Rochester Electric Co). The electrical apparatuses manufactured by Victor were quality constructed and performed well. The units seemed to be painted with black polished lacquer. Metals used were nickel plated and then chrome in the mid to late 1920s. No record of home use apparatuses was found, only physician consumers.

The Victor Electric Corp did not develop new technologies for their batteries and apparatuses, but did supply state-of-the-art apparatuses. The company concentrated on the x-ray and electrical supplies in the twentieth century. No distinguishing features are noted other than those mentioned about the cases, color, signature, and quality.

Faradic Battery

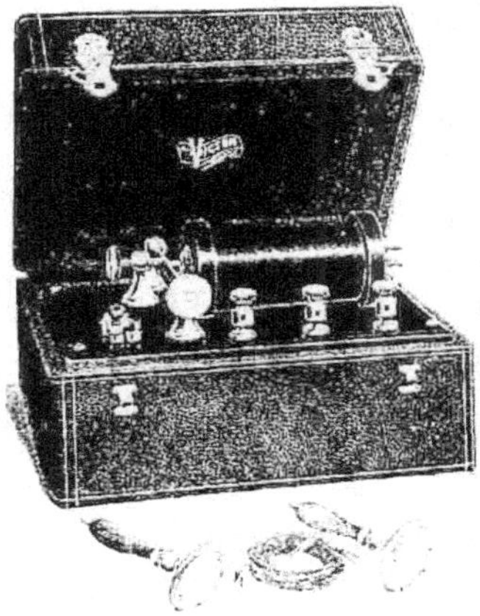

Fig V1. Victor No. 2 Portable Battery[5]

In the mid 1890s and early 1900s, the Victor Electric Corp did make some faradic medical electrical batteries. These faradic batteries formed a series of portable units that were housed in wooden boxes covered with black buckram (leatherette like).

No.2 Portable Battery. This portable unit (Fig V2) has the conventional conduction coil to produce faradic current. The current amplitude is controlled by a sliding metal rod in the induction coil, and a spring lever, adjustable screw contact vibrating interrupter is used to regulate pulse frequencies. This particular unit is powered by dry cells underneath the face plate (hard rubber), has an On/Off switch, and binding posts to connect the patient to combined and secondary faradic currents. The case is covered in black buckram, has a hinged lid, and is secured by two hinged latches and levers. This unit dates around 1900 to 1910.

Combined Current Batteries

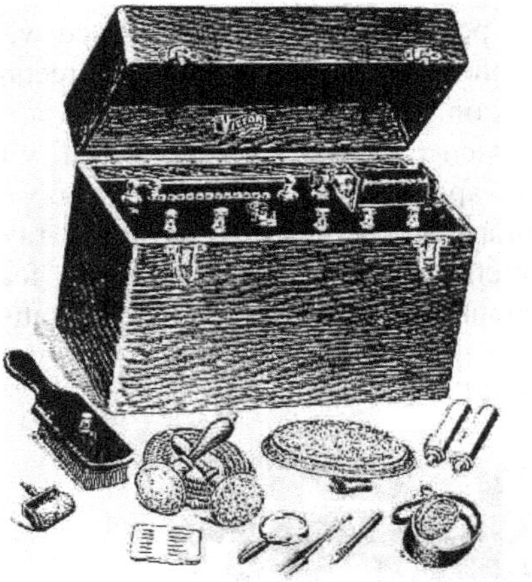

Fig V2. Victor No. 3 Combined Unit[5]

No.3 Combined Unit. The No.3 Combined Unit was another in the series of portable electrical batteries made by Victor around 1900 and continued to at least 1910. The unit has a conventional induction coil with a sliding current controller, and a vibrating interrupter with its adjustable screw contact and spring lever hammer. The galvanic operation also has a sliding metal controller of rheostat. The unit is able to deliver combined faradic and galvanic currents. It is powered by dry cells. The buckram covered wooden case has a hinged lid and is secured in front by two snap latches.

Combined Portable Battery No.5. This unit contained the electrical components of the No.3 unit, but was more elaborate. It was probably made between 1905 and 1909. This unit is capable of providing

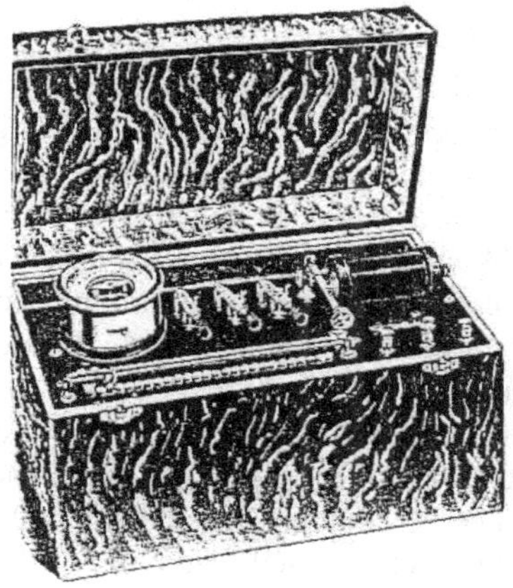

Fig V3 Victor Combined Portable Battery No.5

rapid and slow faradic pulses by two interrupters. The current amplitude of the faradic part was regulated by the sliding rod controller, while the galvanic current amplitude is regulated by a sliding rheostat. The face plate of hard rubber also contains a milliammeter, a current selector switch, an On/Off switch, and three connecting posts. The apparatus is enclosed in a black buckram case and secured by its two snap latches on the front and hinged lid. Dry cells power the unit.

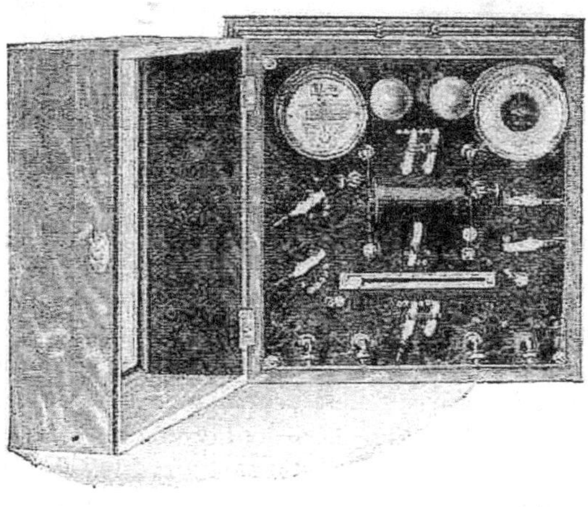

Fig V4. Victor No. 2 Wall Plate[6]

Wall Plates. This No.2 Wall Plate (Fig V4) is a combination faradic and galvanic electrical battery that may have been one of the earliest models manufactured by the Victor Electric Corp around 1895 to 1905. It has a conventional faradic coil that delivers primary and secondary faradic currents. The rheostat for current amplitudes used a sliding scale type of movement that was graduated in arbitrary units. The unit also provides galvanic current along with a combined galvanic and secondary faradic current. Both a milliammeter for galvanic current and a voltage scale for faradic functions are available. A rheotome is present to control faradic pulses along with several lever switches to select and control functions. Lamps (green and red bulbs) are also available for endoscopic light current. By 1918, this unit could be operated by commercial direct current, and with 110 volts it sold for $75.00; and with 220 volts direct current it cost $90.00. The unit also could operate with alternating current if an electrolytic rectifier was added with additional cost. A tiger oak case (17.75 x 17.75 x 10.75 inches) with hinged lid encloses the unit. The lid contains beveled glass (0.25 inch thick x 1 inch bevel) with brass and nickel plated features. A lever latch secures the lid on front of the case. The face plate is marble making the unit heavy.

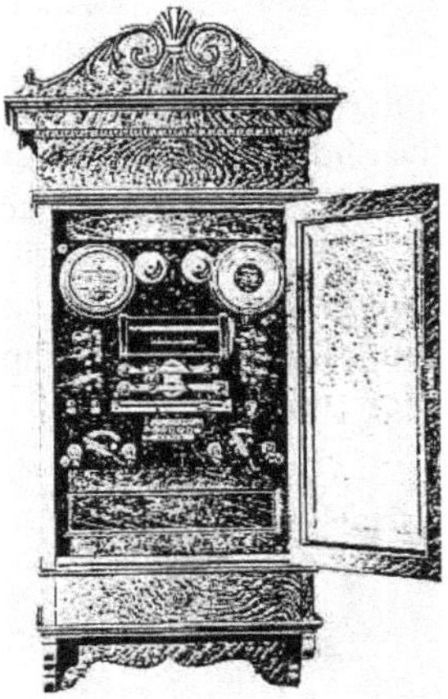

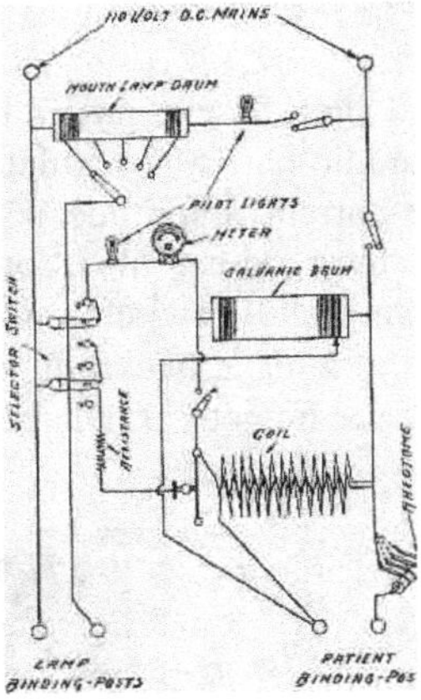

Fig V5. Victor Wall Plate and Circuit Diagram

By 1908, the Victor Electric Corp placed the No.2 wall plate into a cabinet. The cabinet model has the same features of electrical components as the previous unit, but in addition it has a more elaborate enclosure. The cabinet has a glass door that covers the face plate when not in operation. Below the glass door is a drawer for housing the accessories.

The previous combination faradic and galvanic models were updated around 1912 to add sinusoidal current. A direct current motor was added at the bottom of the cabinet of the Wall Plate of Fig V5 to assist in the production of sinusoidal current that was in demand at the time. The cabinet was increased in size over the wall plate so as to rest on the floor. A large glass door covered the face plate when not in operation. Below the glass door was a drawer for accessories. This unit continued to have a conventional type induction coil with the primary coil wound with a few turns of heavy insulated copper wire. Its secondary coil also was wound with copper wire but thinner diameter and many more turns. The

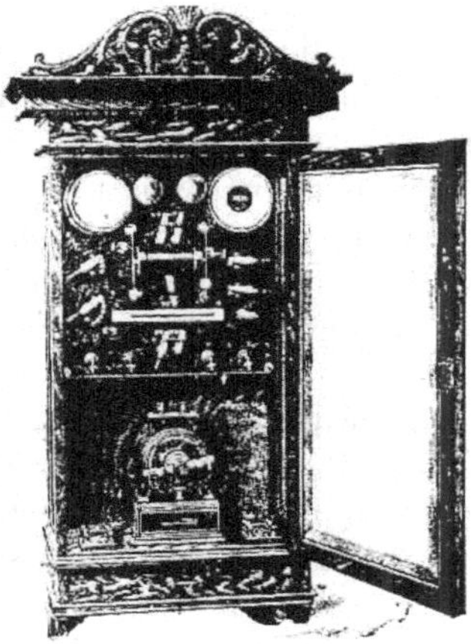

Fig V6. Victor Wall Plate, 1912

electrical components of the Wall Plates of Fig V5 and Fig V6 are identical.

Victor Multiplex-Sinusoidal Apparatus. The Multiplex unit (Fig V7) provided galvanic, surging galvanic, rapid sine, slow sine, surging sine, and muliplex sine currents. The unit could light small diagnostic lamps, and deliver currents for cautery. The Mulitiplex is powered by a DC motor (110 V), but AC is possible when an electrolytic or motor generator is used with the unit. A milliammeter was supplied with the basic unit. The Victor Multiplex was encased in a black steel

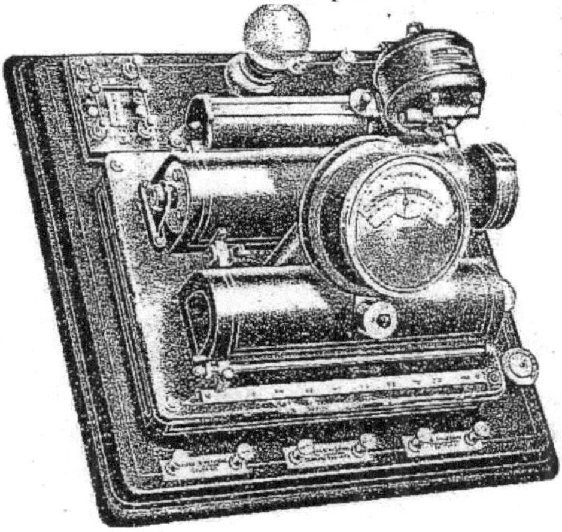

Fig V7. Victor's Multiplex Sine[6]

casing (17.5 x 6 inches), had six connection poles in front of the panel (slow sine, multiplex 5-6), and a metal case covering each of two coils (10.5 x 2.5 inches). The electrical motor connects with these coils to produce sinusoidal currents, a faradic coil is located in back of the unit (6.5 x 2 inches); it contains a light bulb; connecting poles are in the rear; a selector switch with 0 + 2, and two rotating switches for On/Off are also on the face panel. This physician unit was sold from 1909 to 1929. Customers had to contact the company directly for a period of time after 1920 to obtain quotations on the prices of desired equipment. The consumer had the option purchasing the Multiplex unit with or without (table model) a mobile stand.

Combistat. This unit was the multiplex sinusoidal apparatus for electrotherapy combined with additional machinery to increase functions. The Combistat could provide endoscopic light current, cautery currents, nasal drilling, compressed air, suction, pneumatic massage, and vibratory massage. A mobile stand enabled the apparatus to be moved about so as to be available for a variety of medical treatments at different locations. This unit could be purchased in 1918 with fewer or more functions than those cited. The electrotherapeutic aspect of the unit provides galvanic current; surging (ramping) galvanic current; and slow, rapid, and surging sinusoidal currents. The Combistat, similar to the Multiplex Sinusoidal

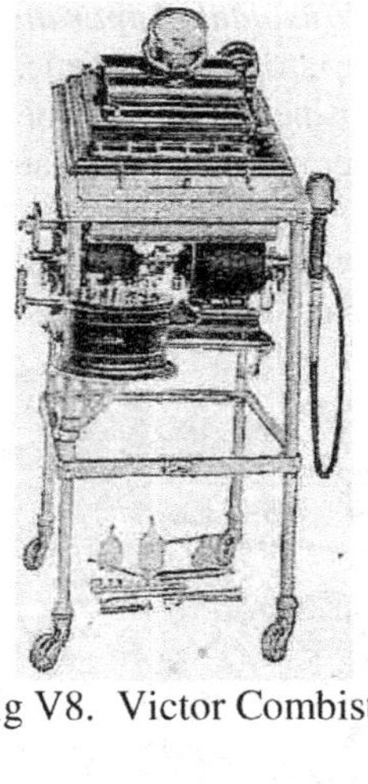

Fig V8. Victor Combistat

Apparatus, was available from 1912 to 1929. The Brooks Denhard Surgical Instrument Co of Louisville, KY[6] (a seller), in 1918 asked the customer to contact the company directly for literature on the unit and price quotations according to the functions desired.

Mutiple Wave Generator. In 1927 to 1929, the Wantz Multiple Wave Generator (Fig V9) was the General Electric X-Ray Corp's (formerly Victor X-Ray Corp) answer to the popular Polysine series by

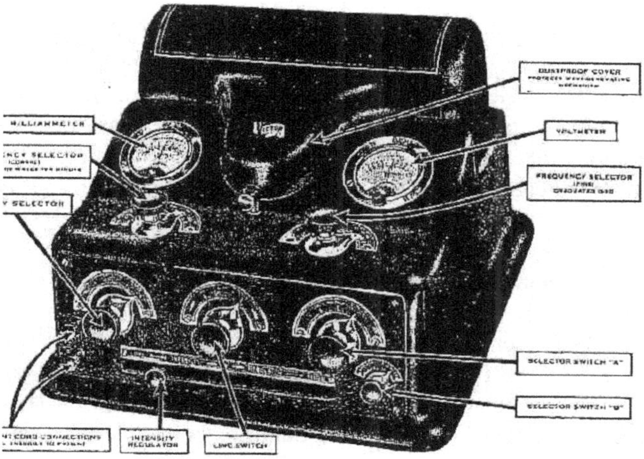

Fig V9. Wantz Multiple Wave Generator

the McIntosh Battery and Optical Co. The Wantz (part of the Victor company's seal, 1910-1915) generator was capable of delivering sinusoidal (slow smooth and rippled), surging galvanic, and galvanic currents. Sinusoidal currents were used mostly to excite muscle and nerve, while galvanic currents were used for ionization, electrolysis, coagulation, and electrodiagnosis. The labels in Fig V9 identify the various functional components of the generator. The metal case is black enameled porcelained steel. This unit is designed to sit on the top of a table or stand (the buyers's option) in the clinic or office of the physician.

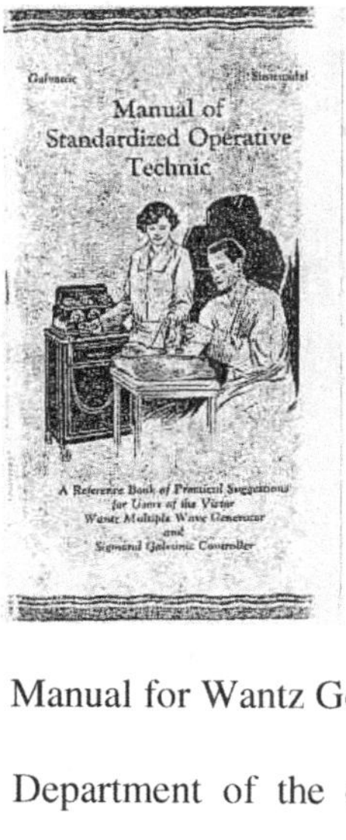

Fig V9A. Manual for Wantz Generator

The Educational Department of the company produced and

published the Manual of Standardized Operative Technic that was a reference book of practical suggestions for physician users of the Wantz Multiple Wave Generator. In addition to the treatment suggestions for physicians the 61 paged booklet contains 20 pages of listings and descriptions of accessories for use with the generator. The booklet accompanied each generator sold by the General Electric X-Ray Corp in 1929.

Summary

The Victor Electric Corp began its manufacture of medical electrical batteries in 1893. Soon after the invention of the x-ray in 1895 the company became involved in that business, too. Although the company continued to manufacture quality medical electrical apparatuses until about 1930, it had become a well known maker of x-ray equipment. Through the 1920s its best electrotherapeutic unit was the Victor Multiplex model. The Victor Electric Corp changed its name to reflect its major concern in 1918 or 1920. Also, the company merged with General Electric only to become completely absorbed by it in 1930. In 1917, the British company was seeking a way to get a good hold into the American x-ray market and it did just that. Before long the Victor name was gone from the company logo. General Electric has it own history of involvement with the manufacture and retail of faradic and galvanic batteries prior to getting into the x-ray business in the United States.

References

1. Dr Alcorn. History: Narratives-Radiology in Illinois. Chicago Radiological Society at the Centennial of Radiology, 1995; (www.chi-rad-sco.org/Illinois.html)

2. Romaine LB. A Guide to American Trade Catalogs 1744-1900. New York, NY, RR Bowker, 1960, pp 235-241

3. Grigg ERN. The Trail of the Invisible Light. Springfield, IL, CC Thomas, 1965, pp 50-80

4. Davis AB, Dreyfus MS. The Finest Instruments Ever Made. Arlington, MA, Med Hist Pub Assocs, 1986, pp 328-330

5. Dugan WJ. Hand-Book of Electro-Therapeutics. Philadelphia,PA, FA Davis, 1910, pp 25, 48, 72, 113

6. Brooks Denhard Sugical Instrument Co, Louisville, KY, Brooks Denhard, 1918, pp 520, 524

CHAPTER 14. WAITE & BARTLETT MANUFACTURING COMPANY OF NEW YORK CITY

Information about Bartlett, one founder of the company, is incomplete, however, Chapter 13 covers the firm and its batteries. Dr Henry E Waite (1848-1916) and Frederick Bartlett (-1905) founded Waite & Bartlett of New York between 1879[1] and 1881[2] or 1882.[3] The Waite & Bartlett catalog of 1901 indicates that 1881 was the founding date.[4] Dr Waite was its president. The company's first location of business was 204 East 23rd Street, and then 202 East 23rd Street in 1884 to 1887.[3] At the time of the company's start Bartlett had been in the same business (Galvano-Faradic Mfg Co) for several years; he brought his experience and innovations to the new company, and he apparently continued to function in both companies until his death in 1905. The company was founded by two friends whose names survived following the death of Bartlett. Bartlett was apparently the technology expert, since he had prior experience with battery designs and their patents. Waite & Bartlett moved to 143 East 23rd St in 1888, and changed the name to the Waite & Bartlett Manufacturing Company in 1889.[3]

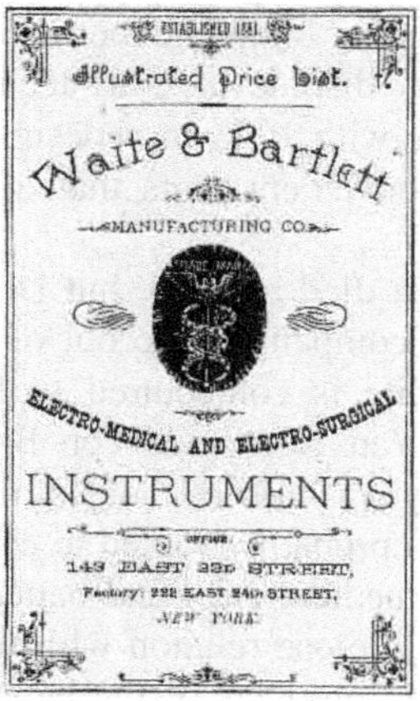

Fig W. Title Page, Catalog of 1901

In 1893, the Waite & Bartlett Mfg Co opened another operation at 222 East 24th Street where it remained until 1898 (108 and 336 East 23rd St), and in 1900 its second location moved to 334 East 23rd Street.[3] From its start in 1881 to 1929, the Waite & Bartlett Mfg Co made quality conventional lines of medical electrical apparatus and accessories. In 1885, Ambrose L Ranney authored the publication Practical Suggestions Respecting the Varieties of Electric Currents and Uses of Electricity in Medicine for the company.

By 1901, the company was well established in manufacturing and retailing x-ray devices, and soon became a leader of that field in the eastern United States. Being a manufacturer and retailer of electrotherapeutic devices for many years made their introduction into the x-ray field very smooth. The company was a leader in medical electrical batteries and using this ingenuity its engineers converted existing high voltage therapeutic devices (influence machines) into powering the glass x-ray tubes. The Waite & Bartlett Mfg Co was one of the most successful manufacturers of the influence (static) machines.[1] These machines were used to power the first x-ray units in the United States from 1896 to 1900 because of their high voltages and their availability.

The company held many patents (viz, x-ray items) with most attributed to the innovations of Dr Henry F Waite, Jr. Waite & Bartlett expanded their business by opening a manufacturing division in Cleveland, OH.[1] Also, in 1901, the company was selling the largest Holtz static electrical machine in existence (Fig W12). In 1902, Dr Waite challenged the Wagner & Co of Chicago over the efficiency of two mica plates versus 10 glass plates for x-ray use. Since x-rays were still in the pioneer stages, designs of competitor models were often challenged in professional journals.[1] Neither clinical experience nor research data were yet available to settle any dispute in x-ray technology. The company's engineers made the best with time to redesign x-ray units into more modern, efficient, and convenient units that eliminated the use of the static influence machine.

Frederick Bartlett died in 1905, but Dr Henry Waite continued using both names as the company's title out of a long friendship. After Bartlett died, Henry Waite is conjectured to have sold the Galvano-Faradic Mfg Co to the Van Houten & Ten Broeck Company of New York. The latter company was also a leader in the making and selling of the influence machines so probably wanted to expand their products with the addition of a line of medical electrical batteries. Van Houten & Ten Broeck appeared to have a close relation with the Galvano-Faradic Mfg Co, since they earlier sold products of the latter firm. The dry and wet cells powering the medical electrical apparatuses were giving way to the use of commercial direct (DC) and alternating currents (AC) in 1905 to 1910 for powering all medical electrical devices. The AC power offered so much more in technology and operational efficiency that electrical cell powered units were being phased out and replaced. The AC powered units could provide faradic, galvanic, and sinusoidal currents more effectively than electrical cell powered units. However, in 1914, the Van Houten & Ten Broeck Company was headed out of business when it went into receivership. The influence machines were also decreasing in popularity at this period of time. First used for therapeutics and then used for powering the x-ray in its early times (1896-1902), the influence machine by 1903 or 1904 was being replaced by machines especially designated and made for x-ray operation. Many products manufactured and sold by Van Houten & Ten Broeck Co were no longer in demand.

From 1905 to 1910 the Waite & Bartlett Mfg Co was located at 113-117 West 31st Street, and in 1912, the company occupied offices at 252-258 West 29th Street. Promotion of electrotherapeutic apparatuses seemed to have decreased or disappeared from the company's advertising literature after World War I. From 1923 to 1929, the company was operating from 53 Jackson Ave, Long Island where their manufacturing plant was located. The company issued mostly pamphlets, leaflets, and flyers from this location in 1923 through 1925. The company was then named the Waite & Bartlett X-Ray Manufacturing Company. At this time the company may have eliminated or at least reduced its product line of electromedical and electrosurgical apparatus, also. Their catalog of 1916 still featured the electrical batteries and machines but the x-ray was now a dominant feature for them and a lucrative business in medicine.

Biography of the Waites

Henry E Waite was a physician graduate from an eclectic school of medicine. Although he was a practicing electrotherapeutist (although the common term used the 19th and 20th centuries, electrologist was used also), and gained a credible reputation as a manufacturer of medical apparatuses, his medical education was not readily accepted by orthodox physicians.[1] His medical background caused him some irritation in 1903 when he applied for membership in the American Electro-Therapeutics Association during its annual meeting (22-24 Sept) in Atlantic City, NJ. The membership committee considered Dr Waite as a manufacturer and a product of an eclectic rather than an orthodox school of medicine. After much discussion the membership committee decided that Dr Waite did not qualify as an active voting member, but did offer him associate membership.[5]

Henry E Waite is said to have been in the Civil War[1] (In 1864 he was just 16 years of age.), was an instructor in electrotherapeutics at the New York Postgraduate Medical School, and was an inventor. Dr Henry E Waite died in 1916.

Of his three sons, one was killed in a train accident in 1910, and the other two sons became associated with their father's business. One son was an electrical engineer and joined the company to make transformers. Henry F Waite, Jr (1874-1946), graduated in 1897 from the New York University Medical School as an orthodox physician. Henry F Waite, Jr, was innovative in the field of x-ray and moved the company more in that direction with company products. He had patents in both the medical electrotherapeutic and x-ray fields. Dr Henry F Waite, Jr, may have been the most innovative American individual in the x-ray field from 1900 into the 1930s. The Waite & Bartlett Mfg Co was among the first and foremost to manufacture the x-ray in the United States.

Henry F Waite, Jr, was responsible for developing the bedside x-ray that was used greatly by the United States Army during World War I. By 1929, age and financial depression were taking a toll on Dr Henry F Waite, Jr, so he sold the company to the Picker X-Ray Corporation of New York. The purchase provided Picker with diversity in medical electrical products, but change also came with the deal. Picker used the Cleveland plant of Waite & Bartlet; developed a Waite & Bartlett division at 30th and Superior Streets, Chicago; closed the manufacturing plant on Long Island, NY; and continued some Waite & Bartlett functions at the New York City facility. Picker never entered the electrotherapeutic apparatus business.

Commonalties of Waite & Bartlett Batteries

The designs of Waite & Bartlett medical electrical batteries were influenced greatly by practicing electrotherapeutists who were renown in that field (eg: Engelmann, Goelet, Morton, Ranney). Thus, the induction coils of the faradic batteries, especially the end caps, up to 1907 or 1910 varied in design from circular to octagonal in shape. The coils were covered by fabric, often of checked pattern. In the box type models the simple sliding metal current controller was used, but in the cabinet models the sledge inductorium was usually preferred.

The rheotomes or frequency control devices vary on the Waite and Bartlett Mfg Co units from the common spring lever, hammer vibrating interrupter to the more elaborate use of two interrupters. In the dual interrupter units, one varied the fast pulses, while another controlled slow pulses.

The Waite & Bartlett Mfg Co promoted the Fuller glass jar cell that has a screw on lid. The cell was usually connected to the electrical circuit of the apparatus by two adjustable screw, pivoting binding posts.

The metal of the electrical components are of heavy nickel plate. The binding or connector posts are of metal adjustable screws. All cases of batteries were well constructed. All in all, the Waite & Bartlett medical electrical batteries were top of the line in construction and quality operation.

The company did not produce as wide a variety of models as did some other companies, but when you combine the large product line of the Galvano-Faradic Mfg Co (owned by Bartlett until 1905) with the products of Waite & Bartlett Mfg Co the product offerings were considerable. The Waite & Bartlett Mfg Co products were aimed mostly toward physician consumers, but the company did include one faradic battery for public consumers. The large cabinet type batteries have a milliammeter located on the top of the unit. The company offered the widest variety of influence machines manufactured in the United States.

The Waite & Bartlett Mfg Co did enjoy a profitable business based on the medical electrical batteries from 1881 until 1905. The interest of the company changed to the x-ray in 1896 and in this field it gained its greatest growth and notable reputation as a manufacturer. The emphasis on the manufacture of the x-ray certainly was influenced by Dr HF Waite, Jr, after joining the company in 1897.

Galvanic Batteries

Plug and Socket. The Waite and Bartlett Mfg Co offered a galvanic battery (Fig W1) that was basically the same in five different sizes that varied by the number of wet cells and the size of the wooden box (case). The basic wooden box came in either polished antique oak or mahogany. The rectangular shaped boxes have a hinged lid that opens from the top to expose the electrical or operational components, and a front door that opens from the right side. The door hides the wet cells, the copper-zinc couples, and the hydrastat when the battery is in operation.

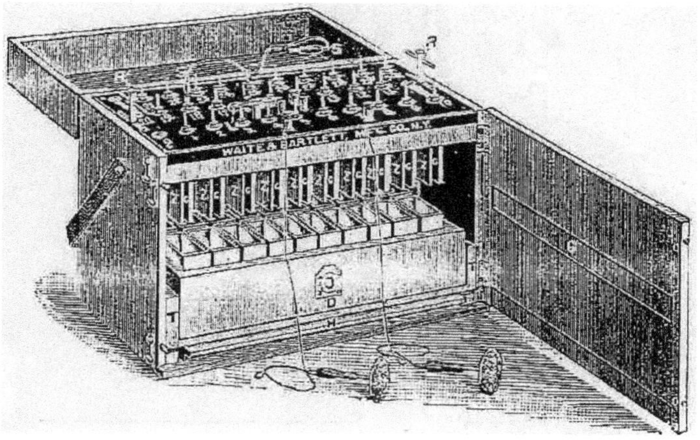

Fig W1. Plug and Socket Galvanic Battery[6]

The wooden box is carried by a leather strap attached to each side. Both the lid and the door are secured by two lever hooks that pivot in and out of a screw. The face plate is hard rubber and contains switches for each number of wet cells, two screw connecting posts, and two lifting rods that screw into the ends of the cell tray and operate to lower and raise the cell tray for operation. A thin board stored on the inside bottom of the box is placed on the door that opens from the right side. The door hides the wet cells, the copper-zinc couples, and the hydrastat when the battery is to be carried. The padded side of the board seals the cells so that fluid does not leak or spill when the apparatus is moved. The AS Aloe catalog of 1893 listed the six-cell unit for $12.00; the 12-cell unit for $20.00; the 16-cell unit for $24.00; the 20-cell unit for $30.00; and the 30-cell galvanic battery for $38.00.

This model of galvanic current apparatus involves five units of varying numbers of wet cells (6 to 30 cells). The galvanic battery was patented in 1887, but probably was first manufactured and marketed in 1888 when Waite & Bartlett changed its name to the Waite & Bartlett Manufacturing Co. The company with the latter name was then located at 143 East 23rd Street in 1889, however, some of these units may bear the former name of the company and its address of 204 East 23rd Street, Chicago, IL. If collectors have a Waite & Bartlett Galvanic Battery of this style and bearing the old address then the unit can be dated to 1887 and 1888.

Faradic Batteries

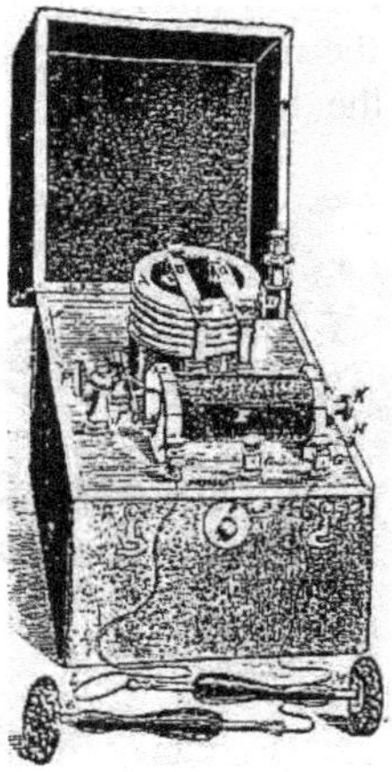

Fig W2. Waite and Bartlett's Family Battery[6]

Family Battery. This faradic battery (Fig W2) was powered by a single wet cell (eg, the Fuller mercury-bichromate jar battery with screw lid and attached elements) housed underneath the face plate, but its top is exposed behind the induction coil for connecting with the circuit. The face plate contained the induction coil that has an octagonal cap at each end; a metal sliding tube current regulator; an adjustable screw spring lever, hammer vibrator type interrupter; two adjustable screw binding posts; three adjustable screw connecting posts; and an opening for fitting the cell jar. The unit is in an oak or mahogany box with a hinged lid, a metal carrying handle on top, and two hook lever latches that pivot in and out of place for locking. The unit sold for $10.00 in the AS Aloe trade catalog of 1893.

Physician's Faradic Battery No.2. This battery is built on the sledge inductorium principle of DuBois-Reymond. It has two interrupters, one delivering slow and one for rapid pulse frequencies, and a manually operated key for controlling pulses in testing nerve-muscle continuity. The unit is powered by one wet cell (Fuller jar) with screw on

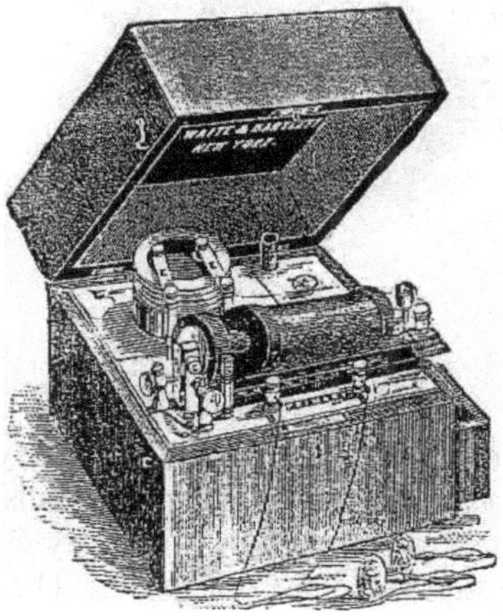

Fig W3. Waite and Bartlett's Physician's Faradic Battery No. 2[6]

lid that joins the circuit by two adjustable screw, pivoting binding posts. The face plate is in three sections: 1) electrical components, 2) cell jar, and 3) accessories with a lid. A lock and key on the front of the box also secures the lid. The front section of the wooden face plate contains the sledge inductorium type of coil to finely control current amplitude. An arbitrary graded scale measures the distance that the secondary coil moves. Two spring lever adjustable screw contacts provide rapid and slow pulse rates. Two screw binding posts connect the patient with the circuitry. The lower right side of the wooden box has a drawer for accessories. The wooden box has a hinged lid that latches on each side by a hook lever and screw. The top of the box has a metal carrying handle. The unit sold for $20.00 in 1893 through the AS Aloe trade catalog.

Engelmann Faradic Battery (Fig W4). The Waite and Bartlett Mfg Co series of faradic batteries included the sledge inductorium design unit by Dr George J Engelmann who was a gynecologist in St Louis, and author of a chapter on induced current in the Bigelow book of 1894.[7] The induction coil of this model was designed for three coils, each wound with different lengths and sizes of wire to give the effect of coarse (for muscle contractions), fine (to treat pain), and medium (for contractions of sensitive muscle) faradic currents. Two coils are stored in slots provided on the face plate and are interchanged when their use is desired. Two

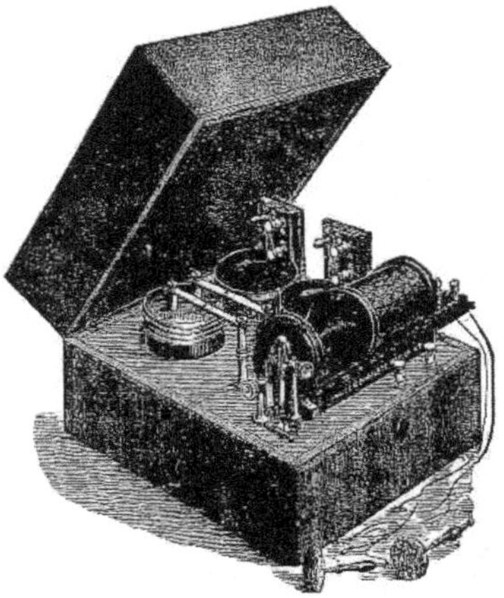

Fig W4. Engelmann's Faradic Battery[6]

adjustable screw spring lever, hammer vibrator type interrupters are present to vary the rates (slow to rapid) of the pulse frequencies. Each coil has its own switch for primary or secondary coil selection, and its own two adjustable screw connecting posts. The unit also has two adjustable screw connecting posts for primary coil current only. The face plate lifts from the wooden case to replace the single cell jar (Fuller battery), and to store accessories. The unit is housed in a wooden box, hinged lid, and secured by a leather strap mounted on each side of the box. The 1893 trade catalog of AS Aloe listed the unit for $40.00. This particular unit was available in 1893 and perhaps earlier.[7]

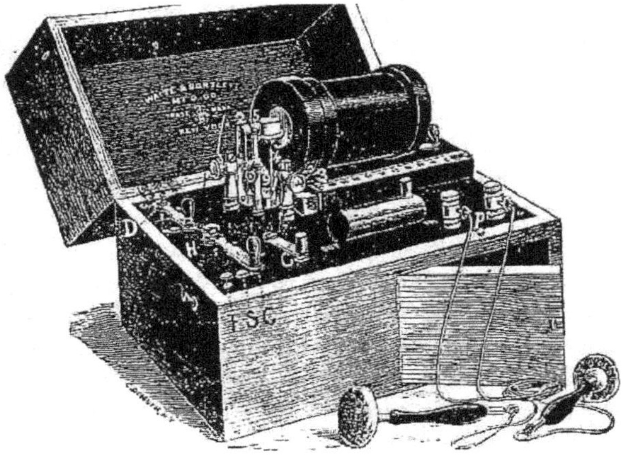

Fig W4A. Engelmann's Faradic Battery

Between 1900 and 1907, the Waite & Bartlett Mfg Co redesigned Engelmann's Faradic Battery that was housed in a wooden box. Like the earlier unit in Fig W4 the operational components were similar. The new model contained an arbitrary scale to measure distance that the secondary coil moved over the primary coil in the sledge inductorium type of faradic coil. The newer model (Fig W4A) has the switches to operate the various windings of the coils relocated, and added a door in the right front of the box to store accessories. The major difference between the two models is that the newer unit uses dry cells rather than wet cells for power. Thus, the company eliminated the inconvenience of the wet cell by 1907 or earlier.

Cabinet Batteries

Goelet Floor Cabinet. This unit is a combined faradic and galvanic apparatus that was marketed by the Waite and Bartlett Mfg Co to provide a less costly unit than the Ranney Cabinet model, $134.00 vs $260.00, respectively. This unit was patented on 15 April 1890. The original unit used 40 Leclanche Gonda porous cup cells that were located on three shelves below the operating components. Rather than a door to hide the cells the Goelet Cabinet has a curtain that slides along a brass rod and rings. The unit has a vertically positioned face plate that contains: a circular switch having metal buttons for corresponding cells and a rotating lever control; a switch that selects the type of current; a

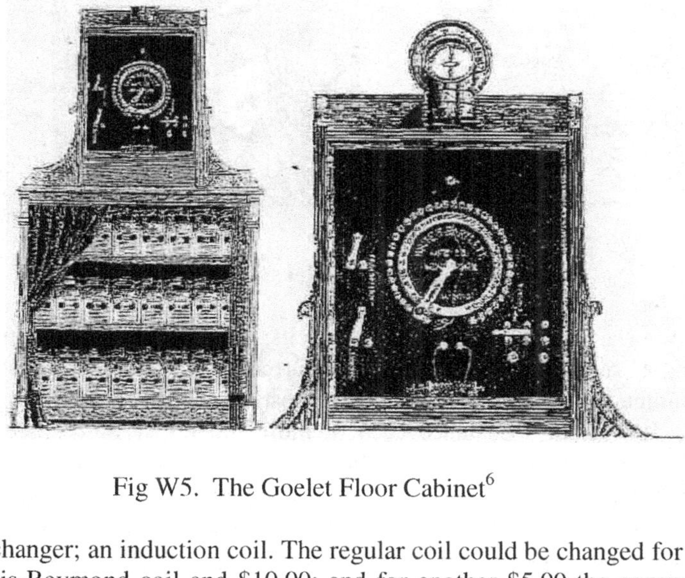

Fig W5. The Goelet Floor Cabinet[6]

pole changer; an induction coil. The regular coil could be changed for the DuBois-Reymond coil and $10.00; and for another $5.00 the consumer could replace the sliding metal current controller with a water rheostat. A Waite and Bartlett milliammeter was furnished with the basic cost and was mounted on the top of the unit. A vibrator for obtaining pulsed monophasic currents from the galvanic circuitry was available for an extra $10.00. The unit was described and displayed in the AS Aloe trade catalog of 1893.

Ranney Complete Office Cabinet. This combination faradic and galvanic cabinet type battery (patented 12 May 1887) of Fig W6 was probably the deluxe model of the Waite and Bartlett Mfg Co product line of electrical apparatuses. The unit came as a cabinet in antique oak or mahogany (69 x 41 x 22 inches), and was shipped as a unit not requiring any assembly. The bottom portion housed the 40 "axo" Leclanche cells on two shelves. Two wooden doors hide the cells, and above it is a full width drawer. The top of this bottom portion holds the vertical or upright wall plate containing the electrical components, and a slide out wooden panel serves as a desk top. A wooden door with glass closes the face plate. On each side of the face plate are beveled glass doors with a small closet. The cabinet has castors for mobility. The face or wall plate (term for large face plates of cabinet batteries) has a current selector capable of

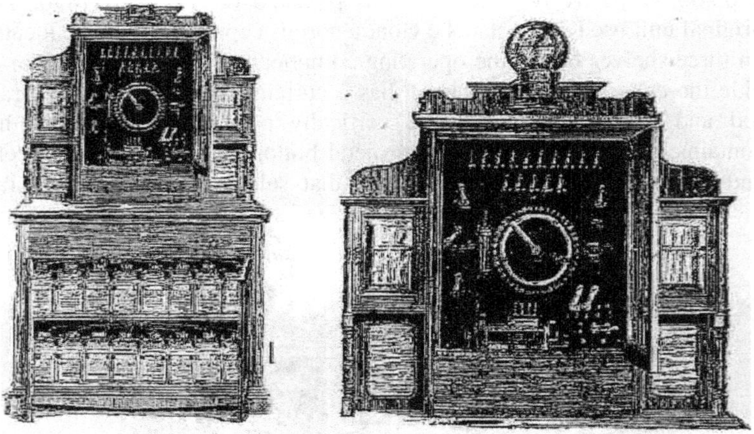

Fig W6. Ranney's Complete Office Cabinet[6]

handling any type or number of cells; an automatic rheotome for monophasic pulses from the galvanic current circuitry; a polarity changer (commutator); a German silver wire rheostat with five coils ranging from 5 to 5000 ohms resistance each; a milliammeter; a water rheostat; a DuBois-Reymond type of faradic coil so that the secondary coil is interchangeable with others to vary the output effects; both a slow and rapid frequency rheotome; and a DeWatteville switch for combined or separate currents. The 1893 AS Aloe trade catalog described and illustrated the unit, and sold it for $260.00. Dr AL Ranney was a practicing physician who also taught at the Post Graduate Medical School in New York City in 1884. He recognized that textbooks of medical electricity did not adequately explain the design and functions of displayed devices.[8] Perhaps from this frustration he designed his versions of the medical electrical battery.

Dr Ranney designed the Complete Office Cabinet in 1887,[9] and the Waite & Bartlett Mfg Co redesigned the cabinet unit to a wall model in 1889. The two units functioned and operated similarly, and both contained the circular dial cell selector of 1887. The cells were external

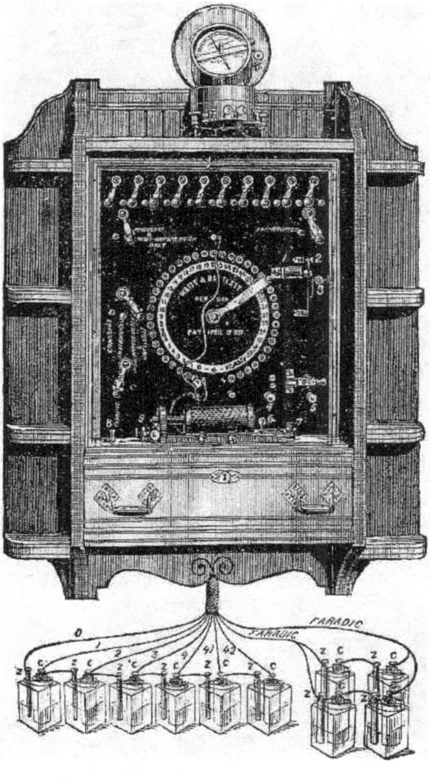

Fig W6A. Waite & Bartlett's Wall Cabinet

to the cabinet that allowed for a more economical, and space saving unit.

In 1889 or 1890, the Waite & Bartlett Mfg Co redesigned the Complete Office Cabinet of Fig W6B[6] with its new Cabinet Battery. Like the first unit of Ranney this model is a complete cabinet. The newer unit contains an updated version of its circular dial cell selector. Various switches are contained on the new Cabinet Battery that specifically control faradic and galvanic currents; constant and interrupted currents; the milliammeter; the faradic interrupter; and the rheostats (faradic and galvanic). Like the other model variations earlier this unit was still powered by wet cells.

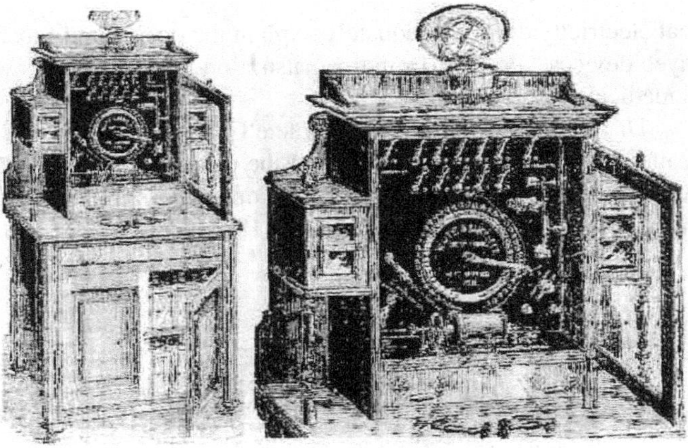

Fig W6B. Waite & Bartlett's Cabinet Battery

Influence Machines

Ranney Charging Machine. This table model of a Wimshurst static apparatus (Fig W7) was used for charging the larger Holtz influence machine or for individual treatment. Humidity during the summer months of July and August in New York City and elsewhere caused moisture in the atmosphere to interfere with the operation of static apparatuses. This charging machine was cranked manually to generate the current sufficient to start the Holtz unit. In 1893, the Ranney Charging Machine was sold by AS Aloe for $66.66.

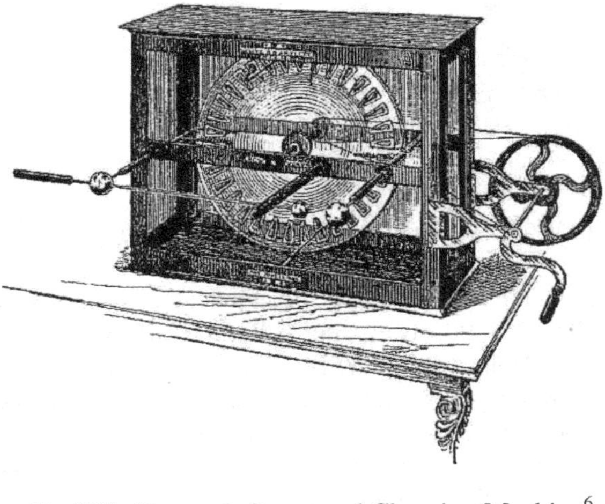

Fig W7. Ranney's Improved Charging Machine[6]

The influence apparatus has two circular discs of plate glass with a spindle axis that allows the discs to be rotated in opposite directions. About 0.125 inches separate the two glass discs. Each disc is attached to a small turning wood (eg, ebonite) pulley. The crank or winch of the large pulley with its two belts drive the glass discs by way of their small pulleys. The crossing of one of the two belts causes the glass discs to rotate in opposite directions. Each disc has 12 or more radiant, sector shaped plates of thin brass glued to them at equal angular distances. At the end of a curved rod is a brush that grazes the brass sector shaped plates of the disc as they rotate. The brass radial, sector shaped plates act as inductors and carriers to act to generate negative and positive charges. The electrodes then collect the static charges for patient treatment.

Holtz Induction Machine. This particular model of the Holtz Induction Machine (Fig W8) was improved (from the original described in the Medical Record of 17 Oct 1885) in 1895 by Professor AL Ranney, MD, for static electrical treatments. Dr Ranney's improvement of 1895 allowed the 1/8 horsepower motor to operate from the power of the added storage battery. The hand crank was used to start the unit and the small motor took over when powered by the storage battery. The unit has six revolving plates of 26 inches diameter, a pair of Leyden jars for collecting and temporarily storing static electricity (early capacitors), and many attachments for providing induced current. The framework came in antique oak or mahogany, and has glass on four sides for view of the operating parts. A hand crank provided the high frequency, slow current amplitude for treatments. A matching wooden insulated platform was included. The framework measures 63 inches high, 36 inches in width, and 72 inches in total length. AS Aloe sold this basic unit with the manual crank for $400.00. For $440.00 the basic unit came with an 1/8

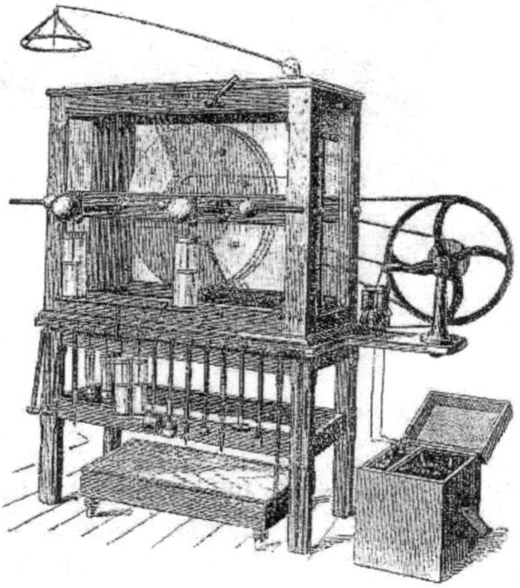

Fig W8. The Holtz Induction Machine and Storage Battery

horse power electrical motor that was powered either by Edison incandescent current (DC) or one Waite & Bartlett storage battery in 1893. The basic unit, including the 1/8 horsepower electrical motor, was sold by the Truax, Greene & Co of Chicago in 1893 for $400.00.

Sometime around 1909 or earlier the Waite & Bartlett Mfg Co redesigned the unit that earlier used a storage battery (Fig W8) to power a small motor for operating the large static apparatus. The newer Holtz apparatus (Fig W9) used a larger motor to operate the static machine. The larger motor used the Edison direct current source. Otherwise the new unit was essentially the same as that of 1893. The influence machines with their circular glass or fiber plates tended to operate to separate the positive and negative aspects of their generated charge and then accumulate it. These machines could generate between 10,000 and 500,000 volts, but only 0.2 to 3 amperes because of very high internal resistances of the apparatuses.

Holtz and Topeler Machine. This machine was invented in 1865 by using principles formed by Alessandro Volta when building his electrophorous unit in the eighteenth century after Varley had modified the electrophorus. The idea was to generate constant electrical charge by revolving a glass disc that was parallel and in the proximity to a charged

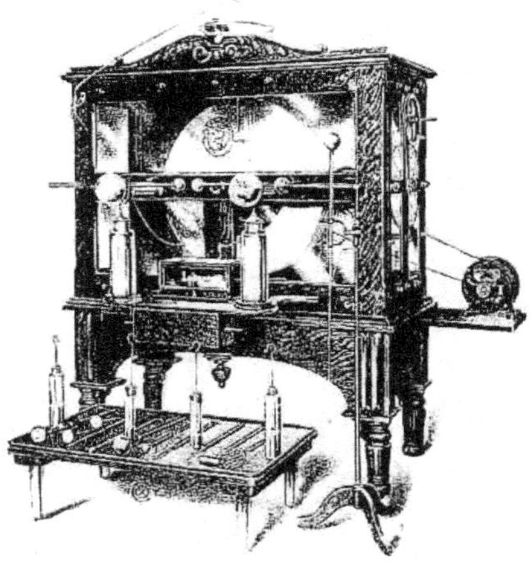

Fig W9. The Holtz Induction Machine and Motor

field. These newly designed static machines were immediately accepted in the United States by electrotherapeutists who found them very powerful. The principle of induction was substituted for friction to produce the influence machine. The Topeler machine was an improvement of the Holtz unit by increasing the number of glass discs or plates, reducing the influence of damp atmospheric conditions, and perfecting the mechanical features of the device. The first improvement was the Holtz-Wimshurst machine, and then came the Holtz-Toepler machine.

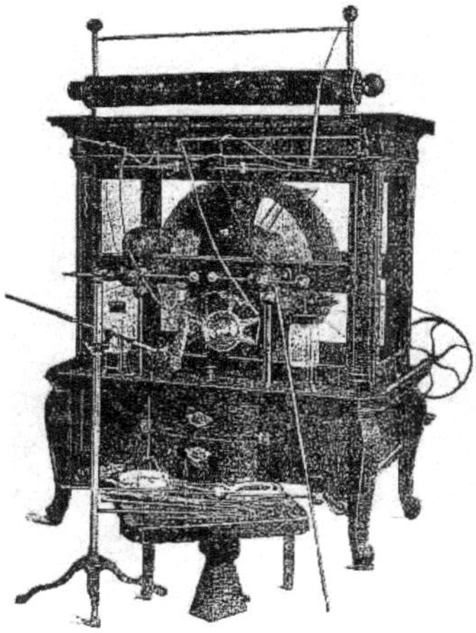

Fig W10. Toepler-Holtz Machine

Characteristics of both the Holtz and the Topeler units are combined in this model. Since influence machines produce very high voltages and very small charges, they were appropriate for use along with a special tube for the first x-rays in 1896. Although this particular unit uses the manual wheel crank to operate, most were designed to use small Toepler or Wimshurst units to produce the initial charge to start the machine. Each stationary plate of the Holtz unit is divided into an upper and lower section and separated by a small horizontal air gap.[9] Each paper sector provides a set of metal points (no discs or brushes). The Toepler unit uses metal discs on one or more sectors, and brushes on the neutralizing rod. The sectors are located between stationary plates or on their external surface, the sectors between stationary plates, or on their external surface. The sectors are provided with metal points that discharge on the surface of the revolving plates. The unit uses fragile glass plates and revolves at high speeds (up to 2000 revolutions per minute).[10]

Morton Machine. The Waite & Bartlett Mfg Co was probably the largest manufacturer of influence machines which were generally large, cumbersome, and expensive. In 1881, WJ Morton, a New York physician, used an influence machine to produce rapid interruptive and graduate current by using a breaker in the circuit with and without condensers (capacitors). He moistened his electrodes to treat patients. He first removed the spark going to the patient but retained all of the physiological effects of the static charge. In his modified version of the influence machine the sparks became a distant feature, while the regulator for timing of the electrical discharges became a dominant feature. A pair of adjustable metallic ball electrodes became the circuit

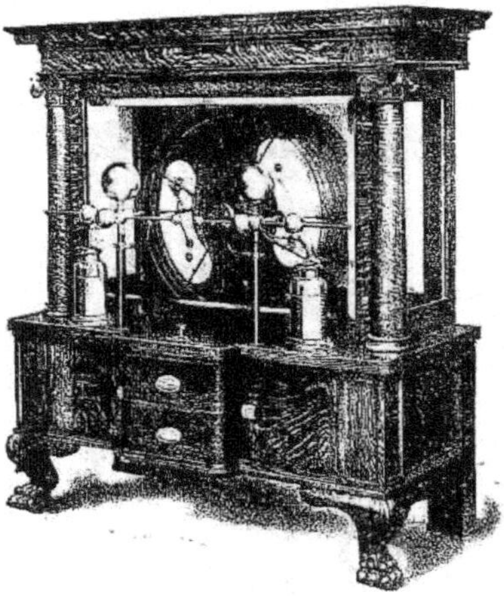

Fig W11. The Morton Influence Machine[11]

breaker. The current produced was in rapid successive equalizations of different potentials of opposite charge condensers (either prime conductor or Leyden jars). Each pulse produced consisted of a large number and range of oscillations or alterations (100,000,000 per second). Nobody could distinguish Morton's current characteristics until 1903 when Manders provided the rationale. Manders stated that the current was undirectional since the impedance of the circuit was so great that it dampened the oscillations that the small capacity condenser produced. Morton's machine was a high frequency current that he applied for patient treatments, and was known as static induced current or Morton current.

Holtz Machine. Waite & Bartlett claimed in 1901 that they had constructed the largest static or influence machine ever. The figure shows the relative size of the unit compared with a man standing next to the unit. The largest Holtz Influence Machine was known to have been popular enough to be sold successfully for a few years. However, by 1901 the giant influence machines were considered an outdated technology for clinical treatments. Static electrical treatments by this form were often ineffective as well as sometime unpleasant to the patients. Because it was bigger and x-rays were new it may have been considered better by some.[12]

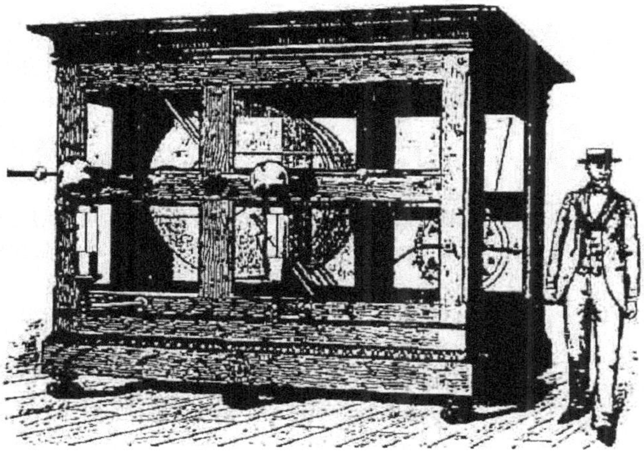

Fig W12. The Largest Holtz Influence Machine
(Courtesy of Radiology Centennial, Inc)

Summary

The Waite & Bartlett Mfg Co succeeded over its 49 years by changing product lines to meet demands of the medical profession. The changes reflect the leadership in the company over time. The company produced quality electrotherapeutic products between 1881 and 1829, but the shift by many physician electrotherapeutists from electrical treatments to the new x-ray field necessitated company changes. The company met these changes successfully until the financial depression of the late 1920s.

A major flaw with the Waite & Bartlett Co was that it never looked into expanding its products to become the dominant manufacturer in its field in the United States. The company never developed a sales force to promote and sale its products nationally. The x-ray was an immediate success in medicine, and by 1903 Waite & Bartlett was only one of more than 200 companies making and selling it.[12]

References

1. Grigg ERN. The Trail of the Invisible Light. Springfield, IL, CC Thomas, 1965, p 71

2. Davis AB, Dreyfus MS. The Finest Instruments Ever Made. Arlington, MA, Med Hist Pub Assocs, 1986, pp 331-332

3. Edmonson JM. American Surgical Instruments. San Francisco, CA, 1997, p 235

4. Catalog of Waite & Bartlett, 1901

5. J Adv Therapeutics. 21:273, 1903

6. Catalog of AS Aloe, St Louis, MO, AS Aloe, 1893, pp 748-753

7. Engelmann GJ. The Faradic or Induced Current; Electro-Magnetism; Electro-Massage, and Instruments. In Bigelow HR (ed). An International System of Electro-Therapeutics. Philadelphia, PA, FA Davis, 1894, pp A117-A184

8. Davis AB. Medicine and Its Technology. Westport, CT, Greenwood Press, 1981, p 19

9. McIntosh H. Practical Handbook of Medical Electricity for Students and Practitioners. Boston, MA, Therapeutic Pub, 1909, p 157

10. Liebig GA, Rohe GH. Practical Electricity in Medicine and Surgery. Philadelphia, PA, FA Davis, 1890, p 221

11. Coleman WF. Electricity in Diseases of Eye, Ear, Nose and Throat. Chicago, IL, Courier-Herald Press, 1912, p 106

12. Sellingtoanemergingprofession.(www.xray.hmc.psu.edu/rci/ss3-4.html6) March2002, p 1

CHAPTER 15. THE ROLE OF THOMAS EDISON AND HIS ASSOCIATES WITH MEDICAL ELECTRICAL BATTERIES

Thomas Edison is a renown inventor and entrepreneur of the nineteenth and twentieth centuries. His innovations involved mostly electricity and as such his laboratory and personnel were expert electricians. Dabbling in medical electrical batteries was an easy step into the manufacturing and marketing fields. The Edison Manufacturing Company of New York developed some excellent electrical cells and electrical components that when juggled could produce medical electrical batteries. Edison's involvement, however, was less then monumental and thus did not impact the field with creativeness or dominate it with volumes of sales.

Because of the Edison name it is fitting that he be included among those that dominated the field of medical electrical batteries. As a collector one can only view his products and those of some associates with passing interest. It is justified, however, to say that Arthur E Kennelly, an Edison associate did have considerable influence in the field of electricity. He was an educator and authority on electricity, and through his consulting work wielded a big stick in forming acceptable and permanent terminology in electricity. He was a frequent figure seen, heard, and highly respected among active electrotherapeutists.

This section presents a small group of noted individuals who were involved with medical electrical batteries, but played a very small role in their ultimate success. This group of men entered the field of medical electrical batteries and exited without carrying a big stick or making a lasting impact. In due respect to these individuals their interest and expertise rested in larger ideals than that of the medical electrical battery.

Thomas Edison

Thomas Alva Edison, the famous American inventor of modern technology, dabbled in the medical electrical battery business. His involvement in the electrical battery business was a natural step since many of his inventions involved electrical components used in the manufacture of the batteries. The medical electrical battery business in the late nineteenth century provided some profit so why not be involved, too.

The Edison Manufacturing Company of New York engaged in making dental and medical instruments that included applications and improvements of the electric cell (eg, Edison-Lalande primary battery in 1889, a storage cell), and medical electrical apparatuses (eg, combination cautery and galvanic cabinet, a cautery unit in 1890-1893).

Thomas Edison's involvement with medical electrical batteries resulted in influencing his son Thomas Edison, Jr, and associates Edwin J

Houston and Arthur E Kennelly. The associates were inventors who worked for Edison on various apparatuses, but than went into their own businesses.

Thomas Alva Edison was the seventh child born to Samuel, Jr, and Nancy Edison of Milan, Ohio, on 11 February 1847. While living in Port Huron, MI, young Edison attended elementary school. His hearing problem led to his being considered a poor student by his teachers, however, when 10 years of age he had a chemistry laboratory in the basement of his parents' home. At age 12 years Edison was working for the Grand Trunk Railway, printing a weekly newspaper, and engaging in laboratory experiments in a freight car. He learned to use the railway's telegraph, and between 1862 and 1868 (15 to 21 years of age) he worked as a telegrapher in the Midwest, South, New England, and in Canada. His work in telegraphy led to his early inventions of a telegraphic repeating instrument, and by 1869 he invented the duplex telegraph and message printer. These latter inventions enabled him to engage in fulltime inventing and its business. (Sahlman R, Strandberg D. Thomas Alva Edison[1]) He went on to become one of the most prolific inventors of the nineteenth and twentieth centuries; a successful businessman, and owner of companies in New York and New Jersey. He died in New Jersey on 18 October 1931.

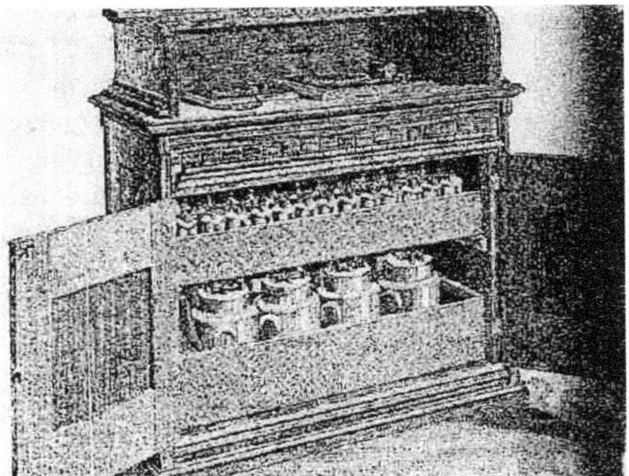

Fig E1. Combination Cautery and Galvanic Cabinet

Combination Cautery and Galvanic Cabinet. The oak cabinet was designed for office use as a cautery and galvanic battery. The cabinet occupies floor space of 46 x 26 inches, and is a roll top desk style. The back is finished wood and has ball bearing casters. The cabinet was designed to accommodate eight Edison-Lalande cells, 50 type A cells (upper tray) for galvanic treatments, and eight M type cells (lower tray) for cautery. The unit has a rheostat, switchboard battery cords, cautery cords. In addition to cautery and galvanic treatments, the combined unit delivers faradic current. Two hinged doors open to expose sliding trays that contain cells for the different operations.

This cautery unit of Fig E2 has three Edison-Lalande cells. Is housed in a wooden case, and complete with cautery equipment sold for $25.00 in the 1893 catalog of Charles Truax & Greene Co of Chicago.

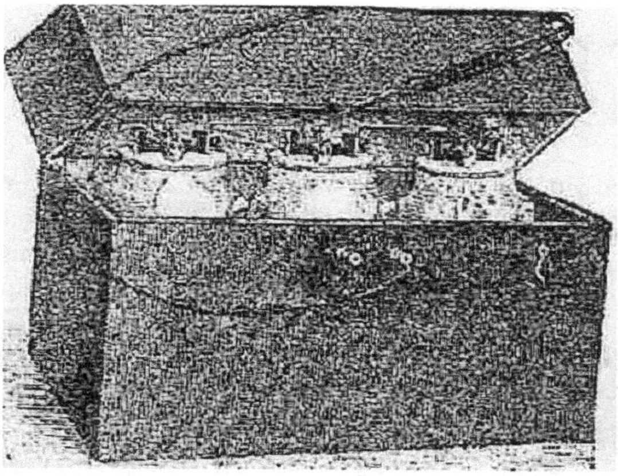

Fig E2. Cautery Unit

Thomas A Edison, Jr

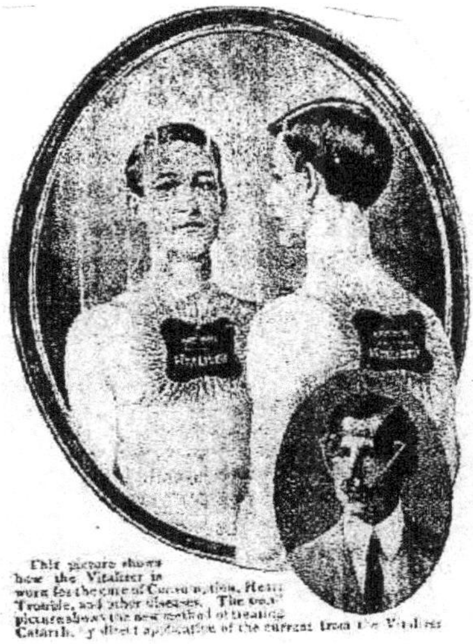

Fig E3. The Magno-Electric Vitalizer

Thomas Edison, Jr, operated The Thomas A Edison, Jr, Chemical Company of New York City (14-16 Stone Street). The company sold the Magno-Electric Vitalizer and advertised in various magazines. The Vitalizer was worn on specific body areas and the head. It was advertised to cure constipation, consumption, catarrh, deafness, defective vision, heart problem, locomotor ataxia, nervous diseases, rheumatism, and paralysis. He advertised in popular magazines (eg, Cosmopolitan) around 1902 and 1903.

Associates

Edwin J Houston

Edwin James Houston was born in Alexandria, VA, on 9 July 1847 and died on 1 March 1914. While teaching at Central High School in a Philadelphia he became a friend with Elihu Thomson who also taught at the same school. Together they formed the Thompson-Houston

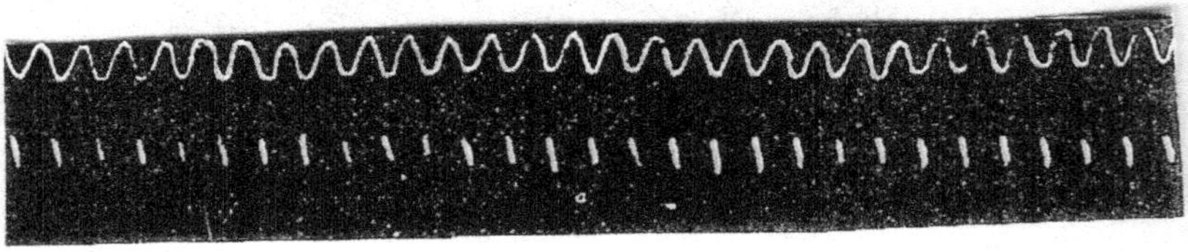

Fig E4. AC from Thompson-Houston Arc Light Coil

company. Tompson and Houston experimented with electricity and in 1881 patented and manufactured arc street lighting. Their work with

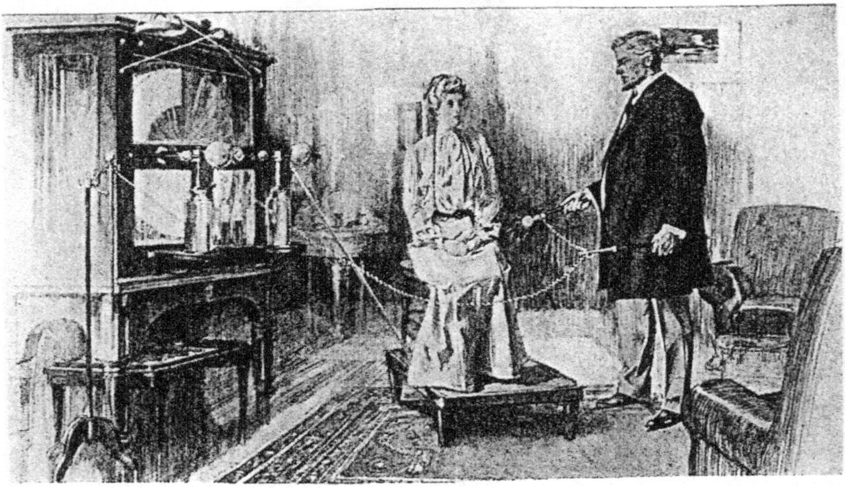

Fig E5. Frontispiece showing a Holtz Static Machine

parallel circuitry enabled lights to be turned on and off individually without involving the whole system.[2] Alternating current of 16,800 times per minute from the coil used by the Thompson-Houston arc light is pictured in Fig E4.

Houston presented his paper "Notes on Phenomena" in 1884 to the first meeting of The Institute of Electrical and Electronic Engineers. He left the company in 1882 to teach fulltime. The Thompson-Houston Co merged with the Edison General electric company in 1892 that formed General Electric. Houston joined AE Kennelly in 1894 to form a consulting company. In 1904, EJ Houston published his book Electricity in Everyday Life. In volume 3 of his book he wrote about the history of electrotherapeutics, electrotherapeutic apparatus and treatment, and electric measuring instruments.

Arthur E Kennelly

Arthur Edwin Kennelly was born on 17 December 1861 near Bombay, India, but was raised in England where he went to elementary school. While working as a telegrapher at 13 years of age he taught himself physics. He became an electrician while working on cable engineering ships between 1878 and 1885. In 1886, Kennelly emigrated to the United States, and joined Thomas Edison as chief assistant for alternating current and electromagnetic studies at the West Orange laboratory. In 1894, Kennelly left Edison to work for the Mexican government in laying cables, but soon joined Edwin J Houston to form their consulting company in Philadelphia. EJ Houston and EJ Kennelly coauthored the book Electricity in Electrotherapeutics, New York in 1896 and 1898. In 1901, he joined the Edison General Electric Co and the General Electric Co of New York as a consulting engineer. Kennelly returned to teaching in 1901 when he became a professor of electrical engineering at Harvard University until 1930. He also taught at the Massachusetts Institute of Technology from 1913 to 1924. He was an exchange professor in France between 1921 and 1924, a research associate of the Carnegie Institution from 1924 to 1930, and a lecturer in Japan in 1931. He discovered a high atmospheric layer of ionized gas that best transmitted radio signals that is know as the Kennelly-Heaviside layer or E region of the atmosphere.[3] Kennelly's medical electrical batteries are of unconventional design. That is, his apparatuses are different than the conventional boxed or cabinet units displayed within this book.

Sinusoidal Apparatus. On the right side of the face plate of the Kennelly Sinusoidal Apparatus with Motor is an alternator that is driven by a small motor (left side) powered by Edison direct current of 110-120 volts. The frame of the alternator is made of laminated iron supported by

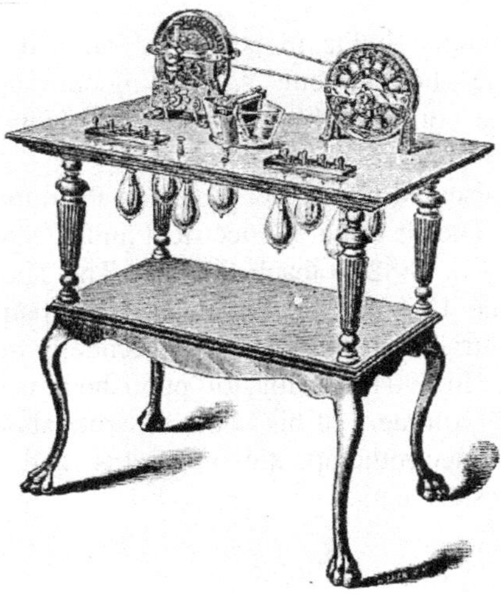

Fig E6. Kennelly Sinusoidal Apparatus with Motor

castings. The alternator has 12 poles; each pole has a spool with two windings of wire. The inner winding of each spool has two layers of fine wire, while the outer winding has two layers of heavy wire.[4]

The inner winding of fine wire is connected in series that forms the secondary coil. Another series is formed by the heavy wire in the outer winding that is the primary coil or field. The continuous primary current is thus transformed into alternating current (AC) in the secondary circuit by driving the armature of the laminate iron discs. By proportioning grooves and projections on the armature the AC becomes a smooth sinusoidal current.[4]

Every revolution of the armature generates 24 alterations that provide 12 periods. The Kennelly unit could achieve 4800 revolutions per minute (115,000 alterations per minute or 1,920 alterations per second).[4] The primary winding of the alternator is powered by 120 volts of direct current that is controlled by a lamp rheostat (underneath the face plate) and operated by a switchboard on the right side of the face plate. This circuit arrangement allows secondary currents to be controlled independently of the frequency.[4]

The lamp rheostat on the left side of the face plate is part of the motor circuit and varies the rate of the motor for control of secondary current alterations. The rheostat in the center of the face plate is connected in shunt with the secondary circuit and varies the amplitude of current applied to the patient. The Figure shows a water rheostat on the face plate.[4]

This unit appears to be two tables, one stacked on top of the other that is of unusual design among American medical electrical batteries. The unit has been traced to 1898 through 1907, but could have been marketed as early as 1894 when Houston-Kennelly consulting company was formed. Kennelly did discuss sinusoidal devices with Dr JH Kellogg in 1893, and apparently did have a unit built (Edison Mfg Co) while still with Edison.

In the mid to late 1890s sinusoidal apparatuses were being marketed, and their designs were either with a permanent magnet or as an electromagnet using a direct current motor. The sources of power for these designs were dry cells for the former and commercial (power grid, direct current) current for the latter. The early units were somewhat bulky. Those requiring dry cells used two to four large acid carbon cells for operating a motor or four or more of the Edison-Lelande cells. So called street current or commercial direct current was the other source for powering these sinusoidal units.

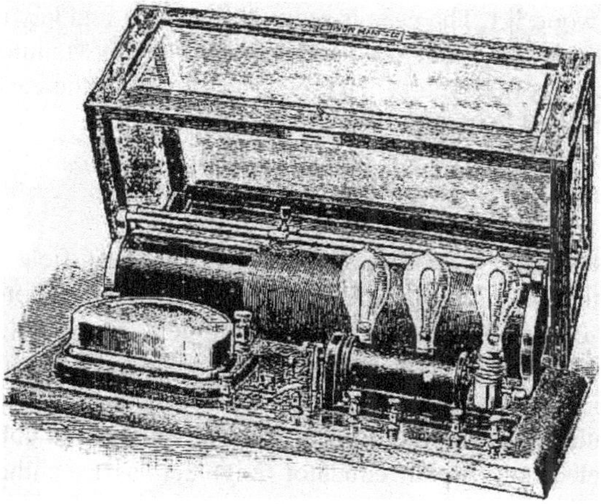

Fig E7. Kennelly Galvanic and Faradic Adapter

Galvanic and Faradic Adapter. Kennelly's Galvanic and Faradic Adapter is a compact apparatus for use with 110 to 120 volts of direct current. This apparatus features a hard rubber cylinder that is wound with designed grooves cut on its face and with several feet of German silver wire that provides very high resistance. On the left end of the cylinder is a very high resistance carbon block that is part of the circuit to offer resistance around 33,000 ohms. The resistance is controlled by sliding the outer part of the cylinder along two rods above and parallel with the cylinder.[4]

A 16 power (cp) lamp is located in the circuit with each wire from the patient to protect against any ill effects from shortening of the circuit. The third lamp (right) has a key arranged in shunt with the resistance. The key, when On, reduces the galvanic current to 60 volts. One milliampere of current is obtained when the binding posts are short circuited when the shunt is operating with all resistance of the rheostat activated in the circuit (moving the sliding contact of the cylinder to the left). When the sliding contact is moved to the right the resistance is decreased that then allows the current amplitude to increase.[4]

Since the lamps decrease current amplitude, a lamp (or lamps) is turned Off with the key. The milliammeter is of Kennelly design (milliammeters were not available in the 1890s to measure AC). A pole changing switch is mounted in the center of the face plate. A faradic coil on the right is also operated by the power grid (street current).[4] The current amplitude from the operating coil was controlled by the DuBois - Reymond sledge inductorium design where the outer coil is moved over the inner coil. Kennelly used the conventional style vibrating interrupter to control the pulse frequencies.

The unit is housed in a glass case that has a wooden base and a hinged glass-wood lid. The case is secured by a lock and key on the front of the base. Kennelly's unit was made by the Edison Manufacturing Co of New York so is believed to have been marketed in the early 1890s. It has been confirmed for 1906.

Summary

This small group of individuals entered the field of medical electrical batteries without decided success. The role of Thomas Edison, Jr, is unclear except for the need for involvement in an area that played on public gullibility and could bring in considerable money. Edwin Houston's contribution was to associate with Edison as a "mucker" and author a popular book in electricity. Arthur Kennelly was outstanding in the field of electricity as an educator, engineer, as an authority of the technology and terminology of electricity. He was renown for his theory of radio waves.

References

1. (www.incwll.com/Biographies/Edison.html), 2003)

2. (www.geocities.com/bioelectrochemistry/houston.html), 2003

3.(www.ieee.org/organizations/history_center/legacies/Kennelly.html), 2003

4. Rockwell AD. The Medical and Surgical Uses of Electricity, new ed. New York, NY, EB Treat & Co, 1907, pp 280-287

PART 3. MANUFACTURERS OF FAMILY (HOME) USE BATTERIES: MAKERS OF HOME SHOCK

The publicity of the effects and popular usage of electrical medical apparatus among physicians during the 1870s and continuing into the 1920s, translated into a demand by the public for electrical treatments in an effort to avoid the fees of the physician. The public wanted a quick fix for medical ills and physical maladies. Manufacturers of medical electrical batteries and apparatuses were of course sensitive to the demands of the public, and always were looking for vehicles to generate more income. Of course medical licensure laws were somewhat lax, as well as the selling of nostrums, patent medicines, and just plain quack devices during this period of time. After all, this was the golden era of the medical electrical apparatuses, and with electricity still in its infancy, without good understanding of its potentials, the batteries were just the ingredient for promised better health. Why not buy an electrical apparatus for $2.95 through the newspaper ads or a mail order catalog that promised an instant cure of all?

This section brings brief histories of a few of the giant makers of home shock. That is, the major manufacturers of medical electrical batteries for the public consumer during the 1870s through the 1920s. Remember, most manufacturers of medical electrical batteries for physicians also appeased the public by offering a "watered down" product line of batteries for home use. Although the competition was very strong, some few companies solely devoted to the public consumer entered the market yet survived for some time. These few companies devoted to the public consumer are the major makers of home shock presented in Part 3.

CHAPTER 16. JH BUNNELL & COMPANY OF NEW YORK CITY

The JH Bunnell & Co of New York City, NY, was a major player in the telegraph business that dominated its manufacturing interest, and it is still in business for that function. The company was also a manufacturer, retailer, and wholesaler of home medical electrical batteries, and a variety of electrical equipment and supplies. The JH Bunnell & Co listed and illustrated its products through its own catalogs as well as through outlets (catalogs, stores) of others. The New No.4 D.D. Home Medical Apparatus of the JH Bunnell & Co is the most widely and frequently seen model of all electrical batteries manufactured for the public consumer.

Biography of Bunnell

Jesse H Bunnell was born in Massillon, OH, in 1843. When he was 11 years of age he delivered telegraph messages, and at 13 years of age he learned to be a telegraph operator. He worked in telegraph offices located in Pennsylvania, and W Virginia from 1859 to 1861. In 1860, when just 17 years old and working in Pennsylvania he forwarded steadily for two hours the last message of President Buchanan to Congress. While telegraphing the message he established a record of an average 32 words per minute.[1]

In 1861, following the attack on Fort Sumter, Charleston, SC, he joined the Union Military Telegraph Service as a telegrapher. The Union corps of telegraphers were civilians[2] who were initially paid $60.00 per month. At first he was assigned to the War Department in Washington, D.C., as a telegraph operator, and where President Lincoln would sometimes go and ask Bunnell for news updates.[1]

In June 1861, he was sent to Annapolis, MD, to establish a telegraphic relay between Annapolis and Washington. In December 1862, Bunnell and 49 other telegraphers petitioned the Government for improved support and pay. When the telegraphers threatened to strike en masse they were countered and accused with an act of conspiracy charge. The telegraphers ended up continuing to serve the Union but also received merit raises, regular transport, and supplies as a result of their political labor actions.[1]

From June 1862 to August 1864, he was assigned to the Army of the Potomac and to the Army of the Cumberland in Tennessee and Georgia. He served in the headquarters of Generals Burnside, McClellan, Rosecrans, Sherman, and Thomas as their personal telegrapher.[2] Exposure to very harsh conditions during the winter of 1864 caused him health problems that resulted in his resignation from the telegraphers corps in August of 1864. While serving as a telegrapher for the Union Army, Bunnell was involved in some of the notable battles of the Civil

War. Bunnell also had observed during the war the few ascensions of balloonists who were wired to send information about enemy troop positions.[1]

Upon his resignation from the Union Army he went to Philadelphia, PA, and became a partner of James Patrick, the successor to Chester, Patrick & Co. The partnership was then called Patrick, Bunnell & Company (manufacturers of telegraphic equipment and electrical supplies) with which he remained from 1864 to 1874.[1] Between 1875 and 1878 he worked for LG Tillotson & Company of New York (manufacturer and seller of telegraph equipment).[1,2]

Late in 1878, JH Bunnell founded his firm as a small manufacturer of bells, buzzers, telegraph keys, and sounders in a shop at 70 Cortland St, NY. (According to EM Kelly the JH Bunnell & Co was founded in 1873 as a manufacturer of communicative equipment, and was first located at 81 Prospect St, Brooklyn, New York[3]) In 1879, he

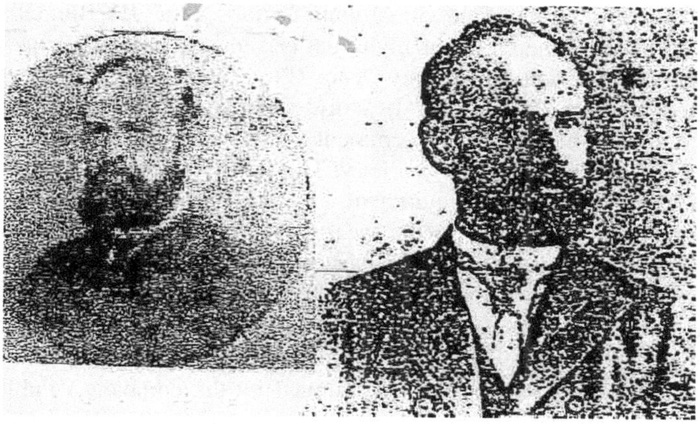

Fig BA. JH BUNNELL[2] At Different Ages

hired Charles McLaughlin as his partner in charge of sales and administration. In just two years he increased his volume of business and gained a national reputation for quality telegraph equipment and supplies so in 1880 he completely reorganized his business to form the JH Bunnell & Co. He then moved to 106-108 Liberty Street (1881 to 1883). Between 1884 and 1889 the company was relocated to 112 Liberty Street. The newly formed JH Bunnell & Co in 1880 increased its volume of manufacturing telegraph apparatus, fire alarm controls, bells, batteries, and miscellaneous electrical equipment (eg, home medical electrical apparatuses).[4]

As the JH Bunnell & Co grew and advanced in technology it moved to various locations in the borough of Manhattan of New York City. From 1890 to 1899, the company office was located at 76 Cortland St, and its factory at 136-138 W 24th Street. The JH Bunnell & Co

Catalogue No. 12 of 1892 gives the address at 76 Cortland Street. The headquarters moved to 20 Park Place, NY, in 1900 and remained there until 1914. Between 1915 and 1924 the company was located at 32 Park Place, NY, and was the address cited in Catalogue No.28 of 1921.[1]

Bunnell introduced several devices into telegraphy that helped advance that field. In 1888, for example, he developed a doublespeed telegraph key called the sideswiper that prevented "glass arms" (carpal tunnel syndrome).[1] Carpal tunnel syndrome is still acquired by workers performing rapid functions with their hands (eg, computer operators, typists, other activities stressing their wrists).

In January 1899, Jesse Bunnell developed a severe cold that his weakened body from the Civil War was unable to fight. On 9 February 1899 (56 years of age) Jesse Bunnell died of heart failure.[1] He was survived by his wife, two daughters, and two sons.[2] He was well known and highly respected during his career as a great telegrapher and entrepreneur in the field of communications. The JH Bunnell & Co telegraph equipment was of high quality and was bought by the United States government over many years (Post Office; military in Spanish American War; World War I; World War II; Cold, Korean, and Viet Nam Wars), the Mexican government and Latin American countries; and the United Kingdom for its military. The JH Bunnell & Co manufactured and sold fire and safety equipment, and then in the 1930s through 1950s commercial radios. In recent years the company has produced fax transmitters and today produces mostly microwave equipment.[1]

Following Bunnell's death, Charles McLaughlin operated the company. In the 1920s JJ Ghegan was made president and introduced many innovations. (This may have been the time when The Home Medical Battery series was discontinued by the company.) Public faith and interest in the medical electrical battery decreased in the 1920s. (The Congress and Food and Drug Administration tightened the laws on sales of medical products to the public, and with these events the profit in such devices was no longer worth the efforts to many manufacturers.–ed) Ghegan was succeeded by JG Dougherty who was then succeeded by his wife who sold the firm in the 1960s to INSO Electronic Products with CJ Meislich as president. JH Jacobs became president of the company in 1989 when it was acquired as a division by MNJ Industrials. Upon the death of JH Jacobs, Matt Jacobs bought and still operates the company.[1]

As noted, the JH Bunnell & Co moved to several locations during its 50 plus years in the borough of Manhattan, NY. In the 1930s, the JH Bunnell & Co moved some of its operation to Brooklyn, NY, but it maintained headquarters at 32 Park Place, NY, for a long period of time. In 1949, while having its general sales office at 215 Fulton Street, Manhattan, NY, it maintained its manufacturing division at 81 Prospect Street, Brooklyn, NY. In the 1940s and 1950s the JH Bunnell & Co was making special communication equipment for the largest communication companies and organizations. In the 1960s (1963 to 1968), all operations of the company were located at 920 Essex Street, Brooklyn. When INSO Electronic Products acquired the company in the 1960s it was moved to 166 Babylon Turnpike, Roosevelt, NY. From 1968 to 1988 the INSO Electronic Products moved to 80 Locust Drive, Kings Park, NY, where it remains presently.[1]

Prior to World War II, JH Bunnell & Co was the major manufacturer of telegraph keys in the United States. During World War II, the company peaked in production and employed 600 workers. Selective telegraph items (eg, keys and sounders) have been manufactured as miniatures to be awarded to individuals (President Eisenhower, Sarnoff of RCA), and sold for personal wear as tie pins and watch fobs.[1] The JH Bunnell & Co manufactured and sold medical electrical batteries mostly for home use. These batteries were developed and sold early in the company's history (1880 to at least 1919).

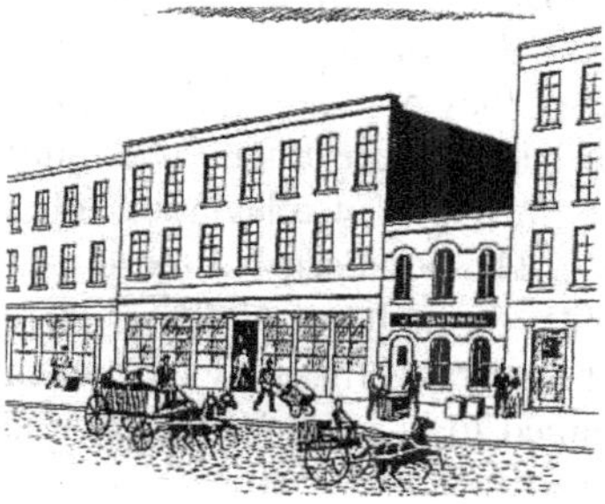

Fig B1. Bunnell Office of 1880[1]

Commonalties of Bunnell Batteries

JH Bunnell & Co apparently made only dry cell powered faradic medical electrical batteries between 1880 and the 1920s. Many of the company's faradic batteries were sold through retailers other than through its own factory. Thus, many of the faradic batteries manufactured by the JH Bunnell & Co do not carry the Bunnell name or logo. Collectors must identify most JH Bunnell & Co batteries by their specific characteristics or commonalties. Units sold directly from the JH Bunnell & Co do usually, however, carry the firm's name on a plate, by recess, or by label.

The end caps on the induction coils are circular and are offset by being slightly larger than the diameter of the coil. Other manufacturers used circular end caps on their coils also, but the batteries of others can usually be identified by other features. The interrupter is the other major identifying feature. The vibrating interrupter and the adjustable screw contact are on the same base mounted at one end of the coil. Most other manufacturers used interrupters that were mounted on the face plate by two or more bases that separated its parts into components rather than as a single unit like Bunnell & Co. The interrupters that control pulse frequencies were mounted by Bunnell in two ways. Some units (viz, The New No.4 Home Medical Apparatus set) have the interrupter mounted vertically to the face plate, while other units made by Bunnell have the interrupters mounted in the usual horizontal fashion to the face plate.

The Home Medical Apparatus Set

Although JH Bunnell & Co made and sold several models of medical electrical batteries, the company specifically manufactured and sold the ***Home Medical Battery*** set that is so commonly seen in antique shops, auction sales, and flea markets. This set consists of two Home Medical Apparatuses: 1) The ***New No.4 Home Medical Apparatus***, and 2) The ***New No.4 D.D. Home Medical Apparatus***. These two battery models have become collector items, and are symbolic of the home use electrical battery. Also, they are very commonplace because of their past popularity with the public consumer. The public bought the Home Medical Apparatuses in hopes of alleviating ailments without incurring the fees of physicians. The popularity of these two particular apparatuses ranged from the 1890s through the 1920s. The first unit was The New No.4 Home Medical Apparatus that may have been introduced in 1880 or 1881 and was continued to at least 1892. The succeeding unit was The New No.4 D.D. Home Medical Apparatus that was introduced in 1892.

Dating the Home Medical Apparatuses may be done by the address on their labels. If Bunnell batteries have the address of 70 Cortland Street on the label inside of the lid they were made from 1878 to 1880. From 1880 to 1884 the JH Bunnell & Co was located at 106-108 Liberty Street, and between 1884 and 1890 at 112 Liberty Street. Many units of JH Bunnell & Co often seen in antique shops have 76 Cortland Street which was the address of the company from 1890 to 1900. During this period of time (1890 to 1900), the signature label (inside lid) of the Home Medical Apparatuses came with or recommended the use of a Burnley dry cell to power the unit. The Burnley dry cell was a standard sized cell (6.25 x 2.5 inches) that was patented on 2 January 1890.

About 1900, the company was using the MESCO (Manhattan Electrical Supply Co) dry cell to accompany these home medical batteries. This recommendation, along with the standard dry cell, also continued while the company was located at its Park Place address (1900-1914).

In the hands of professionals these electrical apparatuses had some value as treatments, although with limits. In the hands of the public consumer the treatments generally were a disappointment. Booklets and manuals accompanying the sale of home units were also of very limited value to the consumer because the booklets promoted the medical electrical battery for cures that could never be realized. Because of the disappointments of the consumer in alleviating a variety of ailments the sales began a gradual decline in the early twentieth century. Yet, the public consumer despite treatment failures was gullible enough to buy these units from the 1880s into the 1920s. The home user most often put aside the battery after several trials. The home batteries ended up in attics, and as a result the electrical medical apparatuses found today are usually still operational, and frequently the wooden boxes encasing the operating components are in good condition because of limited use. These electrical apparatuses are still being found in grand (great) mother's attic.

Collectors are often confronted with missing dry cell cylinders from both of the New No.4 Home Medical Apparatus, and the New No.4 D.D. Home Medical Apparatus. Original buyers probably tried to pawn or sell the nickel plated dry cell cylinder of their batteries believing that they are made of silver. This approach not only did not recoup the cost of the battery, but it lowered the resale price as an antique. If true the original buyer theoretically lost on two accounts, but in reality the cost of the unit or artifact as an antique may have adequately compensated the family of the original buyer.

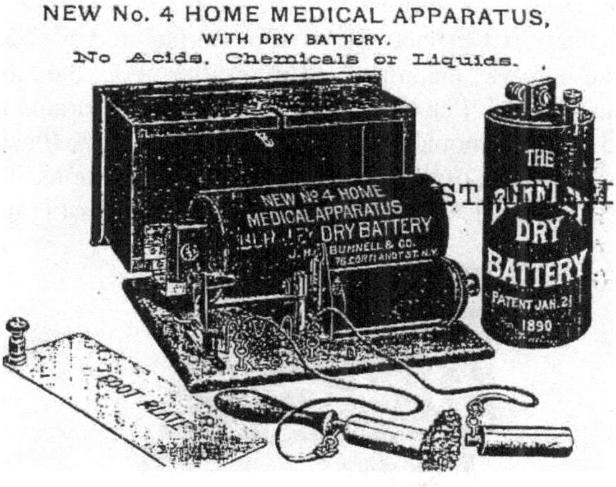

Fig B2. The New No. 4 Home Medical Battery

The New No.4 Home Medical Apparatus may have been introduced as early as 1880, surely by 1890 when the Burnley Dry Cell Battery of standard size (6.25 inches high x 2.25 inches diameter) and patented on 21 January 1890 was used in the Bunnell units. The New No.4 Home Medical Apparatus contains a nickel plated battery cylinder that is hinged at one end so that it could be raised to change the dry cell when exhausted. The nickel plated cylinder is also recessed with

"Burnley pat Jan 1889." The JH Bunnell & Co sold the apparatus including one dry cell for $7.50 from 1880 to 1892. The same device was sold and illustrated in the 1894-1895[5] and 1903-1904[6] catalogs of Montgomery Ward & Co of Chicago for $7.00. An extra battery cost $0.90 and an extra sponge holder was $0.50. An extra metallic hairbrush electrode was sold for $1.25.[7]

The JH Bunnell & Co advertised the unit for both physician and home use, but its major consumer was the public. This No. 4 battery had a single lid, and the base or face panel contained the induction coil, the rheotome (adjustable spring vibrating interrupter), an On/Off switch, and a dry cell and cylinder. The wiring of the electrical circuit was recessed into the bottom of the wooden case, and then covered with buckram (leatherette like) or a fabric. These devices folded into the oak (some were mahogany) box (8.25 x 5.25 x 4 inches with lipped top and bottom) for storage along with the accessories. The apparatus and accessories sold by Bunnell for $7.50 in 1892. This set of home use medical electrical batteries was perhaps the most successfully mass produced apparatuses of all medical electrical batteries.

In 1892, the JH Bunnell & Co came out with an updated or the second version of The Home Medical Apparatus that is known as The New No.4 D.D. Home Medical Apparatus (Fig B3), and was continued to at least 1919. The address of The New No 4 D.D. Home Medical Apparatus has 76 Cortland Street if manufactured between 1892 and 1900. If the unit was manufactured in or after 1900, the label of the unit should read 20 Park Place. The Home Medical Apparatus manufactured from 1915 to 1924 should have the address of 32 Park Place on the label located on the inside of the bottom lid with the directions. The New No.4 D.D. Home Medical Apparatus was probably the most popular electrical

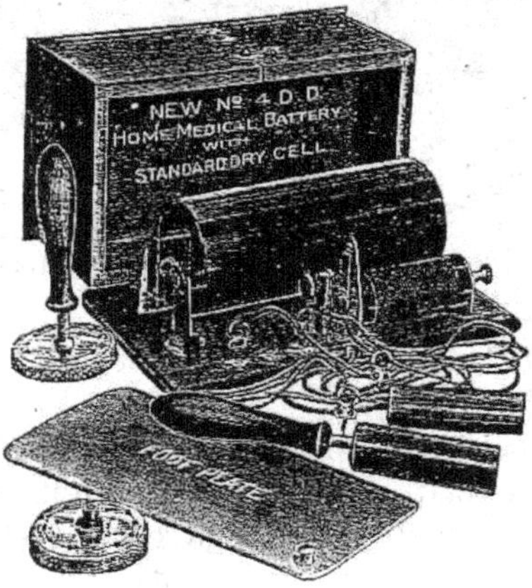

Fig B3. The New No. 4 D.D. Home Medical Battery

battery ever sold for home use. Although not confirmed by any literature of the JH Bunnell & Co, the "D.D." part of the model name may stand for double doors. Double doors or lids are the only major feature of difference between the earlier New No.4 Medical Home Apparatus and the newer New No.4 D.D. Home Medical Battery.

The obvious difference between the two Home Medical Apparatus is that the case of the first or the original New No.4 unit of the 1880s has one lid. One lid meant that both circuit operational components and accessories were contained in a single compartment of the wooden box. Most of these earliest units had mahogany boxes to house their operational components. The latter unit or The New No.4 D.D. apparatus was introduced in 1892. The D.D. unit has two lids rather than one lid, and the "D.D." was added to its name in the signature label on the inside of the top lid. The two lids allowed for two different compartments in the wooden box. One compartment housed the operational components of the apparatus while the other compartment stored the accessories. The latter D.D. model (1892 and later) was issued with either mahogany or oak cases (ca 8.5 x 5 x 4.5 inches with lipped top and bottom). Although mahogany was available in the United States then, it became less available by the 1890s while oak, another hard wood, was available more and probably cheaper than mahogany. Thus, the appearance of one versus two lids, the "D.D." in its name, and the type of wood, mahogany versus oak, are the noticeable differences to the consumer or collector. Both The New No.4 and The New No.4 D.D. apparatus of the late 1890s were often sold with MESCO dry cells. The Burnley battery was associated with Bunnell early on (late 1880s and

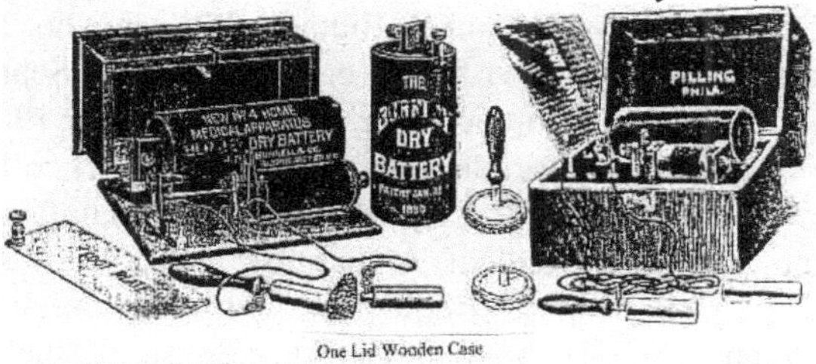

One Lid Wooden Case

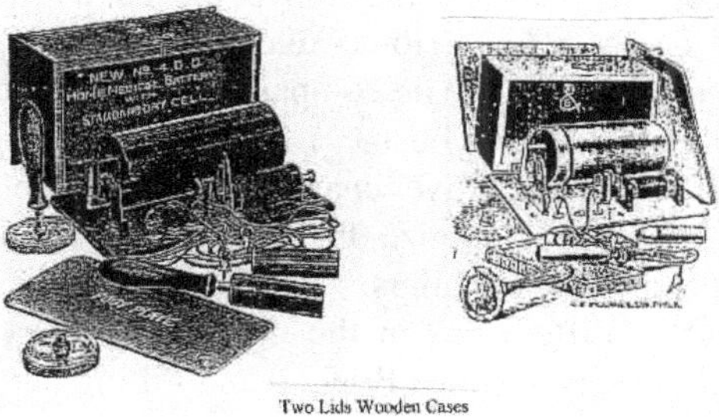

Two Lids Wooden Cases

Fig B4. Bunnell and Pilling Faradic Battereis of The New No. 4 Style early 1890s), but by the late 1890s the MESCO dry cell seemed to have been the choice to accompany By 1904 or 1905, the MESCO dry cell seemed to have been replaced by the JH Bunnell Dry Battery or any standard dry cell of that period of time (1900 to 1920s) as basic issue with each of the No.4 D.D. batteries.

The JH Bunnell & Co and The George P Pilling & Son Co of Philadelphia, PA, manufactured and retailed two models (Fig B4) having almost the same characteristics that collectors must recognize. All models of The New No.4 style were designed for home use. Each company manufactured a wooden box model with one lid, and each made a like version having two lids on their wooden boxes. Although almost similar the electrical components mounted on the face plates of the models have some subtle differences. JH Bunnell & Co originated both the one lid and two lids models. The original one lid No.4 Home Apparatus was designed and marketed by the JH Bunnell & Co in 1880 or 1881, while the comparative model by George P Pilling & Son Co was manufactured and marketed from about 1900 to 1932. JH Bunnell & Co introduced The New No.4 D.D. Home Medical Battery that was similar to its No.4 Home Apparatus in 1892. The New No.4 D.D. Medical Battery was encased in a wooden box having two lids. The Philadelphia Single Cell Battery of George P Pilling & Son Co that is comparable to the New No.4 D.D. Medical Battery of the JH Bunnell & Co was introduced in 1900.

Usually Pilling & Son placed a label or recessed their name into the lid of their electrical batteries for easy identification. Many of these medical electrical apparatuses of exact design and dimensions were manufactured by the two companies (Bunnell, Pilling) who labeled their products using the name of the retailer (eg, George Frye; Sears, Roebuck and Co). This practice of manufacturing and then using the retailers name on the label of the finished product may be confusing to collectors. The JH Bunnell & Co of New York City was the major manufacturer of this particular set of Home Medical Apparatus, however, this particular battery may be found more frequently with other retailers' labels (signatures) than with JH Bunnell & Co because of the company's business practices. JH Bunnell may have played a greater role as a manufacturer of The New No.4 Home Medical Apparatus than it did as a retailer of this particular item. The company did well with this approach in its medical electrical battery business. Because of these trade practices and because of the comparative characteristics of the four different models, collectors must recognize the models by manufacturer traits rather than labels of various retailers.

Besides the differences in the number of lids on the wooden boxes, labels, differences between Bunnell and Pilling faradic batteries of the New No.4 style reside in the design of their induction coils. The JH Bunnell & Co capped the ends of its coils with wooden circular discs or caps, while the George Pilling & Son Co capped the ends of their coils with square wooden discs or caps.

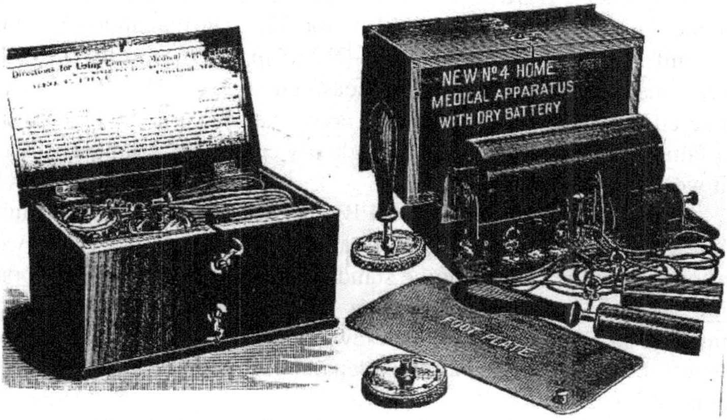

Fig B5. The Frye Label on The New No. 4 D.D. Battery

Fig B5 exemplifies the New No.4 D.D. battery manufactured by JH Bunnell & Co, but retailed with the retailer's name or trade mark on the label of the unit. The retail medical supplier George C Frye of Portland, ME, about the turn of the century, sold a medical electrical apparatus exactly like The New No.4 D.D. (Fig B5, left). Home Medical Apparatus, but labeled it the Congress Medical Apparatus. This unit was offered by the retailer with a MESCO dry cell of standard size. All features of the Congress unit with the Frye label resemble the style of those manufactured by JH Bunnell & Co as the New No. 4 D.D. Home Medical Apparatus. Pilling & Son Co made and marketed two faradic units with the "Congress" title, but these units were not The New No.4 style. The Pilling's Congress models have a unique style of encasement (box), triangular when open. This other style of faradic battery made by Pilling (Congress), but labeled for George C Frye Co (Congress) should not be confused with the New No.4 D.D. unit of Bunnell (see Pilling earlier).

The New No.4 D.D. Home Medical Battery retailed for $7.00 to $10.00 over the years when sold directly by Bunnell. That cost was set with the original apparatus in 1892 and continued among units sold through 1919. The original retail price of The New No.4 Home Medical Apparatus (1880 to 1908) was set as $7.50 by the JH Bunnell & Co in 1892 and was still sold by Bunnell at that price in 1901 according to company catalogs of those years. The apparatus was discounted, however, by the giant mail order retailers Montgomery Ward & Co and Sears, Roebuck and Co of Chicago. The catalog of the Montgomery Ward & Co of 1894-1895 listed the apparatus for $7.50,[5] but the Sears,

Roebuck and Co of 1897 listed the unit for $5.95.[9] The catalog of MESCO of 1900 listed the apparatus for $7.00, while the 1904 catalog of the Montgomery Ward & Co listed the machine for $3.00.[6] The Sears, Roebuck and Co listed the apparatus for $2.95 in its catalog of 1908.[10] This unit illustrated and listed as K 21350 (page 514) in the 1903-1904 Montgomery Ward & Co catalog measured (4.5 x 5.25 x 9 inches), and delivered primary, secondary, and combination currents for physician and family use. Complete with a single dry cell (extra cell cost $0.25) the unit weighed six pounds.[6]

No.4 D.D. Home Medical Battery was the most popular unit of public consumers. The unit was durable, reliable, and not too powerful for home use. The unit used one standard size dry cell. The Electropathic Guide by SM Wells, revised edition 15 of 1899[11] (as did other editions from 1892 to 1919) featured The New No.4 D.D. Home Medical Battery that was considered the most convenient form of medical battery ever produced.

The unit had two lids on its highly polished oak case with a nickel plated handle. The usual case is 9 x 5.25 x 4.5 inches in size, and complete with a dry cell weighs about 5.5 pounds. The upper compartment of the case housed the accessories that included two conducting cords each of four feet length, two tube handle electrodes, two insulating handles (wood) for use with hand or sponge electrodes, two sponge electrodes, and one foot plate. Its lower compartment contains the On/Off switch, rheotome (current interrupter) that hums or vibrates with the switch on, a contact screw that was adjustable to give even and continuous humming or buzzing sounds, and the cylinder to house the cell. All hardware on this unit are characteristically nickel plated. The apparatus provides three different currents. The mildest form of current was from the primary coil (posts 1 & 2); then came the second current from the secondary coil (posts 2 & 3), and finally the combined primary & secondary currents (posts 1 & 3). The apparatus used a standard sized dry cell that could be purchased locally. These standard cells usually lasted from four to 12 months according to the length and frequency of time used in the medical electrical apparatus. The JH Bunnell & Co and its retailers sold the unit for $10.00, an extra cell for $0.50, sponge electrode and handles for $1.50, tube handle electrode was $1.00, and the hair brush electrode for $1.75. A copy of The Electropathic Guide was given with each electrical apparatus purchased.

Dry Cells

The MESCO dry cell was considered to be the most satisfactory and reliable of all available dry cells at the time (ca mid 1890s to1900).[5] The maker and retail resource of the MESCO dry cell was the Manhattan Electrical Supply Company of New York City, NY. This company was a retailer of a wide variety of electrical equipment and supplies, but was the manufacturer of the MESCO dry cell. MESCO did not make The New No.4 or The New No.4 D.D. apparatuses. The company sold these items with its MESCO dry cell. JH Bunnell & Co (both manufacturer and retailer) manufactured some products for the Manhattan Electrical Supply Co (eg, a variety of medical electrical batteries with MESCO labels) and probably through contractual agreement JH Bunnell & Co outfitted many of its Home Medical Apparatuses with MESCO dry cells, and MESCO in turn sold the Home Medical Apparatuses for retail.

The Burnley dry cell was a standard sized battery that was patented on 2 January 1890, made and promoted by the JH Bunnell & Co. This battery was manufactured and sold through Bunnell for use with its medical electrical batteries, bells, alarms, and telephones from 1890 to 1900.

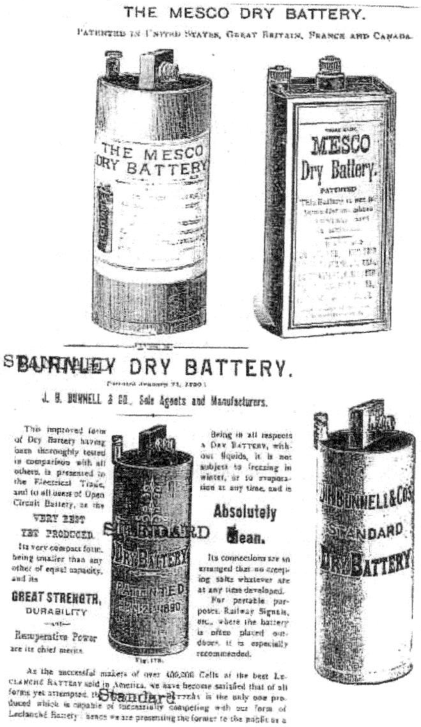

Fig B6. MESCO, Burnley, and JH Bunnell Dry Cells

By 1905, both the Burnley and MESCO dry cells were being replaced by the JH Bunnell & Co Standard Dry Battery (6.25 x 2.5 inches) or any other standard dry cell purchased at any electrical store. The New No.4 units have a nickel plated cylinder designed to hold any standard dry cell of the time period (1890 to 1920s).

Bunnell Literature. The Electropathic Guide was written by SM Wells who was a medical electrician from Beaver Dam, WI. Wells first published his booklet in 1867. The first three editions were titled

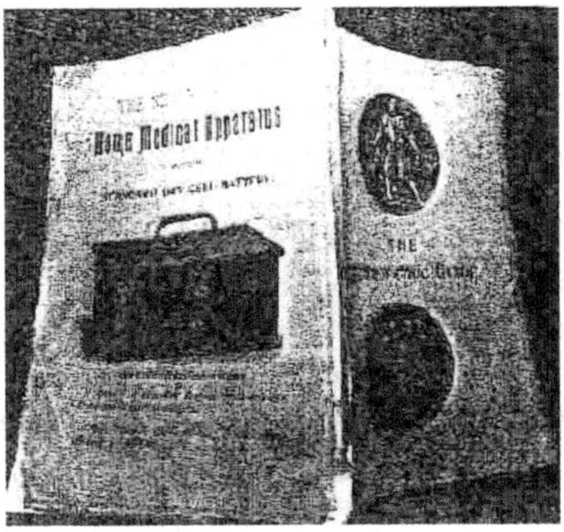

Fig B7. The Electropathic Guide[11]

The Electropathic Guide: Prepared with Particular Reference to Home Practice; containing hints on the care of the sick, the treatment of disease, and the use of electricity. His third edition was published about 1872 (not dated). SM Wells used the title of "medical electrician." His brother, WR Wells, MD, was a physician in Mount Morris, NY, and is believed to have planted the idea and need for a cheap and reliable home use medical electrical battery with instructions. SM Wells may have then taken WR's idea and then designed a battery that met the ideas formed by WR Wells in his books A New Theory of Disease Based Upon the Principle that Man is a Compound Electrical Magnet;...... in 1862 and 1869.[12] In the first edition of SM's book (1867, 90 pp) the "Prof WR Wells Battery" was featured and illustrated. SW Wells who is listed as seller in his third edition of the booklet also sold his booklet for $1.00 each. The Prof WR Wells Battery was manufactured in Boston by Thomas Hall (maker of custom apparatuses). The unique feature of this home use battery is the copper trough wet cell that was made by Thomas Hall but sold under the names of the sellers. The ninth edition (1888) of the guide contained the same long title as the original, and was published in Chicago, IL (see Chapter 3).

SM Wells, and perhaps with WR Wells, lectured prior to publishing his Electropathic Guide. The first edition (1867) states that "In offering this little book to the public…for our pupils, and those who had attended our lectures…"[12] The first edition of the book is hard cover, while those published later for JH Bunnell & Co in the 1890s are paper covered. SM Wells also changed publishers in the 1890s. "Wells lectures in electropathy" were sold for $1.00 as stated in the first edition.

In 1899, the 15th edition of the SM Wells' booklet was published by JH Bunnell & Co of New York City. In 1899, Wells added ...with Full Directions for Treating Over 100 Diseases to the title following the word "electricity" in the third edition. The 15th edition was revised; however, others between 1872 and 1899 must also have been revised. Simple arithmetic indicates that SM Wells published a new edition on the average of every 1.5 years. SM Wells may have begun writing his booklet for the JH Bunnell Co around 1892.

A free copy of the Wells' booklet was given to the customer of the No.4 batteries by the JH Bunnell & Co; otherwise the 100 paged (including advertisements) booklet sold for $0.75 with paper and $1.50 with cloth bindings through Bunnell.

Some statements in the 15th edition of The Electropathic Guide are noteworthy. The booklet avoids technicalities and uses simple terms rather than medical language. On page 13 the name of the battery uses D.D. for discussion, yet pages 14 and 15 that illustrate the battery do not use "D.D," but use "New No.4 Home Medical Apparatus." The author on page 12 states that the unit provides two currents, primary and secondary; yet on page 16 discusses three currents, primary, secondary, and combined. On page 19 the author talks about "unhealthy diseases." Actually, the contents of Wells' book and booklets change little over the many editions (a total of 10 pages that include listing and descriptions of The Home Battery series of JH Bunnell & Co). One could speculate that edition really refers to printing with the many editions. Wells illustrated

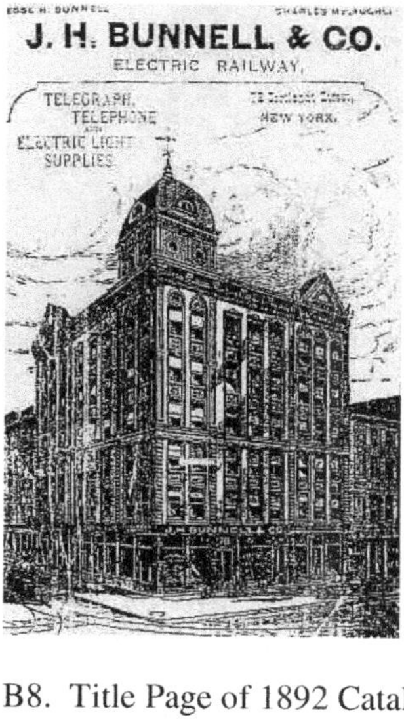

Fig B8. Title Page of 1892 Catalog[7]

only Bunnell products with his 1890s booklets, while the first few editions promoted the Wells' Double-Current Electropathic Instrument (Professor WR Wells Battery); see Chapter 3.

The first edition of the JH Bunnell & Co trade catalog was published in 1881, the 12th edition in 1892, and the 15th edition in 1899. Catalogue No. 12 of 1892 devoted about 40 of 224 pages to cells, medical electrical apparatus, and their accessories. At least 18 different makes of cells were offered that included such notable trade names as: Bunsen, Burnley, Edison, Grenet, Law, and Leclanche. Also, offered in the 1892 Catalogue were a variety of sizes of porous cells, and glass battery jars.[7]

Additional Faradic Batteries & Magnetoelectric Units

The same catalog (1892) illustrated and listed five Home Medical Apparatuses that the company manufactured, and each was numbered and listed. Number 1 was the Home Medical Battery that was powered by a single Grenet wet cell. The complete unit (with cell) sold for $6.50. An extra cell was $2.00 and its replacement elements were zinc at $0.25, and carbon for $0.30 each. Powdered bichromate potash was used to make the cell solution and sold for $0.25 per pound in 1901.

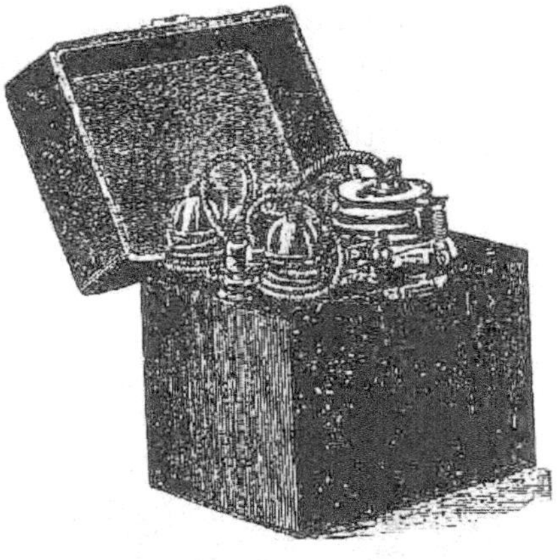

Fig B9. Home Medical Battery, from No. 1[6]

Home Medical Battery. The unit is encased in a wooden box with a self locking device on its front. A metal carrying handle is on top of the box. The unit delivers primary, secondary, and combined currents. The induction coil is underneath the face plate and has a sliding metal current controller. The coil is less powerful than unit No.3. The top of the Grenet type cell is exposed so that connection with the circuitry can be made easily from the top. Slots in the face plate accommodate the handle style electrodes. This unit dates from 1890.

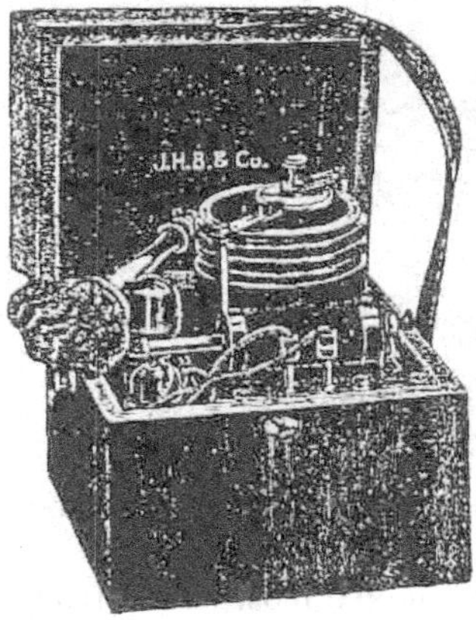

Fig B10. The Home Medical Battery, Improved Form "Number Two"

Number Two. This unit was an improved form of The Home Medical Battery No.1 for $9.00 in 1892.[7] The ability of this faradic battery to provide a power supply for six weeks to three months without having to change the battery solution was a major attraction. Like the wet cell the Fuller mercury bichromate battery of JH Bunnell & Co contained zinc and carbon elements in a porous jar, binding posts, and a sealed rubber top. Both the elements and fluid, however, could be replaced when necessary thus saving the jar and top. This type of cell seemed to be the pivot type between the wet and dry cell batteries. The Fuller battery was superior to the Grenet battery.

The Number Two or The Home Medical Battery provides three currents (primary, secondary, combined) and is encased in a polished walnut box. The hinged lid is secured in front with a self locking device. A leather strap is used to carry the box and is secured on each side of the box. The induction coil is mounted on top of the face plate, and is enclosed at its ends by circular caps. The coil has a sliding metal current controller. Four buttons on the top front of the face plate are available to connect the unit with the subject. Slots are cut into the face plate to hold the handle style electrodes. This unit was first offered in 1890.

Number Three. The unit of Fig B11 was the six currents Home Medical Battery of JH Bunnell & Co. The unit has a triple type induction coil, and was powered by a single hermetically sealed cell (Fuller type). The induction coil is wound to serve as three coils (approach used by J Kidder and McIntosh companies) that were popular briefly but not effective physiologically. The induction coil is mounted on top of the face plate and has circular end caps. The sliding metal current controller

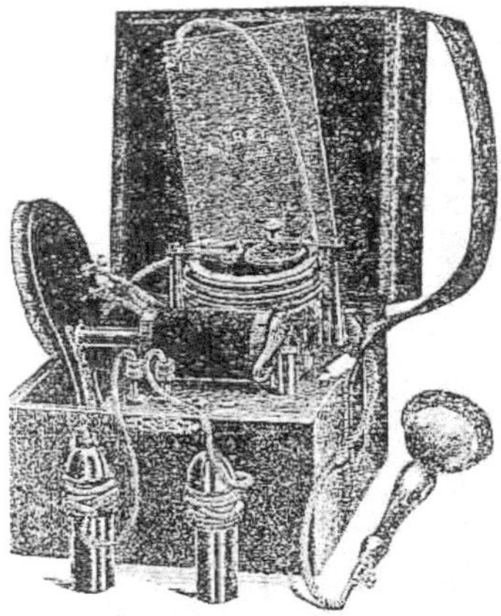

Fig B11. Home Medical Battery, "Number Three"

moves from the left side (unlike most other brands), while the vibrating interrupter and adjustable screw are on the same base on the right side of the coil. Four buttons are available to connect electrodes. Like the Number Two unit this device was housed in a polished walnut box with a hinged lid that is secured by a self locking device. It sold for $14.00; an extra dry cell was $2.00. The Number Three battery was being sold in 1900.[13]

Number 5. This battery (Fig B12) was called The Faraday Battery that contained a standard (6.25 x 2.25 inches) Burnley Dry Cell. The Faradic Battery No.5 complete with the standard dry cell sold for $6.00 in 1900.[10] This is the only battery designed and advertised for parlor entertainment as well as medical care. (The static machines of the 18th century were often used for parlor entertainment in England.) One

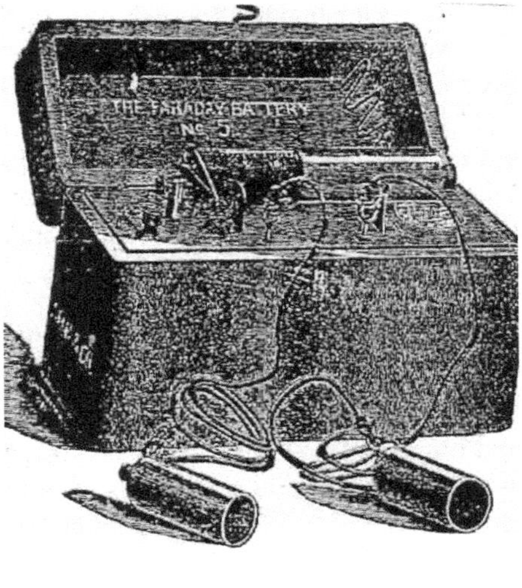

Fig B12. The Faraday Battery No. 5

dry cell powers the unit and is located underneath the face plate. The induction coil is mounted on top of the face plate with its sliding metal current controller located on the outside (rather than inside) of the coil. The vibrating interrupter and adjustable contact screw are on the same base.

The unit is enclosed in a wooden box with a hinged lid that is secured by a single hook latch on front and is carried by a metal carrying handle on top. An On/Off switch is available on the face plate. Two buttons are present to connect the battery with the subject.

No.6 Home Double Power Electro Medical Battery. The JH Bunnell & Co did offer two other small units in its product line of electrical batteries. The No.6 Home Double Power Electro Medical Battery (Fig B13) that sold for $12.00 in 1901[14] used two standard dry cells (extra cell $0.50) that were located underneath the face plate. This particular unit's induction coil provided more current amplitude than other faradic units of the JH Bunnell & Co. The coil was closed by circular end caps at each end and was mounted on top of the face plate. The face plate also contains a reversible pole changing switch, and battery switches for controlling current amplitude (no sliding metal current controller was used). Three buttons are available on the face plate to connect the battery to the patient according to the currents desired. A wooden box with a hinged lid contains the electrical components. A metal carrying handle is on top of the lid, and a key and lock on front secures the lid. The accessories (including an electromedical brush) are

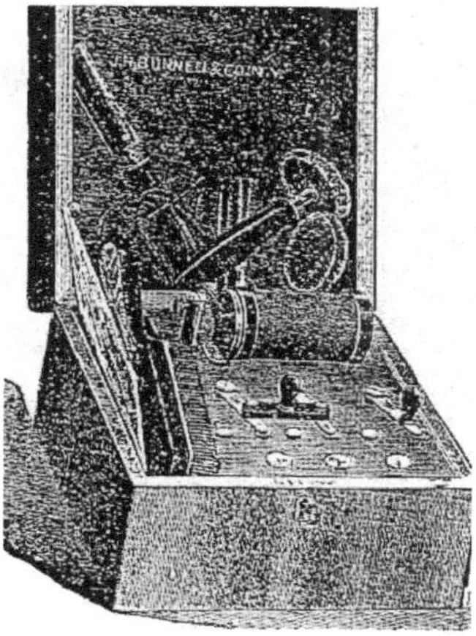

Fig B13. The No. 6 Home Double Power Electro Medical Battery

held in the inside lid and in an open compartment on the left side of the face plate. In 1899, this same No.6 model sold for $15.00. The electromedical brush was especially designed for application with animals in veterinary practices.

Magnetoelectrical Unit. The company sold a novel unit that today could be considered a toy. The "C" type magnetic electrical units with a hand crank has no case but it has a circular oak base of 4.75 inches diameter. Imprinted on the oak base is "Patented April 27, 1897." It sold for $1.00 from 1897 to 1901.[14] On the wooden base is mounted a horseshoe magnet (3.5 x 1.5 x 2 inches). Between the legs of the magnet

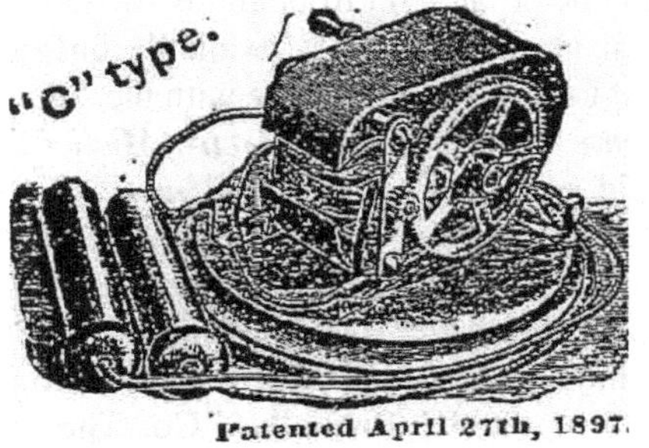

Fig B14. 1897 Magnetoelectrical Unit

is mounted a small coil (1.5 x 0.75 inches) that is rotated by a manually operated crank attached to a brass cogwheel (2 inches in diameter). This little unit can pack a punch, and be packed easily or carried for travel.

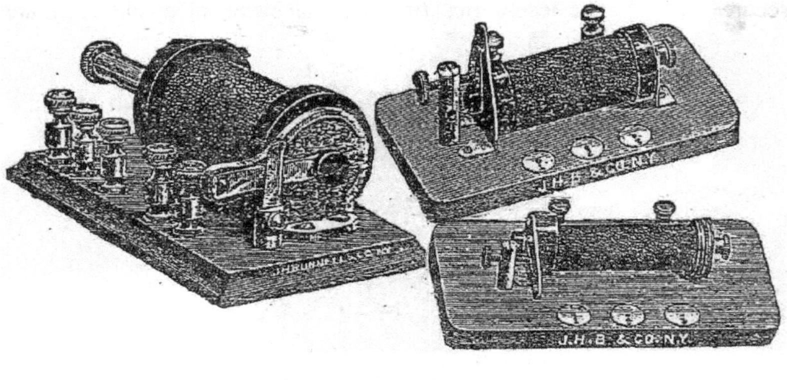

Fig B15. Small Induction Coils

The JH Bunnell & Co illustrated a variety of ***Small Induction Coils*** for $4.00, $3.50, and $3.00, respectively in 1901.[14] Each unit contains a coil with circular end caps, a vibrating interrupter and an adjustable contact screw on the same base, and a sliding metal current controller. Cells to power each unit are located externally to each unit. These three small coils provided the home user basic faradic currents at low costs, and without containers.

Improved Medical Induction Coils. MESCO offered two small induction coils that were slight variations to those cited above. The coil and vibrating interrupters are similar to both units. Only the wooden bases, connecting posts (3), connecting (battery to subject) buttons (2), and costs ($2.40 and $2.00, respectively) differ. All of these medical electrical units were manufactured by JH Bunnell & Co around 1900 to 1905, but were retailed by both the JH Bunnell & Co and MESCO. These two small induction coils differ from the three in Fig B15 by the addition

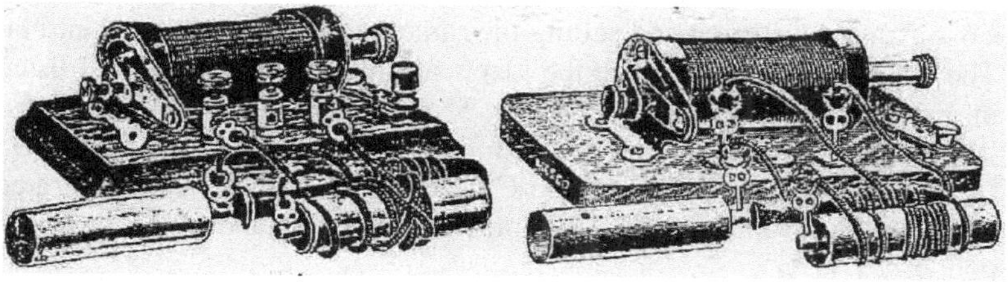

Fig B15A. Improved Medical Induction Coils

of On/Off switches, and variation in the rheotomes. These coils or faradic batteries are operationally similar to the boxed units, but they cut costs that greatly reduced prices to increase conveniences of compactness.

Other Units. The JH Bunnell & Co offered other medical electrical batteries for sale in its 1892 catalog.[7] The Magnetic Electrical Machine (Davis/Kidder type) of Fig B16 was illustrated, and sold for $8.00. This unit is often seen in antique shops and auction sales, and is very popular among collectors. The unit is often represented as being patented in 1854 or 1859, and designed after the well known instrument maker Ari (brother of Daniel, Jr) Davis of Boston and Washington and

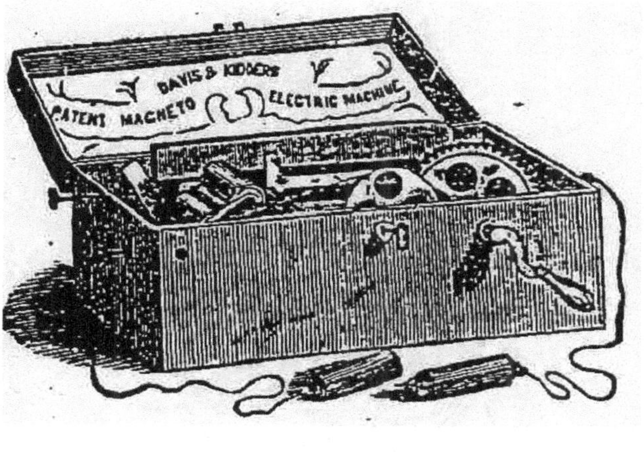

Fig B16. Davis/Kidder Units

financial supporter Walter Kidder of New York City. The Davis/Kidder type of magnetoelectrical machine that was dated 1870 is labeled on the inside of its lid with WH Burnap of New York City as the manufacturer and sole proprietor. Dr Jerome Kidder (manufacturer and retailer of quality electrical equipment for physicians), and frequently confused for Walter Kidder publicly stated that he had no involvement with any medical electrical machines with the name of Davis. The 1892 catalog (p 74) of JH Bunnell & Co was selling the unit as indicated for $8.00. The Davis & Kidder logo was still on the label so assumedly JH Bunnell & Co was manufacturing and selling the same unit that Burnap sold earlier. The same was still true since the identical unit was illustrated and listed in the catalog of 1901 (p 59) for $8.00. Montgomery Ward & Co illustrated and listed the same item for $7.25 in its catalog of 1894-1895 (p 209).[5] The Sears, Roebuck and Co catalog of 1897 (p 478) illustrated and listed the unit for $6.75 complete with cell and weighing 5.75 pounds.[9]

JH Bunnell & Co did illustrate and list No.4 while only listing Nos.5 & 6 medical electrical batteries of Kidder. Since the Jerome Kidder Manufacturing Company was still in business (1865 to at least 1904) when No.12 catalog of Bunnell was published in 1892, it is conjectured that the items were being retailed to attract and solicit business from physicians. The JH Bunnell & Co customarily made and directed its battery business toward the public consumer.[7]

Number 4 was an apparatus advertised as an office and family machine. This unit functions as three coils and delivered variations of six currents. The unit was powered by one sealed cell of the Fuller type, and complete with accessories sold for $20.00.

The ***Number 5*** unit was the same as No.4 but had four coils wound in a single induction coil, and a hydrostat tip cell battery. The

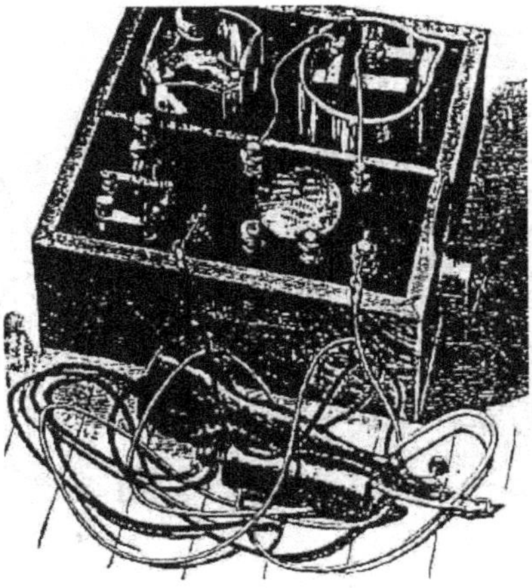

Fig B17. Dr Kidder's Batteries Nos. 4, 5 & 6

windings of the coil were so arranged in various combinations to produce 10 different qualities of faradic currents. It sold for $27.00 complete. Without a tip type cell (patented in 1872) the same battery sold for $24.00.

Number 6, Small Electro-Medical Machine. This unit was the same as the No.4 Kidder machine but smaller in size. Machine numbers 4 and 5 had superior current qualities than this particular unit (No.6). The No.6 machine sold for $15.00.

The different batteries above had varied tappings and windings of the induction coils that the Kidder Mfg Co designed and promoted as something special for clinical treatments. Because they supposedly added versatility in electrical treatments and added manufacturing costs the costs of these units differed (No.4 vs No.5 vs No.6).

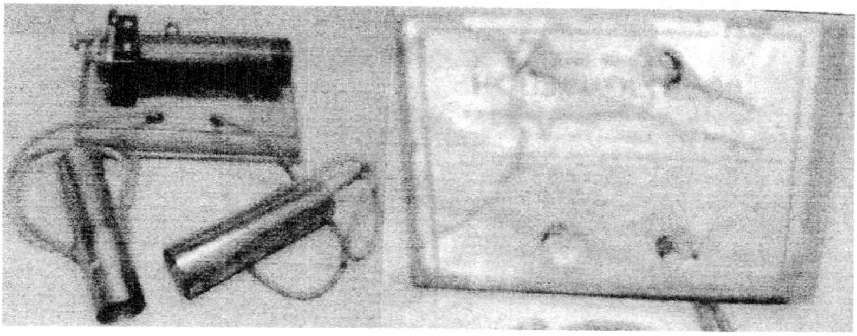

Fig B18. No. 25 Household Coil

Household Coils. Although not illustrated or listed in the JH Bunnell catalog, the manufacture of the No.25 Household Coil is attributed to this company. It probably was made by JH Bunnell & Co for retail by others. This particular unit dates around 1897, and was aimed for treatment of rheumatism and other muscular troubles. A green paper label on the bottom of the cherry base (3.75 x 2.5 x 1.75 inches) contains directions for use, but no date or name of manufacturer. The green printed label covers the circuit wiring. The base has a machined grooved border that serves as the face plate or panel to hold an induction coil (2.75 x 0.75 inches), and an adjustable screw spring leaf type interrupter on one end and closed on the other end. Two connector posts are for electrical cell connections, and the two feet long cords for patient connections are fixed at one end to the circuit, while their other ends are fixed to hand held hollow tube electrodes. This is a miniature induction coil for home use, and since no sliding tube is present to control current amplitude the current is controlled by a step down transformer with 5.84 volt DC input, 2.6 volt AC output (35 to 42% of input), waveform is symmetrical biphasic spikes, 18 mA p/p x 2 ms duration. This unit was illustrated and listed in the 1897 catalog (page 472) of Sears, Roebuck and Co as # 6351[9] without a trademark. A single acid cell or one or two dry cells could power the unit that was designed for portability for travelers. The unit sold for $3.50.

The No.26 Household Coil is exactly the replica of No.25 except that it is mounted on an oak circular base. The coil is a JH Bunnell & Co style induction coil. The current interrupter has both the vibrator and contact screw on the same base as advertised by MESCO in 1900. The faradic current amplitude is controlled by a sliding metal tube. The cylindrical tube electrodes have connecting cloth insulated wires that are

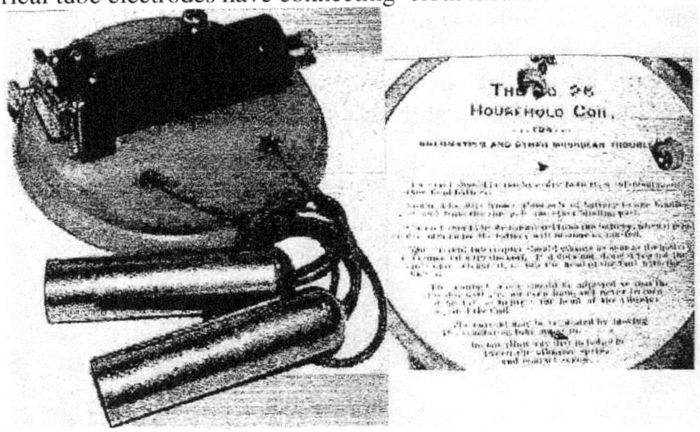

Fig B18A. No. 26 Household Coil

factory sealed at both ends. One end is soldered to the metal electrode and the other end is fixed to the induction coil. This unit is believed to have been manufactured by JH Bunnell & Co in 1897 to 1900 and sold through MESCO. The wording on the paper label pasted on the bottom

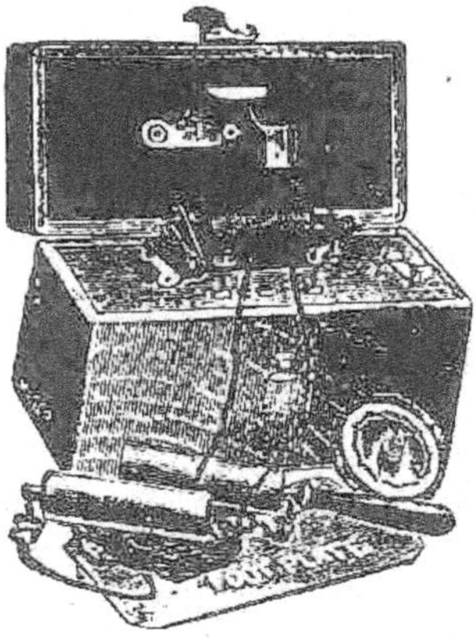

Fig B19. Household Medical Apparatus

of the base reads similarly to that of the No.25 Household Coil.

Household Medical Apparatus Fig B19 illustrates this unit in the 1900 catalog of MESCO.[13] No signature label or plate is attached to this particular apparatus, and the same unit has appeared with the label of "Manufactured by Detroit Medical Battery Co, Detroit, Mich" on eBay auction, the above unit is conjectured to have been made by JH Bunnell & Co for retail by others. MESCO sold JH Bunnell & Co apparatuses without the Bunnell label or signature, and the Detroit Medical Battery Co was a manufacturer and sold this identical unit as the "Elk" battery (see Chapter 17).

The basis for the JH Bunnell & Co identification is the induction coil (2.75 x 0.75 inches) that is covered by a black fabric, and has circular wooden end caps (1.5 dia x 0.38 thick, inches). The circular wooden end caps on coils are a trademark of the JH Bunnell & Co. Other manufacturers had circular end caps but mostly of different materials (eg, hard rubber, metal), sizes, and markings. The above apparatus also has the feature of a one piece interrupter with its adjustable screw spring lever, hammer (new type ca 1900). This unit is in a polished oak box (7.5 x 3.5 x 5.25 inches) large enough for a single dry cell. The wooden box has a hinged lid (1.75 of 5.25 inches height), and a hinged latch with attached hooked lever lock on front. All metal all nickel plated along with the scale (0 to 110 range in increment unit of 10) to measure distance of the sliding tube current regulator. The face plate is matching oak and contains the coil with its metal sliding tube current regulator; an On/Off lever control; and three metal connector receptacles. The 1900 Electro-Therapeutic Hand Book by Trevert illustrated this particular unit for MESCO that sold for $4.00.[15]

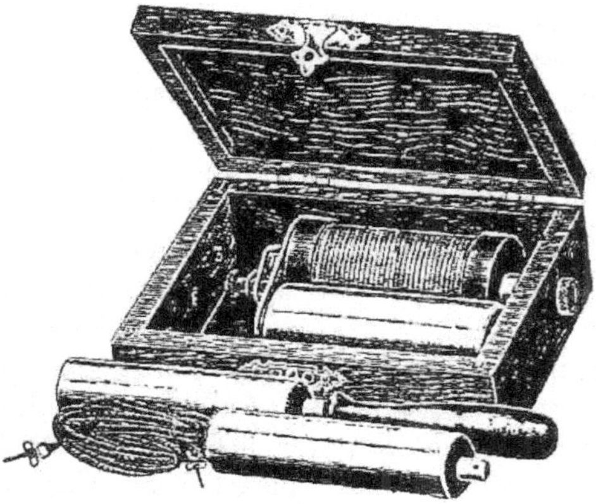

Fig B20. The "Unique" Medical Apparatus

"Unique" Medical Apparatus. The MESCO catalog of 1900 illustrated and listed The "Unique" Medical Apparatus that was probably made by the JH Bunnell & Co (based on design characteristics) for retail by MESCO.[13] The unit is modified after the design by Gaiffe of France. The type of electrical battery is a pocket model that is designed to fit pockets of consumers who travel. The unit has a self contained dry cell housed in a nickel plated tube to power the unit. No face plates are used with this design, otherwise the usual faradic current components are present. The induction coil has a sliding metal current controller that moves from the right side of the cabinet finished oak carrying case (5 x 2.75 x 1.75 inches). The vibrating interrupter and an adjustable contact screw on one base is used. Because of the design (dry cell and interrupter) it is dated 1900. The metal parts are nickel plated. The unit originally sold for $2.50 complete. Replaceable cells sold for $0.20 each.

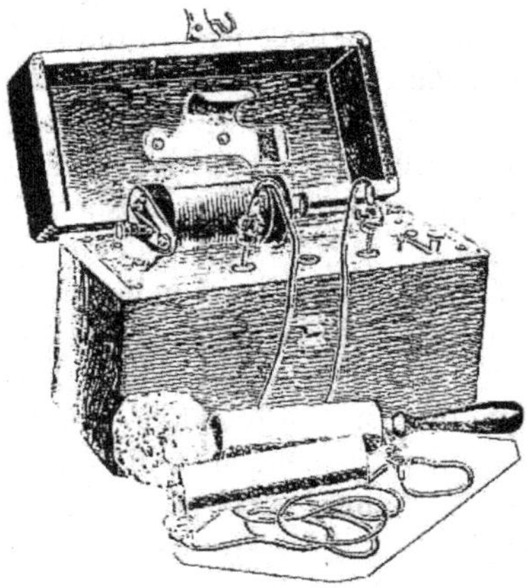

Fig B21. Anti-Doc Medical Apparatus

Anti-Doc. This is a small compact faradic current unit that has been also marketed as Anti-Doc # 6 Medical Apparatus, Elk Medical Apparatus, and without any title. This unit resembles the 1900 version of The Household Medical Apparatus of MESCO. A label or logo only accompanies the unit occasionally, and when it does it is usually on the inside of the hinged lid of the oak box. The oak box has glued corners with a metal carrying handle, and a front lock clasp by a lever hook. The size of the wooden box varies slightly in length (7.5 and 7.6 inches) and width (4.25 and 5.25 inches), but the height is constant (3.5 inches). The unit weighs four pounds and is powered by one standard (6.25 x 2.5 inches) dry cell. All metal are nickel plated. The wooden face plate has an induction coil (2.75 x 1.75 inches) with a sliding metal current controller on its right. The coil is covered by black fabric and enclosed by offsetting circular wooden end caps. It offers primary, secondary, and combined currents. A metal arbitrary scale (10 to 100) is glued on the face plate to measure the distance that the current controller moves. An adjustable screw contact and vibrating interrupter on the same base is mounted on the left end of the coil. The face plate also contains an On/Off switch, and three button outlets to connect the circuitry with the subject. The unit dates from 1902; is advertised in the 1908 Sears, Roebuck and Co catalog;[10] and in the 1900 MESCO catalog a somewhat similar (yet different) unit was cited as The Household Medical Apparatus (Fig B19).[13] The unit is characterized by features manufactured on JH Bunnell & Co faradic batteries. Inside of the hinged lid is a metal clip that stores electrodes when in use. The unit cost $4.00.

Wet Cells. The JH Bunnell & Co either manufactured its own electrical cells or had another company manufacture them for retail for use with its line of medical electrical batteries. In 1894, the company was still selling wet cells in which the glass jars are embossed with "J.H.B. & Co. N.Y." on the side.[16] These three models (top, unequal size) of wet cells are the Lechanche type which during the 1870s to 1900 were perhaps the best available open circuit cell. This wet cell was designed by Leclanche of France between 1865 and 1867. The cell used a solid depolarizer in which zinc in diluted sulfur acid and platinum are surrounded by peroxide of lead. The solution is put into a porous cup set

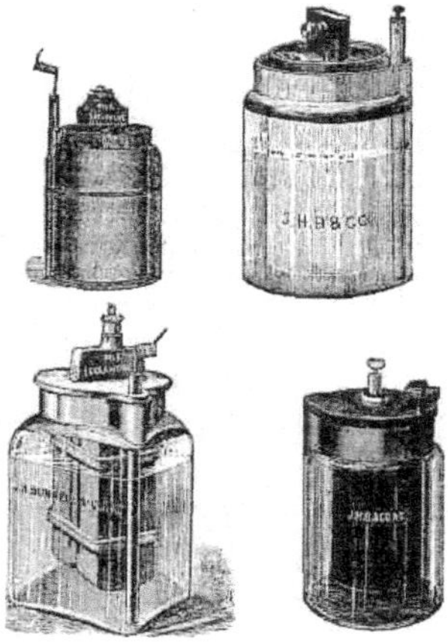

Fig B22. Wet Cells by JH Bunnell & Co

in the glass jar, and when first activated delivered 2.4 volts, but within 30 minutes with load the force dropped to 1.4 volts. A zinc rod is located near the edge of the jar while the carbon plate is in the center surrounded by a lead cast holding it as a binding post.

Summary

JH Bunnell founded his firm in 1878. The JH Bunnell & Co was a major manufacturer of telegraphic equipment and supplies. In additional to telegraphic items the company manufactured medical electrical batteries for home use. The New No.4 D.D. Home Medical Battery was perhaps the most successfully marketed battery in the United States. This particular battery is commonly seen wherever medical electrical batteries are sold. The company manufactured medical electrical batteries to be sold by retailers throughout the country. As a result of the company's business practice to make its batteries for others to sell, the identification today of the JH Bunnell & Co origin is often difficult for the collector. The success of this company has been sufficient enough to survive time and it still exists today as a division of MNJ Industrials.[1]

References

1. Jacobs J. JH Bunnell & Co. Past, Present, Future. Antique Wireless Assoc Conf, Rochester, NY, 1994; correspondence 2000; (http://Fohnix.metronet.com/~nmcewen/bunnell.html)

2. Obituary Note. The late Jesse H Bunnell. Electrical World 18 Feb 1899; (http://wwav.com8080/bunnell/)

3. Kelly EM. The Business Founding Date Directory. Scarsdale, NY, Morgan & Morgan, 1954, p 19

4. JH Bunnell & Co, Inc. New York, NY, Bunnell Telegraph Apparatus-Standard of the Globe, No 73, 1918, pp. 3-5

5. Catalog of Montgomery Ward & Co. Chicago, IL, Montgomery Ward, 1994-1995, p 209

6. Catalog of Montgomery Ward & Co. Chicago, IL, Montgomery Ward, 1903-1904, p 514

7. Catalogue No.12. New York, NY, JH Bunnell & Co, 1892, pp 48-82

8. Electro-Therapeutic Catalogue, ed 18. Chicago, IL, McIntosh Battery Optical, 4 1897

9. Catalog of Sears, Roebuck and Co. Chicago, IL, Sears, Roebuck, 1897, p 478

10. Catalog of Sears, Roebuck and Co. Chicago, IL, Sears, Roebuck, 1908, p 206

11. Wells SM. The Electropathic Guide. New York, NY, JH Bunnell, 1899, pp 13-17, 100

12. Wells WR. A New Theory of Disease Based Upon the Principle that Man is a Compound Electrical Magnet. Rochester, NY, Steam Press of CD Tracy, 1862 (ed 2, 1869)

13. Catalog of MESCO, New York, NY, MESCO, 1900

14. Catalogue No.14. New York, NY, JH Bunnell & Co, 1901, pp 54-59

15. Trevert E. Electro-Therapeutic Hand Book. New York, NY, MESCO, 1900

16. Bleyer JM. Galvanism. In Bigelow HR (ed). An International System of Electro-Therapeutics. Philadelphia, PA, FA Davis, 1894, pp 260, 266-267

CHAPTER 17. DETROIT'S MEDICAL BATTERY COMPANIES

Two different companies in Detroit at different times engaged in the manufacture of medical electrical batteries. Both companies targeted the family or home use market. Both companies were small in operation and sales volume, and each business was relatively short lived. Chapter 17 presents the Detroit manufacturers and their batteries.

DETROIT ELECTRICAL WORKS

Little is known about this company's involvement in the medical electrical battery business. In 1876, there was a Detroit Electrical Works that was a builder of railways, and later of telegraph systems. In 1880, the Detroit Electrical Works was listed and described in Industries of Michigan as manufacturers of and dealer in telegraph and various electrical apparatuses and supplies. The company was a dealer of the Western Electric Manufacturing Co that accounts for the telegraph and telephone phases of the business. Detroit businessmen GM Balch, JS Newberry, J McMillan, and WA Jackson (manager) were officers, founders, and proprietors of the company. Around 1884 or earlier, the company had $10,000.00 capital stock with a then healthy outlook. The company's office was located at 98 Griswold Street and its brick and stone building at 44-46 Woodbridge Street was the factory. At that time the company employed 30 people. The company's products were sold throughout Michigan and major cities in the United States.[1]

In 1888, the company was located in a large three storied building at 7th and Woodbridge Streets. At that time the company was listed as a manufacturer of burglar alarms, general electrical apparatus, medical electrical batteries, telephones, and telephone supplies.[2]

According to the Michigan State Gazetteer & Business Directory for 1891-1892, the company was expert in the industrial application of electricity, Rae's electrical railway system, electrical power plants, and electrical motors. The company, in addition to consultation and design in electrical matters, manufactured annunciators, electrical bells, burglar alarms, and general electrical supplies. Officers of the company in 1891-1892 were: H McMillan, president; WA Jackson, vice president; W H Wells, secretary; CA Benton, manager of the railroad department; FB Rae, electrical engineer and designer of the railway system bearing his name; and L Warfield, general manager. The office of the company was located on the SW corner of Woodward & Baltimore Avenues.[3(1891-92,488)] In 1892, the company built Detroit's first electrical trolley line on Jefferson Street.[4]

The directory of the City of Detroit for 1895 listed the company at 1457 Woodward Ave, and its trustees as L Warfield and WA Jackson. Other owners of the business may have sold their interests to Warfield and Jackson between 1890 and 1895. In 1895, the Detroit Electrical Works went out of business and lost its charter.[1] The Michigan Gazetteer & Business Directory for 1895 cited the company's address as Woodward Avenue at the Railroad Crossing.[3(1895)]

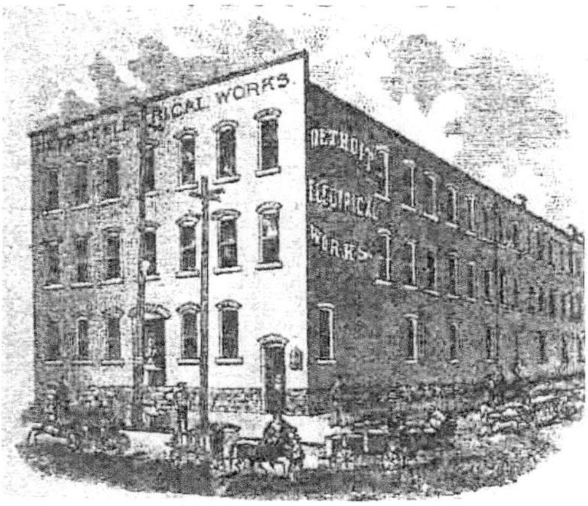

Fig D1. The Detroit Electrical Works Building in 1888

The Detroit Electrical Works' medical electrical batteries, the Universal Faradic Batteries, were advertised for sale in the catalog of Charles Truax & Greene Co of Chicago in 1893. Although the Detroit Electrical Works was manufacturing medical electrical batteries in 1888, the only date and models are confirmed for 1892. The Universal Faradic Batteries (Nos.1 & 2) are the two confirmed batteries. One can speculate that the limited selection was available from 1888 to 1895. Since the span of time for making medical electrical batteries is short, it is also speculated that the Universal Faradic Batteries were the only models made, and are not commonly seen in antique shops or on Ebay auctions.

Commonalties of Batteries

No commonalties exist for faradic battery models manufactured by the Detroit Electrical Works. The Universal Faradic Battery No.2 has characteristics that resemble the New No.4 Home Medical Apparatus that was manufactured by the JH Bunnell & Co of New York City from 1881 to 1890 or 1892. The end caps of the induction coil are circular; the spring lever vibrating interrupter is parallel to the face plate that is unlike most faradic current models, but similar to those of the JH Bunnell & Co. One end of the nickel plated cylinder is fixed to serve as an axis while the other end is lifted to remove the exhausted dry cell. The oak case is rectangular shaped, while that of the New No.4 Home Medical Apparatus has a lid and bottom that form lips or overhangs (flared).

Universal Faradic Battery No.2. The Detroit Electrical Works manufactured two faradic batteries in 1892 that could be purchased through the catalog of the Truax, Greene & Co of Chicago. Pictured is the No. 2 model that is enclosed in a finely finished wooden case (9.25 x

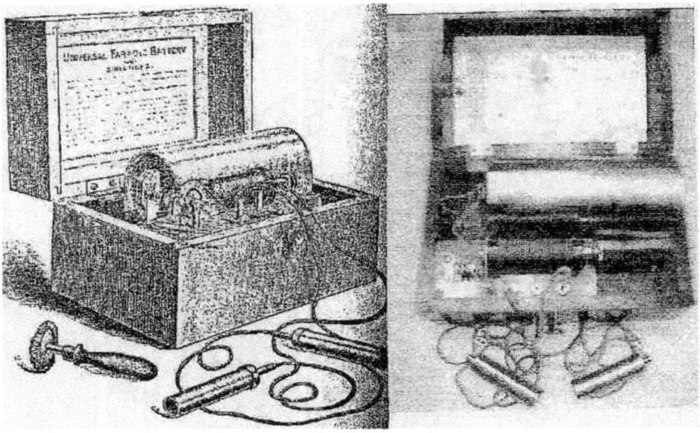

Fig D2. Universal Faradic Battery No. 2

5.75 x 5.38 inches) with glued grooved corners. The face plate is black lacquered wood with a small open compartment on its right for accessories. The honey tone oak case is modeled like the earlier JH Bunnell & Co unit of 1881 to 1890 with its single rather than two lids but without the lipped bottom. The model has an automatic cut-out lock that shuts off the unit when not in use to save the life of the cell. The model was designed for family use, but the manufacturer stated that physicians would also find it convenient to use. The No.2 model is similar in design and operation to the New No.4 Home Medical Battery of JH Bunnell Co of New York that was also marketed in 1892. The single dry cell is enclosed in a nickel plated cylinder that is raised from one end to permit easy removal of a single No.6 dry cell (standard cell in the 1890s). The raised cylinder is then lowered to connect the battery to the circuit. Unlike the New No.4 Home Medical Battery of JH Bunnell that has a completely encased battery cylinder, the cylinder of the Universal Faradic Battery No.2 does not completely enclose the battery. The cylinder is open on the bottom that rests on two wooden foundations, and is not part of the electrical circuit. The battery connects with the circuit by two insulated wires. Directions for operating the unit are glued to the inside of the lid. Electrodes and silk connecting cords were included with the basic model, but a nickel plated foot plate was an additional cost. The faradic coil has a sliding metal current controller, and an adjustable screw spring hammer vibrating interrupter that is similar to that on the Elk model. A lever switches On/Off functions, and three connecting buttons offer primary, secondary, and combined currents. The carrying handle is made of sturdy metal that rolls up and down (lever style), and is located on top of the lid. The lid is secured by a sturdy metal screw latch.

The Universal Faradic Battery No.2 of the Detroit Electrical Works, although having similarities to models made and sold by the JH Bunnell & Co and the George P Pilling & Son Co of Philadelphia, does differ. The case of the Universal Faradic Battery No.2 differs from the lipped box of the New No.4 Home Medical Apparatus by having a conventional rectangular shape. The circular end caps of the induction coil of the Universal model differ from the similar model manufactured by the George P Pilling & Son Co which has square end caps.

The Detroit Electrical Works also made and sold the No.1 Universal Faradic Battery (not shown) at a lower price than the No.2 model. Model No.1 was similar in function to that of No.2, but its cell was located in a different position that causes the wooden case to be larger and square shaped. Both units were designed for home use.

Summary

The Detroit Electric Works is best known for its building of electrical systems and electrical railways locally. The medical electrical battery business was a very small portion of its involvement in electrical matters, telephones, and telephone supplies. Although the firm may have operated since 1876, its tenure with medical electrical batteries was short lived (1888-1895). Although not confirmed, the Universal Faradic Batteries No.1 and 2 of the Detroit Electric Works may have been manufactured for them by the JH Bunnell & Co of New York City for the Detroit firm to retail. The Detroit Electric Works did, however, have the manufacturing capabilities to enter its own products on the market at the time.

THE DETROIT MEDICAL BATTERY COMPANY

The Detroit Medical Battery Company, the second manufactory of medical electrical batteries in the city was not a satellite or directly formed from an existing company (ie, the Detroit Electrical Works). Personnel associated with this company differed from those of the Detroit Electrical Works. The Detroit Medical Battery Company was not listed in the directory of the City of Detroit until 1902. The company was apparently founded in 1901 and listed in the directory as soon as it was possible, 1902. The address of the company in 1902 was cited as 6 Walker Block with F Wardell as its general manager. Information on the company is also supported by the 1903 issue of the Michigan State Gazetteer & Business Directory.[3(1903,p576)] In 1905, the company was functioning from 1311-1313 Majestic building, and the officers were then FC Badgley, president; HH Mallory, vice president; RA Oliver, secretary; and WF Harkness, treasurer. The 1905 Michigan State Gazetteer & Business Directory cited F Wardell as treasurer and general manager.[3(1905,p752)] The officers of the company changed in 1907 to EC Harkness (president & general manager), WF Harkness (secretary), and WC Seely Jr (treasurer), and moved to 906 of the Majestic building.[3(1907,p670)] The personnel listed for 1907 remained stable through 1909.[3(1909,p563)] Although still located at 906 Majestic building, CW Tousley (spelled Tonsley in 1910) assumed the position of president in 1909. AP Wood was both president and manager in 1911 which indicates the business may have been sold in 1910 or 1911.[3(1911,p548)] Although still listed at 906 Majestic building in 1912,[4] the Detroit Medical Electrical Battery Company was not listed in the directory of the City of Detroit after 1912, nor in the Michigan State Gazetteer & Business Directory for 1913.

According to an advertisement of 1902 the Detroit Medical Battery Co was located at 935 Walker Block. In an advertisement of 1905 the company listed its address as 390 Majestic building, Detroit. The Detroit Medical Battery Company is believed to have been a small firm, yet the company advertised itself as a manufacturer and dealer. The disagreement in locations of the company (directory vs advertisement) for 1902 and 1905 suggests that the business was small enough to pick up property and move within a building, and street to street. Five electrical battery models have been traced to the company, and features of two of these medical batteries can be traced to the design of manufacturer JH Bunnell & Co of New York City. Possibly the Bunnell batteries in question were not patented or the Detroit Medical Battery Co was allowed to make similar batteries or Bunnell manufactured the two electrical batteries in question for the company that then sold them with its signature.

Commonalties of Detroit Medical Batteries Co

The commonalties of this company are mixed. The mixed characteristics involve the Elk Faradic Battery with another company, but the features of the Detroit Medical Battery Co's Portable and Two-Cell Faradic Batteries are unique to this manufacturer. The Elk Faradic Battery is an exact copy of the "Anti-Doc Medical Apparatus" of MESCO (believed to have been made by the JH Bunnell & Co of New York City). The battery was marketed in 1905 by MESCO and by the Detroit Medical Battery Co about the same period of time.

The Portable and the Two-Cell Faradic Batteries have their induction coils nickel plated. The rheostats are also nickel plated as well as all of the electrical components on both units. The number of nickel plated items is an exceptionally unique characteristic of batteries manufactured by the Detroit Medical Battery Co.

Batteries

Elk Faradic Battery. This unit is smaller (7.5 x 3.5 x 5.25 inches) than most faradic batteries with a single dry cell. The lid is hinged with a hinged latch with a locking lever on the front of the oak box, and a metal carrying handle on the top. Inside of the lid is a thin nickel plated clip for containing the accessories. The top of the wooden face plate has a fabric covered induction coil with circular wooden end caps (Bunnell style) that are larger than the diameter of the coil. On the left end of the coil is a vibrating interrupter with an adjustable screw, and on the right end of the coil is a sliding metal controller that are nickel plated. Three metal buttons on the right front of the face plate are used to select the three currents (primary, secondary, combined). The patient is connected to the unit by cloth insulated wires connecting the battery to the electrodes. An On/Off lever is located on the right side of the face

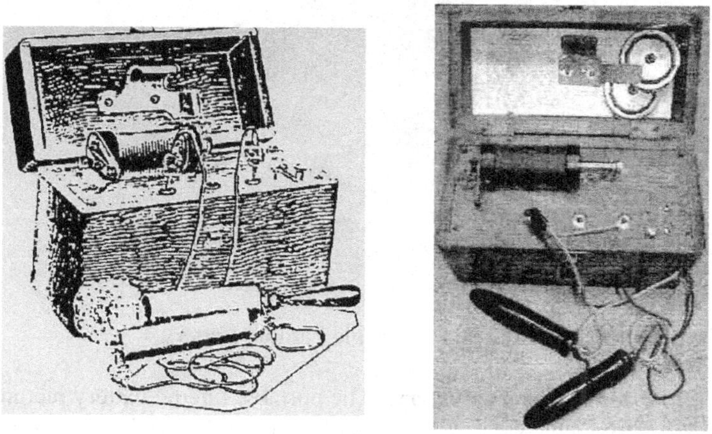

Fig D 3. Elk Faradic Battery

plate. The Elk Faradic Battery was still being manufactured in 1925 that raises further doubts about the Detroit Medical Electrical Battery Co being the manufacturer. As is known, devices that were not patented were fair products for manufacture and sale by competitors of the time, and this was certainly common practice.

This particular unit has also been seen by the author having the above "Elk" label that is similar to a model described and sold by George P Pilling & Son as the "Elk" unit in 1900. The George P Pilling & Son company used square end caps on their induction coils so this Elk Faradic Battery was unlikely to have been manufactured by Pilling.

Collectors must recognize that the signature plates and signature data on the directions label are often those of retailers who insisted that manufacturers place their name on products that they sold. The prime example of this situation is that of Montgomery Ward & Co, and Sears, Roebuck and Co of Chicago. Neither company was a manufacturer of their products, but retailed items made for them, and with their names on the items. In some cases the retailers may even have insisted on specific characteristics in the design of the medical electrical batteries that they sold. In some models the designs ordered by the retailer are uniquely different from other marketed electrical batteries by the maker.

In 1904 through 1906, The Detroit Medical Battery Co, through an advertisement, promoted its book (booklet), Cure Yourself by Electricity,[6] in anticipation of the World's Fair in St Louis, MO, that year. The book was free to anyone requesting it.

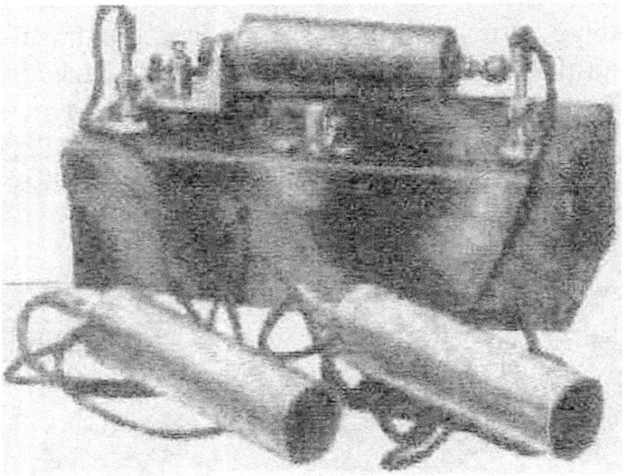

Fig D 4. Portable Faradic Battery

Portable Faradic Battery. The portable faradic battery pictured in the advertisement was available in 1904 for $1.95, and an individual could try it for a trial of 30 days. The advertisement promised positive effects from electricity for many diseases and physical problems. The coil on the battery is a nickel plated cylinder and at its ends are the customary sliding metal current controller and vibrating interrupter. No case is available for this small portable unit designed for the traveler and family. A single cell operates the unit, and it is encased underneath the face plate.

A similar advertisement of 1905 offered the booklet Cure Yourself by Electricity free by written request to the company. The electrical battery in Fig D4 (available in 1904) was available for $1.95 and was pictured in the advertisement. This battery was suppose to cure insomnia, kidney and liver malfunctions, and rheumatism. The battery could be used for electrical baths, beauty treatments, and massages. The booklet listed the electrical batteries sold by the Detroit Medical Battery Co that ranged in price from $1.95 to $11.65.

Two-Cell Faradic Battery. In 1904 to ca 1910, The Detroit Medical Battery Co marketed a golden oak case (book style; 9.38 x 12 x 4.75 inches) containing the No.2 Home Battery (Fig D5) designed to deliver both faradic and galvanic currents for home use. A lever latch on front of the case secures the lid that has four brass clips to contain electrodes. Units were supplied with the booklet Cure Yourself by Electricty. All components are mounted on the thinly nickel plated face plate. This is perhaps the only American made medical electrical battery that has a nickel plated face plate. The components include an induction coil in which a nickel plated shell or cover serves as a secondary coil over the fabric covered primary coil (DuBois-Reymond principle). The induction coil is positioned with the width (front to rear) of the case rather than the usual location along the length of the case. The front of the coil has a unique dial or disc type of rheostat (nickel plated). On top of the dial is a small knob connected to a sliding (racheted) metal current controller that operates by turning the small knob over the dial. The dial has etched numbers (arbitrary units) ranging from 0 to 200 with a revolving pointer. The pointer moves with the small knob and the moving coil. The other end of the coil has an adjustable screw vibrating hammer, interrupter.

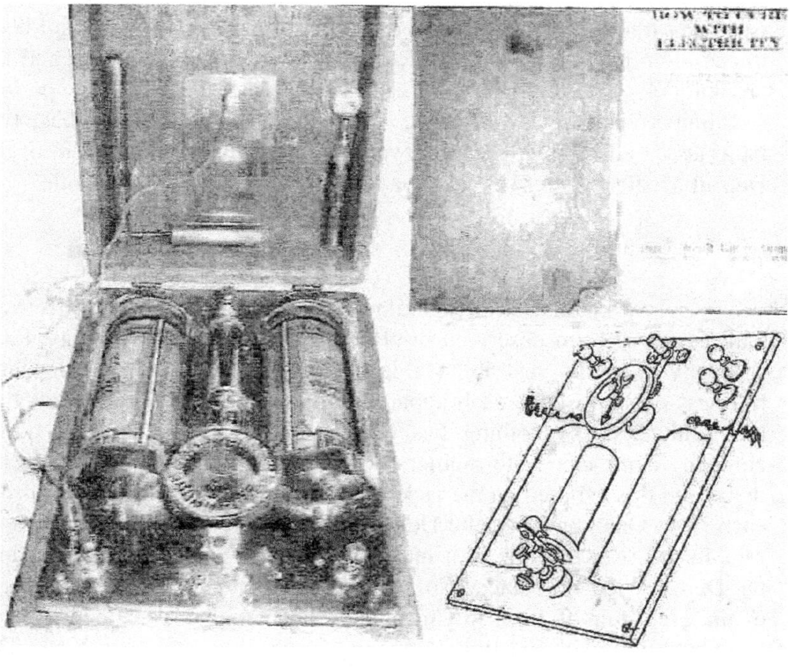

Fig D5. Two-Cell Faradic Battery and Manual

Two standard dry cells power the unit. The dry cells are contained underneath the metal face plate in separate tin trays. The top of each dry cell is exposed to the operator. Three binding posts serve for current selection and connection with the patient. The single post (lower right) serves as a universal post for all connections, while the two posts at lower left serve to provide either faradic or galvanic currents. An On/Off lever switch is located in front of the disc. (see diagram lower right in Fig D5). All electrical components are nickel plated as well as the semicircular slots for holding the two dry cells.

No.1 Home Battery. The company also made a No.1 Home Battery (not shown) similar but cheaper in cost to that of the No.2 battery. The No.1 unit did not have the elaborate racheted coil, dial, pointer arrangements for current control. The No.1 unit uses a sliding current controller from the coil; the top of the coil is covered with fabric that has markings from 10 to 100 in arbitrary units for movement of the secondary coil over the primary coil. It has two dry cells for power, a nickel plated face plate and coil cover, and also dates from 1904.

The latter two units shown are different than those of all other medical electrical batteries produced in the United States in that period of time. The nickel plated induction coils on the two units; and the location of the coil and the nickel plated rheostat of the No.1 and 2 Home Batteries, make these units unique. This small firm apparently did not issue any trade catalog for its products. Also, the company has not been traced after 1912. Because the electrical batteries of Figures D4 and D5 are uniquely different from others manufactured at the same time period, the company apparently did some of its own manufacturing of these two batteries. No data have been uncovered to clarify this predicament of the Detroit Medical Battery Co being a manufacturer or retailer or both.

Summary

Two small Detroit manufactories dealing in medical electrical batteries have been described briefly because of limited findings. Each company lasted for just about a decade, changed locations during their business existence, and each apparently had limited product models that had limited sales. Nothing has been found that suggests that either company contracted with retailers to manufacture electrical batteries for them, and this is based on the lack of commonalties among batteries from each firm. One company, the Detroit Electrical Works, evolved from an established firm dealing with industrial electricity. The other company, the Detroit Medical Battery Co, seemed to be formed to take advantage of the great fair of 1902 in Chicago. Neither company seemed to have competed well with existing companies of Chicago and New York. The artifacts from these two Detroit companies are not commonplace in the antique market with the exception of the Elk Faradic Battery. Both companies aimed their products for the public consumer for home use. One company exited in the nineteenth century, while the other entered and exited in the early twentieth century.

References

1. Edwards R. Industries of Michigan, City of Detroit: Historical and Descriptive Review-Industries, Institutions, Commercial and Manufacturing Advantages. New York, NY, Historical Pub Co, 1880, p 135

2. (http://store5.yimg.com/I/scripophily-1685-38138641)

3. Michigan State Gazetteer & Business Directory. Detroit, MI, RL Polk, 1891

4. (www.Google.com);(http://detnews.com/history/trolley/trolley.htm)

5. (Mark Bowden, Burton Hist Coll, Detroit Pub Lib. Correspondence 6 Jly 02).

6. (www.Google.com);(www.uiowa.edu/~english/profpage/blandon/tlucht/advert1.html)

CHAPTER 18. SIGNAL ELECTRIC MANUFACTURING COMPANY OF MENOMINEE, MI

The history of companies in Menominee making medical electrical batteries is presented in Chapter 18. Some medical electrical apparatuses often bear a signature (trade name) on a paper label attached to the inside lid of the box. The label may indicate that the unit was made by the Signal Electric Manufacturing Co of Menominee, MI. The units by Signal are often stated by sellers as being of 1902 to 1912 vintage. This company's history is rich, but its involvement with medical electrical batteries seems limited. Records involve the company with only four models of medical electrical batteries. Although only four models of batteries can be traced to the Signal Electric Mfg Co, two of these four units were big sellers among the American public. The frequency of the batteries seen in antique shops and on eBay auctions attest to the apparent popularity of these units for home use in the early twentieth century.

In 1892, the Menominee Electric and Mechanical Company on 13th Street, Menominee, MI, was founded by Henry Tideman. Tideman was born in Germany and educated at Heidelburg University before coming to the United States. He was a former employee of Thomas A Edison, and when with Edison he probably worked with condensers (capacitors), electromagnets, rheostats, batteries, and Wheatstone bridges for telegraphic equipment. The Edison Manufacturing Co of New York was marketing two medical electrical batteries at the time Tideman was working for Edison. He must of known about their electrical components and functions. In 1892, Tideman's company produced crank telephone generators, switches, and telephones. Later (1893) the company made electrical fans, medical electrical batteries, and small motors. Electrical desk and bank fans were major items manufactured by the Menominee Electrical and Mechanical Co between 1908 and 1919. Medical electrical batteries with a signature plate bearing the Menominee Electric Co have not surfaced, at least in recent years with a signature label for that early period of time.[1] Although not documented, Signal may have been used as the logo for the medical electrical battery by Tideman prior to the name of Signal being used as the name of the company after 1919. Identification of some products (eg, fans, medical electrical batteries) manufactured by the Menominee company were not labeled with the company's name until sometime around 1910 to 1912.

The Michigan State Gazetteer & Business Directory for 1895 lists the company as having $30,000.00 capital; J Flesheim (pres), JM Opsahl (vice pres), E Daniell (sec & treas), and H Tideman as manager. The company appeared to be doing well in business by 1899 when it employed 85 people.[2] The company was located at 514 Park Avenue. The president of the Menominee Electrical and Mechanical Co, Joseph

Fleshheim. committed suicide in February 1900. Mr Fleshheim was facing personal financial problems, and even considered filing for bankruptcy prior to his death. He was an elected state senator of Michigan, also.[2]

In 1901, the name of the company changed to the Menominee Electrical Manufacturing Company, and was then located on Broadway at the corner of Park Avenue. Also, the Directory for 1901 contained an advertisement that listed electrical batteries as one of the company's products.[3(1901,pp1257, 1260)] The Michigan State Gazetteer & Business Directory for 1903 listed the company's manufactured products as telephones, general electrical supplies, telephone switchboard drops, telephone motor generators, magneto generators, and all telephone apparatus. LC Harmon was president, AD Gibbs was vice president, H Tideman was secretary, and MS Harmon was treasurer of the company. The location and company officers remained the same through 1918.[3(1901,p1260)]

The original building of the Menominee Electric and Mechanical Co burned in 1904, so the company functioned for awhile in Marinette, WI, just across the Menominee River from Menominee, MI. When the new Menominee plant opened in 1906 the company added more telegraph instruments and wireless radio devices to its product line.[5]

This company produced items that apparently were popular enough to turn a creditable profit for that period of time. The Menominee Electric Co was sufficiently successful over the years to absorb the local automobile manufacturing business of the Dudley brothers and their Dudley bug.[1]

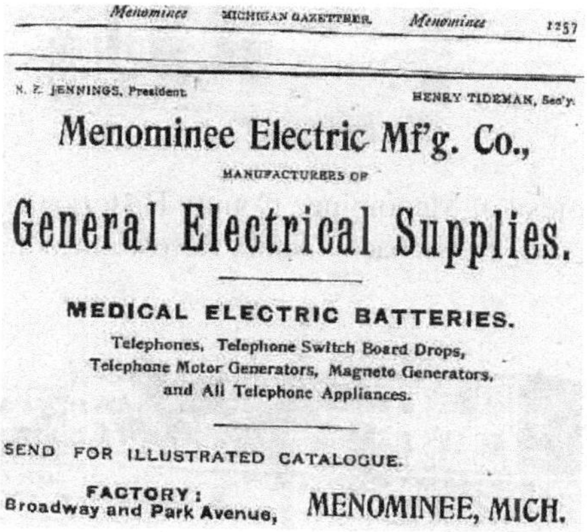

Fig S. Company Advertisement, 1901

The Menominee Electric Manufacturing Co in 1901 advertised its medical electrical batteries, along with telephone apparatuses in the

Michigan State Gazetteer & Business Directory.[3(1901,p1257)] The company at that time issued an illustrated catalog of its products. No evidence has surfaced for a trade catalog being issued by the Signal Electric Manufacturing Co.

In 1919, Henry Tideman (as secretary) decided to move his electric company to Cairo, IL, and did not manufacture medical electrical batteries any longer. The pending move of the company of course was expected to impact negatively on the small community of Menominee. The longtime director of finance of the Menominee Electric Co, Charles Hammond, was able to convince Henry Tideman to give him an option on the purchase of the manufacturing plant. After negotiations, and a down payment Tideman agreed to the sale of the plant. Hammond began to solicit financial help from businessmen in the community, but at first was unable to raise enough money to complete a quick settlement. After a 30-day delay the deal became history. Hammond's group of businessmen were successful in buying the plant and necessary equipment to get started. Tideman moved his business to Cairo in October 1919, and the very next day after leaving the Signal Electric Manufacturing Company of Menominee was reorganized, incorporated, and in operation.

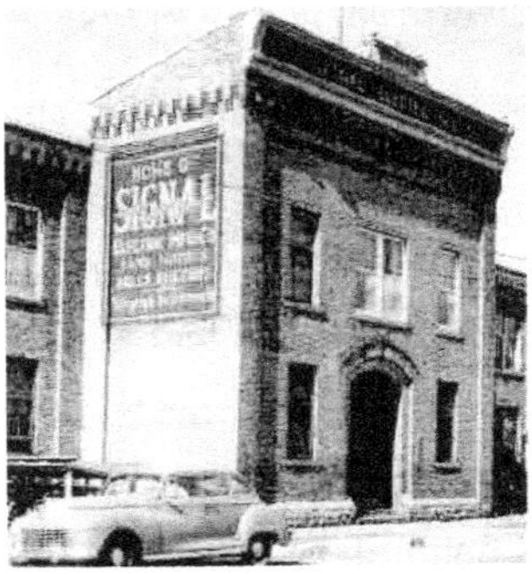

Courtesy of Menominee County Historical Society, Inc
& Michael J Anuta Research Center

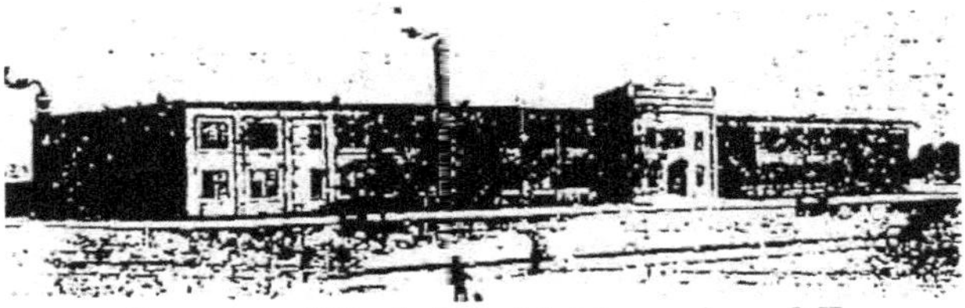

Courtesy of Eagle Herald, Menominee, MI

Fig S1. Signal Electric Company, 1922 and later

The company was then locally owned and operated by individuals (John Henes jr, president; Othmor Henes, vice president and general manager) of Menominee, MI.[5] CE Hammond was the secretary and treasurer of the new company in 1919 that remained in the location of the Menominee Electrical Manufacturing Co on Broadway at the corner of Park Avenue.[3(1921-1922,p1229)] The new owners, Henes brothers, were not able to manufacture electrical fans for five years (1925) because of a contract agreement with Tideman with the sale of the business.[2]

In 1920, The Signal Electric Company's major product was the radio equipment for wireless operations around the world.[5] The company produced kits for the "Signola" brand radio crystal set. Additionally, the company manufactured electrical bells for home use to fire alarms, portable electrical hand tools, small motors, telegraph instruments and accessories (until about 1934), and medical electrical batteries.

The new company did well in 1920, but the business slumped for nine months in 1921. The work force of the company was reduced to 48 employees in 1921. Suddenly in 1922, business increased tremendously. The company made three thousand dollars more profit in the first three months of 1922 than it did in all of 1921. The radio business was doing well under the brand name "Signola." The Signal Electric Mfg Co continued to make telegraph keys into the 1930s. The company began operating the low powered local radio station WFLB with local talent.[1] Eventually, federal regulations forced the closure of the local radio station.[5]

By the end of 1922, the company had installed nineteen thousand dollars of updated equipment that it paid in full. One hundred ninety-five employees were working shifts that covered 20 hours per day. At that time the company was capitalized at $125,000.00 and had a sizable reserve in the bank.[1] The Signal Electric Co was even shipping some of its manufactured products by means of the Ann Arbor Car Ferry Line of the Detroit, Toledo and Ironton-Ann Arbor Railroad Co. The car ferry operated on the Great Lakes, and loaded in Menominee at the docks that connected with a railroad line.[6]

The plant made all phases of the products it sold. Expert mechanics worked drill presses, lathes, specialty machines; a finishing and varnishing room was present; cabinet making and hand rubbing was part of the plant; metal parts were enameled and baked; and silk was wound to insulate copper wires (for induction coils of medical electrical batteries and radio tuners). Valuable specialty tools were hand crafted at the plant, labeled, indexed, and when not in use were stored in a vault.[1]

The company had distribution centers in the United States, three offices in Canada, and single offices in China, Australia, Hong Kong, London, Japan, and New Zealand. Both Montgomery Ward & Co, and Sears, Roebuck and Co of Chicago, IL, were major retailers for the company. The double, and three-cell medical electrical batteries that were advertised and sold by Sears, Roebuck and Company' catalogs and stores in 1908 were manufactured under the name Signal Electric Co for home use.[1]

In 1904, OG Tradewell wrote the 32-paged booklet Medical Electricity at Home that was copyrighted and published, and used by the Signal Electric Co to provide its consumers complete directions for curing and relieving diseases by the use of electricity. The booklet by OG Tradewell accompanied each medical electrical battery sold by and for

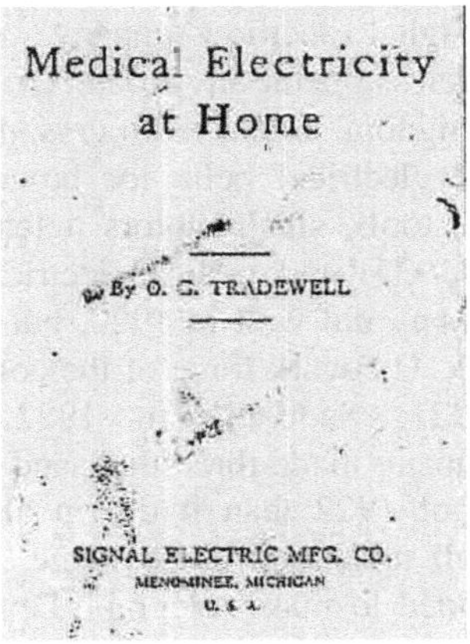

Fig S2. Medical Electricity at Home by OG Tradewell

the company.[7] This publication allows the conjecture that the Electric Co of Menominee made medical electrical machines for home use that were then copied by Signal Electric Co in and after 1919, or that the Signal Electric Co placed its name on a booklet after 1919 that had been published in 1904.[8] An unexplainable problem, however, occurs in the history of the company. The booklet of 1904 carries the name of the Signal Electric Company yet no company by that name was listed in the City Directory of Menominee until 1920 or the Michigan State Gazetteer & Business Directory until its issue of 1919-1920,[3(1921-1922,p1229)] the first listing after the company was incorporated in 1919. No records have surfaced to explain the dates of the Signal Electric Co prior to 1919, but the booklet exists and medical electrical batteries made with that name were illustrated, listed, and sold from the mail order catalogs of Sears, Roebuck and Co of 1904 to 1908. It is conjectured that the Signal name was used by Henry Tideman in 1901, 1904, and 1908 for the medical electrical batteries manufactured by the Menominee Electric and Mechanical Co.[4] Mail addressed to the Signal Electric Co no doubt was given to Tideman and his company. Perhaps the Signal Electric Co was only officially recognized when Tideman sold the company in 1919 and the Signal Electric Co was incorporated. Thus, Tideman apparently used the Signal name prior to the time that the name of the company was changed.[4]

All medical electrical batteries manufactured by Signal Electric Co and sold through Sears, Roebuck and Co were accompanied by Medical Electricity at Home by OG Tradewell, directions on the inside lid, and by Directions for Operating Our Medical Batteries by Sears, Roebuck and Co. The Three-Cell Medical Electrical Battery retailed by Sears, Roebuck and Co and manufactured by the Signal Electric Mfg Co is the only twentieth century American electrical battery having the wheeled rheotome. Also, the unit contains a nonessential polarity changer.

In 1923, the company was using the name Signal Radio & Electric Corp, and in 1926 it used Signal Electric Manufacturing Company for promoting its radios. Two medical electrical batteries were manufactured by the company in 1937[4] when consumer interest in medical electrical batteries for home use had waned. Sears, Roebuck and Co had also dropped most of its medicine and nostrums from its catalogs by that time. Interest in the wireless radio business of the company began to decline by the early 1930s so the company changed its major product line to desk and ventilating fans. The radio business was soon phased out. The company's business peaked in the 1930s with the electrical fans, and operated with more than 500 employees making 30,000 desk fans and 20,000 ventilating fans each year.[5] In 1937 and 1938, the north wing of the plant was constructed to allow expansion of products. From 1935 to 1940, the company was specializing in small horsepower motors of various types. The company expanded its plant in both 1935 and 1940.[4]

In December 1952, the Signal Electric Manufacturing Co was sold to King-Seely Thermos Co of Ann Arbor, MI. William H Calley became the vice president and general manager of the King-Seely plant of Menominee. The company now produced portable electric hand tools and small electrical motors. In 1955, the Menominee company expanded with an additional wing built in 1954, however, in the late 1950s the plant had labor problems and strikes that caused loss of revenue. The strike caused Signal Electric Co to lose its major customer so the King-Seeley Thermos Co closed its Menominee plant in 1964, and sold it to the Vernco Company of Tennessee. The Vernco Co in November began making automotive parts, filters for air conditioners, and motors for fans and humidifiers.[4]

Sears, Roebuck and Company of Chicago became the company's major customer and retailer for the Vernco products. Between 1969 and 1977, many additional items were manufactured in the plant (eg: vacuum cleaners for home and shop use, hair clippers, engraving tools, soldering guns, gear reduction motors). In December 1977, the Vernco Company was sold to the Emerson Electric Company that still operates the plant in Menominee, MI.[4] The Emerson Electric Co has expanded products and buildings, but is closing in 2005.[2]

Commonalties of Signal Batteries

No identifying features peculiar to the Signal Electric Company's batteries are noted. Features peculiar to competitor designs appear in Signal units. Signal Electric Co or the associated retailers (Sears, Roebuck and Co) have their signatures printed on the labels of these units. The Three-Cell Medical Battery by the Signal Electric Co is the only twentieth century American electrical battery to have a wheeled rheotome, and to have survived into the 1920s. Both the Three-Cell and the Portable Double-Cell Faradic batteries are still seen in antique shops and on the eBay auctions. The conclusion is drawn that both of these batteries were popular among public consumers to realize present day exposures. The faradic coil designs are often different by the various manufactures but the Signal Electric Co used both circular and square end caps on its coils to render it without unique features for identification.

Faradic Batteries

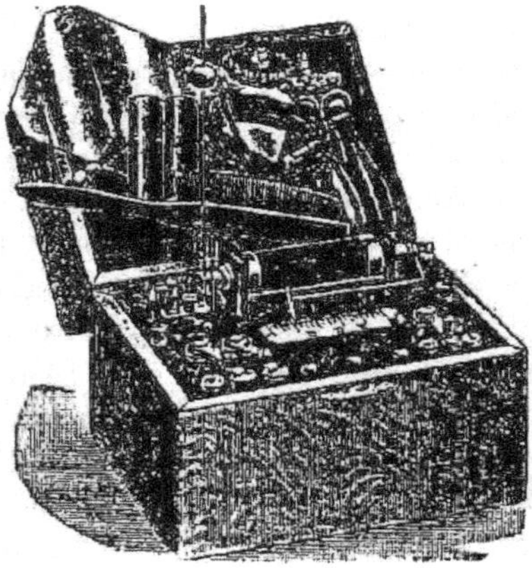

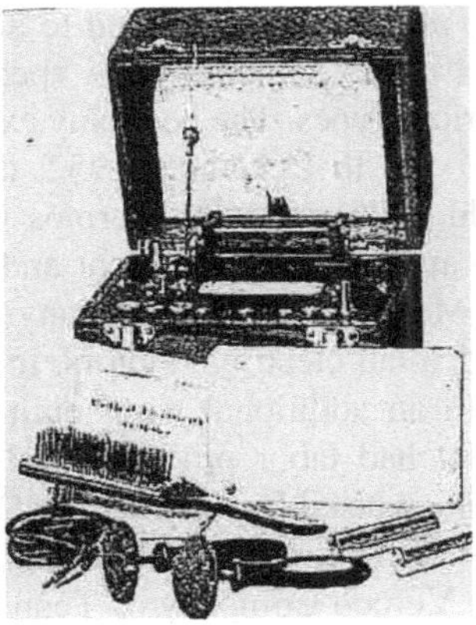

Fig S3. Portable Double-Cell Faradic Battery

Portable Double-Cell Faradic Battery. This unit was manufactured by the Signal Electric Co around 1901. The unit was advertised and sold by Sears, Roebuck and Co of Chicago, and was illustrated in its 1908 catalog.[8] Sears, Roebuck and Co called the unit the Double-Cell Medical Battery in its catalog and sold it for $6.80 that year. It weighed 10 pounds when shipped. The unit is cased in a polished walnut, box (8.75 x 6.25 x 8.25 inches) with dove tailed glued corners. The box has two hinges, a metal carrying handle on top, and two snap latches on front to secure the lid. Inside the lid is a hinged metal lid that encloses an area for storing the accessories, and also a paper label with directions.

The face plate is painted black wood covering an area underneath for two standard sized dry cells. The face plate has an induction coil (4 x 1 inches) on the right rear area. The fabric covered coil has square (1.5 inches) black painted wooden end caps (much like that of Otto & Sons Co, and GP Pilling & Son Co), two metal connecting rods joining the two caps (much like that of McIntosh, and Galvano & Faradic Mfg Cos), and a metal sliding tube current controller at the right end of the coil. A wire pointer is attached to the current controller to give a measure of its distance when moved over a metal scale plate that is in front of the coil and ranges from 0 to 400 (arbitrary units). All metal on the unit are nickel plated. Also, on the face plate is an adjustable screw spring lever, hammer vibrating interrupter; an Off lever control on the right that also switches to an one or two- battery operation; three metal receptacles for connecting the subject to primary, secondary, or combined currents; and a double lever control joined (left side) to reverse current polarity. (Note: faradic or alternating current has no polarity effects on body chemistry like galvanic current) At one time (1908) the wooden box had a self locking device on the front of the case. The double snap latches on the front probably were supplied on later models (ca 1919 to late 1930s) of medical electrical batteries.

The Portable Double Cell Faradic model was still being made in February 1937.[4] At that time the unit sold for $12.00, and weighed six pounds. Tradewell's booklet was still accompanying this unit in 1937.

Three-Cell Medical Battery. Sears, Roebuck and Co sold a three-cell unit through its 1908 catalog that cost $9.95. This unit was manufactured by the Signal Electric Co of Menominee, MI. The unit was housed in a polished oak box with hinged lid, tongue and groove glued corners, a metal carrying handle on top, and two hinged snap latches on the front. Inside the lid is a wooden hinged compartment to store accessories. A front bottom drawer slides in and out for housing three standard sized dry cell batteries. The face plate is black painted wood that contains the fabric covered induction coil (4 x 1 inches) with square (1.5 inches) black wood end caps joined by two metal rods (like that of McIntosh) from cap to cap. To its right is an adjustable screw spring lever, hammer vibrating interrupter or rheotome for faster pulses. To its left is a four-stared wheel rheotome (developed in the 1830s and 1840s by Clarke, Page, and Palmer) for slow pulse frequencies. The wheeled rheotome was a device first used in 1838, but had subsequently been replaced by 1908 with the adjustable screw, spring leaf vibrating interrupter adjacent to the induction coil. Thus, the wheeled rheotome on this particular battery was a gimmick for the Sears, Roebuck and Co customers. No other medical electrical battery in the United States in 1908 had a wheeled rheotome.

A circular fixed carbon (graphite) rheostat (4 inches dia) with a centered rotating lever control is centered on the face plate. On the left is a lever control and four metal buttons to select the desired number of cells, and to the right is a double lever joined control to reverse current polarity (of alternating current?). Two adjustable screw connecting posts are also located on the front-center of the face plate.

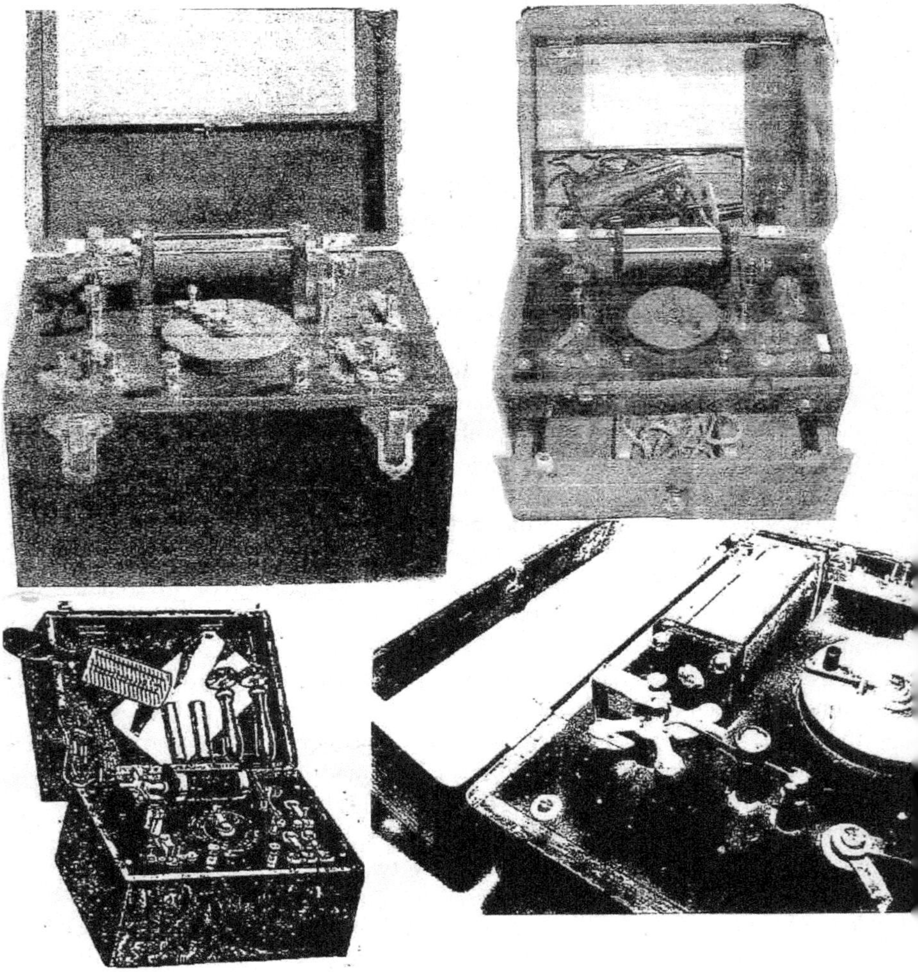

Fig S4. Three-Cell Medical Battery

The oak box of the pictured unit measures 10.9 x 7.75 x 4.9 inches and has the two hinged snap latches on the front. The size of cases housing the Three-Cell Medical Battery may vary from unit to unit. The size difference may indicate a difference in dates of manufacture. The earlier units are slightly larger than the older units. Decreasing wooden box sizes of a particular electrical battery over time was not unusual by companies in an effort to reduce manufacturing costs. The unit's case illustrated by the 1908 catalog of Sears, Roebuck and Co measures 11 x 8 x 8 inches and has two hooked latches on the front of the box. Otherwise models of the Three-Cell Medical Battery dating from ca 1904 to the 1930s are similar in design and function but their boxes differ in size. Another difference between cases is that the model to the left in Fig S4 enclosed the cells underneath the face plate by lifting the plate from the case. The case on the right in the Figure has a drawer with divisions for each cell. In 1908, the shipping weight of the complete units was 18 pounds.

The Three-Cell Medical Battery was discontinued by Signal Electric Co in late 1936 or early 1937. At the time of being discontinued the unit sold for $16.50, weighed eight pounds, and its oak case measured 10.75 x 8 x 9.5 inches. It is a popular collector's artifact.

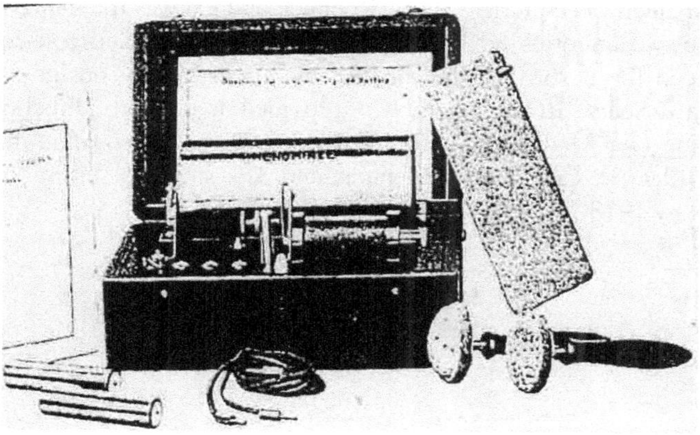

Fig S5. Single Cell Medical Battery

Single Cell Medical Battery. This single cell unit resembles that made by the JH Bunnell Co of New York City. It was probably marketed in 1919 and continued to at least 1937. The rectangular-shaped battery has a single hinged lid (like Bunnell's before 1892), a nickel plated cylindrical holder for a standard sized dry cell. The holder pivots by its connection to the right side of the face plate to lift up for replacing the cell. The faradic coil has circular hard rubber end caps. A common adjustable screw spring lever vibrating interrupter is attached to the left end of the coil while a sliding metal current controller is to its right end.

Three connecting buttons allow for primary, secondary, and combined currents to be delivered to the patient. In 1937, the unit sold for $8.50, weighed five pounds, and the mahogany case measured 9 x 5.25 x 4.75 inches.

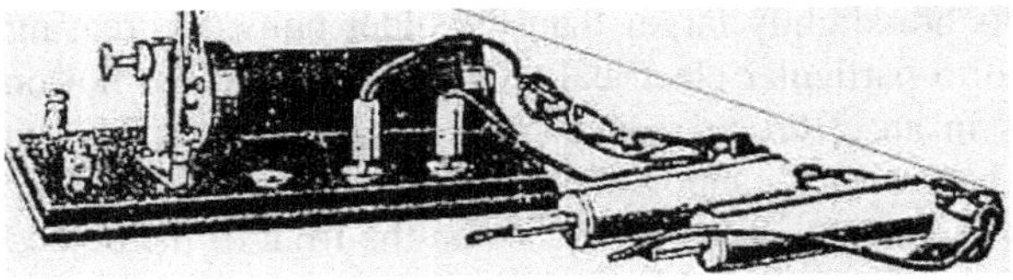

Fig S6. Medical Coil

Medical Coil. This small simplistic designed faradic coil of Fig S6 was mounted on a mahogany base. The base housed the screw adjusted spring lever, hammer interrupter, two binding posts for one external dry cell connection, and three button connections for providing primary, secondary, and combined currents. A sliding metal current controller operated from the right end of the coil. This one pound unit sold for $3.50 when it was discontinued in late 1936.[4]

The Signal Electric Co apparently manufactured four to six medical electrical batteries. Sears, Roebuck and Co was the major retailer of these two batteries for the Signal Electric Mfg Co and consequently influenced the destiny of the medical electrical battery business of the company. Sears, Roebuck and Co provided a booklet Directions for Operating Our Medical Batteries with each of these two units made by Signal Electric Co. Sears, Roebuck and Co stopped selling medical devices by 1918.

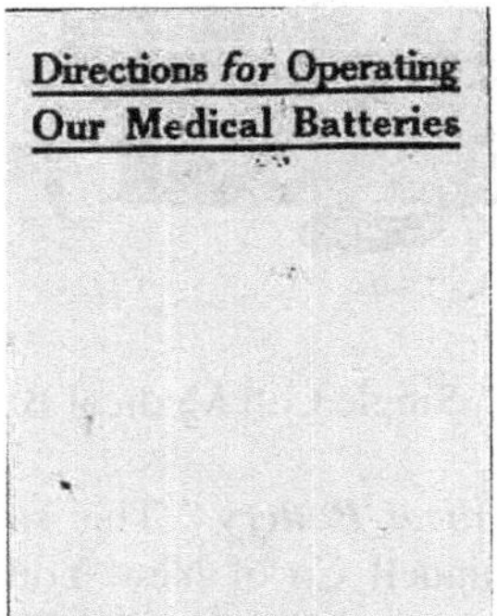

Fig S7. Directions for Operating Our Medical Batteries

Single Cell Faradic Battery. Another medical electrical battery attributed to the Signal Electric Mfg Co in 1904 is similar in design to the popular home use units manufactured and marketed by JH Bunnell & Co and George P Pilling & Son Co. This unit like the two others sold by Sears and Roebuck Co was accompanied by the booklet written by OG Treadwell. Also, like the two other units (Figs S3 and S4) the unit was sold in 1904 or 15 years prior to the founding of the Signal Electric Mfg Co. The Menominee Electric and Mechanical Co was the existing company that marketed the Signal products in 1904.

Like the single cell home battery of Bunnell (New No.4 D.D.) and Pilling (Faradic Home Medical Battery) this single cell unit by

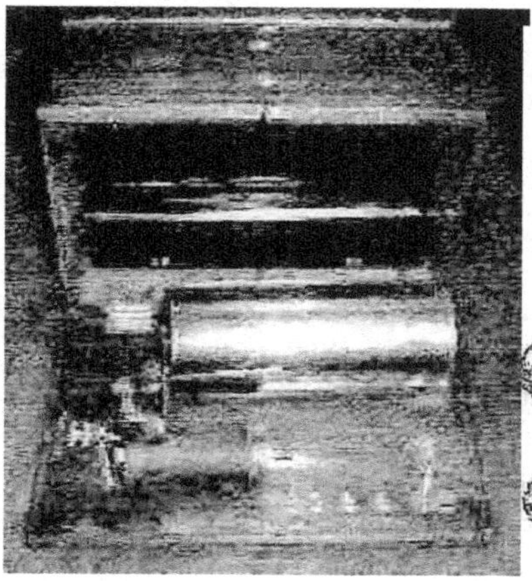

Signal Model

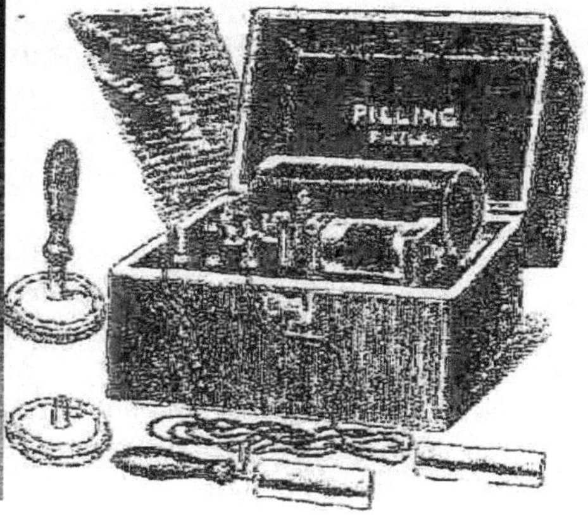

Pilling Model

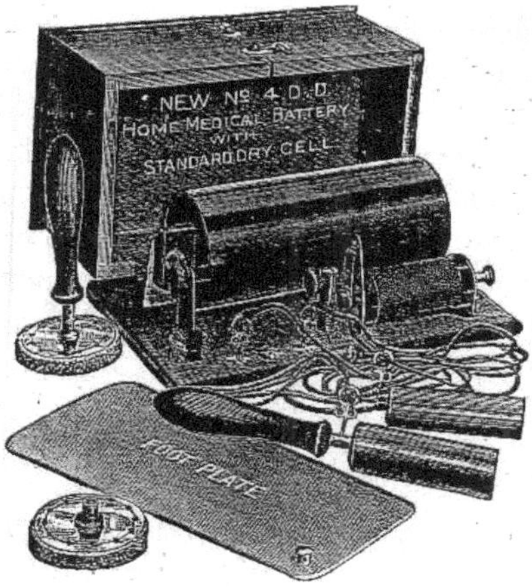

Bunnell Model

Fig S8. Single Cell Faradic Battery of Signal, Pilling, and Bunnell

Signal contained the nickel plated cylinder that rolls upward for cell replacements, and for holding the then standard 1.5 volt cell. The induction coil has circular end caps with a sliding metal current amplitude controller.

The faradic pulses are controlled by the adjustable screw, spring hammer vibrating vibrator. Three button connecting posts are also mounted on the wooden face plate for delivery of primary, secondary, and combined faradic pulses to the patient. The case has two lids; one for exposing the electrical components during operations and another lid for entry into the storage compartment for accessories. Placement of the electrical components on the face plate are slightly different than the Bunnell and Pilling units. The coil is located to the left on the Signal model rather than right side of others.

Summary

The Signal Electric Manufacturing Co has a long and colorful history for a small company. It was founded in 1892 as the Menominee Electrical and Mechanical Co, and in 1919 it was reorganized and incorporated as the Signal Electric Mfg Co. The company's name survived for 33 years until it changed again. The Signal Electric Mfg Co was best known for its manufacture of telegraphic and telephone apparatuses, accessories, and wireless radios.

The medical electrical battery business began with the Menominee Electrical and Mechanical Co around 1904. The name Signal Electric Mfg Co was apparently used with these early batteries that were sold mostly through Sears, Roebuck and Co. During the production of medical electrical batteries by the company just four models have been identified. Two batteries, the Portable Double-Cell Faradic and Single-Cell Medical Batteries, were popular enough with the public consumer to survive after 1937, and these two models are frequently seen today in antique shops and on eBay auctions. Another of Signal's batteries, the Three-Cell Medical Battery, was also popular among public consumers to have survived until almost 1937. This model is unique and is easily identified by its star-wheel rheotome.

References

1. Donnell BW. Signal Electric Has Big Boom in Business. Menominee, MI, Menominee Herald-Leader, Vol xxv, No. 88, Friday evening, April 14, 1922, pp 1-2

2. (www.mari.net/~jcallow/signal/history.htm)

3. Michigan State Gazetteer & Business Directory. Detroit, MI, RL Polk

4. J Callow: Personal Correspondence. Menominee Historical Society (and excerpts via Emerson Electric Co). Menominee, MI, 11 Apr 2002

5. History of Signal Electric Company, Menominee, MI. Menominee County Historical Museum Archives; (http://www.mari.net/~jcallow/Signal/history.htm), 2002, p 1

6. (www.eagleherald.com/lar0317.htm)

7. Tradewell OG. Medical Electricity at Home. Menominee, MI, 1904

8. City of Menominee Centennial Corp (ed). The Past with Remembrance....the Future with Longing 1883-1983, Dallas, TX, 1983, p 30 (courtesy of Spies Public Library, Menominee, MI.)

9. Catalog of Sears, Roebuck and Co. Chicago, IL, Sears, Roebuck, 1908, p 206

CHAPTER 19. VOLTAMP ELECTRIC MANUFACTURING COMPANY OF BALTIMORE

The Voltamp Electric Manufacturing Company made and sold medical electrical batteries for home use, toys, and small motors. Three companies appear closely entwined with its history: the Voltamp Electric Manufacturing Co itself, the Chloride of Silver Dry Cell Battery Company, and the Charles Willms Surgical Instrument Company. All three companies were located in Baltimore, MD, very near each other (Voltamp Electric Mfg Co and Chloride of Silver Dry Cell Battery Co), and one (Willms Surgical Instrument Co) as a proprietary operation located a few blocks from the other two. Chapter 19 presents the products and history of the Voltamp Electric Manufacturing Company.

Mr Manes E Fuld (1863-1956) was the president and owner of the Voltamp Electric Mfg Co, and in 1897 he additionally assumed the role of general manager of the Chloride of Silver Dry Cell Battery Co. In 1897, Manes Fuld not only took over management of the Chloride of Silver Co, but also founded the Voltamp Electric Mfg Co in the same year or perhaps in 1896. This action provided him with control of a manufacturing potential for the Voltamp Electric Mfg Co, a home consumer division, as well as the continued operation of an established physician consumer company, the Chloride of Silver Dry Cell Battery Co. The Voltamp Electric Co probably designed and went into production with its medical electrical batteries sometime in 1896, since Voltamp sold its Portable Faradic Unit through the catalog of Sears, Roebuck and Co of Chicago in 1897. Voltamp also wholesaled its batteries to many other retailers who in turn had their names placed on the products. Collectors need to keep this in mind when identifying and dating their artifacts. Only a few manufacturers of solely family or home use batteries existed compared with the many retailers of medical apparatuses and supplies.

Patents for components of its electrical batteries (viz, Fuld current regulator) were given in 1899. Publication of its Faradic Hints or the Faradic Current in the Treatment of Disease booklet for inclusion with the sale of the medical electrical batteries was copyrighted and first published also in 1899.[1] The booklet Faradic Hints...... served the purpose of an instruction manual and as a catalog for the company's product line of faradic electrical batteries. When the company marketed its galvanic batteries of 1900 the booklet was modified to include some information about galvanic current and eliminate the faradic products. The title of this second version was Faradic Hints:The Faradic Current in the Treatment of Disease; The Galvanic Current in the Removal of Superfluous Hair, Facial and Other Blemishes (see Fig VE16).

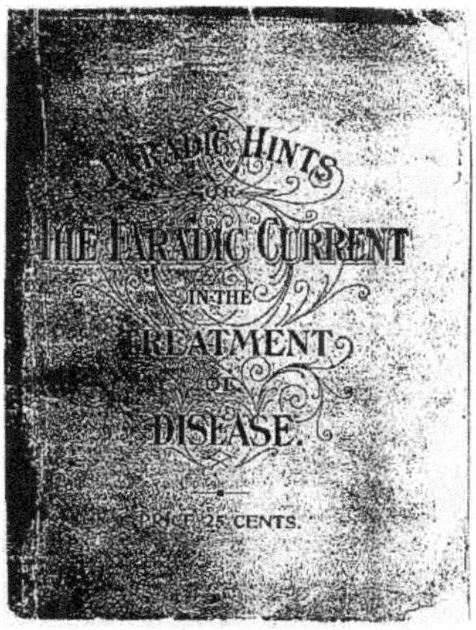

Fig VE1. Voltamp's Faradic Hints

Charles Willms at different times had a role with each of these three companies (Charles Willms Surgical Instrument Co, the Voltamp Electric Mfg Co, and the Chloride of Silver Dry Cell Battery Co). Charles Willms was owner of his own surgical instrument and supply business located at 300 North Howard Street about two or three blocks away from the other two companies. Willms, while still running his own business, was also the general manager of the Chloride of Silver Dry Cell Battery Co from 1890 to 1897, and while there in 1894 patented the Willms Current Controller or disc style rheostat that carried his name. Willms is believed to have been the first to adopt ideas of Charles Wheatstone of England into controlling current flow in the medical electrical battery. The Willms Current Controller became a standard component of some batteries of the Chloride of Silver Dry Cell Battery Co after 1894. He seemed to have been associated with Fuld at the Chloride of Silver Dry Cell Battery Co and Voltamp Electric Mfg Co after 1897, perhaps as a consultant.

In addition to manufacturing and selling a variety of medical electrical batteries, Voltamp Electric Mfg Co made and sold toy electrical trains from 1903 to 1923. Manes E Fuld made his first toy train in 1897 for his youngest son. Family and friends liked the toy electrical train so much that he decided to manufacture and market them in 1903, and when he did the company sold out of stock shortly after being advertised locally. His train business was aimed toward local wealthy consumers rather than national sales. Fuld designed the trains after the local Baltimore & Ohio blue trains and the United Railway street cars of Baltimore,[2,3] and perhaps after some aspects of The New York Central Railroad.[4] He made mostly steamers for two-inch rail track. Each model produced contained fine details; the trains were painted blue, and the streetcars were painted red and lettered in white for "United Electric."

The trains had bronze bearings, cast iron wheels, sheet metal bodies, copper and brass trim, and gold leaf decals. The trains were expensive for those times, $57.00 for one set, and some locomotives selling for $35.00 each (some of these units sold for $2,500.00 or more in year 2000 as collectors' items). His early trains were powered by Voltamp dry cells connected in series. The dry cells also powered carbon lights. At first he used a solenoid or induction coil like that used for his medical faradic electrical apparatuses as a controller of the toy trains. He also used rheostats to control power of the trains. Fuld in 1908 invented transformers and many other pieces of equipment such as a remote control transformer, and an automatic coupler, but he never patented his toy inventions.[2,3]

Fuld never did a large business with his toy trains. He was content to sell them locally and advertise in only a few catalogs that are now rare collectors' items. Fuld never did national business like his competitors of that time (American Flyer; Carlisle & Finch; Ives; and Lionel), but he excited many children in Baltimore when Christmas time arrived.

Lionel was the dominant manufacturer and marketer of toy trains at the time. Lionel was the first toy train company founded earlier (1901) by Joshua Lionel Cowen. Cowen kept a very close watch on the toy train business, and in 1905 he took action against his competitors with a marketing strategy in which he stated publicly that other companies were duplicating Lionel and selling them cheaper. He claimed that only Lionel trains were durable (Time has proven that Lionel has endured in the toy train business.) Also in 1905, Lionel did $8,000.00 of business that was its best year up to that date.[4] Carlisle & Finch sold their business in 1915,[4] and in 1922 or 1923 Fuld sold his Voltamp toy train business to Boucher, Inc of New York.[2,3]

Dry Cells. The Voltamp Electric Mfg Co continued to make electrical products like its chloride of silver dry cells (absorbed from Chloride of Silver Dry Cell Battery Co), small motors, and animated toys. Fuld maintained his office at 408 North Paca Street (near Paće St) and his factory at the rear on Jasper Street (near Pierce St).[2,3]

The Voltamp Electric Mfg Co in 1899 offered a large number (12) of faradic coil medical electrical batteries for public consumers' home use. The company recommended some batteries for both physician and home use, but its business was dominantly with the public rather than the professional. Five of its units (No.1 through No.5) used the company's special sized dry cell (5.25 x 2 inches, patented 27 June 1899) that was smaller compared with the standard dry cell (6.25 x 2.5 inches). Both sized cells delivered 1.0 to 1.5 volts each. The company thought that customers preferred the smaller sized dry cell to the larger one because of its compactness and its convenient size. Seven of the company's faradic units (No.6 through No.13) used the standard sized dry cells. In 1904, the No.14 faradic unit was added to its product line. Two small portable coils without cases were sold, and both could use either sized dry cell. Voltamp did not use the chloride of silver dry cell in its medical electrical batteries for home or family use. Voltamp also offered a Six-Cell Galvanic Unit in 1899 to 1904 and later. The company continued in business at least until 1928 and perhaps later. Voltamp, however, may have been a victim of the economic depression of that time.

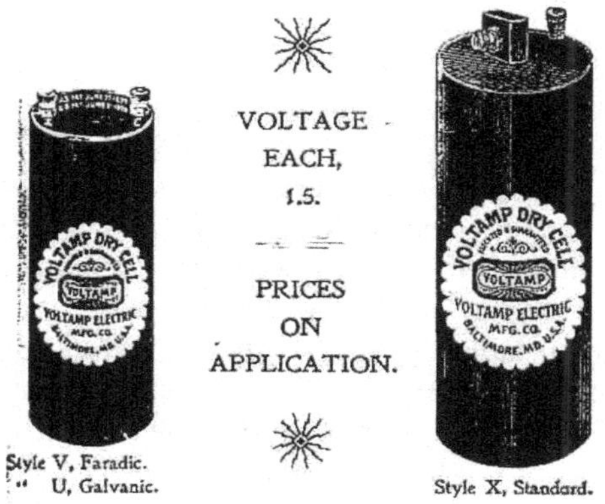

Fig VE2. Voltamp Dry Cells

Consumers had a choice of the medical electrical machines according to battery size, each battery delivered 1.0 to 1.5 volts. The size of the electrical batteries (in addition to the numbers) dictated the overall size of the wooden box encasing the faradic coil unit with its appendices. That is, the units using the smaller dry cells were smaller in overall size (box or case) than those using the standard dry cell. The Voltamp Electric Co named each of its medical electrical batteries for consumer selection and identification. Units using the smaller sized dry cells (5.25 x 2 inches) were called: Home Comfort, No.1; Solace, No.2; Relief, No.3; Samaritan, No.4; and Little Gem, No.5. Those electrical machines using the standard sized dry cells (6.25 x 2.25 inches) were labeled: Majestic, No.6; Olympia, No.7; Fireside, No.8; Imperial, No.9; Crown, No.10; Invincible, No.11; and the Champion, No12. The electrical machines using the two different sized dry cells were paired by their number of cells and performance. Number 1 matched No.7; No. 2 matched No.11; No.3 matched No.12; No.4 matched No.6; and No.5 matched No.8. The number of cells varied from one to two in 1899, and their electrical output varied accordingly. By 1904, the company offered the Monarch, No.14 Battery with four standard sized dry cells.

Voltamp Emblem. An emblem is printed on Voltamp's induction coils, and the emblem contains the words "Voltamp" in its

Fig VE3. Voltamp Emblem

center. The words “Voltage,” “Amperage,” “Trade,” “Mark” appear in the corners of the emblem from the upper left to the lower right, respectively.

Commonalties of Voltamp Batteries

Specific identifying features unique to the manufacturer’s product lines can be observed. Voltamp enclosed (capped) each end of its induction coils with raised 0.38 inch wide circular caps of black wood or hard rubber (or gutta percha). The Voltamp faradic batteries No.2, 3, 11, 12, 14, and the bath cabinet plate have the Fuld Current Regulator that is embossed on the hard rubber disc. Each apparatus has a name on its lid along with the directions. Face plates of the boxed apparatuses are black painted wood. The boxed faradic electrical apparatuses have a yellowish colored paper label glued on the inside lid, and this label has the company’s printed signature. Voltamp always cited a hand written serial number on the paper label of each medical electrical battery. It was the only company to use the “Fuld Current Regulator.”

The exception to the stated commonalties was when Voltamp manufactured medical electrical apparatuses for other retailers. Often the name and address of the retailer was cited on the yellowish colored paper label on the inside of the lid rather than that of Voltamp, the manufacturer. In some cases of retailer models the induction coil was labeled “professional” rather than “Voltamp.” In some cases the coil was not labeled, but these units remained Voltamp style (circular end caps of wood or hard rubber enclosing the coils, materials, and size). All Voltamp faradic batteries, except No.14 the Monarch (ca 1904), are dated from 1899.

Faradic Batteries

Home Comfort Battery. The unit of Fig VE4 delivers three currents (primary, secondary, and combined); is housed in a cherry box (8 x 5 x 5.38 inches) with a hinged lid and a leather strap as a carrying handle; single throw On/Off switch; and a single dry cell underneath the black painted wooden face plate. The patient is connected by electrode wires joining a combination of two button type connectors. Directions for use and company signature were printed on a yellowish paper label and glued inside of the lid.

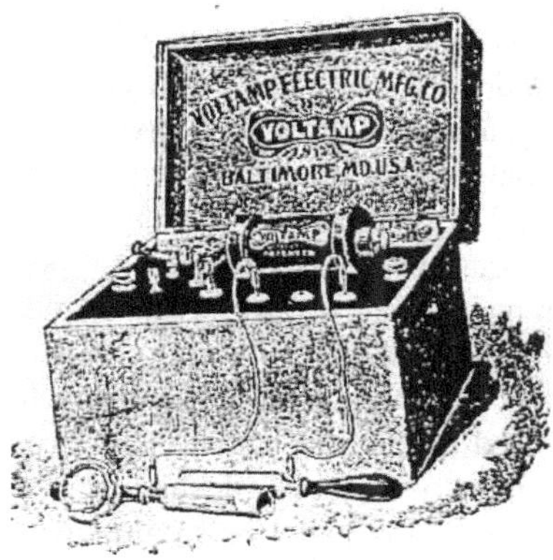

Fig VE4. No. 1 Home Comfort and Olympia No. 7[1]

The Home Comfort unit matched exactly in design and size with the No. 7 Olympia. The difference between the two batteries was that the Home Comfort used one small Voltamp cell (5.25 x 2 inches) for power, while the Olympia used one standard dry cell (6 x 2.5 inches). Voltamp Electric Mfg Co did not list prices of its electrical product line in its 1899 booklet, but in the catalog of 1904 it sold the No.1 Home Comfort model for $7.00.

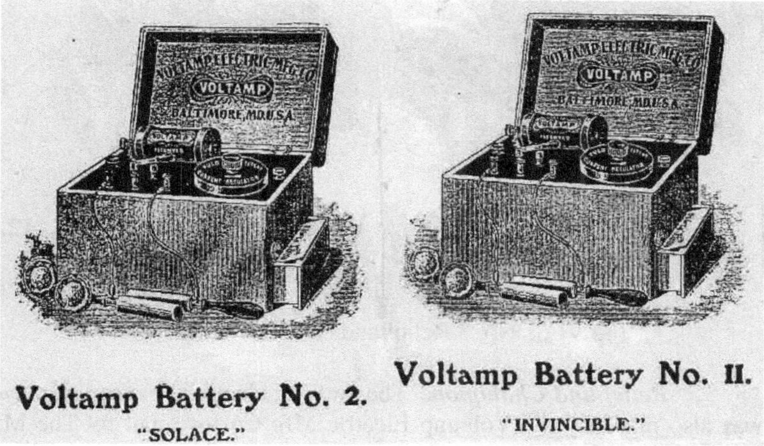

Fig VE5. No. 2 Solace and No. 11 Invincible[1]

Solace and Invincible. The No.2 faradic electrical battery was powered by two small Voltamp Electric Co dry cells, and is therefore larger than the No.2 and No.11 batteries. It is housed in a stained cherry box (9.25 x 5.5 x 7 inches). The corners of the box are dovetailed and glued. The box is carried by a leather strap attached to the sides. Inside of the lid is a yellowish paper label that includes directions and signature. The bottom right side of the box has a drawer (1.5 x 4.5 x 8.5 inches) that houses accessories, and is secured by a pivoting nickel plated disc (0.75 inches). The face panel is black painted wood with three adjustable screw connector posts (1, 2, 3); the primary current is obtained from posts 1 and 2; the secondary current is obtained from posts 2 and 3; and the combination current is obtained from posts 1 and 3. The left rear of the face panel has an adjustable screw spring interrupter to regulate current frequencies, and an induction coil (3.5 x 1.5 inches) labeled "Voltamp" with each end closed by circular caps of hard rubber. Between the coil and front three connector posts is a lever type throw switch for On/Off, and on the right side of the panel is a Fuld Current Regulator (rheostat patented by Fuld in 1899) with a circular control knob (1 inch).

The No.2 Solace matched exactly with the No.11 Invincible except that it used two small batteries for power while the Invincible used two standard sized cells. In 1904, the No.2 and the No.11 model each sold for $10.00.

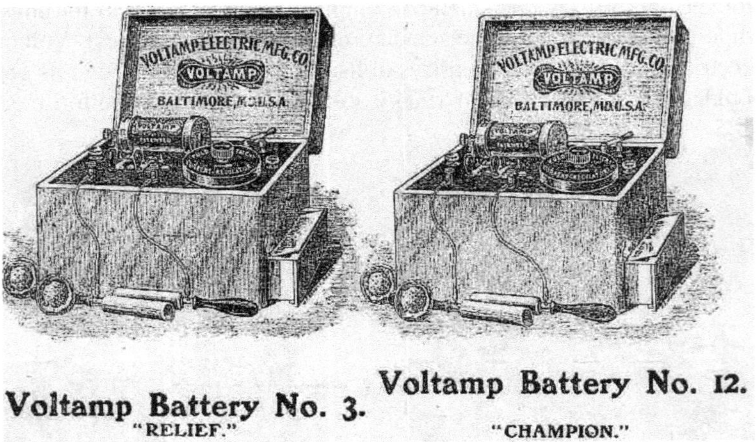

Fig VE6. No. 3 Relief and No. 12 Champion[1]

Relief and Champion. The medical electrical battery displayed was also made by the Voltamp Electric Mfg Co for retail by The Max Wocher & Son Co of 19-23 West Sixth Street, Cincinnati, OH. This is another battery that exemplifies a manufacturer's product under a different signature, than that of the retailer or seller. This faradic unit was housed in a walnut box (10.38 x 6.38 x 7.75 inches) and has a metal carrying handle on top. The right side of the box has a drawer (about 9.5 x 5.5 x 1.5 inches) for accessories. The face panel is black painted wood secured by four metal screws. The face panel contains an induction coil (3.75 x 1.75 inches) sealed at each end by a raised circular cap or sleeve of wood or hard rubber (gutta percha); on left of the coil is an adjustable

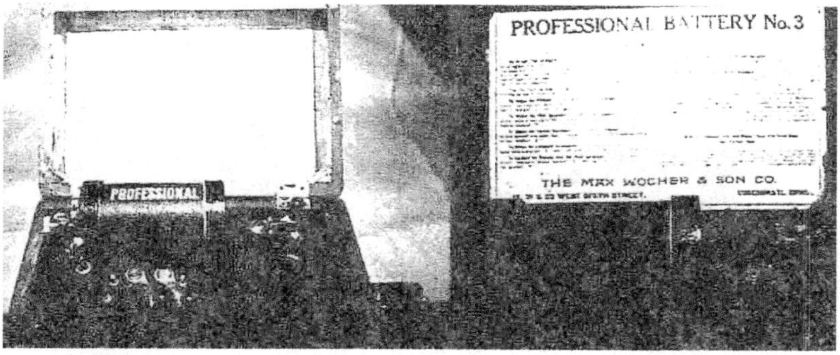

Fig VE 6A. Professional Battery No. 3, Max Wocher

screw spring type of interrupter; two lever controls with four buttons ("1, 2, 3, 4") for five currents; N and P connecting poles; an On/Off lever control; and a Fuld Current Regulator ("pat Jan 10, 1899 & Mar 27, 1899") with a fixed circuit unit with rotating knob (1 inch). This faradic battery delivers five current variations. This unit is powered by two small dry cells of 1.5 volts each, and was also sold by Montgomery Ward & Co through its catalog in 1903,[6] as was the No.12.

Differences occur between the No.3 retailed model by the Voltamp Electric Mfg Co and that manufactured for retail by Max Wocher & Son Co of Cincinnati. Both wooden boxes are constructed with tongue and goove glued corners. The box for the unit sold by Wocher is cherry and smaller (9.25 x 6.25 x 7.75 inches), hinged lid with a metal carrying handle on top and latched in front with a hook lever. The unit retailed by the Voltamp Electric Mfg Co is of walnut and larger (either 10.25 x 6.25 x 8 or 10.38 x 6.38 x 7.75 inches), hinged lid with a carrying leather strap mounted on each side. The actual dimensions of the walnut box may vary somewhat from the company's advertisements. Both face plates are black painted wood secured in the corners by four wood screws. The size of the face plates differ. That of Wocher is smaller (8.5 x 5.5 inches) than that sold by Voltamp Electric Mfg Co (9.5 x 5.5 inches). The face plate contains an induction coil (3.75 x 2 inches) covered by black fabric (labeled "Professional"), and sealed by hard rubber circular end caps; and a Fuld Current Regulator. The On/Off controls differ. The Wocher unit has a lever control, while that of Voltamp Electric Mfg Co has a single throw (knife) switch. Although a larger case, the Voltamp Electric Mfg Co used two small dry cells and the Wocher unit used two standard sized dry cells to power the units. Both units use the yellowish paper label but differ in signature information. The Voltamp Electric Mfg Co unit sold for $15.00 in 1904. The units date from 1899 to at least 1928. The possibility exists that the Wocher unit was made about 1904 because of its smaller case and cheaper On/Off control than that of the Voltamp Electric Mfg Co unit that was made in 1899.

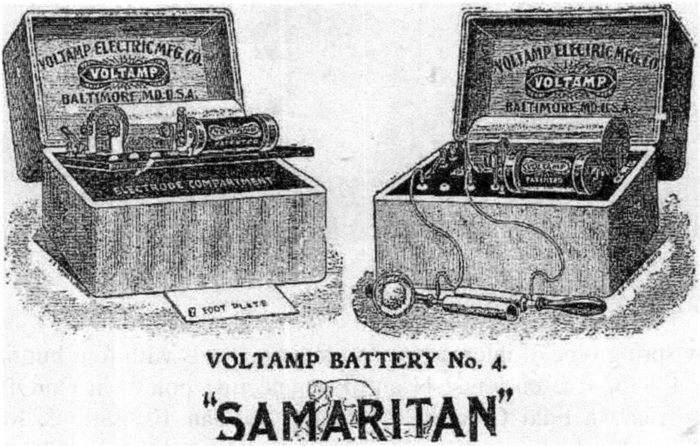

Fig VE7. No. 4 Samaritan

Samaritan. This unit is encased in a cherry box, and a hinged lid with a leather carrying strap mounted on the sides. It has a "nonshort" circuiting switch that prevents a closed circuit when the lid of the box is shut (protects the dry cell); a dry cell underneath the black painted wooden face plate that pivots (latched) to open for accessories; delivers primary, secondary, and combined currents; and is powered by a single small Voltamp Electric Mfg Co cell.

No.4 Samaritan matches the No.6 Majestic in design, but differs with the Majestic No.6 in box size (8.25 x 5.25 x 5 inches, No.4 vs 8.75 x 5.5 x 5.38 inches, No.6), and cell size, small vs standard, respectively. The No.4 unit sold for $8.00 in 1904.

Little Gem and Fireside. The Little Gem, No.5, that uses a single small Voltamp Electric Mfg Co dry cell (underneath face plate) is exactly the same as No.8, Fireside, in design and box size, but differs from No.8, Fireside that uses a standard sized dry cell for power. These units sold for $5.00 each in 1904, but were available in 1899.

The Little Gem, No.5, is the smallest of the boxed faradic batteries in the Voltamp Electric Mfg Co line. It uses one small sized dry cell for power; is housed in a cherry or oak box (8 x 3.75 x 5 inches) with hinged lid containing directions and signature on a yellow paper label; and leather carrying strap with mounting pins on each side. The black, painted wood face plate contains the induction coil with a sliding tube current controller; an adjustable screw spring lever, hammer type interrupter; a lever On/Off control; lever control to obtain primary, secondary, or combined currents; and three connecting posts.

The Little Gem electrical medical battery was illustrated and

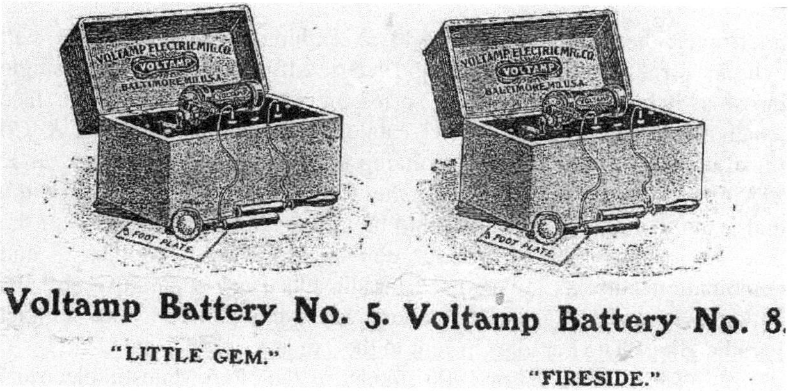

Fig VE8. No. 5 Little Gem and No. 8 Fireside

listed as # 6353 in the 1897 (page 473) catalog of Sears, Roebuck and Co.[5] In the catalog the Little Gem was encased in a polished oak box (4.5 x 4.75 x 7.75 inches), complete with its one dry cell it weighed 5.5 pounds, and cost $5.75 (extra dry cell cost $0.70). The oak box was thus used from 1897 to 1904 when the Little Gem, No.5, and the Fireside, No.8, were encased in cherry boxes.

Majestic. The Majestic, No. 6 faradic battery of the Voltamp Electric Mfg Co (Fig VE9) was sold also through the mail order catalog of Montgomery Ward & Co in 1900. The unit is encased in a cherry box (8.13 x 5.13 x 5 inches) with directions and signature printed on the paper label inside lid. The label shows patent dates of January 10, 1899 and September 15, 1900. The face panel is the customary Voltamp Electric Mfg Co black painted wood that contains the induction coil (3.5 x 1.25 inches, marked "Voltamp"); an adjustable screw spring type

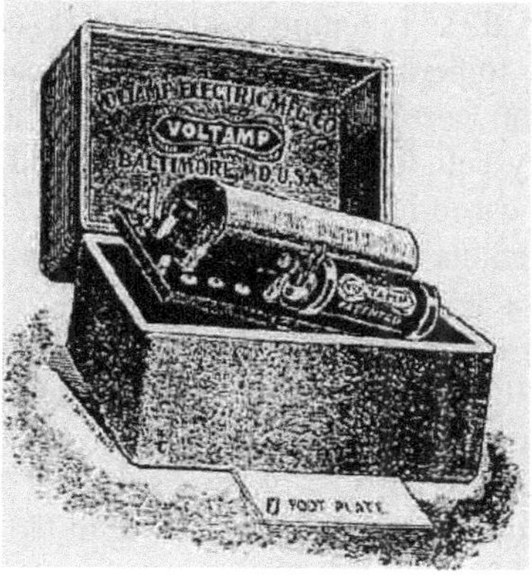

Fig VE9. No. 6 Majestic

interrupter; three connecting posts (1, 2, 3); hinged nickel plated dry cell cylinder for a single small Voltamp Electric Mfg Co dry cell; and a single throw switch for On/Off. Accessories are placed underneath the face panel that lifts easily. The 1903 catalog of Montgomery Ward & Co illustrated and listed the No.6 Voltamp unit, without a trade mark, as K 21354, and sold it for $3.75.[6] This unit has a "nonshort" circuit switch that is automatically thrown open to break the circuit when the lid of the box is closed. The Majestic delivers primary, secondary, and combination currents. Like other faradic electrical apparatuses by the Voltamp Electric Mfg Co this battery was accompanied by the booklet Faradic Hints: The Faradic Current in the Treatment of Disease."

The later (1905 or 1906) model of the No.6 Majestic electrical battery has some minor design changes from the earlier units (pre 1905). The No.6 unit was named the Majestic when retailed by Voltamp, and the No.6 Household Medical Battery when retailed by Montgomery Ward & Co. The dovetailed cherry box contains changes. Pre 1905 wooden boxes have a carrying strap that was mounted from each side, while the later units (after 1905) have a nickel plated carrying handle mounted on the top. The earlier boxes (pre 1905) do not have a locking device on the front, but the later models (after 1905) have a pivoting hook lever latch on the front. The overall size of the box remained the same for each design, but the division between lid and base differ. The pre 1905 box divides evenly (2.75 inches each) between lid and base, while the 1905 box divides with a larger lid (3.12 inches) than base (2.38 inches). The face plate with its components were also the same in all No.6 models, but the method of reaching the dry cell differ. In the pre 1905 models the face plate is raised by pivoting screws from one end of the box. In the models of 1905 and later the face plates raise by having pivoting screws from the sides on the rear side of the box, and is secured by a small catch. In 1904, these two units sold for $8.00 each.

Imperial. The Imperial (Fig VE10) is a small unit and less powerful than others that were also designed for home use. It uses a single standard sized dry cell for power that is located underneath the face plate. The unit is encased in an oak box (8.75 x 5.25 x 5.25 inches) with hinged lid and directions and signature on the paper label glued on the inside lid; and has a leather carrying strap. In all other electrical faradic batteries made by the Voltamp Electric Mfg Co the black, painted wooden face plate is flush to the lower electrode wires joining a combination of two button type connectors. Directions for use and company signature were printed on a yellowish paper label and glued inside of the lid portion of The opened box, but with No.9 the face plate is recessed to the opened box. The face plate contains the induction coil with its sliding tube current amplitude controller, an On/Off lever control, and three connection buttons for primary, secondary, and combined currents. This unit sold for $8.00 in 1904.

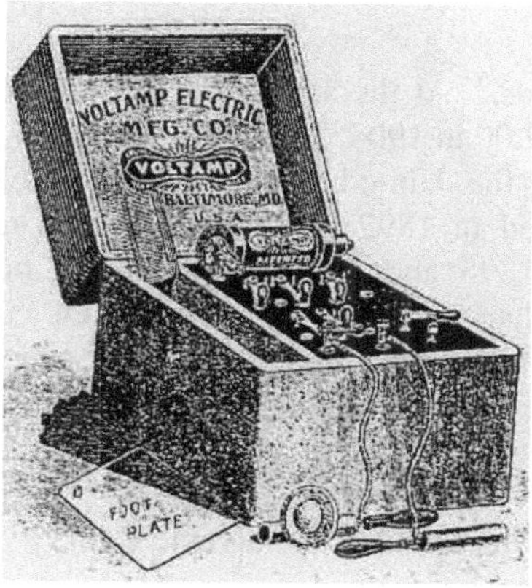

Fig VE10. No. 9 Imperial

Crown. This electric faradic battery uses two dry cells for power and provides higher current amplitudes than other models of the Voltamp Electric Mfg Co; the cells are located underneath the face plate.

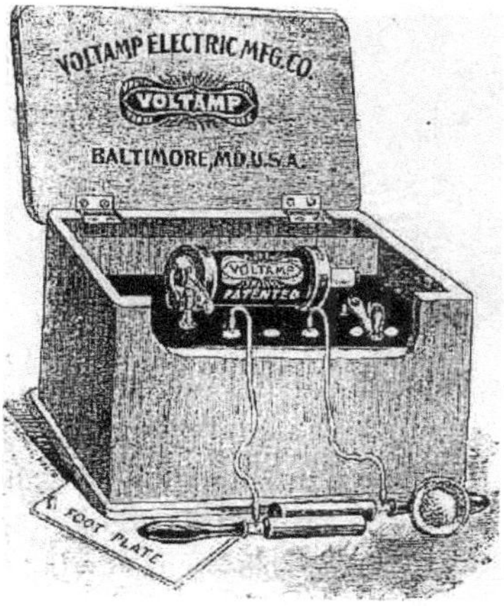

Fig VE11. No.10 Crown

The black, painted wooden face plate contains the coil with its sliding tube controller; a coil selector for primary, secondary, and combined currents; a pole changer, a cell selecting switch; a single throw On/Off switch; and two screw connecting posts. The wooden box enclosing the unit is 8 x 8 x 5.63 inches. Because of its power this unit was recommended for veterinary uses. Although the polished cherry box (6 x 5.25 x 5.25 inches) shown by Montgomery Ward & Co was for home use, and was smaller than that shown by Voltamp, The Crown Family Battery had the other characteristics of Voltamp. Montgomery Ward & Co of Chicago sold the unit through its 1903 catalog for $3.50 and it weighed 2.25 pounds.[6] At the same time the Voltamp Electric Mfg Co sold the unit for $12.00 in 1904.

Patents in the United States on the above faradic electrical batteries were issued in 1892 to 1901. Similar patents were issued in England between 1895 and 1900.[1] These dates bring the company's alleged founding date of 1896 in question. Of course items can be patented prior to their actual marketing dates, and perhaps the patents were made with the Chloride and Silver Dry Cell Battery Co by M Fuld who activated some later with Voltamp.

Combination Faradic and Galvanic Battery

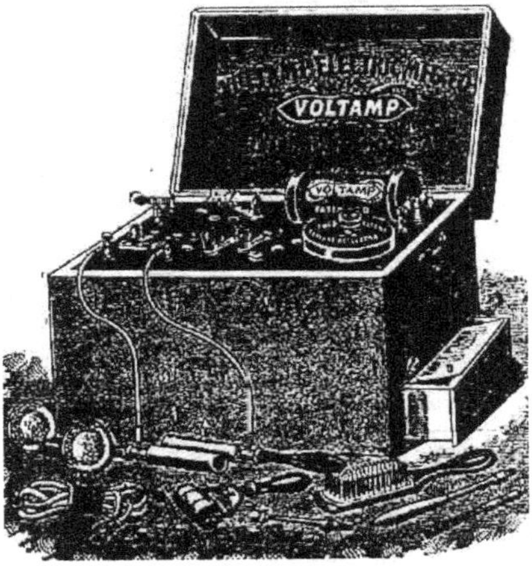

Fig VE12. No. 14 Monarch

Monarch. This electrical faradic and galvanic battery of Fig VE12 by the Voltamp Electric Mfg Co was built between 1899 and 1904 for multipurpose uses (veterinary, children, faradic, or galvanic) because of its quality. Four standard dry cells powered the unit and were kept underneath the face plate. The unit is encased in a wooden box (11.5 x 8.25 x 8 inches) with hinged lid. The unit is carried by a leather strap anchored on each side of the box. The lower right side of the box contains a drawer for accessories. The black, painted wooden face plate contains an induction coil with a double high tension secondary coil; a pole changing switch; a single On/Off throw switch; a coil selector switch, two adjustable screw connecting posts; and a Fuld Current Regulator. This model sold for $20.00 in 1904.

Miscellaneous Models

Bath Cabinet Plate. A bath cabinet plate consisting of a faradic coil especially designed electrical unit for use in galvanic-water baths was offered by Voltamp. In 1904, the Voltamp Electric Mfg Co offered the Bath Cabinet Plate that was similar to the No. 3 Battery. The Bath

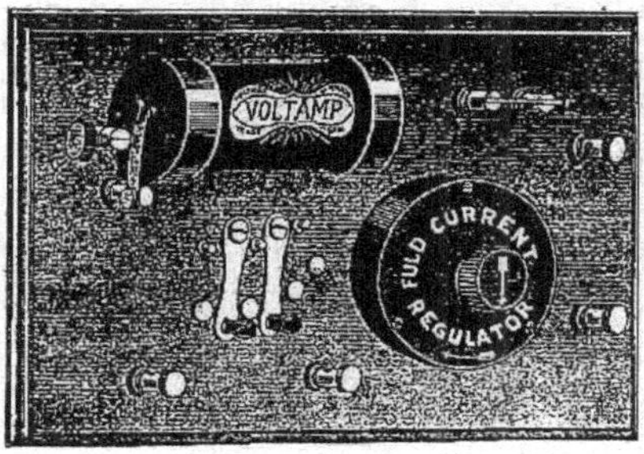

Fig VE13. The Bath Cabinet Plate

Cabinet Plate, mounted on the wall or top of a table, was designed and built for use in a bathtub. Two dry cells (either size) were needed to power it. Accessories differed from the No.3 Battery by having longer conducting cords, and electrodes for the head and foot of the tub. The unit sold for $15.00 in 1904.

Portable Faradic Unit. The Voltamp Electric Mfg Co made a small portable faradic coil mounted on a polished mahogany base (4.51 x 3.13 x 0.25 inches). This particular unit has "Voltamp" stamped into the bottom of the walnut base, but without a trade name like other medical electrical batteries of Voltamp Electric Mfg Co. The coil (2.13 x 0.75 inches) is mounted on the wooden base by a fixed square (1.13 inches) black painted wooden block on its left end. Also, on the left end of the coil is an adjustable screw spring vibrating type interrupter to control pulse frequency. A nickel plated hollow tube slides over the top of the coil's core to control current amplitude. Two nickel plated posts for cell

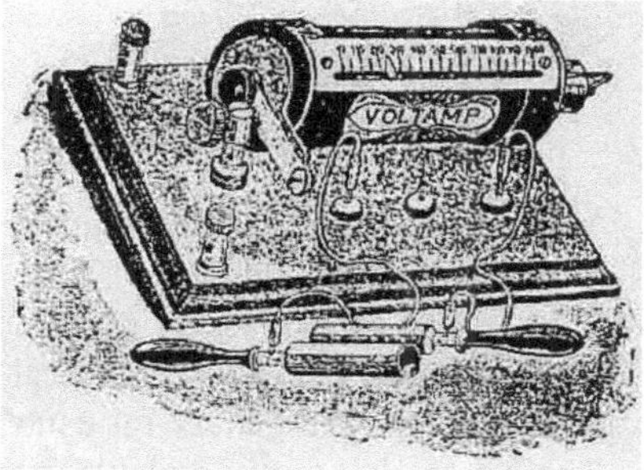

Fig VE14. Voltamp Small Portable Faradic Unit, Faradic Coil

connection (1.5 volts dry cell) is on the left, while the two connecting cords to the patient are attached directly to the circuitry that is underneath the base. The two one foot long patient connecting cords each leave the base through nickel plated buttons, and are fixed to hand held electrodes that are not removable. The unit pictured dates from 1899 to 1905, and in 1904, this model sold for $2.50. This coil is really the same as the Home Comfort No.1 and the Samaritan No.4, but without a box enclosure. It is the equivalent of the operational components of the other two units that sold for $10.00 and $8.00, respectively. Unlike the other faradic batteries by Voltamp, the coil has an arbitrary scale that registers a value when the sliding tube of the current controller is moved in and out of the induction coil. The wiring of the circuitry is underneath the base of the wooden block and is covered by a fabric.

Hairbrush (not pictured)

For consumers who have scalp or hair loss problems the Voltamp Electric Mfg Co's Farado Masseur was available. It is a hairbrush equipped with a self contained cell and faradic coil.

Galvanic Batteries

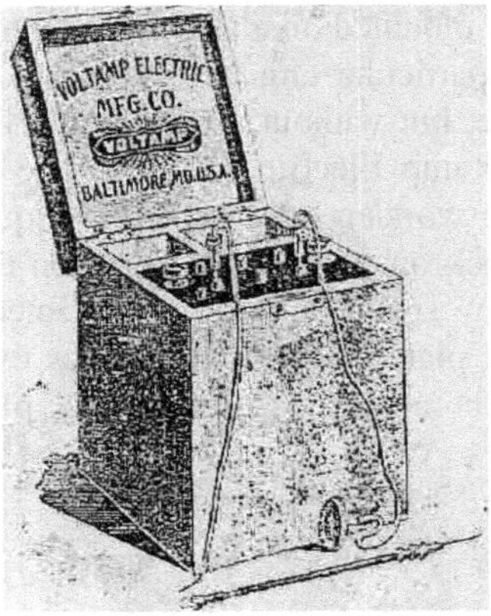

Fig VE15. Voltamp Six Cell Galvanic Battery

Six-Cell Galvanic Battery. In addition to the Voltamp Electric Mfg Co's wide selection of faradic coil electrical apparatuses, the company offered a six-celled galvanic battery for cautery and chemically affected treatments. This unit is housed in a cherry box (6.63 x 5.63 x 6 inches) with a hinged lid. The box is carried by a leather strap. The black, painted wooden face plate contained six buttons connecting posts arranged in series so that one to four dry cells can be used simultaneously. Two screw nuts secure the face plate that rests on top of the standard sized dry cells. The galvanic battery was designed for treatments requiring a small amount of direct current (eg, removal of superfluous hair). In 1904, the unit cost $10.00. The unit dates from 1899.

Galvanic Battery. Voltamp marketed another six cells galvanic battery for home use in 1900. This model (Fig VE16) contained six dry cells of special size (4 x 1.625 inches, smaller than those of Fig VE2) that were patented in 1899 in the United States and Great Britain. The cells are housed underneath the face plate and connected in series on a removable rack. The face plate is black painted wood and holds six spring clips for accessories, two adjustable screw binding posts, and a six stud cell selector switch. The cherry box (11.5 x 5.25 x 3.75 inches) is hinged with two box-button type latches on front to secure the lid. A metal carrying handle is also on the front. All metal are nickel plated. Inside of the lid contains the characteristic yellow/black label of the Voltamp logo, address, and patent dates.

Each galvanic battery was accompanied by a booklet Faradic Hints, The Faradic Current on the Treatment of Disease; The Galvanic Current in the Removal of Superfluous Hair, Facial and Other Blemishes. The 32 paged booklet contains five pages on the galvanic current and its applications for removal of naevi, port wine marks, birth marks, moles, warts, and similar growths. An eye/head type of magnifying piece was among the accessories.

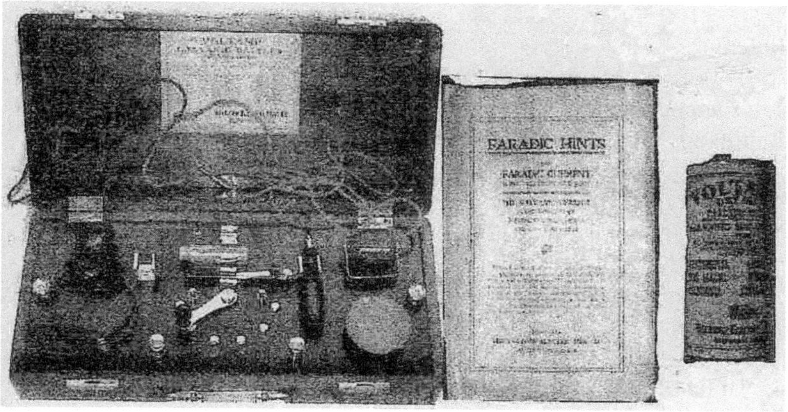

Fig VE 16. Galvanic Battery, Booklet, and Dry Cell

Summary

Voltamp electrical medical batteries were sold through medical supply companies that used their own labels or signature plates; eg, G Frye, Portland, ME; Sibley Mfg Co, St Paul, MN (Improved Sibley

Battery No.11, with a Voltamp coil and Fuld rheostat, 1899); Max Wocher & Son, Cincinnati, OH; and others. The mail order giants Montgomery Ward & Co, and Sears, Roebuck and Co of Chicago sold Voltamp medical electrical batteries. The outlets for the Voltamp batteries once formed a formidable list.

All Voltamp Electric Mfg Co medical faradic batteries were accompanied by the booklet Faradic Hints or Faradic Current for the Treatment of Diseases or the galvanic version for galvanic batteries that provided basic electrical information, electrical treatment of a wide variety of diseases and ailments, and descriptions of its product line. The Voltamp Electric Mfg Co medical electrical batteries appear to have been made in 1897 (portable coil), 1899 for models No. 1 through No.13, and in 1904 for the Monarch No.14.

This company, directed toward the family consumer business, was formed in 1896 or 1897 by an individual who also operated a manufactory doing the same function, but directed toward the physician consumer. Both the Voltamp Electric Mfg Co and the Chloride of Silver Dry Cell Battery Co had several patents. The latter company made only medical electrical batteries and accessories whereas the former company additionally engaged in the manufacture of toys and motors. The home use or family battery products were of many designs, and sold well enough to be commonplace today in the antique markets. The company seemed to disappear in the late 1920s when economic times were poor and the demand for the batteries was waning with the public.

References

1. Faradic Hints or The Faradic Current in the Treatment of Disease. Baltimore, MD, Voltamp, 1899, 1904, pp 25-41

2. Roth AO. I remember the old Voltamp electric trains. Baltimore, MD, The Baltimore Sun, 22 Dec 1957

3. Stump W. A railroader with 800 trains, but no track. Baltimore, MD, The Baltimore Sun, 1 Jan 1956

4. Hollan R. All Aboard, Rev. New York, NY, Workman Pub, 2000, p 40

5. Catalog of Sears, Roebuck and Co, Chicago, IL, Sears, Roebuck, 1897, p 473

5. Catalog of Montgomery Ward & Co, Chicago, IL, 1903, p 514

CHAPTER 20. PG WILLIAMS MANUFACTURING ELECTRICIAN OF NEW YORK CITY

Percy G Williams of New York City, founded his company in 1880. The company has many artifacts for the collector's quest, however, several are rare even though offered in 1905. The products and history of the PG Williams company are reviewed in Chapter 20.

The company has been identified by different names; that of PG Williams Manufacturing Electrician, and after 1904 that of PG Williams Electro Medical Battery Co (Williams Electro-Medical Battery Co, and Electro-Medical Battery Co of New York). In 1905, his catalogue listed the company simply as Percy G Williams. The company had at least five different addresses during its existence; the earliest was 1679 Broadway (1880s); and followed by 82-84 West Broadway; 12 Vesey Street (perhaps 1892-1900); in 1904 it was located at 6 Barclay Street; and perhaps as late as 1920 the company was located at 12 Jersey St. The company is known to have published 25 yearly catalogues from 1880 to 1905 (viz, <u>ElectroMedical Batteries and Instruments</u>).

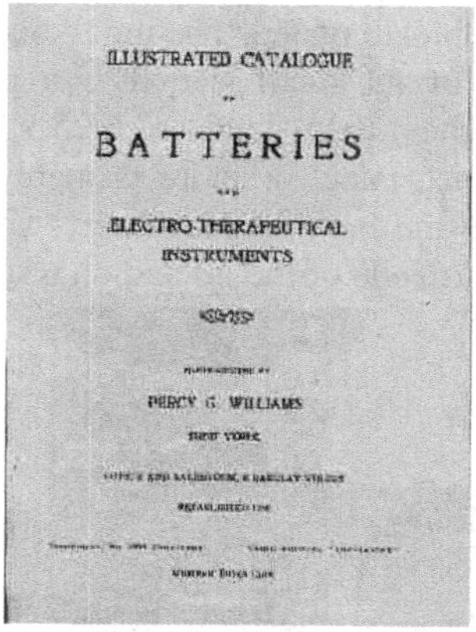
ILLUSTRATED CATALOGUE

BATTERIES

ELECTRO-THERAPEUTICAL INSTRUMENTS

PERCY G. WILLIAMS

NEW YORK

Fig W. Catalogue of Batteries, 1905

Although not verified, Percy G Williams was purported to have been a Vaudeville actor and theater owner in New York City during the 1870s and 1890s. He supposedly became a physician, as was his father, and manufacturer of medical electrical batteries. PG Williams was not listed as a physician in New York in Polk's 1904 Medical Registry.[1]

Commonalties of the PG Williams Batteries

The paper labels citing directions and the company's signature inside of the lid of the Williams' home use batteries used contrasting colors (red with white ink, black with yellow ink, light green with black ink). The models of the medical electrical batteries having a specific name (eg, Red Cross) were for home use and their quality supports that contention, these were first made prior to 1900. The induction coils of the Williams faradic electrical batteries were covered with different materials (eg, colored black or red fabric, nickel plate). The end caps of Williams' faradic batteries were square blocks. Williams' batteries have a metal plate logo bearing his name and address.

In the Williams' 1905 catalogue, many batteries were made for physician use and their quality improved compared with his home use batteries. Metal components were also improved; for example, the binding posts were adjustable screw types rather than button holes.

Faradic Batteries

Red Cross Faradic Battery. Williams' Improved Red Cross Faradic Battery is housed in a small polished oak box (7 x 5.25 x 6 inches) that has a metal carrying handle on top of the case, and is secured in front by a hinged type clasp that has a pivot L shaped lever that locks. All metal on the unit are nickel plated. The unit is judged to be of 1900 to 1919 vintage. Because of its small size it was powered by a single smaller (eg, 5.25 x 2 inches) than standard (6.25 x 2.25 inches) dry cell placed underneath the face panel or more probably a standard dry cell was placed externally to the box. The signature was located on the red paper label (directions) inside of the lid and on a small yellow colored

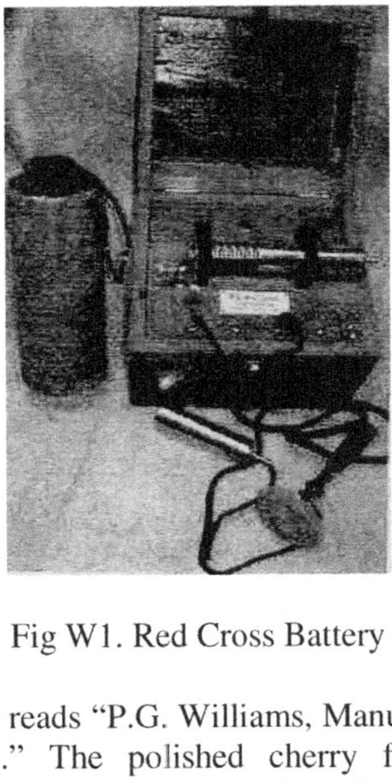

Fig W1. Red Cross Battery

hard rubber plate that reads "P.G. Williams, Manufacturer, 6 Barclay and 12 Vesey St., N.Y." The polished cherry face panel forms two compartments. The rear compartment has a lid (6 x 1.6 inches) with screw handles. The lid can be removed to place most accessories into the compartment. The larger panel (6 x 3 inches) contains the operational components: induction coil (3 x 0.75 inches) with 1.25 inches square black painted wood block or cap at each end. To the left end of the coil is an adjustable screw spring leaf hammer type interrupter that controls frequency and to the right end is a hollow tube (3.25 x 0.75 inches) that slides over the coil to control current amplitude. When the tube moves away from its stationary position the scored scale on the coil is seen (marked 10 to 100 with range of 0 to 110 arbitrary units). Four buttons used for connecting electrode cords to the patient are on the front part of the panel and marked A, B, C, and D to direct the primary, secondary, and combination currents. On the right front of the face panel is a lever switch and two buttons for Off/On control. A foot plate is housed underneath the face plate along with perhaps a small sized dry cell. The unit is accompanied with an eight paged booklet Directions for Using Williams' Batteries that provides suggested treatment for a wide variety of diseases and ailments. Since two addresses are part of the manufacturer's signature on the red paper label ("6 Barclay–12 Vesey"), this model is dated around 1900 to 1904.

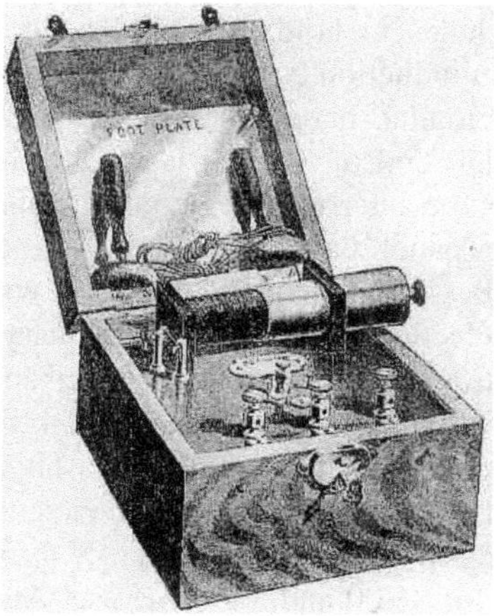

Fig W1A. Faradic Battery No. 1

In 1905, the Red Cross unit was also the ***Faradic Battery No.1*** for physicians. It used two dry cells for power. The No.1 was housed in a polished quartered oak box (8 x 9 x 6 inches) with a metal carrying handle on top of the hinged lid, and two lever catches on front along with a boxed button type lock on fromt. The face plate is black slate with On/Off switch, and three binding posts for patient connection. The coil has a metal sliding cover to control current. The secondary coil is wound with 1500 feet of fine wire to provide smooth currents, and a spring hammer vibrating interrupter is on the left of the coil. The fabric of the coil is printed with a scale to show movement of the coil cover in current control. Accessories are kept in the lid. This unit cost $10.00.

Perfection. The Williams' Perfection Electro-Magnetic Battery (Fig W2-A) delivered five currents while powered by one Grenet type wet cell. A cherry box (6 x 6 x 6.5 inches) housed the contents of the unit. The box was secured by a hinged type latch on the front, and has a metal carrying handle on top. Inside of the lid are directions and signature data of "PG Williams, Manufacturing Electrician, 12 Vesey St, NY." Based on its use of a Grenet wet cell the date of this pictured unit (Fig W2-A) is around 1892 or before. The Grenet wet cell was composed of a circular green glass jar (base of 3.5 x 3.5 inches with narrowing neck 2.25 inches), bimal (pat 1830-1920) made with a casting mold. Top of the Grenet cell is a hard rubber disc (2.25 inches) constructed to seal the jar that contains three elements (1 zinc 1.25 x 1.38 inches between 2 carbon elements, 0.88 x 1.38 inches each), and a metal lifter for the zinc element. The cell lid has a small nickel plate "Williams' Perfection Battery." The wet cell is set underneath the face panel with its top exposed to connect to metal connectors wired with the circuit under the face panel, and to operate the lifter. The face panel is matching wood of the case that has two holes to hold the metal hand held hollow tube electrodes. It contains an induction coil (3.75 x 0.75 inches) covered with red fabric, and with circular hard rubber ends or caps of different diameters; and on the left end of the coil is an adjustable screw spring leaf, hammer vibrator type interrupter to control pulse frequency. The front part of the face panel has four holes with eyelets or button connectors labeled (A, B, C, D) for joining electrical wires or cords to the patient with current selections marked (AB=primary; BC=secondary; CD=combined, very strong; AC=combined, mild; and BD=combined, very mild). The electrical wire or cord connections to the patient provide a fixed current amplitude; no sliding tube or rheostat was supplied with the model. The consumer could replace the zinc elements for $0.25 each by contacting the company at 12 Vesey Street, NY, where in 1892 the company sold this unit for $5.00 and for home use. Also, some cases for The Perfection Battery in 1892 measured 5 x 5 inches. (Note: The German Electric Co occupied 12 Vesey St at one time. It sold batteries.)

Prior to or about 1900, dry cells were replacing the inconvenient and problematic wet cells of approximately the same voltage (1.5 V). Addressing this issue of wet versus dry cell advantages, Percy G Williams apparently redesigned the Perfection Battery twice (B, C for identity), about 1900 to 1904, to remain competitive.

The second generation of the Williams Perfection Battery was redesigned from the original pictured in Fig W2 that was powered by a single Grenet wet cell. The second model (B) differs from the original by its case and induction coil. Model B is encased in a quarter sawn oak box

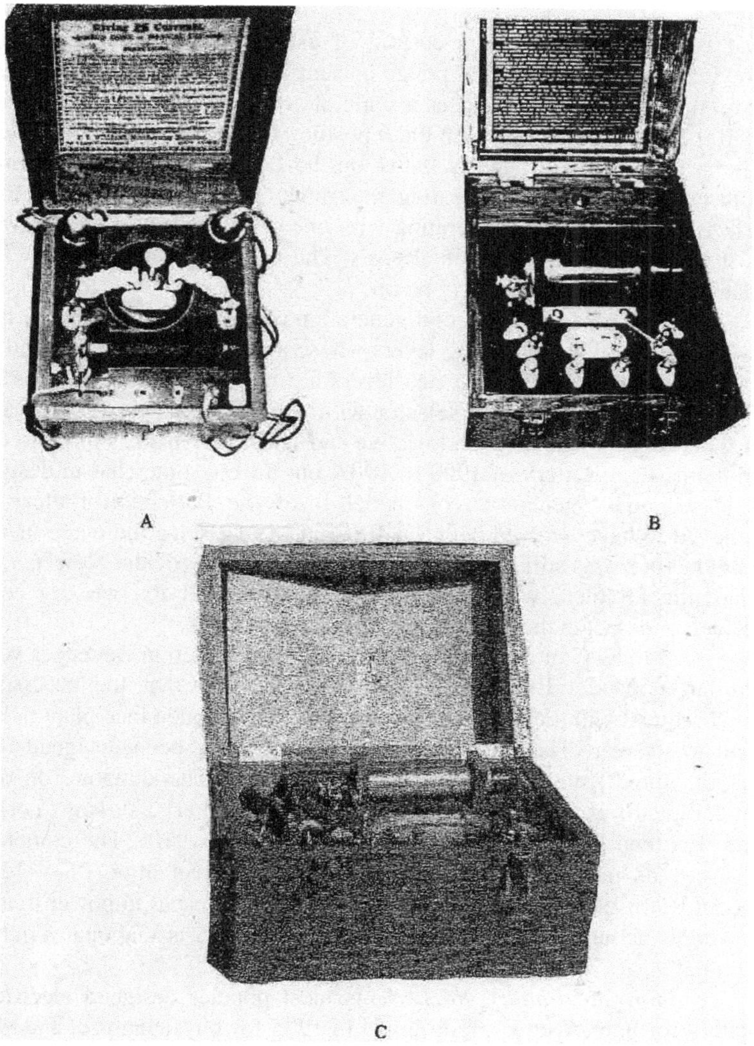

Fig W2. Perfection Battery; A, B, C

(9 x 8 x 6 inches) that has a hinged lid that is secured on the front of the box by two snap latches. The tongue and groove corners are glued. On top of the box is a metal handle with the company's name etched. An accessory compartment with a wooden lid is located behind the black slate face plate.

Although the inside of the lid has a label giving the directions for operation, a separate signature plate (customary of Williams) is mounted on the slate face plate ("P.G. Williams, 6 Barclay Street, New York"). Model B has square hard rubber end caps on the induction coil that is a departure from its custom of using circular end caps on all previous models. The nickel plated current controller when pulled away from the primary coil discloses a scale of arbitrary units ranging from 0 to 100. The further away from the 0 position the more current amplitude. The scale is a type of fabric. Also, on the face plate is a conventional adjustable screw spring vibrating interrupter, a lever On/Off switch, a selector lever switch for operating with one or two cells, and four screw post type connectors or terminal posts. The metal parts are thinly nickel plated, and terminal posts may be tin.

The model B or second generation of the Perfection Battery has two horseshoe-like collapsing levers whose axes are mounted on another rectangular bar. When these two levers are positioned they serve as an On/Off switch, and current selector with connecting posts A, B, C, and D. This concept and function to active and select currents is similar to the Williams Dial Battery of 1900 to 1902, but differs somewhat in design. This secondary generation or model B of the Perfection Battery is believed to have evolved between 1902 and 1904, since the name of the manufacturer was still "Williams Manufacturing Electrician, New York." The unit complete weighs about four pounds with its two dry cells located underneath the face plate.

Model C or the third generation of the Perfection Battery is very similar to Model B. Model C differs from B in that the accessory compartment with lid is located to the left of the wooden face plate rather than to its rear. The model C is believed to have been designed and manufactured sometime between 1910 and 1920. The signature on this model identifies the "Williams Electro-Medical Battery Co. New York," and was then located at 6 Barclay Street (1905 to 1910). The company changed its name and relocated to 6 Barclay Street after 1904. Like model B, this model C uses two dry cells (1.5 volts each) to power it, and it weighs about four pounds. The case of model C is mahogany rather than oak.

Faradic Battery No.3. This most popular designed electrical battery for home use was redesigned in 1905 for physician use, and was the Faradic Battery No.3. The case was quartered oak with dovetailed glued corners (9 inches square); hinged lid has a metal carrying handle. The lid is secured by two hinges latches having lever hooks on front. The unit operated with two standard dry cells to provide high tension (voltage). The slate face plate contains three adjustable screw binding posts, a pole changer, On/Off switch, cell selector, coil, and adjustable spring hammer vibrator (slow and fast pulses) that does not hum. The coil fabric is marked in arbitrary units of 0 to 100 for recording current control by a sliding metal cover. The secondary coil is wound in sections with 3000 feet of No.36 wire (section 1 tapped at 700 ft, 2 at 1800 ft, and 3 at 3000 feet). All metal are nickel plated. Accessories are stored on inside lid. It cost $20.00 in 1905.

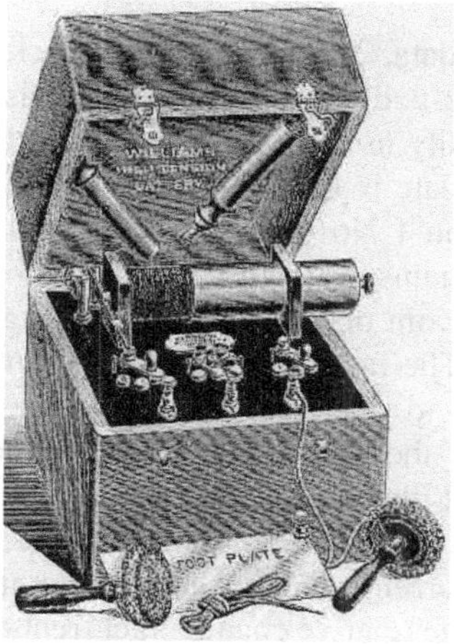

Fig W3. Faradic Battery No. 3

Dial Battery. The Williams' Dial Electro-Magnetic Battery (Fig W4) is uniquely different from batteries of other manufacturers. The original design of the Dial Battery may have been designed for coin operation by PG Williams and AW Roovers, but when manufactured by 1892 it was advertised for home and medical use. The PG Williams,

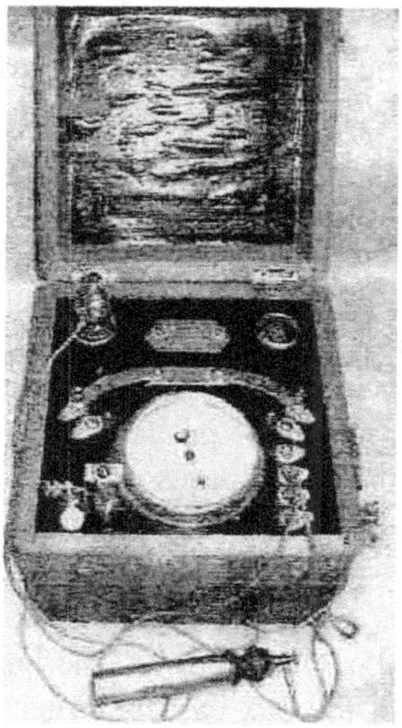

Fig W4. Dial Battery

manufacturing electrician, company was then located at 12 Vesey Street, New York. As customary, it is housed in a golden oak box (7.88 x 8 x 7.75 inches), secured with two hinged latches in front, and a metal carrying handle on top. Inside of the lid has a paper label with directions and company signature data. The face panel is black slate for units built from the 1880s to 1902 and later for some models. Units built in the 1890s to the 1920s usually used black polished hard rubber. In this unit pictured the slate face plate is flush with the bottom portion of the box. The unit was patented on 1 November 1887 (patent number 372,441 is on the dial face). Williams originally intended for the Dial Electro-Magnetic Battery to be coin operated when applying for his patent on 6 May of the same year. The face panel displays a circular dial marked in arbitrary units from 50 to 600. and with a needle to indicate current amplitudes. Underneath the face panel is the induction coil (4 x 0.5 inches) that has a nickel plated tube core that works with a set of gears (cogged wheel commutator) and the dial meter on the above panel. When the sliding metal tube current regulator moves out and in the dial of the meter turns to indicate the relative change in current amplitude. This gear and dial meter arrangement is the only American made medical electrical battery having this component. (The Two-Cell Faradic Battery of the Detroit Medical Battery Co had a cogged dial for amplitude control but differed from this Dial unit) On the right side of the box is a disc latch to secure the nickel plated tube core that when pulled and pushed operates both needle indicator of the dial and controls current amplitude. Two dry cells were housed underneath the face panel and powered the unit. This unit sold for $10.00 in 1892, and was considered a more powerful battery then The Perfection Battery.

The lower left side of the face plate has an adjustable screw spring interrupter that is different with the spring going under the face panel to the coil; two levers formed like a horseshoe and adjacent to the dial meter serve as an On/Off switch on the left, and on the right are connecting posts (A, B, C, D) with button holes for nickel plated cord connectors. Two metal framed holes hold hand held, hollow tube electrodes. The unit displays directions with the address of 6 Barclay Street, NY on a paper label inside of the lid. This model appears to have been the deluxe unit of the Williams product line. A 1902 advertisement by the PG Williams Mfg promised cures or relief from several physical conditions, and a free inspection after payment was made. The unit cost $12.00 in 1902.

The PG Williams Co also produced a variation of its Dial Battery around 1902 to 1905. This model of the Dial Battery is similar to that described above except the oak case is larger (10 x 8 x 6 inches) to accommodate a compartment to the left of the face plate. The compartment holds accessories, and has a removable wooden lid that is flush with the face plate to cover the accessories. The wood case also has a metal lock device on the front. The PG Williams Co's signature plate lists its last address as 1679 Broadway, NY. Because of the accessory compartment and larger case the unit was pricier than the Dial Battery shown in Fig W4.

The Dial Battery of PG Williams was accompanied by the booklet Suggestions and Directions for Treating Disease with Faradic Currents of Electricity.[2] This booklet was written by JJ Mackey, MD. (Dr Mackey graduated from Bellevue Hospital Medical School, New York City, in 1882, and practiced at 220 Bergen, Brooklyn, NY.[1]) The contents of the 29 paged booklet contained treatment precautions, electrical treatment for a wide variety of ailments (asthma to skin disease), electrical baths, general electrization, female complaints, directions for care of the machine, and description of its flexible back electrode. Directions for operating the Williams batteries included the arrangements with the button connectors and their polarities: A & B primary (A negative, B positive); B & C secondary (B positive, C negative); A & C combined (A positive, C negative); C & D strong (C negative, D positive); and B & D mild (B positive, D negative). This booklet is believed to have been first published in 1900.

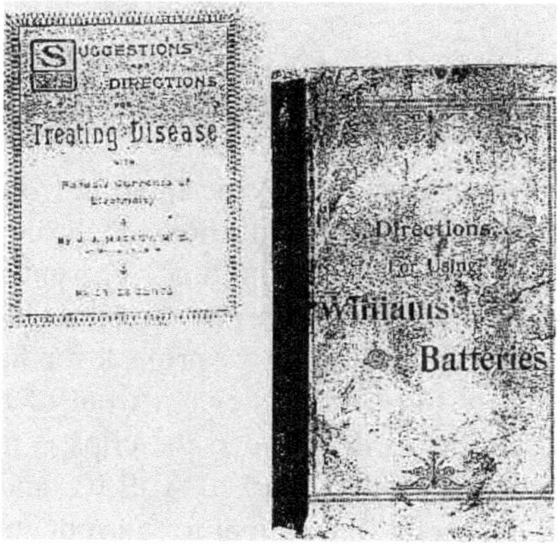

Fig W5. Williams' Booklets

Williams also had another booklet Directions for using Williams' Batteries.[3] This booklet is an abbreviated version of Dr Mackey's booklet with its eight pages. It may have been the original booklet for accompanying the Williams' electrical batteries, and possibly published in 1899. The contents include: directions for operating the batteries, electrical treatment of many conditions, general "electrization," and foot bath.

20th Century Battery. Although the Williams' batteries were mostly small built units and for home use, the smallest unit was perhaps the Williams' 20th Century Battery, 12 Jersey Street, NY. This faradic unit is dated about 1920, the date the company located at 12 Jersey Street. The encased unit is in a golden oak box (7.75 x 3.75 x 5.75 inches), secured by a hinged type latch with a pivoted lever lock on the front. Inside the lid are directions and signature data with printed white ink on red paper. The black painted wooden face panel is flush with the bottom of the box. The face panel contains an induction coil (3 x 0.75

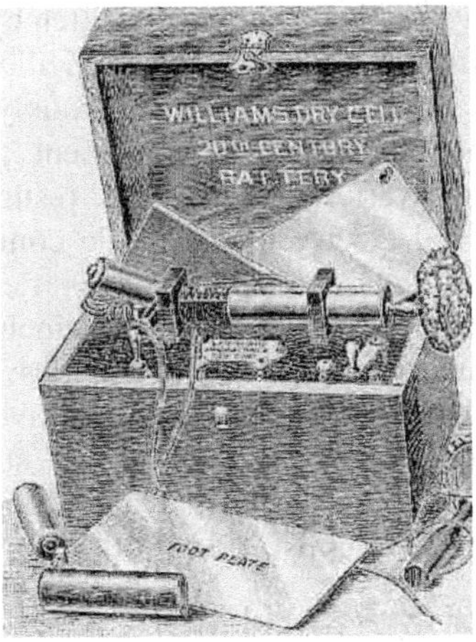

Fig W6. 20TH Century Battery

inches) with a white printed arbitrary scale ranging from 2 to 100. The scale can be visualized when the sliding hollow chrome plated tube is slid over the coil to control current amplitude. The ends of the coil are black wooden blocks (1.5 inches square) as mounts. On the left side of the induction coil is an adjustable screw spring lever hammer, vibrator type interrupter to control pulse frequency. In front of the coil are two metal clips that hold the dry cell; between the clips is a signature plate "PG Williams." Four metal buttons marked A, B, C, and D on the front part of the face panel connect to the patient for current combinations, and to the right is a lever control for On/Off. The then standard size dry cell was placed underneath the face panel. It cost $6.00 in 1905.

Faradic Battery No.2. This faradic battery was shown in Williams' 1905 catalogue, and was designed for physician use. The battery was enclosed in a polished quartered oak case (12 x 3.5 x 10 inches) that has a hinged lid with a leather carrying handle on its front. The lid has two nickel plated hinge clasps and a lock on the front. The unit operates by two standard dry cells. The face plate is wood; it contains a selector switch that also serves as On/Off switch, three binding posts with adjustable screws, a spring hammer adjustable vibrating interrupter, and a coil. The induction coil is wound with No.22 wire, and the secondary coil is wound with 1500 feet of No.36 wire. The fabric over the secondary coil is marked with scale ranging from 0 to 100 arbitrary units. A nickel plated cover slides over the coil to control current. Accessoris are stored in a separate small box. The unit is accompanied with Dr Mackey's booklet, and sold for $12.00.

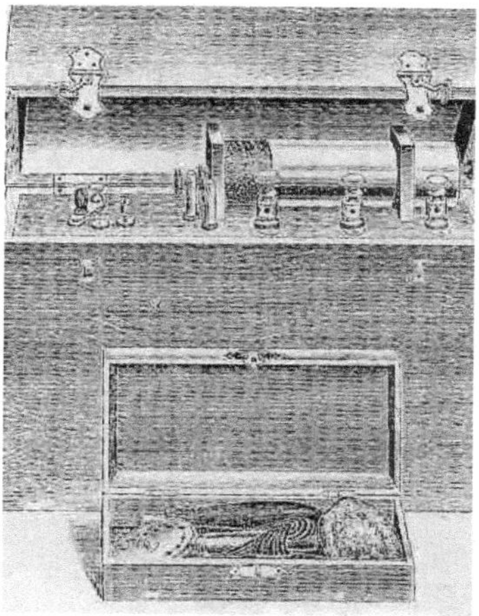

Fig W7. Faradic Battery No. 2

Wall or Table Plate No.4. The No.4 faradic unit was a Faradic Wall or Table Plate for physician use. The induction coil, selector and On/Off switches, three binding posts, and coil are mounted on slate face plate. The coil is exactly like that used in batteries No.1 and 2. The components are mounted on a polished quartered oak base (14 x 10 inches). One standard dry cell is mounted on each side of the face plate. The unit cost $12.00.

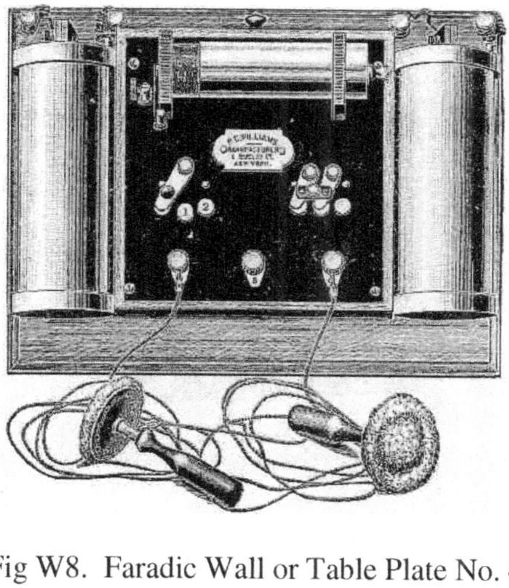

Fig W8. Faradic Wall or Table Plate No. 4

Galvanic Batteries

Williams offered four galvanic batteries for physician uses. These galvanic batteries included a nine cell, 24 cells, 28 cells, and a cautery unit. The galvanic units were used to treat facial blemishes, remove superfluous hair, and strictures.

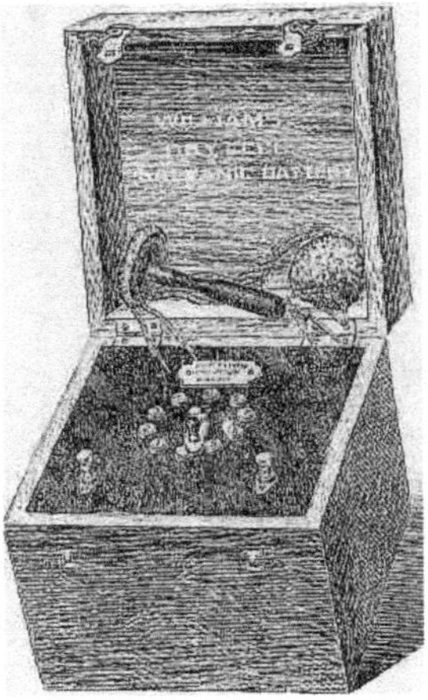

Fig W9. Nine Cell Galvanic Battery

Nine Cell Galvanic Battery. This galvanic unit came in a polished quartered oak box (8 inches square), hinged lid with two hinge latches, and a metal carrying handle on top. The black face plate is slate and contains a cell selector switch with contact buttons for activating any number of the nine cells, and, two binding posts. Accessories were stored on the lid; it cost $10.00, and weighed 12 pounds.

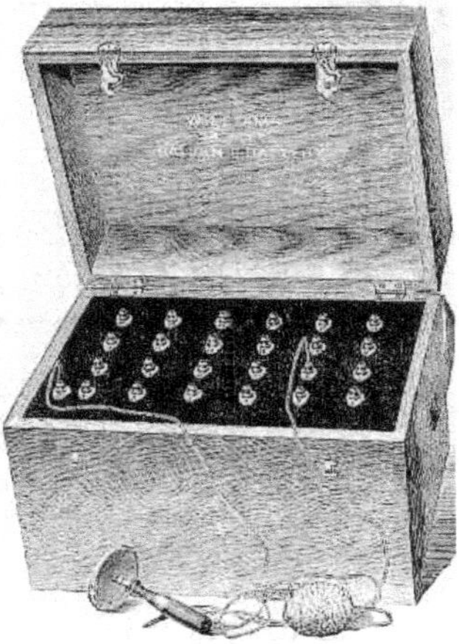

Fig W10. Twenty-four Cell Galvanic Battery

Twenty-four Cell Galvanic Battery. Like the other Williams' batteries this unit is housed in a polished quartered oak box (13 x 9 x 9 inches) with a hinged lid, leather carrying strap is mounted on each side, and two hinged latches on front to secure lid. The face plate is slate and contains 24 binding posts numbered consecutively for physician cell selection. Cells of this unit are two inches square with a height of four inches. This $18.00 unit weighs about 30 pounds.

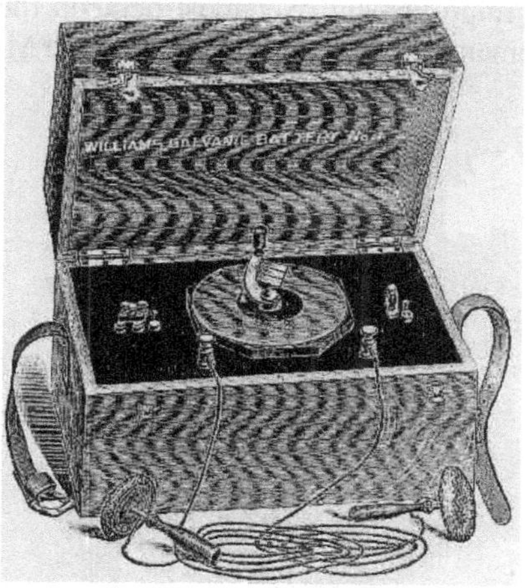

Fig W11. Twenty-eight Cell Galvanic Battery No. 1

Twenty-eight Cell Galvanic Battery. The 1905 catalogue of Williams described and illustrated the Twenty-eight Cell Galvanic Battery No.1 that deviated from previous battery designs of the company. This battery used the octagonal (graphite) shaped rheostat. The 15 x 9 x 9 inches quartered oak box contained the 28 cells that were 4 x 2 inches each, and located underneath the slate face plate. The unit is equipped with a pole changer, an On/Off switch, and two binding posts (adjustable screws). The basic unit cost $20.00 but when a milliamperemeter was added it cost $30.00. The choice of meter ranged from 0 to 100 MA ($10.00) or range of 0 to 400 MA and 0 to 20 mA.

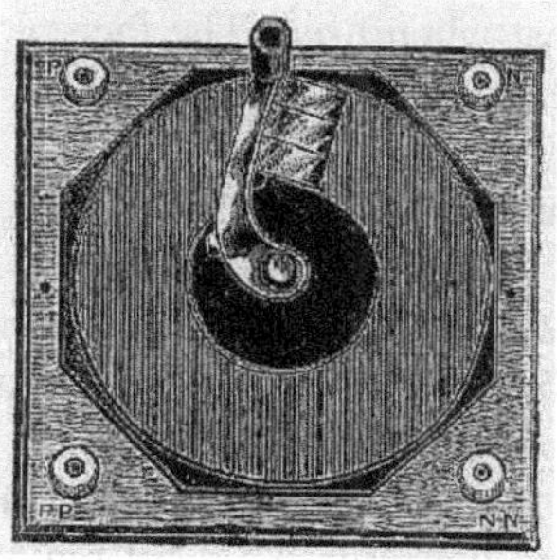

Fig W12. Graphite Shunt Rheostat

Rheostat. The shunt type rheostat of Fig W12 was on a block of slate that had graphite injected to form one surface of graphite. The radial arm carries spring contacts to vary the resistance when rotating over the slate/graphite surface. The shunt form avoids the failure to cut out current or unwanted shocks to the patient over the range of 0 to full voltage. This function was an improvement over most octagon rheostats in 1905, and until the development of the MacLagan unit by the McIntosh company.

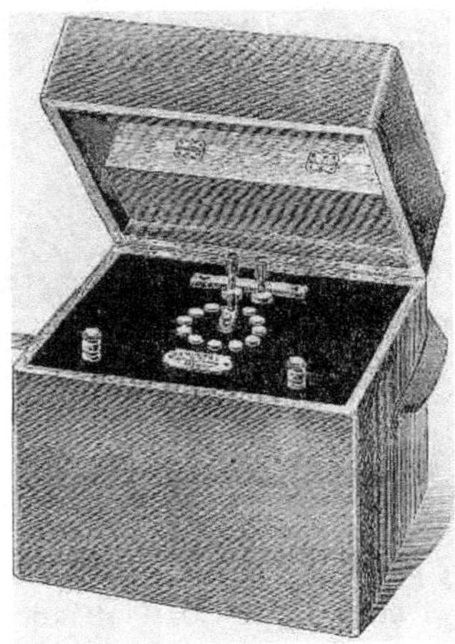

Fig W13. Galvano-Cautery Battery No. 1

Galvano-Cautery Battery. PG Williams always kept prices low to physicians buying electrical batteries, and only dealt in cash transactions. Thus, this unit was among the lowest priced Galvano-Cautery batteries on the market in 1905. Its cost was $10.00 with six dry cells, $12.50 for nine cells, and $15.00 for 12 cells. It resembles the Nine Cell Galvanic Battery of Fig W9 closely. The unit operated with standard dry cells (6.25 x 2.5 inches). A German silver rheostat is placed between the cells and binding post. The cautery electrodes were heated from cherry red to white heat when used. The face plate is slate and enclosed in a quartered oak box.

Combined Faradic and Galvanic Batteries

Combined Faradic and Galvanic Battery. This unit is housed in a rather large oak box (11 x 9 x 9 inches) that is carried by a leather strap anchored on each side of the case. The lid is secured by two metal spring latches on the front of the box. Inside of the lid is a paper with directions for operating the unit. A nickel plated signature plate on the face reads "P.G. Williams Manufacturer, 6 Barclay Street, New York." The accessories are stored underneath the face plate as are two dry cells.

The secondary current is operated by sliding a nickel plated controller over the primary coil. The primary coil is covered by a black fabric that has an arbitrary scale (0 to 100) to indicate amplitude when moved out

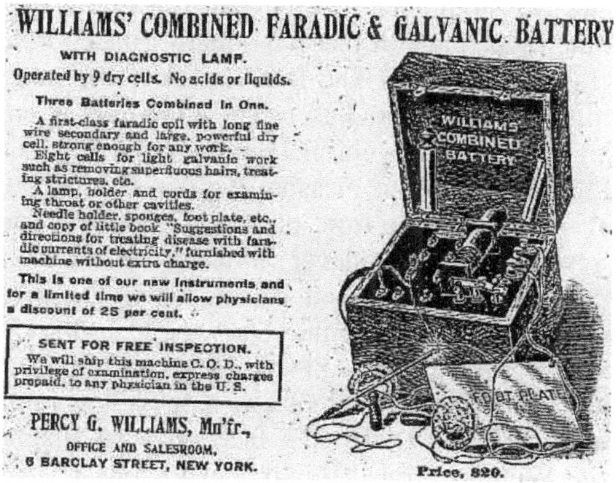

Fig W14. Combined Faradic and Galvanic Battery

and in each end of the induction coil has a square hard rubber block to secure it to the face panel. The induction coil is mounted parallel to the sides of the box rather than in the common position parallel to the length of the box. A switch enables faradic or galvanic currents. Three adjustable screw posts are available for faradic functions while eight small posts are available for galvanic functions. The unit is believed to have been manufactured in the 1880s, although the advertisement was in 1904.

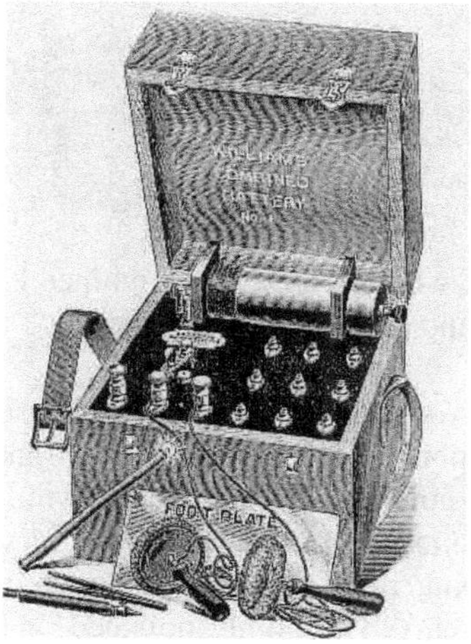

Fig W15. Combined Faradic and Galvanic Battery No 1

Combined Battery No.1. This unit (Fig W16) is an oak boxed battery that delivers faradic and galvanic currents. The hinged lid of the box is secured by two hinged latches on front of the box. The box is carried by a leather strap anchored on each side. The face plate is slate and contains the induction coil that has square wooden blocks or caps at each end of the primary coil. The faradic part is the same as the No.1 faradic unit of Fig W1A. Faradic current amplitude is controlled by a sliding tube over the coil. The coil is fabric covered and its top is marked in graduated arbitrary units to measure the distance that the metal tube has moved over the coil. The front portion of the coil is adjacent to the adjustable screw contact, spring lever vibrating interrupter. Three binding posts are available for faradic and galvanic currents, while a selector switch allows for faradic or galvanic currents. One dry cell powers the faradic currents, while eight cells (4 x 2 inches each) power the galvanic operation with each being used simultaneously with any number of cells. All cells are located underneath the face plate. A diagnostic lamp is included, since Williams aimed this model for physician use. The unit cost $20.00 in 1904, but was probably new in 1902 or 1903.

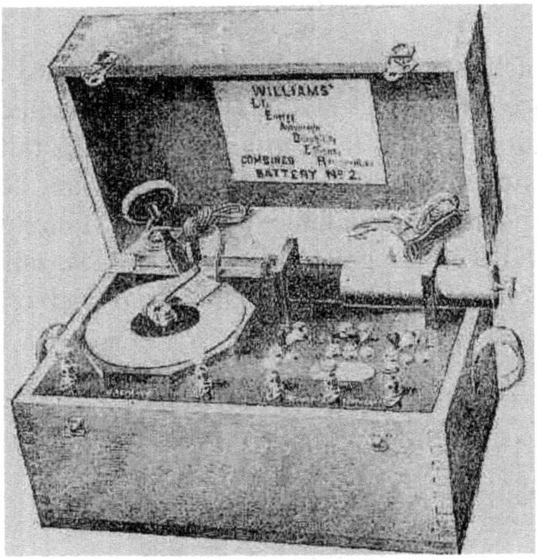

Fig W16. Twenty-eight Cell Combined Faradic
and Galvanic Battery No. 2

Twelve Cell No.2 Battery. Williams considered this unit (Fig W17) as a high grade portable battery. The 14 x 8 inches slate face plate contained a secondary coil wound of long fine wire, a graphite rheostat, switches for On/Off control, a pole changer, and a selector switch. Five adjustable screw binding posts are for galvanic, primary faradic, and secondary faradic currents. The highly polished quartered oak box was 15 x 9 x 9 inches. The corners of the box are dovetailed and glued. The hinged lid has two hinged latches in front. A leather strap is used to carry the unit. It cost $25.00 without a milliamperemeter and $35.00 with a meter, and it weighs 38 pounds. Two dry cells operated the faradic function while 26 dry cells (4 x 2 inches each) powered the galvanic part. Each cell was 1.45 volts.

The 12 cell combined faradic and galvanic battery (Fig W17)

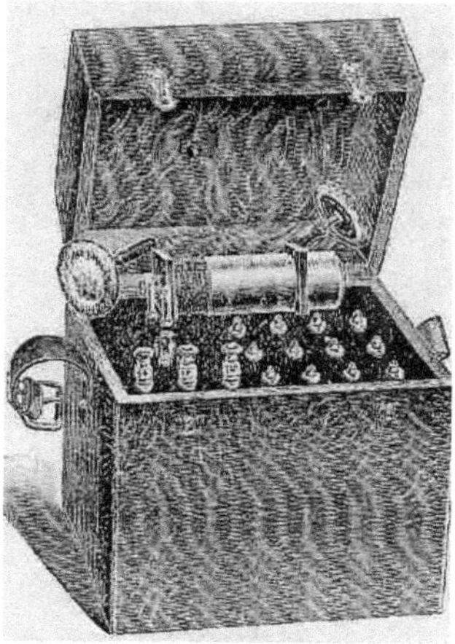

Fig W17. Twelve Cell Combined Faradic And Galvanic Battery No. 3

used standard dry cells rather than the special 4 x 2 inches cells of the company's other units. The secondary coil is wound by 1500 feet of fine wire. A sliding metal cover over the coil controls current and the operator can record the amount of the movement (0 to 100 scale). The vibrating interrupter is an adjustable spring hammer for smooth and even pulses at various rates. Eleven dry cells operate the galvanic part independently from the faradic operation. All nickel plated metal are mounted on a slate plate enclosed in a polished quartered oak box (11 x 11 x 10 inches). A leather strap carrying handle is mounted from each side. The box is hinged and has two hinge latches on front. The unit has a diagnostic lamp, a booklet by Dr Mackey, and cost $25.00 in 1905.

Combined Faradic and Cautery Battery No.1. This battery was used for faradic treatment, cautery, and lighting a diagnostic lamp. The faradic function uses a primary coil wound with No.22 wire, and 1500 feet of No.36 wire for the secondary coil. Two large dry cells operate the faradic function. Ten cells operate the cautery function so that medium to white heat can be reached. The coils, switches for On/Off control, selection of operation, five binding posts, and a galvanic button rheostat are mounted on a slate face plate (10 x 8 inches). All metal are nickel plated and enclosed in polished quartered oak box (11 x 9 x 11 inches). The 12 dry cells measure 7 x 2.5 inches each (large size). The basic cost was $20.00 but with extra cautery electrodes the cost was $25.00.

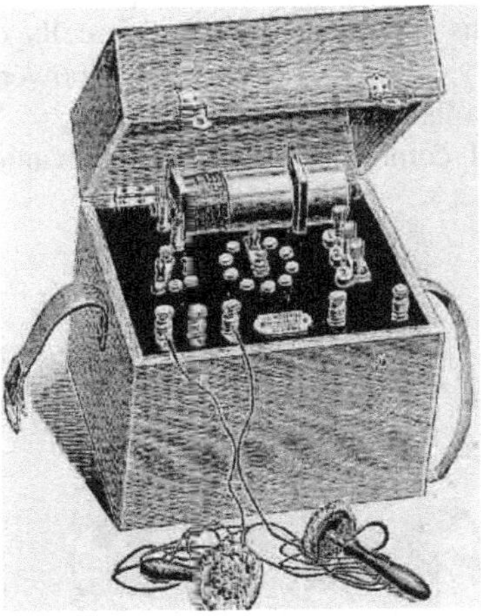

Fig W18. Combined Faradic and Cautery Battery No. 1

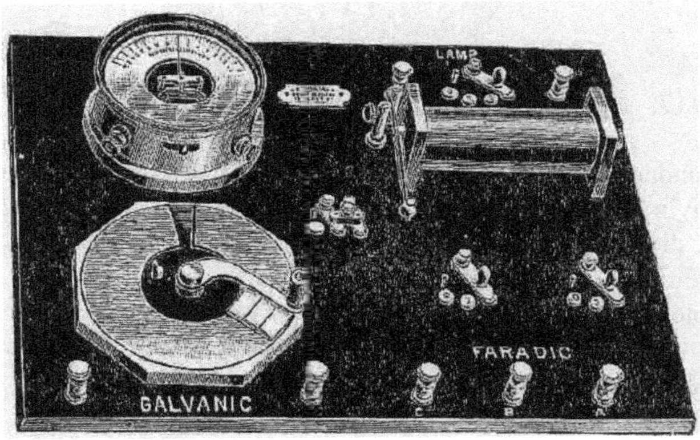

Fig W19. Faradic and Galvanic Table or Wall Plate No. 5

Table or Wall Plate No.5. This combined instrument has a slate plate (18 x 14 inches) that contained a high tension coil, and a secondary coil wound with 3000 feet of No.36 wire and could be tapped by a selecting switch for controlling three lengths of wire. An adjustable rod and ball regulates faradic current pulses. The face plate has a pole changer, switch to control the current for lighting a diagnostic lamp, a graphite rheostat, shunt milliamperemeter, and five adjustable binding posts. The unit could not be operated by commercial or grid current sources. Options were available to adjust its cost at $30.00 or $40.00.

Cabinet Battery No.8. This combined faradic and galvanic model that in addition to serving as a battery also is a stationary office cabinet. The cabinet is made of figured quartered oak with paneled sides and top (28 x 21 x 17 inches). The physician was given a choice of a paneled oak cover for $55.00 or a beveled plate glass cover for $60.00 in 1905. The cabinet was rubbed down with polish and antique finish. A sliding drawer is available on the right side to store accessories. The unit is powered by 48 dry cells. The slate face plate (18 x 14 inches) holds a high tension induction coil (same as Faradic Battery No. 3, Fig W3), a

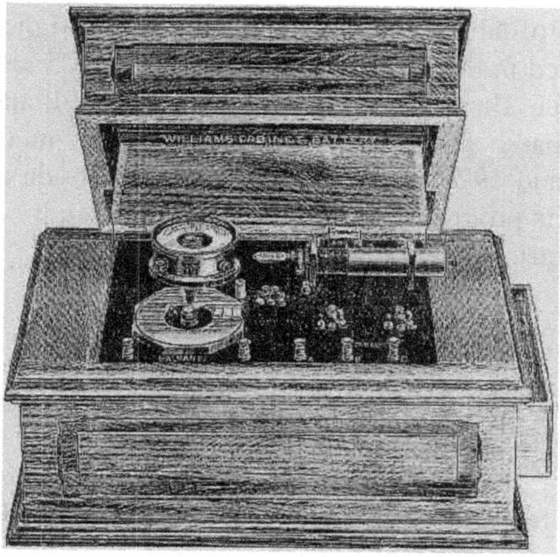

Fig W20. Cabinet Battery No. 8

switch for tapping the coil at different lengths, a cell selector and pole changer, an octagon graphite rheostat, and a shunt milliamperemeter for galvanic current. Also, on the face plate are five binding posts (2 galvanic, 3 faradic), and two posts for a diagnostic lamp. The unit also provides cautery functions and $5.00 would buy special cautery devices.

Percy G Williams company also imported medical electrical batteries for retail in 1905. The imported units were the Galvanic and Faradic Table or Wall Plate No.6 ($35.00), Wall Plate in Case No.7 ($60.00), Galvanic Plate No.1 ($16.00), and Faradic Switch Board No.8 ($16.00). These units were imported from the McIntosh Battery and Optical Co of Chicago, and are illustrated and described in Chapter 4, McIntosh Battery and Optical Co.

Summary

Like other companies of the medical electrical battery industry, the PG Williams Mfg Electrician often moved its business location. Since the industry was mostly low profit and competitive, companies were constantly seeking the best quarters to function at an economical and competitive level. PG Williams is judged to have been a profitable business for about 30 or 35 years. This length of time may have been a career for Percy Williams and it apparently ended like so many others when economic times became difficult in the 1920s.

Most of the seven known medical electrical battery models for home use that PG Williams manufactured are commonly found today in antique shops and on eBay. Using this as a criterion of success the present day volume of batteries of PG Williams Mfg Electrician found in the antique market helps to support the contention that the PG Williams business was profitable. The electrical batteries designed for physician use and displayed in the company's catalogue of 1905 are not commonly found in antique shops or eBay auctions. PG Williams was a small manufacturer that began in 1880, but most of its models were made between 1900 and 1920. The company issued 25 trade catalogs over as many years of its product line, and did not engage in products other than the medical electrical battery.

References

1. Polk RL. Medical Register and Directory of North America. Baltimore, MD, RL Polk, 1904, pp 50, 2875

2. Directions for Using Williams' Batteries. New York, NY, William, ca 1900

3. Mackey JJ. Suggestions and Directions for Treating Disease with Faradic Currents of Electricity. New York, NY, Williams, ca 1900

PART 4. SELLERS OF HOME & PHYSICIAN SHOCK MACHINES

Manufacturers of medical electrical batteries for both physician and home (family) use frequently made units for agents or distributors (retailers). The retailers often wanted their own label or signature plates placed on the product lines that they sold, and manufacturers accommodated their requests. Today's collector of these apparatuses is confronted with the dilemma of who was the real maker of a particular medical electrical battery. Some retailers even claimed to be the manufacturer or sole proprietor of the item when in fact the item was manufactured by another company, and wholesaled with the retailers name. This book is outlined to separate manufacturers from the retailers, and the manufacturers are separated according to their dominant sale interests (eg, physician vs home use). Of course some manufacturers who sold dominantly to physicians also sold electrical batteries on a lesser scale for home or family use. Manufacturers of home use electrical batteries sold commonly inferior quality units when compared with those sold for physician use.

This section presents some of the most frequent seen names of sellers associated with the medical electrical batteries of either physician or home use or both. There were, of course, medical suppliers all over the United States, but the antique market seems to repeatedly offer artifacts of electrical batteries of a certain few companies. The firms presented herein are those either spotlighted from the literature, or their labels are most often on the items because of their previous sales volume.

CHAPTER 21. THE GIANTS

1. The AS ALOE COMPANY OF ST LOUIS, MO

The first of the giant retailers is presented in Chapter 21. Sadoc and Nancy Aloe along with their son Albert immigrated from Edinburgh, Scotland, to New York City in 1854 where Sadoc set up business as an optician.[1] His son Albert Sidney Aloe (1841[1(B)] or 1842[2,3]-1893) became a seaman in 1856 sailing around Cape Horn before reaching San Francisco where he left sailing to become a lens grinder in an optical shop. After one year in San Francisco he moved to South America to work as a mechanical engineer while building a sugar mill.[1] Around 1860[1(H),2] or 1862,[4(205)] he settled in St Louis, and opened his shop for making quality engineering and surveying instruments[2] or optical items.[4(205)] AS Aloe opened his individually operated shop at 24 North Fifth Street (corner of Chestnut),[4(205)] or at the corner of Third and Olive Streets,[1(H)] St Louis, MO.

His father, Sadoc[1,2] or Saddock,[4(205)] joined Albert in 1864[4(205)] or by 1865[1,2] through 1867[1,2] at 300 Olive Street (corner of Third St),[4(205)]

St Louis, to make instruments together as S Aloe & Son. The business offered the making of and selling of magnifiers and telescopes;[1] field, opera, and spy glasses; microscopes; spectacles; and stereoscopes.[2]

From 1867 to 1875, AS Aloe again worked alone as an optician, and maker of mathematical instruments at 206 North Fourth Street,[4(205)] and his business was known as the AS Aloe Company.[2] He engaged The Blunt Co of New York as a major seller (outlet) of his instruments between 1868 and 1872. During this period of time, he also made and sold carriage odometers.[2] Thus, early on Aloe was a manufacturer and retailer. Over time AS Aloe became a major retailer in the United States.

AS Aloe hired David Prince[1,4(205)] (Louis H Prince[2]) to work for him sometime before 1872.[2] Prince first appears in the St Louis Directory in 1869 as a stencil cutter, as a salesman in 1878 and then in 1879 and 1880 as a clerk for AS Aloe.[1] Prince was a cousin of Albert's wife (he married Isabella Prince in 1863),[2] or cousin of AS Aloe or son-in-law to William H Hernstein.[1] Parsons and Elgin state that Prince lived with Hernstein in 1872 and in 1884 moved with him from Pine Street to Laclede Avenue.[1] In 1872, Aloe displayed his drawing, optical, and survey instruments at the Cincinnati Industrial Exposition, and this exposition apparently laid the ground work for the expansion of his business. In 1873, Prince set up a branch of the AS Aloe Company in Cincinnati, OH.[2] About 1876, LM Prince issued a catalog on vision. He was listed as an optician in Cincinnati, OH.[3]

In 1876, William H Hernstein joined the AS Aloe Co as a partner; and at that time the office was at 206 North Fourth Street, and the factory to manufacture surgical instruments was located at 311 North Fourth Street.[1] The name of the company changed to Aloe & Hernstein in 1876 to 1880.[1(B),4(205)] Not until Hernstein joined the company did AS Aloe begin making surgical instruments.[4(311-312)] The Hernstein name (Hermann Hernstein) was associated with medical instrument making during the time period of the Civil War. William H Hernstein appeared in the 1874 St Louis Directory as a druggist.[1] In 1876, AS Aloe decided to expand his instrument line by retailing various brands, and manufacturing and selling of mathematical instruments.[2]

In 1879, the Aloe & Hernstein Co published an illustrated catalog advertising their line of surgical instruments; apparatuses, and hospital and office furnishings for physicians.[5] The company's name changed in 1880 to Aloe, Hernstein and Co,[1] and included Prince as a principal (but not in the title) in the company.

By 1883, the Aloe, Hernstein and Co advertised themselves as the largest instrument store in the United States. The company offered items such as: transits for engineers and vernier transit compasses; engineer's Y level; compasses for miners; universal eclimeter; surgical instruments; electrical instruments like bells, batteries, and medical apparatuses; and annunciators for cottages and hotels as well as other related items. The company's catalog of 1885 showed that it occupied a four-story building in St Louis,[2] and about that time (or 1883) introduced the medical electrical battery for sale. The AS Aloe Co did not manufacture its own medical electrical batteries, but sold those of several manufacturers for home and physician use.

In 1885, the company's name changed again to AS Aloe Co when William Hernstein and David[1,4(205)] (Louis[2]) Prince left Aloe to form their own company as importers and manufacturers of surgical, optical, and electrical instruments at 317 North Fourth Street. Their business location was across the street from the AS Aloe Co.[1(M)] In 1887, the splinter company changed its name to Hernstein & Prince Surgical & Optical Company, but then the name in 1889 and 1890 became H Hernstein, surgical instruments at 710 Olive Street. Hernstein returned to the AS Aloe Co by 1891 to become a clerk and manager until 1898.[1] Meanwhile in 1885, the AS Aloe Co was managed by Albert Sidney and son Sidney A; while sons Louis P, and David B Aloe were salesmen.[4(205)] Alfred, the youngest son, made a career in the United States Army.[1(H)]

Probably in the early to mid 1880s, Albert S Aloe divided his company into three specialized departments. The optical department manufactured and retailed optical equipment; the photo department manufactured equipment for photographers; while the surgical department manufactured and retailed surgical instruments.[1] The entire business operated from the address at Fourth Street.

The catalog of 1890 lists the AS Aloe Co at the corner of Fourth & Olive Streets. The catalog illustrated, priced, and advertised superior surgical instruments, physical supplies, and hospital furnishings. This catalog contained 1946 pages.[3] Also in 1891, the company published its number four supplemental catalog having 378 pages, and an index.[3] The 1893 catalog of 1069 pages was the sixth edition listing the prices of instruments. The catalog was illustrated and advertised the company as having superior surgical instruments and supplies, and hospital furnishings.[5] The number of pages of its catalogs is a crude measure of the company's growth and success.

On 30 June, 1893, Albert S Aloe died.[1,2] During his lifetime in St Louis he was a very prominent individual. He was very active in several organizations in which he held offices at various times. Examples of organizations that he was a member of were: Benevolent and Protective Order of Elks, Legion of Honor, Masonic Order, and Order of Odd Fellows.[1]

Immediately upon Albert S Aloe's death the company may have been run briefly by Mrs Albert S, Sidney A, Louis P, and David B.[4(205)] By late 1893 or early 1894, control of the company was given to Louis P Aloe (1867-1929).[1,4(205)] Louis was born in St Louis and attended the Stoddard School, Wyman Institute of Alton, and Washington University.[1]

The AS Aloe Co continued to prosper under the direction of Louis Aloe. The AS Aloe Co was incorporated in 1893 after AS Aloe's death. Louis Aloe moved the surgical department to 1921 Olive Street[1] because of its growth. The other departments remained at their previous location, however, Louis soon moved the company to an eight-story building. The company was advertised as the largest laboratory supplier in the United States. Louis, like his father, was also civic minded so he contributed much money and service time to the city of St Louis.[1]

Louis became a civic leader in St Louis while running the AS Aloe Co. He was active in the Business Men's League and held office in the National Association of Surgical Dealers of the United States and Canada, and the Columbian Club. He became involved in local politics in numerous ways: Young Republicans, Republican State Committee, Board of Election Commissioners, National Republican Conventions, Board of Aldermen, and once even acting mayor of St Louis.[1]

AS Aloe's name was continued on the company's letterhead until 1895. The company's letterhead of 1895 shows that Louis was president and treasurer, David B was vice-president, while a non-family member (TD Benjamin) was the secretary.[1]

Sometime after 1894[1] to 1897, the AS Aloe Co was located at 415 North Broadway and advertised as technical opticians, surgical and mathematical instrument makers.[4(205)] Its catalog of 1894 had 1071 pages.[3] In 1895, the AS Aloe Co's catalog illustrated, priced, and advertised superior surgical instruments, physical supplies, and hospital furnishings. Like its catalog of 1891, this catalog was also cited as edition six with 1071 pages.[3] According to the catalog's Preface, the company only sold state-of-the-art medical electrical apparatuses and accessories, outdated equipment was removed from the catalog. The Aloe catalog of 1893 carried: 1) electrolytic, 2) electromagnetic, 3) electroscopic, 4) electrosurgical, and 5) electrotherapeutic equipment. AS Aloe Co was then serving as agent for such companies as: Dawson, Edison, Galvano-Faradic Mfg Co, the Jerome Kidder Mfg Co, The Law Battery Co, Leclanche Battery Co, The McIntosh Battery and Optical Co, EB Meyrowitz, Piffard, Smith & Shaw, Vetter, and Waite & Bartlett. Thus, the Aloe catalogs had a very wide variety of medical electrical products for sale as the world's largest store of its kind. In 1895, the AS Aloe Co was offering electrical converters (direct to alternating currents) with some of their apparatuses for consumers living in towns with electricity, while continuing to offer apparatuses powered by electrical cells for those consumers living where city electricity was not yet available. Because of the many batteries shown in Aloe catalogs individual desciptions and illustrations are cited throughout this book.

About late 1896 or 1897, keeping up with the latest technology, Aloe sold x-rays built by Fessenden Mfg Co, Pittsburgh, PA. The x-ray units used a conventional coil patented by Reginald Fessenden (1866-1932) who taught physics at the University of Pittsburgh.[6]

The location of the company in 1898 to 1900, and for many years thereafter was 517 Olive Street. Aloe's products were very acceptable to health consumers as measured through sale volumes.[3]

In 1903[2] or 1905,[1(B)] the AS Aloe Co was claiming to be the largest instrument company in the world. According to Parsons and Elgin the Aloe advertisements of 1905 exaggerated its commercial status; however, the AS Aloe Co may have been the largest retailer of mathematical and surveying instruments, and allied goods west of the Mississippi River at that time.[1]

The AS Aloe Company in 1912 published its catalog as the 16th edition. In this same year fire destroyed the firm's office, however, the company continued to operate smoothly and soon rebuilt.[1] The company supplied the United States Army with electrical and surgical devices in 1918 during World War 1. That same year the company published a booklet entitled What Electro Therapy Means to the Physician.[3] The AS Aloe Co was then manufacturing and selling medical electrical machines that were powered by alternating current.

In the 1920s the Aloe Company capitalized at $1,000,000.00 and had 350 employees. The AS Aloe Co had branches in Chicago, IL; Kansas City, KS; and Los Angles, CA.[2] The AS Aloe Co headquarters was located at 1819-1823 Olive Street, St Louis, MO, according to its catalog of that year. An Aloe bulletin numbered 123 was published in 1926, and an additional catalog was issued in 1927. In 1928, the publication was called the Opportunity Bulletin as it was also in 1929.[3] During the 1920s, Aloe was selling quality polysine electrical machines for clinical use. These units were mostly manufactured by the McIntosh Battery and Optical Company of Chicago.

In 1927, Howard F Baer, husband of Isabel, one of four daughters (Clarable, Isabel, Louise, Viola) to Louis and his wife, moved from Charleston, WV, to St Louis to join the AS Aloe Co when Louis B Aloe became ill. In 1929, Louis Aloe (father-in-law) died, and Howard Baer was given control of the AS Aloe Co. He had the responsibility of saving the company during the financial depression. Howard Baer was apparently an astute business person because he saved the company by selling the optical and photo departments, but keeping the surgical department as the company by 1930. He then developed and expanded the surgical instrument and supply aspects of the AS Aloe Co to national prominence.[1] The Frank S Betz Co of Chicago was bought in 1937.[1]

The hospital catalog of 1949 listed the AS Aloe Co at 1831 Olive Street, St Louis, MO,[3] The Aloe Company may have subsequently been divided and sold as two separate divisions. The laboratory supply division was sold to Curtin-Matheson, and the medical division was sold to Sherwood Medical Industries.[2] In 1959, the final business of the AS

Aloe Co was brought to an end when it was sold and incorporated into the Brunswick Corporation.[1]

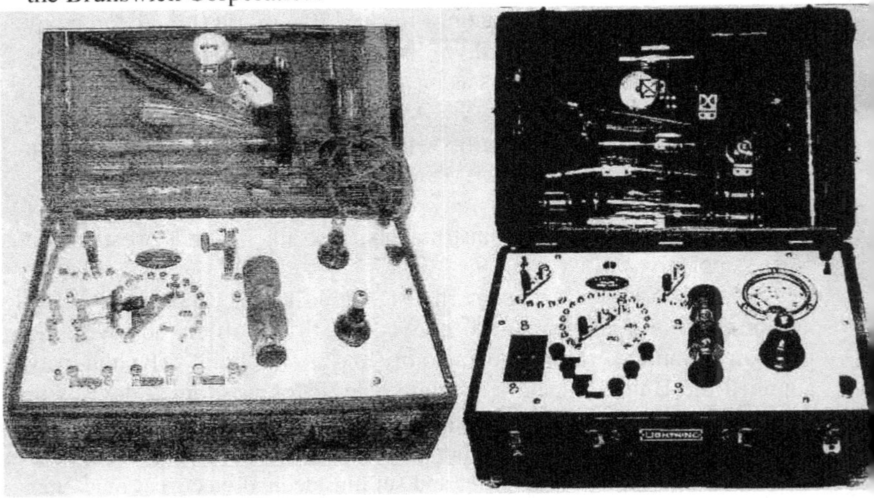

Fig A. The Lightning

Lightning. One of Aloe's most popular medical electrical apparatuses among physicians around 1918 through the 1920s was the "Lightning," an electrical high frequency model. Two versions were offered with some varying features. The "Lightning" was manufactured by the FS Betz Co of Chicago, IL, that made and sold electrical apparatuses for retailers under a different name such as that of the retailer; eg, AS Aloe Co. AS Aloe Co was a retailer of but never a manufacturer of medical electrical batteries.

The major difference between the two versions of the "Lightning" was the meter for measuring milliamperes of the galvanic (cautery) current circuit located on the face plate. The earlier of the two models does not contain the meter (left). Thus, the earlier model without the meter is dated about 1918, while the unit with the meter is dated about 1922. The latter model (right), in addition to having a meter, also has fewer control switches, otherwise the two models function similarly. The earlier model has a double throw switch for On/Off control whereas the latter model with its meter has a button switch for the same function. Both models have a lever/button switch to the rear left that serves as a rheostat to control current flow to the apparatus. The lever/button switch located in rear-center is for fulguration (for destroying tissue by electricity/ lightning form). The large double lever/button switch controls the current amplitude to the separate functions of cautery (destroys tissue by burning via galvanic current), diagnosis (x-ray), sinusoidal (alternating pulsed currents), and ozone.

The spark interrupter is located right-center on both models and is adjusted by a screw to control high frequency oscillations used with the glass violet electrodes. The glass violet electrodes are used for treating body parts and areas such as nasal, throat, eye, spine, orifices, and scalp. Both models have Tesla and d'Arsonval coils for high frequency functions affecting muscular and physiological responses, and warming (diathermy) responses, respectively.

One early Lightning unit was No.9086 that was powered by 110 volts and 60 Hertz alternating current. This particular unit was quite heavy because its face or base plate was white marble. The unit has an Aloe signature plate mounted on the marble, and another plate with "Lightning" mounted on the outside front of the case. The case consists of wood (white pine) covered with black buckram or leatherette, and wood corners that were dovetailed and glued. External corners of the case are steel reinforced. The case has a leather carrying handle. The inside of the lid is covered with green velvet, and stores 12 accessories. Concealed underneath the marble face are three coils (1 induction coil 5.5 x 1.75 inches) for sinusoidal current with a primary and secondary stationary coils. The other two coils (6 x 1.5 inches) boost voltage for cautery and x-ray functions; each coil is sealed at the ends, and each is connected with multilayered plate magnets.

This unit was built on the closed core transformer principle of d'Arsonval to provide maximal output. The unit functioned to provide high frequency current to power x-rays, fulguration, cautery, ozone, diagnostics, and sinusoidal current. The marble face contained two high frequency poles that spark across 4.25 inches (center to center), but serve to connect with a heavy glass x-ray tube; an On/Off double throw switch; a 20 control studs or buttons with "S/D;" another control switch marked "E/K cranyon;" and an adjustable screw to double coils.

The Lightning units each weigh about 34 pounds, and were designed as multipurpose electrical apparatuses for physician uses. Each unit when sold was accompanied by a booklet of instructions for installing and operating "Lightning": The Aloe Electro-Therapeutic Cabinet.This 55 paged booklet provided such information as basic electricity; installation instruction; explanation of controls; treatment instructions for a variety of physical conditions and ailments by miscellaneous high frequencies; diathermy; fulguration (electro coagulation); sinusoidal currents; diagnostic hints; listings and prices of cautery, diathermy, glass, fulguration, and miscellaneous electrodes; ozone generator; and accessories.[7]

The Lightning units are popular among collectors because of their impressive spark discharge from the Tesla coil. An example of this electrical discharge can be seen in Chapter 2, Fig 16.

Summary

The AS Aloe Co was founded in St Louis in 1860, and although it was divided into two divisions in 1946[2] business was continued until the Brunswick Corp bought the company in 1959.[1] During this period of time, the company manufactured engineering, optic, surgical, and surveying instruments. Although the company began selling medical electrical batteries extensively in 1883 or 1885, it never manufactured them. The AS Aloe Co retailed medical electrical batteries of several manufacturers. Most often the medical electrical batteries sold by the company maintained the identity of the manufacturer; eg, Galvano-Faradic Mfg Co, Jerome Kidder Mfg Co, and Waite & Bartlett. The "Lightning" was a high frequency multipurpose electrical apparatus made by the FS Betz Co of Chicago for sale by the AS Aloe Co under the Aloe signature. This particular electrical apparatus is often found in antique shops and on eBay auctions. Collectors like the unit because of its sparking device that is dramatic when in operation. The AS Aloe Co was at one time one of the largest medical apparatus suppliers in the world.

References

1. Parsons HA, Elgin RL. The St Louis Makers of Surveying Instruments Since 1830, pp 3-5, 9, 2000; (http:www.surveyhistory.org/ St_l); from (B) Bedini SA. Collector's Corner. Professional Surveyor, 5:52, 1985: (H) Hyde W, Conrad HL (eds). Encyclopedia of the History of St Louis, New York, NY, Southern Hist, 1889, pp17-18: and (M) McGuire JM. The Man Who Can't Say No, St Louis Post-Dispatch, 29 Oct 1989, Sec F, p 14

2. Warner DJ. The A.S. Aloe Instrument Business. Rittenhouse 34:62-64, 1996

3. Davis AB, Dreyfus MS. The Finest Instruments Ever Made. Arlington, MA, Med Hist Pub, 1986, pp 37-38, 263

4. Edmonson JM. American Surgical Instruments. San Francisco, CA, Norman Pub 1997

5. Romaine LB. A Guide to American Trade Catalogs 1744-1900. New York, NY, RR Bowker, 1960, pp 235-241

6. Grigg ERN. The Trail of the Invisible Light. Springfield, IL, CC Thomas, 1965, pp 50-80

7. Instructions for Installing and Operating, "Lightning," The Aloe Electro-Therapeutic Cabinet. St Louis, MO, AS Aloe, (no date), pp 1-55

2. MANHATTAN ELECTRICAL SUPPLY COMPANY OF NEW YORK CITY

Little is known about the Manhattan Electrical Supply Co (MESCO), although one of its retail products, The Home Medical Apparatus No.4, is commonplace among collectors of medical electrical apparatuses and seen often on eBay auctions, and antique shops. This section presents what is known about the company and its products.

MESCO was established around 1880, and at one time LG Pacent was proprietor.[1] The first catalog of record for this company was its number 16 (ca 1896 to 1900). The 78 paged catalog has no title nor cited date.[2] The No.16 catalog listed and priced general electrical supplies that the company manufactured and retailed (eg, the MESCO dry cell). In 1900, the company issued its 22nd edition trade catalog advertising its product line. The company was apparently successful in manufacturing and selling a wide variety of electrical apparatuses and accessories, but MESCO was not a manufacturer of medical electrical batteries. The medical electrical batteries sold by MESCO were manufactured by others.

The MESCO cell that often accompanied the medical electrical batteries sold by JH Bunnell & Co and the Manhattan Electrical Supply Co was manufactured by MESCO. The company had facilities for grinding carbon and pulverizing manganese, molding the plates or elements, making the zinc cups, and finishing the dry cells. MESCO

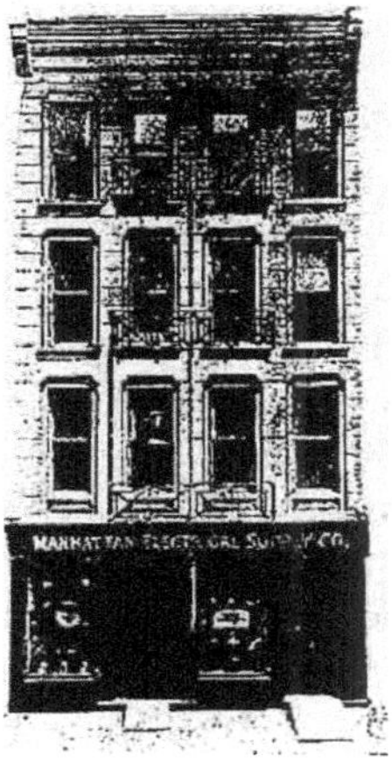

Fig M1. MESCO Building in New York, 1900
(Courtesy of Bob Alexander, Clarkston, MI)

advertised that they engaged in the process of making the cells, and maintained that their process kept the costs of their cells low.

In 1900, offices of the company were located in New York, NY, and Chicago, IL, and factories were located in Jersey City, NJ, and Ravenna, OH. New York City was headquarters (17 Park Place and 14 Murray Sts at various times), and the Chicago office was located at 188 Fifth Ave. The building of Fig M1 in New York operated from 32 Cortland Street, and served as office, salesroom, and supply center. The MESCO building located at 15 Exchange Place, Jersey City, NJ, was dissolved by unanimous consent of the company on 12 December 1916,[3] although an advertisement dated 1931 has been attributed to MESCO.[2]

Cells. The company seemed to offer any and everything electrical such as a large line of telegraph instruments (keys, senders, sounders), relays, transmitters, and systems for intercommunication. This 750-paged illustrated catalog and price list (22nd edition) offered galvanic batteries, magnetoelectrical generators, galvanometers, induction coils, magnets, books on electricity that were mostly instructional for 'how to make.' Books on medical electricity were offered but the selection was very limited. The Manhattan Electrical Supply Co sold the MESCO (1900 to 1905), and the Red Seal (1905 to 1910) cells with its medical electrical machines for home use. Although this company made the dry cells, it apparently maintained close ties with manufacturer JH Bunnell & Co. The JH Bunnell & Co did make telegraphic equipment and supplies, and medical electrical batteries. Many features of MESCO apparatuses resemble those of the JH Bunnell & Co. The two companies had a close relation in business, therefore, the obvious conclusion is that JH Bunnell & Co manufactured many models of medical electrical batteries sold by MESCO

Literature. Dr Edward Trevert in 1900 (perhaps in 1890s) authored a 96-paged booklet Electro-Therapeutic Hand-Book, NY,[4] published by and issued by the Manhattan Electrical Supply Co (MESCO) to consumers of its medical electrical machines. The methods of electrical application, treatment of diseases by electricity, vibration, and electrical massage are discussed in the booklet. This booklet contained nine pages of illustrated apparatuses and accessories that included: The New Home Medical Apparatus No.4 (exactly like that of JH Bunnell's unit of 1901,[5] and sold by Montgomery Ward & Co in its 1904 catalog,[6] and Sears, Roebuck and Co in its 1897 catalog[7]); the Apollo medical electrical apparatus; The Household electrical battery; and the Double Cell Medical Apparatus. The term "Electropathic guide….." was used in the booklet that is the title of the booklet issued by JH Bunnell and was written by SM Wells. Dr Edward Trevert, a New York physician, also authored several books on various technologies from 1890 (Experimental Electricity) to 1902 (The ABC of Wireless

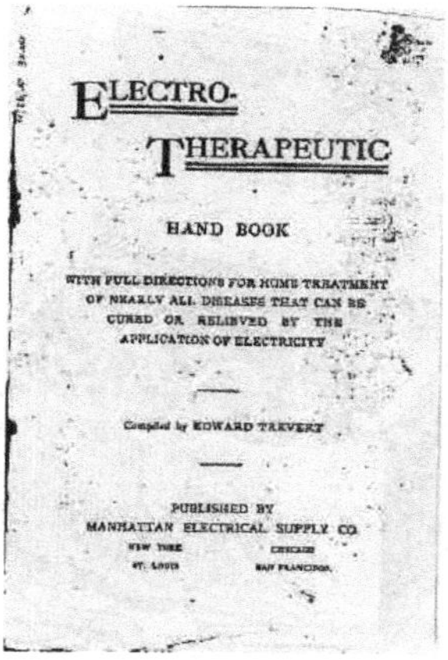
ELECTRO-
THERAPEUTIC
HAND BOOK
WITH FULL DIRECTIONS FOR HOME TREATMENT OF NEARLY ALL DISEASES THAT CAN BE CURED OR RELIEVED BY THE APPLICATION OF ELECTRICITY
Compiled by EDWARD TREVERT
PUBLISHED BY
MANHATTAN ELECTRICAL SUPPLY CO.
NEW YORK CHICAGO
ST. LOUIS SAN FRANCISCO

Fig M2. Electro-Therapeutic Hand-Book

Telegraphy). In 1892, he wrote and published Practical Directions for Armature & Field-Magnet Winding, and in 1896 Something About X-Rays for Everbody. His books were published in Lynn, MA, through Bubier Publisher. This latter book is a guide to x-ray construction and its experiments, and may be his most well known publication.

Faradic Batteries

The eighteenth edition of the MESCO catalog was published between 1900 and 1902. This particular catalog featured three faradic electrical batteries that apparently did not sell well enough to survive and be featured in the catalog of 1905. The three models featured in the 1902 catalog were the Excelsior, the Little Giant, and the Petite Medical Apparatuses.

Excelsior. This unit was powered by a single dry cell that is housed underneath the hard rubber face plate. This model is believed to have been manufactured in 1900 by the George P Pilling & Son Company of Philadelphia and sold with the MESCO signature. The square wooden end caps on the induction coil are characteristic of the Pilling models, and the Excelsior resembles the Manhattan Medical Apparatus in Fig M9 that was manufactured in 1903 (also by GP Pilling & Son Co). The Excelsior's face plate is recessed below the level of the wooden case (approximately 8 x 3.5 x 5.25 inches) to allow the flat hinged lid to close. The face plate houses the coil, the spring lever hammer vibrating interrupter, the sliding metal current controller, three button style connectors for current selection and patient contact, and an On/Off lever switch. A very narrow open space at the rear of the face plate offers some storage for electrodes and wires. A metal foot plate is attached to the inside of the lid for storage. These features are very

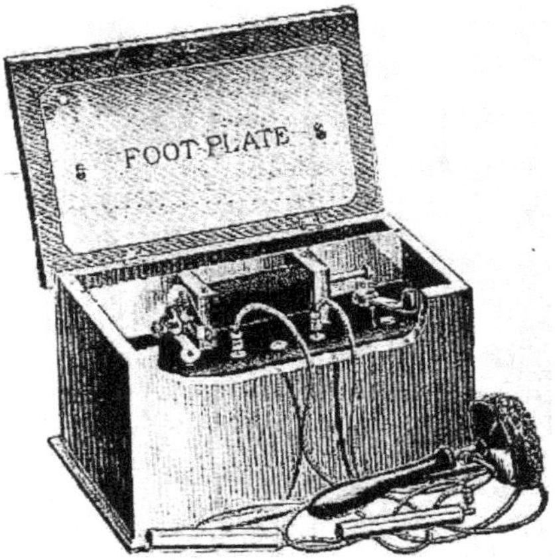

Fig M3. Excelsior Medical Apparatus
(Courtesy of Bob Alexander, Clarkston, MI)

similar to those of the later model, the Manhattan Medical Apparatus. The case has a lip footing extending out from the bottom beyond the case. The case is also cut out in the front that is rather unique among home use electrical batteries made in the United States. All metal are nickel plated. In 1900, the Excelsior sold for $6.00. It was designed for family use, and was promoted for its absence of a wet cell for power.

The difference between the Excelsior and the Manhattan Medical Apparatus is the size of the case. The Manhattan Medical Apparatus of 1903 replaced the Excelsior by a larger oak case. The Manhattan unit is one inch wider than the Excelsior to provide a small compartment for accessories, and to house two dry cells underneath its face plate. The glued corners of the Manhattan unit are dovetailed.

Little Giant Medical Apparatus. This faradic unit was made between 1900 and 1902 by the JH Bunnell & Co of New York. The oak case (6 x 4.13 x 3.5 inches) has a sliding wooden lid (like a cheese or fish box), and may be the only one like it manufactured in the United States. The face plate is recessed, covers a single dry cell, and houses the induction coil. The coil has circular end caps characteristically like JH Bunnell & Co units. The left end of the coil has a spring lever hammer vibrating interrupter, and the right end of the coil has a sliding metal current controller. Two circular holes are cut in the face plate to store the circular handle style electrodes. Three button type connectors are on the face plate to connect with the patient and select current types. An On/Off lever switch is provided. All metal parts are nickel plated. The unit cost $2.50 around 1902, but was not listed or illustrated in the 1905 catalog of MESCO.

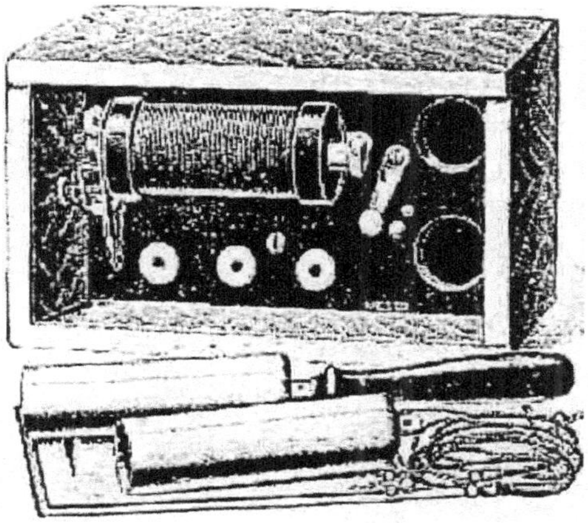

Fig M4. Little Giant Medical Apparatus
(Courtesy of Bob Alexander, Clarkston, MI)

Petite Medical Apparatuses. These units include a small circular metal faradic battery, and separately an electrical hairbrush that also uses the small circular battery. The manufacturer is unknown because of its unique and different characteristics. These units were apparently unpopular enough for MESCO to discontinue them before 1905.

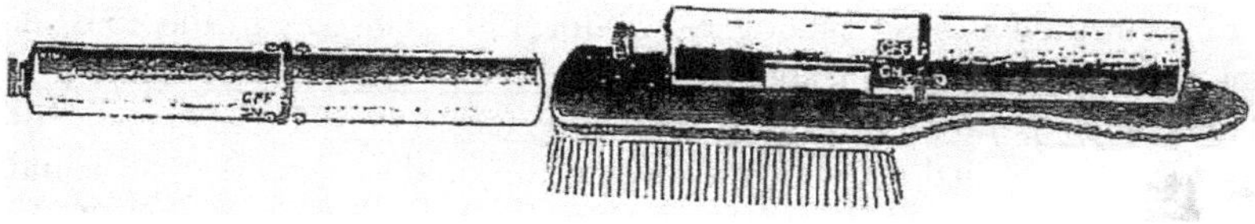

Fig M5. The Petite Medical Apparatuses
(Courtesy of Bob Alexander, Clarkston, MI)

The Petite Medical Apparatus is a tiny (6.5 long x 0.88 diameter, inches) electrical medical battery resembles a pen type flashlight of today. The case is a nickel plated shell that contains the coil and cell. On one end is a metal sliding current controller, while the On/Off switch is centered outside of the case. The On/Off switch is twisted or rotated for operation. A threaded hole is located at the other end of the cylindrical case to connect to the patient. The special cell was designed for this particular unit and measures 2.5 x 0.5 inches. The unit sold for $3.00 between 1900 and 1902, and was not available in 1905 by MESCO.

MESCO also sold the Petite Medical Apparatus with a Special Hairbrush Electrode. This unit is the combination of the Petite Medical Apparatus and a hairbrush that used the Petite battery for its electrical source and operation. This electrical hairbrush contains an induction coil, dry cell, and a hand electrode. The On/Off operation works by rotating part of the circular shell; the operation is shown in a small window. The hairbrush is about 8.9 inches long. The complete unit weighs less than one pound, and sold for $4.50 in 1900.

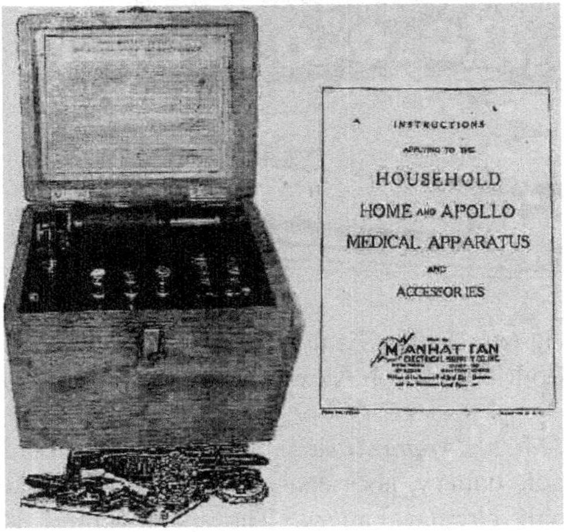

Fig M6. The Apollo Medical Apparatus

Apollo Medical Apparatus. The Apollo was not displayed or priced in the MESCO catalog No.21 for 1905, but was in the 1910 (? later) accompanying manual Instruction Applying to the Household Home and Apollo Medical Apparatus and Accessories. These versions of the Apollo unit had circular end caps on their induction coils that would resemble and indicate its manufacture by JH Bunnell & Co for MESCO.

The Apollo Medical Apparatus is housed in an oak box (9 x 8 x 7 inches) with a hinged lid. The lid has a self locking device on the front. The oak box has dovetailed and glued corners and a metal carrying handle on top. Instructions for the unit's operation are glued inside of the lid. The hard rubber face plate contains the induction coil (faradic current) that has a metal sliding current controller on its right, and a spring lever hammer vibrating interrupter on its left. A single and double lever switch along with three patient connecting posts, and an On/Off lever are also on the face plate. The dry cell is underneath the face plate. The unit weighs seven pounds, and the metal is nickel plated. After 1910, MESCO published a separate instruction booklet to accompany its Apollo and Household (Anti-Doc, Fig M8) Medical Apparatuses rather than use their Electro-Therapeutic Hand Book.

Home Battery No.4. The No.21 catalog of MESCO for 1905[8] listed company offices in New York, and Chicago with its factory in Jersey City, NJ. This catalog listed six faradic home batteries and one galvanic unit. The double lid (2 compartments faradic battery Home Medical Apparatus No.4 (Fig M7) was illustrated and described on two pages of the catalog. This unit was manufactured by JH Bunnell & Co.

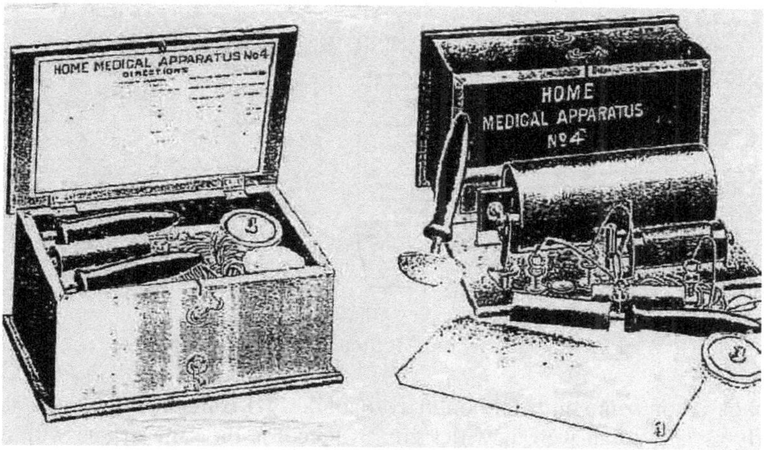

Fig M7. Home Medical Apparatus No. 4

It is encased in a mahogany or oak box (9 x 5.25 x 4.5 inches), metal carrying handle on top, and two lever latches on front of the box. One compartment held the accessories while the other contained elements of the circuitry. The elements were the hinged nickel plated cylinder for holding a single standard sized dry cell (6.25 x 2.5 inches); the spring lever, hammer vibrating interrupter with its separate adjustable contact screw; three buttons for patient connections with primary, secondary, and combined currents; and an On/Off lever. This unit was replacing the old No.4 D.D. unit; was listed as No.2204; and sold for $10.00.

Anti-Doc Medical Apparatus. This unit was described and sold as No.2215 and $4.00 in the 1905 MESCO catalog.[8] This company sold medical electrical batteries just like the "Elk" type of Detroit Medical Battery Co (still selling in 1925), but did not label them or provide a signature. This is an one dry cell (housed under the face plate) unit contained in a polished oak box (7.5 x 3.5 x 5.25 inches) with the face plate made of matching wood. Some units have dovetailed glued corners on the oak boxes. The box has a hinged lid, a metal carrying handle on top, and a hinged latch with lever on front to secure the lid. On the inside of the lid is a metal fixture for holding electrodes and wires. The face plate contains the functional elements such as the induction coil that is covered with black fabric and enclosed by black circular wooden end caps (Bunnell style) and having a sliding metal current controller. It contains an armature and vibrating parts (patented 30 Dec 1902 and

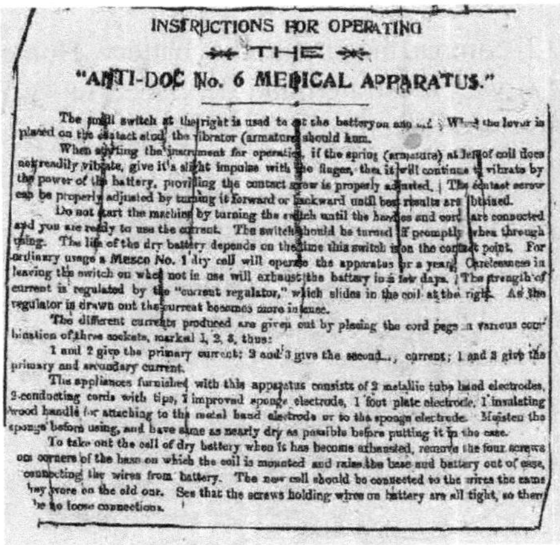

INSTRUCTIONS FOR OPERATING

THE

"ANTI-DOC No. 6 MEDICAL APPARATUS."

The small switch at the right is used to put the battery on and off. When the lever is placed on the contact stud the vibrator (armature) should hum.

When starting the instrument for operation, if the spring (armature) at left of coil does not readily vibrate, give it a slight impulse with the finger, then it will continue to vibrate by the power of the battery, providing the contact screw is properly adjusted. The contact screw can be properly adjusted by turning it forward or backward until best results are obtained.

Do not start the machine by turning the switch until the handles and cord are connected and you are ready to use the current. The switch should be turned off promptly when through using. The life of the dry battery depends on the time this switch is on the contact point. For ordinary usage a Mesco No. 1 dry cell will operate the apparatus for a year. Carelessness in leaving the switch on when not in use will exhaust the battery in a few days. The strength of current is regulated by the "current regulator," which slides in the coil at the right. As the regulator is drawn out the current becomes more intense.

The different currents produced are given out by placing the cord pegs in various combination of three sockets, marked 1, 2, 3, thus:

1 and 2 give the primary current; 2 and 3 give the second... current; 1 and 3 give the primary and secondary current.

The appliances furnished with this apparatus consists of 2 metallic tube hand electrodes, 2 conducting cords with tips, 1 improved sponge electrode, 1 foot plate electrode, 1 insulating wood handle for attaching to the metal hand electrode or to the sponge electrode. Moisten the sponge before using, and have same as nearly dry as possible before putting it in the case.

To take out the cell of dry battery when it has become exhausted, remove the four screws on corners of the base on which the coil is mounted and raise the base and battery out of case, connecting the wires from battery. The new cell should be connected to the wires the same they were on the old one. See that the screws holding wires on battery are all tight, so there be no loose connections.

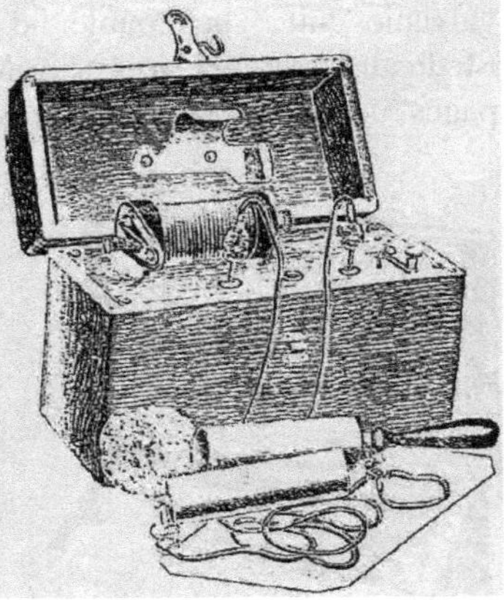

Fig M8. Anti-Doc Medical Apparatus

embossed on some units, although available on JH Bunnell & Co units as early as 1890) that were new designs arranged on the same frame with a contact adjustable screw and fixed to the coil. Adjacent to the coil on the face plate is a recording metal scale graduated in arbitrary units to measure distances of the current controller; three metal buttons for connecting the subject to the unit and selecting primary, secondary, or combined currents; and an ON/OFF lever. The 1902 patent featured a new type of vibrating interrupter, the spring hammer riveted to nickel plate over one end of the coil (rounded ends). The vibrator and contact screw are on the same base that is attached to the induction coil. The unit was listed as No.2215 and sold for $4.00 in 1905. In 1910 and later, this same unit was listed as No.2215, but was labeled the Household Medical Apparatus, and sold for $9.50. The unit was accompanied by the 96 paged booklet Electro-Therapeutic Hand Book.

Manhattan Medical Apparatus. This is a two cells faradic unit housed in a polished oak box (8 x 4.5 x 4.5 inches) with glued dovetailed corners. This unit operated also with one standard sized (6.75 x 2.5 inches) dry cell. The lid of the box is hinged; has a metal carrying handle on top, and a lever latch on front. All hardware are nickel plated. The black painted face plate is recessed in the box and is separated by a nickel plate to form a compartment for accessories. The face plate contains: the induction coil, covered with black fabric, and enclosed by square wooden end caps (PG Pilling type and probably made by that company); the coil has a sliding current controller; three buttons to connect the subject to primary, secondary, or combined currents; the one piece vibrating and contact adjustable screw vibrator is on units made in 1903 and later, while those made earlier (eg, 1900) have the two piece contact adjustable screw and the spring lever hammer type vibrator; and an ON/OFF lever control. In 1905, the unit was listed as No. 2225 and

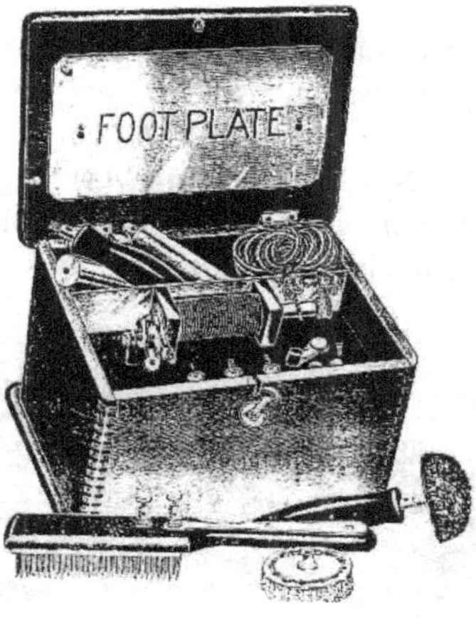

Fig M9. Manhattan Medical Apparatus

sold for $12.00. The unit was not listed by MESCO in 1910 and later.

Unique Medical Apparatus. This unit is a small faradic battery housed in a wooden case (5 x 2.75 x 1.75 inches), and has a hinged lid with a lever latch on front. The unit is small enough to be placed in one's large pocket, and was designed after that of Gaiffe of France. The case contains a nickel plated cylinder to enclose the special MESCO cell (3 x 1.25 inches). Adjacent to the cell cylinder is the induction coil, covered

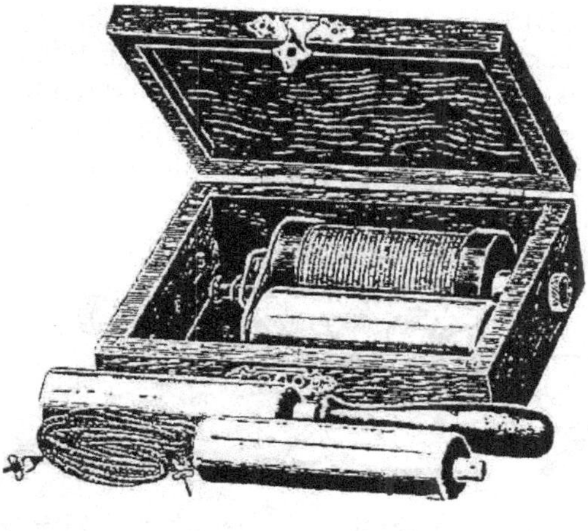

Fig M10. The Unique Medical Apparatus

with black fabric, and contains a sliding current controller that is pulled and pushed from the right outside of the case. The coil is closed by circular end caps (JH Bunnell & Co style, the manufacturer of the same unit The "Unique" Med App, Chapt 16, Fig B20) and fixed to a single plate containing the vibrator. The accessories are placed in the case with the electrical components. This No.2202 unit sold for $2.50 in 1905, and replacement cells were $0.20 each.[8] The coil of this unit is the same as that for the Anti-Doc No.2215 unit (Fig M8).

Improved Medical Induction Coil. This small faradic battery is powerful for its size having a coil size usually found on larger units. The

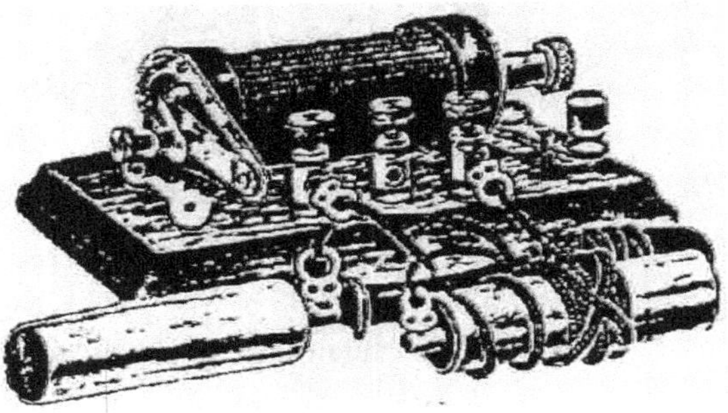

Fig M11. Improved Medical Induction Coil

coil is mounted on a finished and polished oak base that is beveled on each side. The unit contains three connecting posts to allow for primary, secondary, or combined currents; no wooden case is provided with this small unit that sold for $2.40 in 1905 without dry cell and as No.2234. The coil design (circular end caps) was manufactured by JH Bunnell & Co (Chapt 16, Fig B15A). The vibrator is the single vibrating unit on the same plate as the contact adjustable screw (invented in 1902). The coil is covered with black fabric and is similar to that advertised by Bunnell in 1901[5] with the exception that this 1905 version has the one piece vibrating parts. Bunnell's 1901[5] version has the two pieces vibrating parts and contact adjustable screw.

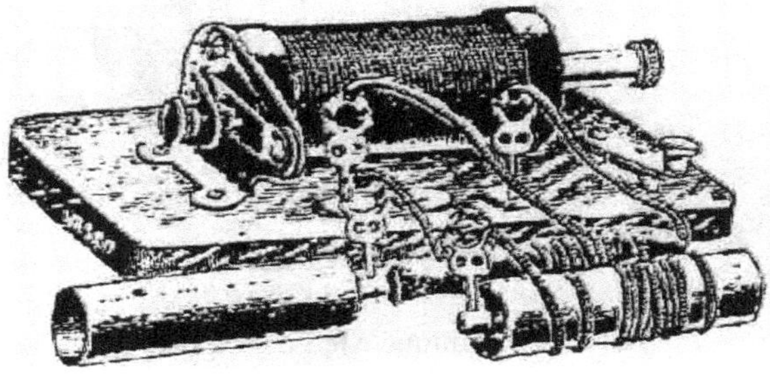

Fig M12. Standard Medical Induction Coil

This unit is similar in size to that of the Improved Medical Induction Coil presented (Fig M11), but is less refined. The consumer had a choice of wooden bases made either of mahogany or oak that was straight on all sides as a plain rectangle. This unit had three buttons for connecting the subject to the machine for either primary, secondary, or combined currents. No wooden case or electrical cell was furnished at the unit price of $2.00 and listed as No.2235. Some wooden bases bore the signature of MESCO embossed on one side of the base. The induction coil was covered with black fabric, had circular end caps (JH Bunnell & Co is the manufacturer, Chapt 16, Fig B15A), and a sliding current controller. The connecting cords or wires could be detached from the buttons on the base, and the electrodes.

Galvanic Battery

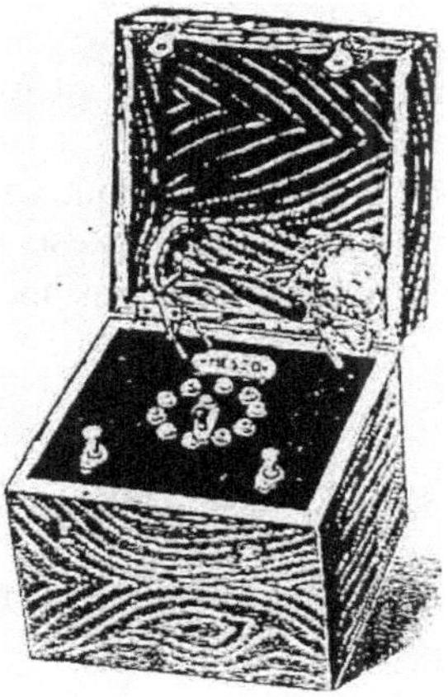

Fig M13. Galvanic Battery and Epilation Outfit

This galvanic battery (Fig M13) is contained in a polished oak box (8 x 8 x 8 inches) that has a metal carrying handle on top, and two lever, hinged latches on the front. The polished slate face plate has two screw connecting posts, and 10 buttons (0-9) for selecting dry cells controlled by a rotating lever. The galvanic unit was designed for removing superfluous hair (epilation), facial blemishes, and strictures at home. The unit contained nine standard dry cells, was listed as No.2231, and sold for $10.00 complete in 1905.

This unit resembles in some features the galvanic batteries made by Galvano-Faradic Mfg Co (Chapt 7, Fig G16). The Galvano-Faradic Mfg Co also made a similar styled unit for the Brooklyn Dry Battery Co (Chapt 22, Fig B1).

Summary

MESCO had a long successful business life as a manufacturer of electrical cells, and retailer of many types of electrical apparatuses, accessories, and supplies. Its electrical apparatuses included telegraph and telephone units. The JH Bunnell & Co was a major manufacturer of medical electrical batteries that were made for and sold by MESCO. Likewise, JH Bunnell & Co reciprocated business with MESCO by using MESCO and Red Seal dry cells in its medical electrical batteries.

In 1905, MESCO was still manufacturing and selling the MESCO dry cell.[8] This cell came in many sizes, both cylindrical and rectangular shapes. In 1910 and later, the company had offices in New York, Chicago, St Louis, and San Francisco. The company in 1910 was also manufacturing and promoting the Red Seal dry cell rather than the MESCO cell, as well as telegraph equipment. The Manhattan Electrical Supply Co may have been doing business in 1929, but records are not readily available after 1910.

MESCO issued many trade catalogs of its product lines. Many of the medical electrical battery models that it sold under its name or without signatures are available today in antique shops and on eBay. The volume of MESCO units available today suggests that the company was successful in selling the units to the public consumer for home use.

References

1. (www.zianet.com/sparks/sparkmakers2.html)

2. Davis AB, Dreyfus MS. The Finest Instruments Ever Made. Arlington, MA, Med Hist Pub, 1986, pp 37-38, 213

3. Keane CP, Emmerich HJ (eds). Marvyn Scudder Manual of Extinct and Obsolete Companies, Vol 1. Marvyn Scudder, New York, NY, 1926, p 724

4. Trevert E. Electro-Therapeutic Hand-Book. New York, NY, MESCO, 1900

5. Catalog of JH Bunnell & Co. New York, NY, Bunnell, 1901

6. Catalog of Montgomery Ward & Co. Chicago, IL, Montgomery Ward, 1904, p 514

7. Catalog of Sears, Roebuck and Co. Chicago, IL, Sears, Roebuck, 1897, p 473

8. Catalog of Manhattan Electrical Supply Co. New York, NY, MESCO, 1905

3. MONTGOMERY WARD & COMPANY OF CHICAGO

The Montgomery Ward & Co of 600-618 W Chicago Ave, Chicago, IL, was established in August 1872[1] by Aaron Montgomery Ward (17 Feb 1843-7 Dec 1913) and two of his employees.[2] His first mail order business was located at Clark and Kinzie Streets. He started with $2,400.00[2] or $1,600.00[3] to start the mail order business for rural America. Initially, the Ward Company listed 163 products and prices on a single page of paper (8 x 12 inches) that was mailed to potential customers.[2] His brother-in-law, Thorne, joined Ward in the company that

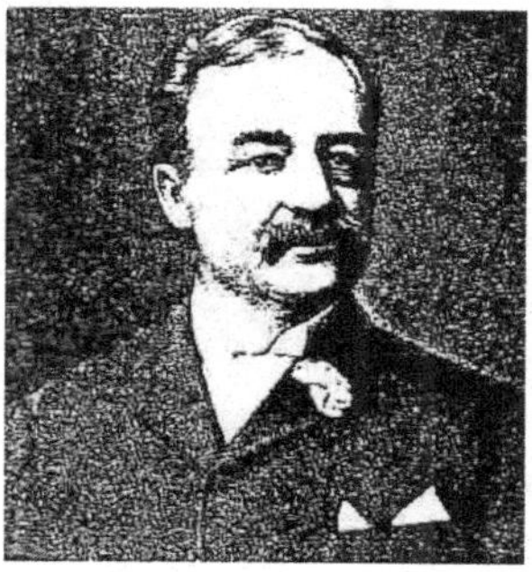

Fig MW. A Montgomery Ward

began to grow into a profitable business. In 21 years the company had a capital and surplus of two and one-half million dollars. The company by the 1880s became a major retailer and the first major mail order firm in the United States, and in 1894 it began selling the medical electrical batteries of several manufacturers. Along with his marketing success Montgomery Ward became civic minded and contributed much money to preserve the waterfront in Chicago.[2]

In 1894, the Ward catalog (page 209) illustrated and listed The Crown Family Battery that sold for $3.50 (top right); and the Alpha Family Battery for $5.00 (manufactured by FG Otto & Son, 2nd top right); Smith & Shaw Portable Battery for $7.00 (right, 4th from top); the New No. 4 Home Apparatus with the Burnley nickel plated cylinder cell holder (manufactured by JH Bunnell Co; right, 3rd from top) sold for $7.00; the Magnetoelectrical Battery (Davis/Kidder type; right, 5th from top) sold for $7.25 (then manufactured by JH Bunnell & Co); and The Family Battery was $10.00 (right, bottom).[4] Prices for the New No. 4 Home Apparatus were reduced to $3.00 in the 1904 edition (p 514). The price reduction of this particular unit may have been the result of competition in medical electrical batteries, but more likely because the mail order business was a discount operation, and was selling the unit close to cost. In 1904, the Voltamp No.6 faradic battery sold for $3.75 (p 514 of the Ward catalog). Also, in this same year Montgomery Ward &

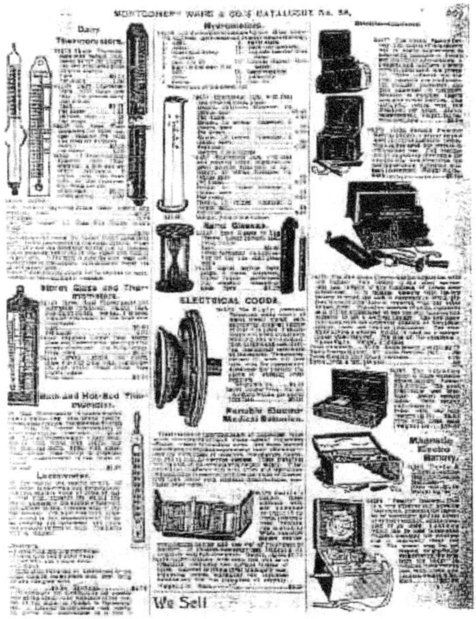
ELECTRICAL GOODS
We Sell

Fig MW1. Catalog of 1894-1895

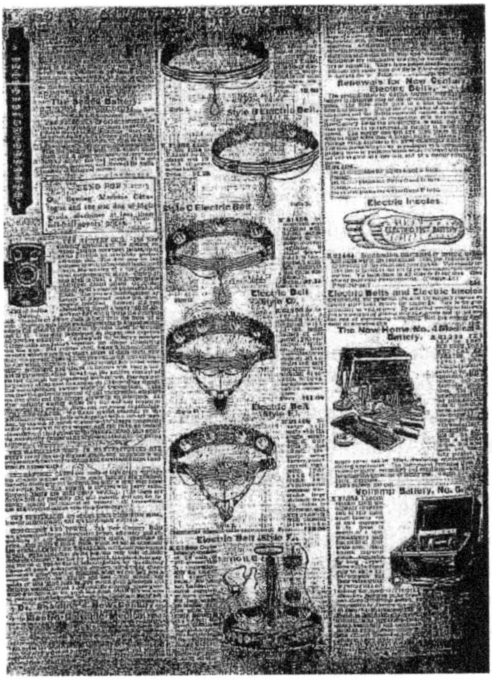
Electric Insoles

Fig MW2. Catalog of 1904

Co initiated the "satisfaction guaranteed or your money back" policy.[2]

Summary

Montgomery Ward & Co was a major competitor of Sears, Roebuck and Co also of Chicago. The Ward catalog of 1909 and 1910 devoted nine pages to drugs and patent medicines, but advertisements were more restrained than those of Sears, Roebuck and Co. Montgomery Ward & Co advertised its products as remedies rather than cures as did Sears, Roebuck and Co. Montgomery Ward &Co advertised that the buyer received pure medicine as guaranteed by the Food & Drugs Act of 30 June 1906.[5] The Food and Drug acts placed restrictions on marketing of medicine and nostrums, and reduced blatant abuses. Many medicines and electrical apparatuses could no longer be sold directly to the public without a physician's prescription. The margin of profits for the company was also affected.

Montgomery Ward was still selling, although a reduced volume, some patent medicines in 1911.[5] The public liked trade names, and a popular item sold by Montgomery Ward was electrical belts. The Heidelberg electrical belt was very popular for several years.[5] The sale of medical electrical batteries through catalogs also faded in the early twentieth century. Medical electrical batteries were not being sold through Montgomery Ward & Co catalogs by 1912. The catalog business ended in 1985, and the remainder (stores) of the firm closed in 2001 to end 128 years of retailing.[6]

References

1. Davis AB, Dreyfus MS. The Finest Instruments Ever Made. Arlington, MA, Med Hist Pub Assocs, 1986, pp 337

2. (http://www.lib.niu.edu/ipo/ihy000441.html); (via www.google.com).

3. Graham DK. From the publisher. Antiques & Collecting, Chicago, IL, Feb 2001, pp 12, 74

4. Catalog of Montgomery Ward & Co. Chicago, IL, Montgomery Ward, 1894-1895, p 209

5. Emmet B, Jeuck JE. Catalogues and Counter: A History of Sears, Roebuck and Company. Chicago, IL, U Chicago Press, 1965, pp 104, 249, 254, 414

6. (http://www.chipublib.org/004chicago/timelinfe/mtgmryward.html)

4. SEARS, ROEBUCK AND COMPANY OF CHICAGO

In 1886, the RW Sears Watch Co was founded in Minneapolis, MN, by Richard W Sears (1863-1914) who had previously worked in several different businesses. In 1887, Sears moved his watch business to Chicago,IL, and hired a watchmaker, Alvah C Roebuck. The business was located on 925 Herman Street.[1] In September, 1893, the business was named the Sears, Roebuck and Co, and the mail order catalog was started for watches and jewelry. Its first catalog was issued in 1893 that was cited as the "Consumer's Guide for 1894." Alvah Roebuck retired in 1895 because of poor health, and in that same year Juluis Rosenwald became vice-president and directed the catalog activities. The name of the company remained the same. The first catalog of general merchandise by the Sears, Roebuck and Co was introduced in 1896. He wanted to bridge the gap between the industrial east and the rural midwest farmers for purchasing clothing, equipment, and medical items. Also in 1896, the company moved to a new building of six stories with a basement. Its illustrated trade catalog of 1896 began listing and pricing the sale of patent medicines, and various nostrums. Nostrums in the first edition catalog only described the items. In 1897, illustrations of the nostrums began in the Sears' catalog, and the medical electrical batteries of different manufacturers were described, illustrated, and priced.[2,3(102)] The Capital battery (manufactured by FG Otto & Son) was sold for $4.50; the New No.4 Home Apparatus with the Burnley nickel plated cylinder cell holder (manufactured by JH Bunnell & Co) was listed for $5.75; The Climax (manufactured by FG Otto & Son) was $4.00; and the Magnetolectrical apparatus (then manufactured by JH Bunnell & Co) was sold for $6.75.

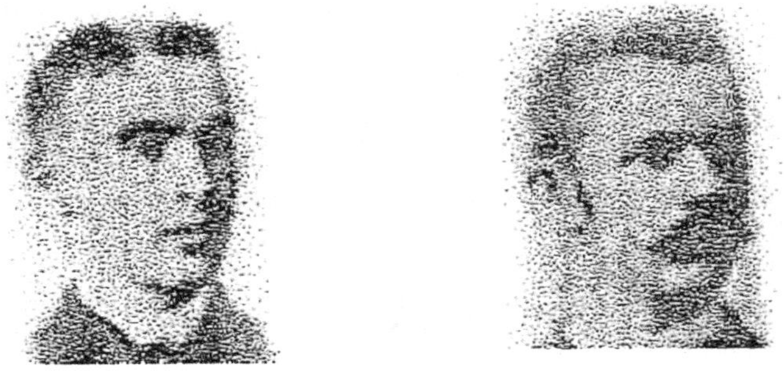

The Fig SR. Richard W Sears, Alvah C Roebuck

The company's trade catalog expanded from 322 to 507 pages in 1898. Sears soon became the largest mail order store in the world. The outstanding growth of the company, in part, was related to the post office and railroads that provided free delivery and parcel post to rural America, and to volume buying by the Sears, Roebuck and Co.[4] business continued to prosper enough to expand with a plant in Texas in 1906, and in that same year a new plant and office building opened on the West side of Chicago. Sears, Roebuck and Co then became the largest business building in the world.

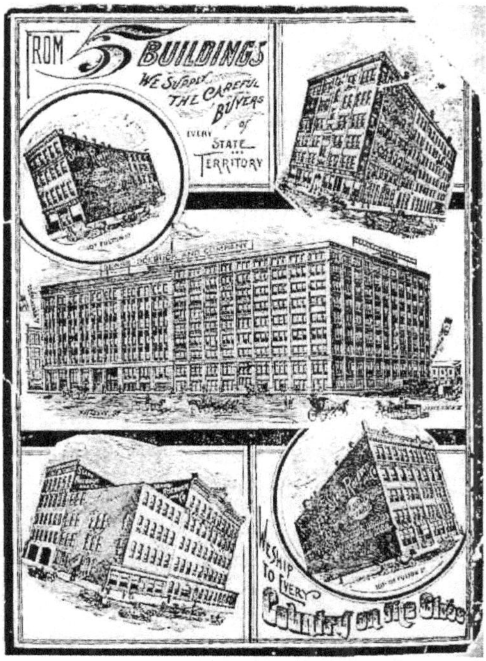

Fig S1. Catalog of 1897

The Induction Coil #6351 shown in the 1897 Sears catalog[2] was designed for the traveler as a portable unit having a hard wooden base (5.75 x 2.75 inches). It is comprised of an induction coil with a sliding metal tube current controller. Since the ends of the coil are capped with wooden circular sleeves, it is believed to have been manufactured by JH Bunnell & Co of New York City. The base also contains an adjustable screw spring lever, hammer vibrating type of interrupter, two metal adjustable screw binding posts, and two metal adjustable connecting posts to the patient. The unit was powered by one dry or one wet cell, not included with the price of $3.50.

Patent medicines were a big sale item before 1860, but after the Civil War they became even larger sale items. By 1865, proprietary medicine advertising was so popular that it was covering half of the lineage in many newspapers. Sears, Roebuck and Co and others took advantage of this public demand for medical items and delivered them through their catalog product lines. Conditions were inviting all kinds of health aides for public consumption.

Medical schools in the United States could not turn out enough physicians to meet the health needs and demands of the public. Harvard Medical School in 1870, for example, could not hold written examinations in medicine because most students could not write well enough. The largest portion of population in the United States lived too far away from the nearest physician, and only a minor portion of people could afford the fees of physicians. Thus, golden opportunities for charlatans and quacks were present, and, of course, the public had leanings for self treatments and medicines.[3]

In 1898, electrical belts covered two pages in the Sears catalog, but patent medicines needed eight pages. In the 1899 catalog, the patent medicines coverage grew to nine pages. Sears offered electrical rings in 1896 as a cure for rheumatism, but they were discontinued in 1898. The electrical belts were much more successful in sales than the electrical rings, and occupied two full pages of the catalog in 1899 and 1900.[3(103-104)]

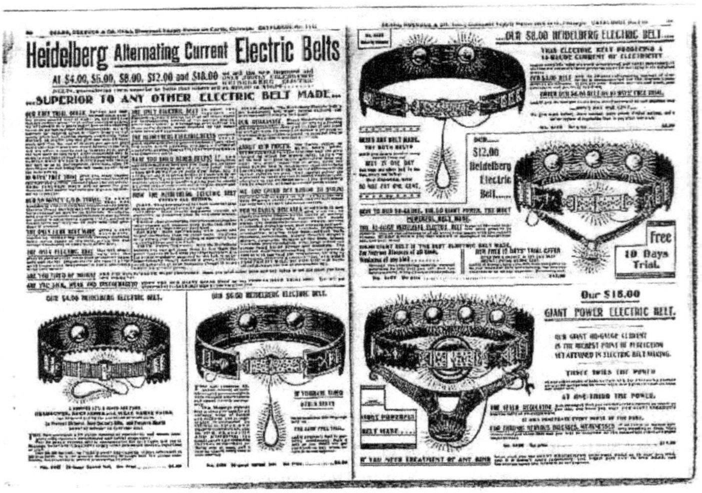

Fig S2. Catalog of 1902, Batteries, Rings, Belts

The popular "Giant Power Heidelberg Electrical Belt" with the advertisement "In a month you will be a new man" was priced at $18.00 (what a deal for fantastic health).[3(414)] The public liked trademark names, so items were often given names (eg, Heidelberg electric belt, and Voltamp's individual names for its medical electrical batteries). The electrical belts reached their heyday in the catalog of 1901 with three pages of coverage. By 1903, electrical belts dropped to a single page, and in 1905 the belt dropped out of the catalog of Sears, Roebuck and Co.

Sears went for electricity, however, in a big way. Sears advertised electrical insoles for shoes to help people with poor circulation

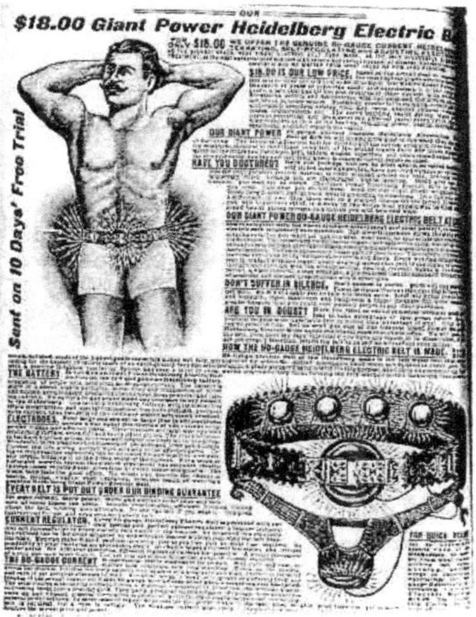

Fig S2A. The Heidelberg Electric Belt, 1902

and cold feet. A battery plaster replaced the electrical ring and electrical belts. Battery plasters were aimed for women with bad backs and menstrual problems, rheumatism, and kidney and muscle pain in their backs.

In 1900, Sears was selling dental products, but was dominantly directing its mail order catalog for medicines to physicians as well as home consumers in 1902. By 1901, patent medicines were selling so well for Sears that they replaced the space previously allotted for jewelry and watches. The Sears catalogs were offering popular medical products, and making exaggerated claims as offered in newspapers and magazines of the time.

Sears did, however, warn buyers to see physicians if the patent medicine purchased did not help their condition. However, Sears contracted and retailed medicines from manufacturers without knowing the ingredients of the product.[3(247-249)]

Medical electrical apparatuses continued to be sold in the catalog of 1902 (edition 5, p 44). The Sears catalog of 1903 showed a lot of surgical instruments and physician supplies. By 1905, nostrums sold by Sears occupied five pages of their catalog. Medical electrical batteries and supplies were continued for sale in the Sears catalogs of 1904 to 1918.[3(102-104)]

In 1906, the Pure Food and Drug Act was passed that began to restrict exaggerated and unfounded claims, and misrepresented patent medicines. The Act also introduced an educational campaign to help consumers select medical products with some confidence and creditability. As a result of the medical educational plan the public began to be more selective in its buying of nonphysician recommended medical products. Later amendments to the Act of 1906 also made manufacturing of patent medicines and nostrums more restrictive, and again the public reacted by being more selective in its buying of medical products through the catalogs. These responses of course affected the medical electrical battery usage and sales. Sears increased its scrutiny of products and the upgrading of their quality around 1908.[3(299)]

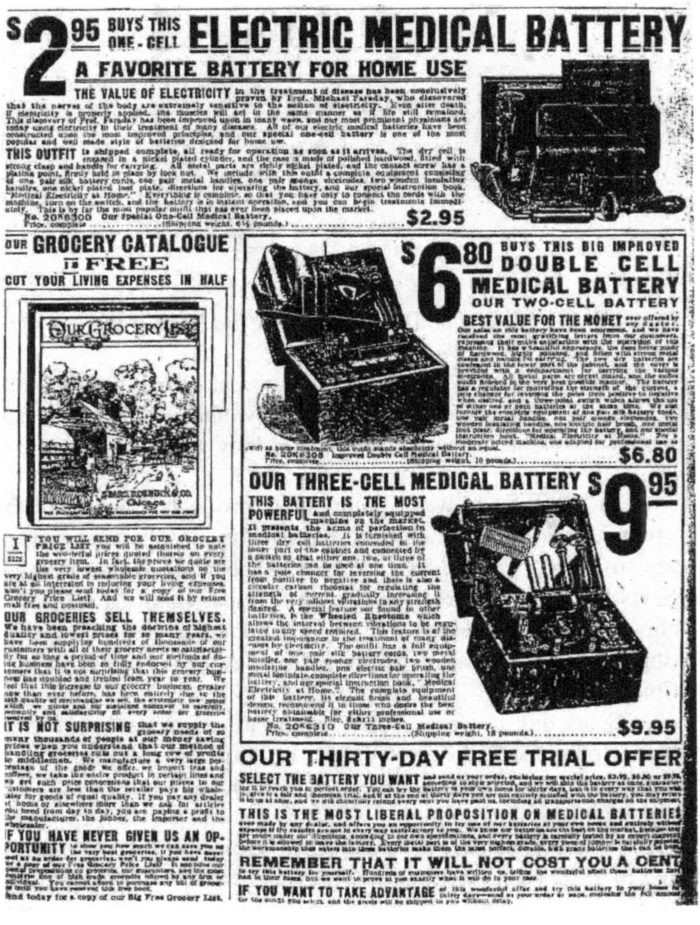

Fig S3. Catalog of 1908

In 1908, Sears, Roebuck and Co devoted only one page of its catalog to three medical electrical batteries. The one cell Electrical Medical Battery ($2.95), the Double Cell Medical Battery ($6.80), and the Three Cell Medical Battery ($9.95) were illustrated, described, and priced on page 206 of that catalog. These three batteries were manufactured by the JH Bunnell & Co (Chapt 16, Fig B3, top), and by the Menominee Electric Company of Menominee, MI (see Signal Electric Mfg Co, Chapt 18, Figs S3 & S4), for the Sears, Roebuck and Co. The three-cell unit was also available in the catalog of 1906.

Summary

Richard Sears started his watch and jewelry business in 1886, but expanded into a mail order business offering general merchandise in 1895. Sears, Roebuck and Co is still doing business today but the company stopped its mail order catalog in 1993. Medical electrical batteries were a small part of the Sears, Roebuck and Co catalog business between 1896 and about 1910 when the company began phasing out its patent medicines and nostrums. Sears, Roebuck and Co never offered many batteries in any one catalog; the company listed only a few in each year's catalog and by 1908 three batteries were shown and described. During the time period that medical electrical batteries were listed and described in its catalogs, some models carried the name and brand of the manufacturer while some were made for Sears, Roebuck and Co with the manufacturer's identity absent. Booklets accompanying the batteries sold by Sears, Roebuck and Co carried the Sears name and address. The company served as a discount retailer for the sale of medical electrical batteries. Examples of manufacturers of medical electrical batteries that sold their products through Sears, Roebuck and Co were: JH Bunnell & Co of New York, Signal Electric Mfg Co of Menominee, MI, and Voltamp Electric Mfg Co of Baltimore.

The patent medicine department was among the most profitable division for the Sears, Roebuck and Co since it operated in 1896 through 1912 or for a 16 years span of time. During this period of time, Sears, Roebuck and Co exaggerated product claims in their catalog presentations. Although Sears started to scrutinize its products in 1908, it was not until 1911 that they really began to clean up their advertisements and improve policy on their patent medicines.[3(247-249)] Sears, Roebuck and Co began to eliminate some patent medicines and nostrums in 1911. The catalog of 1912 contained one less page of patent medicines than did the catalog of 1911.[4] By the end of 1912, Sears was beginning to drop their involvement with patent medicines and with some nostrums.[3(247-249)] The catalog of 1913 dropped its listing of home remedies and provided an explanation "Why We Have Discontinued Patent Medicines."[4]

Patent medicines were eliminated from Sears, Roebuck and Co catalogs in 1913 when the company became more aware of the accuracy and creditability of the products and manufacturers' claims. Advertisements in their catalogs began to provide the truth about products illustrated and listed, such that improvements were noted in 1918.[3(247)]

References

1. Kelly EM. The Business Founding Date Directory. Scarsdale, New York, NY, Morgan & Morgan, 1954, p 112

2. Catalog of Sears, Roebuck and Co. Chicago, IL, Sears, Roebuck, 1897, p 473

3. Emmet B, Jeuck JE. Catalogues and Counters: A History of Sears, Roebuck and Company. Chicago, IL. U Chicago Press, 1965, pp 102-104, 247, 249, 299, 414

4. (http:www.sears.com/sr/misc/sears/about/public/history/)

5. MAX WOCHER & SON COMPANY OF CINCINNATI

Maximilian Wocher started his business in Cincinnati, OH, as a cutler, but founded his instrument making business in 1837[1] or 1838.[2] In 1840, his shop was located on Walnut Street (between 4th and 5th), but between 1842 and 1852 he was located at College Street (corner of George and Plum Sts). He again moved in 1853 to 11 College Street. He became a very successful businessman in Cincinnati by time of the Civil War. His shop was moved by 1855 to the site of the Ohio Medical College (105 6th Street between Vine and Race) where it helped him gain business among the physicians. The Max Wocher business remained at this location until 1869. In 1861 through 1863, he advertised as a surgical and dental instrument maker, and was making surgical instruments for the Union during the Civil War period. In 1870, Max Wocher became Max Wocher & Son when his son Louis entered the business. Max Wocher and Henry S Hoeller were, however, the principals between 1870 and 1874. In 1876, the company began to import surgical and dental instruments in addition to their own manufacture.[2]

Max Wocher died in 1883, and in 1895 the ownership of the business went to Max Schmidt and Henry S Hoeller.[2] The new owners continued to use the well known trade mark of Max Wocher & Son.

The City Directory of Cincinnati of 1876 shows Max Wocher & Son Co as "Manufacturers and Importers of Surgical and Dental Instruments," located at 106 West 6th Street.[3] In 1891, the company's office and salesrooms were located at 29-31 West 6th Street, while its factory and enameling department were at 609-611 College Street. The company in the same year issued a 318-paged illustrated catalog and

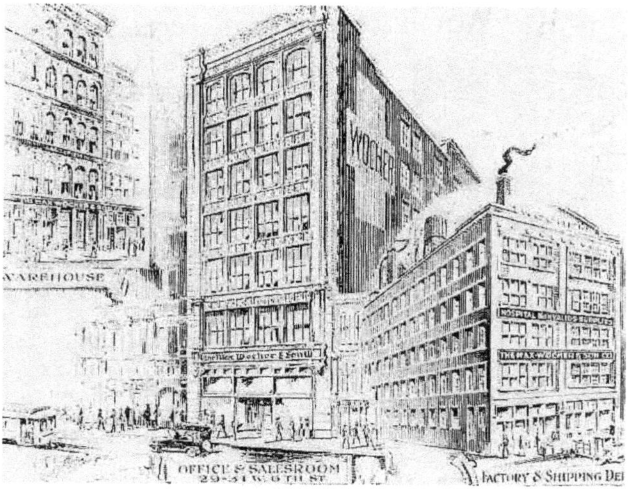

Fig W1. Warehouse, Office, Factory

price list for surgical instruments and orthopedic apparatuses. About 1895, the company used the phrase "Quick Service Our Motto" in its catalog. Manufacturers of medical electrical batteries sold apparatuses and accessories through Max Wocher & Son, but placed the name and address of Max Wocher & Son Co on the label inside the lid of their particular units. Page 375 of the catalog of 1905[4] illustrated and listed the price of two such batteries. The McIntosh Professional Combination Galvanic and Faradic Battery was listed for $45.00 with reduced prices when fewer cells were supplied to power the unit. This particular unit was manufactured by the McIntosh Battery & Optical Co of Chicago for the Max Wocher & Son Co. Cells ranged from 12 to 30 in numbers. The No.2 Professional Faradic Battery was sold for $16.00, and provided three currents (primary, secondary, and combined). The No.2 unit was manufactured by Voltamp Electrical Mfg Co of Baltimore, MD, and contained the Fuld rheostat. Some manufacturers retained their names and logos on batteries sold by Max Wocher & Son Co.

The Max Wocher & Son Co reorganized in 1895 when new owners took over the business. In 1896 the company had its office and salesroom located at 23 West Sixth St, while its factory and warehouse was at 611 College Street, Cincinnati, OH. Also about 1896, the company issued the "Second Edition" of an illustrated catalog and price list of surgical instruments, orthopedic apparatus, trusses, elastic hosiery, electrical batteries, microscopes, hospital and laboratory supplies, office furniture, and rubber sundries. The 533 paged catalog listed medical electrical batteries and accessories on at least 60 pages. The wide variety of medical electrical items included: medical electrical batteries with wet cells, dry cells, storage cells, and cautery; magnetoelectrical machines of

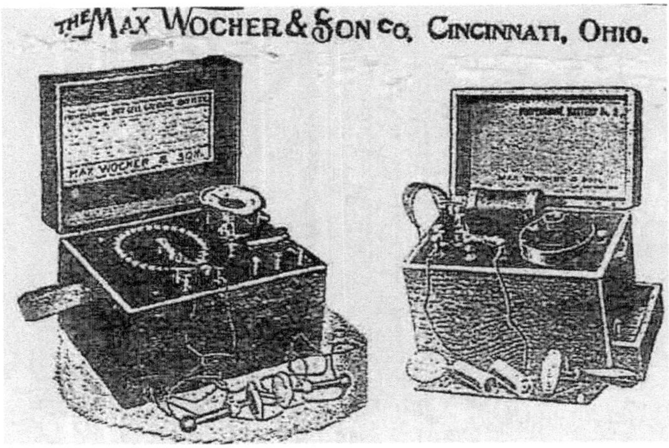

Fig W2. Units with Wocher Label

the Davis-Kidder type; and electrical belts. These products were made by Chloride of Silver Dry Cell Battery Co, Otto Flemming, Gaiffe of France, Galvanic-Faradic Manufacturing Co, Kennelly, Jerome Kidder Manufacturing Co, McIntosh Battery & Optical Co, JC Vetter & Co, and Waite & Bartlett Manufacturing Co.

The third edition of the company's illustrated trade catalog contained 55 pages, and was issued in 1900. It indicated that the company was a manufacturer, importer, wholesaler, and retailer of surgical instruments, orthopedic apparatus, trusses, elastic hosiery, medical electrical batteries, microscopes, hospital and laboratory supplies, office furniture, and rubber sundries. Wocher & Son Co probably manufactured some instruments and furniture, but never manufactured medical electrical batteries. Their advertisement would suggest that they manufactured medical electrical batteries, but rather they had their signature placed on some batteries made by other companies that are listed above.[1]

By 1903, the company was selling veterinary instruments, books, drugs, and turf goods. The sixth edition catalog (518 pages) was issued in 1904. The company was using 21-23 West 6th St as its address in 1904.

In 1910, a special edition catalog offered sundries and furniture for the hospital and surgery. The catalog for 1919 (114 pages) showed that the company had added apparatuses for experimental work, and research adopted to the needs of medical schools, hospitals, and research institutions. Instruments for eye, ear, nose, and throat were added in 1937.[1]

The newspapers of Cincinnati from time to time provided news coverage of local corporations of which Max Wocher & Son Co was featured at different times. In 1938, the Wocher Co introduced a lamp for killing germs in surgery, and before long the lamp was being used during surgery for light. In 1940 and 1941, the company was starting its second generation of business and the plant increased its production for the war efforts. In 1942, the company experienced labor problems but survived to move to different facilities at Price Hill on York Street.[1]

In 1948, the company manufactured Bowie knives, and in 1949 it honored its employees of 50 years. Also, in 1949, the company sold its furniture plant. In 1950, the company celebrated 113 years of business and was said to be the oldest company of hospital supplies in the United States.[1] On 2 November 1978, Wocher & Son Co closed its retail store on 10 West Seventh Street, Cincinnati. At the time of the closing the company had completed 141 years of business. It announced that it planned to open a larger store, but the Cincinnati City Directories listed Wocher & Son Co from 1876 to 1978 (102 years). No information could be obtained about the company after 1978.[1]

As mentioned during its business years, the company did not manufacture medical electrical batteries. The company served as a regional seller of various medical electrical batteries of manufacturers like: Chloride of Silver Dry Cell Battery Co of Baltimore, MD; McIntosh Battery & Optical Co of Chicago; and Voltamp Electric Manufacturing Co of Baltimore, MD.

Summary

Maximilian Wocher started as a cutler but evolved into the instrument making business in 1837 or 1838. Through expansion the business became a large retailer of hospital, medical, and surgical apparatuses and supplies. In 1870, the business became the Max Wocher & Son Co when his son joined him in the firm. Sometime in the 1890s the company sold medical electrical batteries made by several different companies. Some medical electrical batteries were made by various manufacturers for the Max Wocher & Son Co to sell using the Wocher name or signature on the models, while the company also sold batteries of other manufacturers having the makers name or signature remaining on their products. Max Wocher died in 1883 and the company was sold in 1895. Medical electrical batteries were apparently sold by the company into the 1920s. The company sold off some assets in the mid twentieth century, and closed its doors in 1978. This giant retailer of hospital, medical, and surgical apparatuses and supplies remained in business for at least 141 years.

References

1. Public Library of Cincinnati and Hamilton County, OH, (courtesy of Depts of History and Genealogy, and Rare Books per Patricia M Van Skaik, head)

2. Edmonson JM. American Surgical Instruments. San Francisco, CA, Norman Pub, 1997, p 249

3. Directory of Cincinnati, OH, 1876, p 1030

4. Catalog of Max Wocher Co. Cincinnati, OH, 1905, p 375

CHAPTER 22. THE LOCAL SELLERS

Local sellers are selective retailers of medical electrical batteries whose businesses were on a smaller scale than those described as Giant Sellers. The difference between local and giant sellers is based on the volume of medical electrical batteries encountered in antique shops and frequency on the eBay auction. This section limits the number of local sellers to four examples. Every large city had one or more retailers of medical electrical batteries; some could be considered regional by their volumes of sales.

Examples of retailers not presented are: Codman and Shurtleff of Boston, Leach and Green of Boston; EF Mahady Co of Boston; Smith and Shaw Electric Co, and George Tiemann & Co of New York; Whitail Tataum Co, and Truax, Greene & Co of Chicago.

1. BROOKLYN DRY CELL BATTERY COMPANY

The company operated under two different names: the Brooklyn Dry Cell Battery Co, and the Brooklyn Battery & Instrument Co, Inc, and was a retailer rather than a manufacturer of medical equipment. The company under both names was located at 991 Madison Street, Brooklyn, New York. The style of their known medical electrical batteries appear to be 1898 to 1904 vintage.

Galvanic Battery. The Brooklyn Galvanic Battery was a quality unit built for direct current use in treatment and cautery. This battery was powered by six dry cell batteries labeled as Brooklyn Dry Cells, and was built for physician use. The batteries in this particular apparatus appear

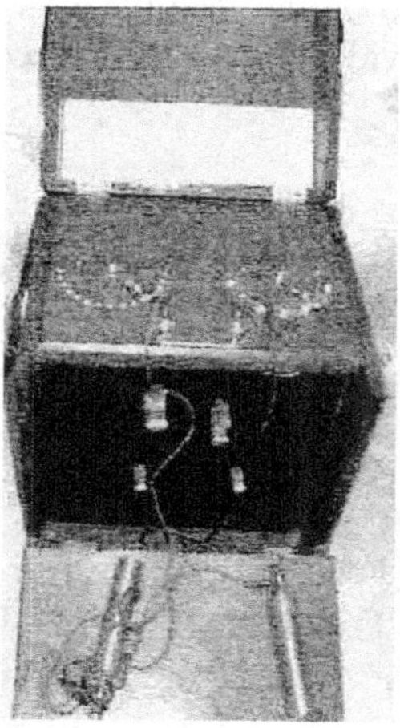

Fig B1. Galvanic Battery

the same as the Burnley dry cells of 1897. The positive or carbon pole is about one inch wide and the negative or zinc pole is the standard threaded screw variety seen on later standard dry cells for both poles. The Galvanic Battery has similarities of workmanship and design of the galvanic apparatus built in the 1890s by the Galvano-Faradic Manufacturing Co of New York, and is conjectured to have been manufactured by this latter company. The operator used a lamp connected to the unit to test the power. The lamp lighted when the six cells were at full power.

Another medical electrical battery with a Brooklyn Medical Battery Co label appeared exactly like The New No.4 D.D. Home Medical Apparatus of the JH Bunnell & Co from 1892 to the 1920s. The difference in the two faradic units is that the Brooklyn Medical Battery Co was powered by two Red Seal dry cells (MESCO), and produced 10 currents. Although its Two Cell, Ten Currents, Faradic Battery was advertised as a physician unit, this author believes its quality was more suited for public consumers.

Two-Cell New Current Faradic Battery. The Brooklyn Dry Cell Battery Co also sold a two dry-cell faradic battery (Fig B2). The cells were located underneath the wooden face plate. The wooden face plate matched the oak case. The wood case is hinged with a metal carrying handle on top and is secured in front by an engraved metal lever clasp. Instructions for operating the unit are glued inside of the lid. The induction coil, mounted center-rear of the face plate, has a sliding current controller (left), and an adjustable screw spring lever vibrating interrupter (right). The coil is covered by black fabric and has circular hard rubber end caps. An On/Off lever switch along with five button type current patient connectors are also on the face plate. A small open space to the right of the face plate provides for storage of accessories. The design of

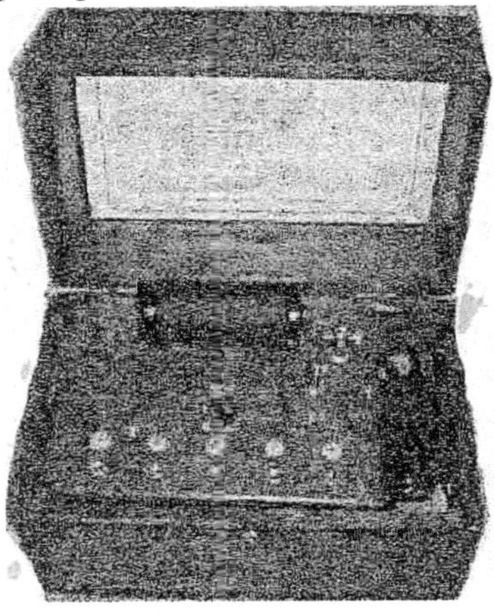

Fig B2. Two-Cell New Current Faradic Battery

the unit is similar to those manufactured by the Galvano-Faradic Manufacturing Co of New York in the 1890s.

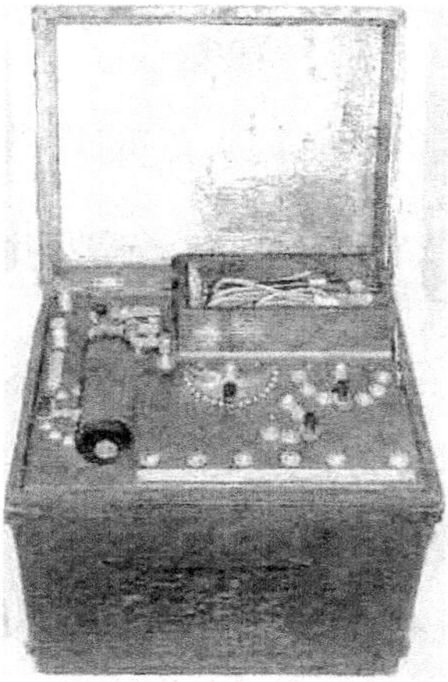

Fig B3. Combination Cautery, Faradic and Galvanic Battery

Combination Cautery, Faradic, and Galvanic Battery. The unit of Fig B3 of the Brooklyn Dry Cell Battery Co was perhaps the deluxe unit sold by that retailer. Like the others offered by the company, this unit also contains features designed and manufactured by the Galvanic and Faradic Manufacturing Co of New York.

The oak case (11.5 x 9 x 11 inches) is hinged with a metal carrying handle. The lid contains directions for operating the unit. Twelve dry cells are housed underneath the wooden face plate. The induction coil (circular end caps) is mounted along the width of the face plate (most are mounted along the length). Control switches for selecting the function are to the left as are the two patient connecting posts for cautery. Six metal connecting posts are located on front of the face plate to connect the patient to a combination of faradic currents. The unit has a vibrating hammer type rheotome for control of faradic pulse rates. A lever switch rotates over buttons that serve as a rheostat for each of the faradic and galvanic current functions. An On/Off switch is located on front center of the face plate. An unusual box like storage compartment for accessories is located on top of the face plate. All metal electrical components are nickel plated. A latch secures the lid on front of the case and the corners of the box are reinforced by metal angles mounted on the exterior of the case. The unit weighs 40 pounds complete with cells, and dates from about 1895 to 1900.

Summary

The Brooklyn Dry Cell Battery Co is believed to have been a

small retailer of medical electrical batteries in the 1890s and early twentieth century. The two batteries featured are similar in construction and style to have been manufactured for the company by the Galvano-Faradic Manufacturing Co of New York.

2. GEORGE C FRYE COMPANY OF PORTLAND, ME

The George C Frye Co of 203 Congress Street, Portland, ME, opened an apothecary shop in 1866. He remained at this address until 1868 when he moved the business to the corner of Franklin and Congress Streets. He moved again in 1869 to 186 Congress Street and then in 1875 to 320 Congress Street.[1]

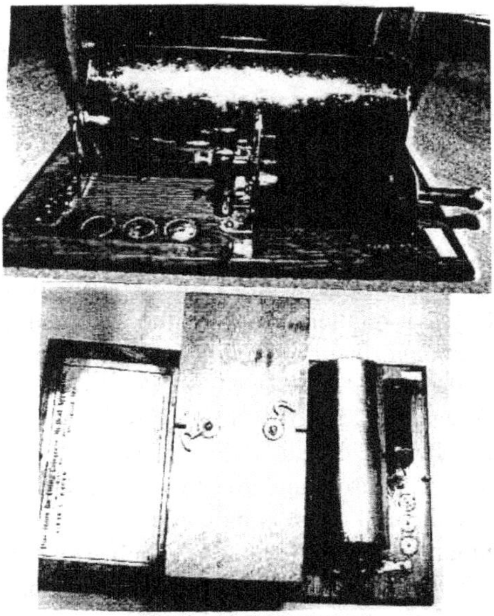

Fig F1. New Home No. 4 D.D. Battery

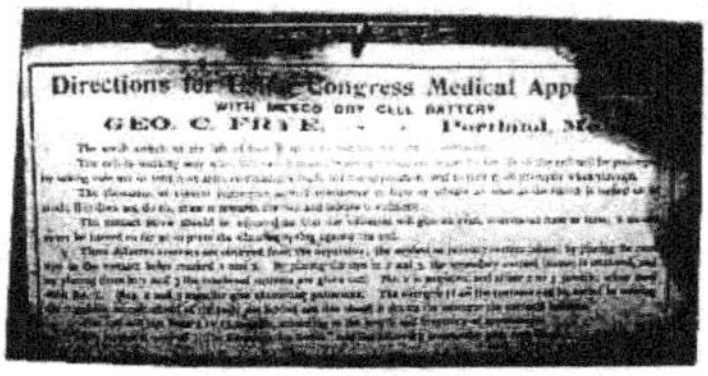

Fig F1. New Home No. 4 D.D. Battery

In 1881, the company issued a catalog (177 pages) of electrical batteries, orthopedic appliances, and surgical instruments. This catalog also contained 20 pages of advertisements involving products of other companies[2] that implies that Frye would buy items not stocked for customers while making some profit on the transaction. This also implies that he did catalog business before Sears, Roebuck and Co. In 1883, another catalog was published by Frye Co that illustrated electrical batteries, orthopedic appliances and supplies, and surgical appliances and instruments, as well as hospital and surgical supplies.[3] In 1900, Frye Co only published a Bulletin of surgical instruments that was four pages in length, and it was printed in double newspaper size. At this time the company was again located at Franklin & Congress Streets. A later catalog of surgical apparatuses and instruments showed that George C Frye, the druggist & apothecary[2] was still operating from his address at 320 Congress St in 1904.

No other records were found on this once flourishing medical and surgical supply company that also sold medical electrical batteries of several manufacturers. The George C Frye Co may have once sold the Demming Faradic Battery that bears the cities of Portland, ME, and Providence, RI, on different batteries of the same model and trade name. George C Frye Co sold medical electrical batteries for family use that have his signature on the item. Collectors might think that Frye was the manufacturer of the particular artifact, but he was a retailer only in medical electrical batteries. His signature appears on electrical batteries made by Pilling & Son of Philadelphia, and Voltamp Electric Mfg Co of Baltimore.

Summary

The George C Frye Co was a successful business in New England for medical and surgical apparatuses as well as medical electrical batteries. Being an apothecary he ventured into the various medical and surgical items much like pharmacists do today. Medical electrical batteries bearing his signature but manufactured by other companies for his retail are frequently found in antique shops and on eBay auctions. Surgical instruments bearing his name are collector items.

References

1. Edmonson JM. American Surgical Instruments. San Francisco, CA, Norman Pub, 1997, p 194

2. Davis AB, Dreyfus MS. The Finest Instruments Ever Made. Arlington, MA, Med Hist Pub Assocs, 1986, pp 137-138

3. Romaine LB. A Guide to American Trade Catalogs 1744-1900. New York, NY, RR Bowker, 1960, pp 235-241

3. CHARLES WILLMS SURGICAL INSTRUMENT COMPANY OF BALTIMORE

The Charles Willms and Company was both a manufacturer and business retailer in Baltimore starting in 1869. His earliest known location (1871) was 113 North Howard Street. From 1871 to at least 1889, surgeons from the Johns Hopkins hospital bought instruments and supplies from the local firm. Charles Willms' transactions with the local surgeons soon made him well known nationally and internationally. He moved his business to 79 North Howard Street in 1879. In 1887, he located his business to 224 North Howard St,[1] and then finally in 1890 to 300 North Howard St

The Baltimore City Business Directory of 1881 to 1892 listed Chas Willms & Co, 300 N Howard, under Surgical and Dental Instruments. The same city directory for 1888 listed Charles Willms & Co (Chas Willms), surgical instrument manufacturer, 224 N Howard).[2] (He may have had the office and store separate from his factory in the same city block.).

The Charles Willms & Co issued trade catalogs before 1885 (503 pp) for such items as: laboratory equipment, orthopedic apparatus,

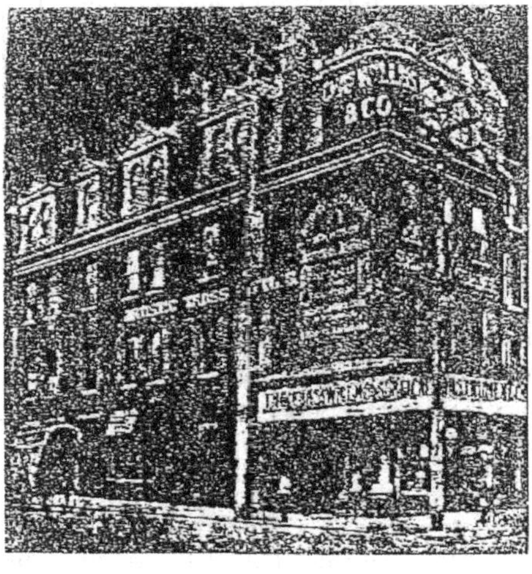

Fig W1. Building of the Willms & Co (courtesy of Smithsonian Institution Libraries, Washington, DC)

apparatus,office furnishings, and surgical instruments. In 1895, the Charles Willms & Co catalog (503 pp) contained price lists for physicians' and surgeons' instruments and supplies, orthopedic apparatuses, elastic hosiery, trusses, hospital supplies, microscopes, and a wide variety of other items. Forty pages of the catalog were devoted to medical electrical batteries, while 28 pages showed Chloride of Silver

Dry Cells of Baltimore, MD, for which Willms was its general manager in 1890, and whose machines featured the Willms patented rheostat. The Charles Willms & Co catalog of 1905 was the same as that for 1895 except for the increased number of pages to 365.[3] Willms had a policy that he would match prices of other manufacturers'items shown in their respective catalogs. The Charles Willms office, factory, and salesroom were all housed in the same building in 1905.[3]

In 1893, the company's name changed from the Charles Willms and Co to the Charles Willms Surgical Instruments Company. It continued to be located at 300 North Howard Street.[1]

Willms apparently invented his circular rheostat around 1885 when associated with the Chloride of Silver Dry Cell Battery Company of Baltimore (a short distance away from his store). At the same time he was the owner and manager of the Charles Willms & Company. After inventing his rheostat the device bore his name on several models of

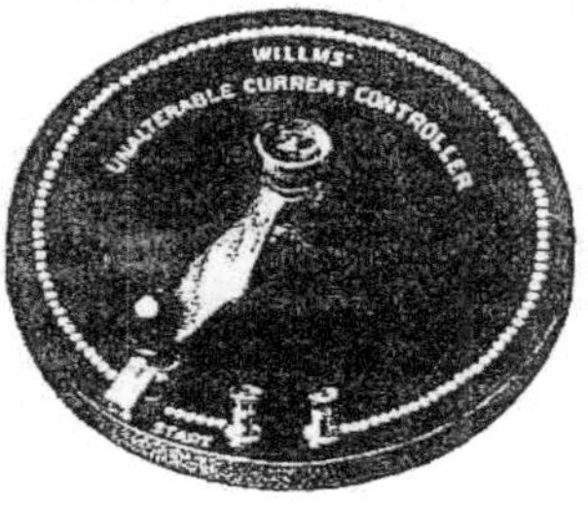

Fig W2. The Willms Rheostat

medical electrical batteries of the Chloride of Silver Dry Cell Battery Co after 1886. From 1890 to 1897 Charles Willms was the general manager of the Chloride of Silver Dry Cell Battery Company in addition to owning and managing his surgical instruments company.

Summary

The Charles Willms Surgical Instruments Co is listed here at a local manufacturer and retailer of medical and surgical apparatuses and supplies, although at one time he was both nationally and internationally known for his fine surgical instruments. His early business in surgical instruments centered mostly with surgeons of the Johns Hopkins Hospital in Baltimore. His medical and surgical supply business flourished in Baltimore and Maryland. The medical electrical batteries retailed by the Charles Willms Surgical Instruments Co retained the signature of their manufacturer, thus no batteries bear the Willms signature. His major outlet for medical electrical batteries was through The Chloride of Silver Dry Cell Battery Co of Baltimore which he managed from 1890 to 1897.

A disc or circular type rheostat bears his name and patent data, and was used on several models of batteries made by The Chloride of Silver Dry Cell Co. His rheostat was innovative in 1886 when first introduced, and at that time he had professional contacts with several individuals who later were involved with him and the battery company.

References

1. Edmonson JM. American Surgical Instruments. San Francisco, CA, Norman Pub, 1997, pp 196, 292

2. The Baltimore City Business Directory, Baltimore, MD, 1881-1882, 1888;Correspondence with Enoch Pratt Public Library. Baltimore, MD, 2000

3. Catalog of The Charles Willms Surgical Instrument Co. Baltimore, MD, 1895, p 503

4. Bleyer JM. Galvanism. In Bigelow HR (ed). An International System of Electro-Therapeutics. Philadelphia, PA, 1894, 238-239

PART 5. THE EPILOGUE

Just like most fads the medical electrical battery and its popularity, especially with the public consumer, was a passing or temporary approach to self care. Electricity in specific forms, however, spanned a very long period of time in medicine. The first treatment by static electricity was given by Christian G Kratzenstein of Germany in 1745, and continued with galvanic, faradic, and sinusoidal currents into the 1930s by physicians. The golden years for physicians' hands-on involvement in the United States were between the 1870s to World War I (1918). Peak years were the 1880s and 1890s for physicians, and the 1890s to the 1930s for the family or public consumer. These years are not exact because the fad did not start one day or end on a specific day. As previously stated, several factors intervened to alter the momentum of the so called electrical cures by medical electrical batteries.

During the so called golden years, the physician giving the treatments with medical electrical batteries were known by various terms. Terminology varied with electrologist, electrician, electrotherapeutist, electrotherapist, electroradiologist, physical therapist, and physiatrist. In the 1920s, electro was generally dropped from identity for all physicians using the medical electrical batteries.

Medical electrical batteries in the United States were designed by specific manufacturers in mass after 1870, and often design changes were made sparingly over the next 35 to 40 years or lifetime of a particular battery. Some design changes occurred more frequently within some small companies; an example of such change was the Perfection Battery of the small PG Williams Co of New York City. This particular faradic battery for home use was redesigned three times in about a dozen years. The prototype cell that powered faradic and galvanic batteries changed in the 1890s to about 1900 when the dry cell replaced the wet cell. The faradic battery that dominated electrotherapeutics between 1872 and 1890s also changed in 1900 when sinusoidal current started to replace the more noxious current of the induction coil. The sinusoidal units required an electrical motor to generate the alternating current so the basic design of the faradic battery of the late 1890s was changed to up date units with the state-of-the-art technology. The updated technology or evolution of the faradic apparatus design is best followed in the McIntosh Battery & Optical Co of Chicago. This company was a leader in electrotherapy through the years because of its products and it survived all manufacturing competition of medical electrical batteries during the first third of the twentieth century. During this period of time the collector is confronted with changes from cell power, commercial direct current, to commercial alternating current, changes in accompanying motors, the addition of meters to measure, to vacuum tubes, and changes in containers (wood boxes to buckram to porcelain to metal to plastics). The disappearance of the traditional induction coil, the vibrating interrupter (rheotome), to electronc time switches, decreased weight and in some cases size of units, but also there were increases in full complements or components and accessory devices. The current amplitude control changed from the sliding metal tube over the coil to the octagonal disc to the circular disc rheostat to vacuum tubes and switches.

Several casual factors can be listed as contributing to the demise in popularity of the medical electrical battery after the illusion that the mystical phenomenon, electricity, promised cures for stubborn and resistant ailments and diseases. Contributing factors to the demise were:

1. The discovery of the x-ray in 1896 immediately attracted physicians (electrotherapeutists) who were knowledgeable in the physics and technology of electricity,

2. In the early twentieth century the federal government enacted laws that restricted what could be claimed about medical products and enforced the manufacturing quality of devices,

3. Both medical professionals and public consumers realized that exaggerated claims by manufactures and clinicians were frequently yielding poor results,

4. The development of injectables (medicines and method of delivery) replaced galvanic current, electrolysis, and iontophoresis (induced medicine by electricity),

5. Specialties in medicine improved education, licensing laws, quality of practice, research, and scope of practice that then changed the field of medicine, and

6. Medical specialtists and licensing laws delegated many previous physician only functions to nonphysicians. A prime example of this delegation was the use of medical electrical batteries for patient care by nonphysician physical therapists prior to, during, and after World War I.

Each factor added to the demise of the medical electrical battery in medicine. In spite of the several casual factors contributing to the so called downfall of the medical electrical battery the use of galvanic or direct current and alternating currents continue to be used in the field of medicine.

Physical therapists are the major users of electrical currents (direct and alternating) in the clinic along with chiropractors, and sports trainers. Galvanic current is used to induce medication in body areas with inflammation. Alternating currents, for example, are used to control pain, pace hearts and lungs, improve function in patients with spinal paralyses, and in sports medicine.

With time and research the electrical current has become more directed to specific functions. In the golden years little research was conducted, while clinical observation and trials prevailed with arbitrary discretion and without controls. Testimonials of consumers in advertisements played a heavy role in inducing the gullible public into the use of home designed medical batteries.

The control of pain or TENS (transcutaneous electrical nerve stimulation) is probably the single major use of the medical electrical battery today. The electrical units used in these treatments are customarily prescribed by the physician and physical therapist. The treatments are usually started by medical professionals in the clinic or office and then given to the patient to use on an outpatient basis. The benefits of such electrical treatment is recognized by health care insurers.

Medical needs continue to dictate research with the use of medical electrical batteries, while engineering and manufacturing constantly strive to meet the needs uncovered by research and clinical trials.

The complete history of the medical electrical battery in the twentieth century awaits publication. Excerpts of their use in the twentieth century have been published by specific interest groups. Also, this book is not all inclusive of manufacturers and retailers of medical electrical batteries between 1870 and the 1920s. Such names as Barclay Mfg Co, Fischer, Law, Meyers, EB Meyrowitz, JG Vetter, and Weinhagen have not been discussed as manufacturers, nor have the retailers Codman and Shurtleff, Leach and Green, Smith and Shaw, George Tiemann & Co, and Truax, Greene & Co. These companies surely played a role in the American business of medical electrical batteries, but escaped the computer this time around.

INDEX

D

E

N

S

T

U

W

Made in the USA
Monee, IL
05 November 2026

67811486R00285